D1443731

EVALUATION, TREATMENT AND PREVENTION OF MUSCULOSKELETAL DISORDERS

VOLUME ONE—SPINE

4th Edition

H. Duane Saunders, MS PT
Robin Saunders Ryan, MS PT

with guest authors

James R. Beazell, MS, PT, OCS, FAAOMPT, ATC

David A. Groom, BAppSc (Physio), GDMT

Gregg Johnson, PT, FFCFMT

Andy Kerk, PT, OCS, CFMT, ATC

Michael Koopmeiners, MD

Steven L. Kraus, PT OCS MTC

Allyn L. Woerman, MMSc, PT

The Saunders Group, Inc.
4250 Norex Drive
Chaska, MN 55318
www.thesaundersgroup.com

Evaluation, Treatment and Prevention of Musculoskeletal Disorders
Volume One—Spine
4th Edition

The Saunders Group, Inc.
4250 Norex Drive
Chaska, MN 55318
www.thesaundersgroup.com

Library of Congress Control Number 2004091469

ISBN Number 1-879190-12-5

Copyright 2004 by The Saunders Group, Inc.

Edited by Robin Saunders Ryan, MS PT

Cover Design by Audrey Fletcher-Price, A-Design Ltd

Text Layout by Peter Gold, KnowHow ProServices

Printed in the United States of America

H. Duane Saunders, MS PT
CEO/President
The Saunders Group, Inc.
4250 Norex Drive
Chaska, MN 55318
duane@thesaundersgroup.com

Robin Saunders Ryan, MS PT
Chief Operating Officer
The Saunders Group, Inc.
4250 Norex Drive
Chaska, MN 55318
rsaund@thesaundersgroup.com

James R. Beazell, MS, PT, OCS, FAAOMPT,
ATC
University of Virginia
HealthSouth Sportsmedicine and Rehab
545 Ray C. Hunt Drive, Suite 210
Charlottesville, VA 22903

David A. Groom, BAppSc, GDMT
Musculoskeletal Physiotherapist
Auburn Spinal Therapy Centre
126 Auburn Rd
Hawthorn, VIC 3122
Australia
dgroom@auburnspinal.com

Gregg Johnson, PT, FFCFMT
Institute of Physical Art
43449 Elk Run
Steamboat Springs, CO 80487
gvrt@cmn.net

Andy Kerk, PT, OCS, CFMT, ATC
Body Mechanics
807 N. Jefferson Street
Milwaukee, WI 53202
andy@BMechanics.com

Michael B. Koopmeiners, MD
Medical Director
HealthPartners WorkSite Health
8100 34th Ave South
Minneapolis, MN 55435
MBKoopmeiners@Healthpartners.com

Steven L. Kraus, PT OCS MTC
Physiotherapy Associates
2770 Lenox Road, Suite 102
Atlanta, Georgia 30324
stevekraus@mindspring.com

Allyn L. Woerman, MMSc PT
CEO/Member
Adult Rehabilitation Therapies, PLLC
4905 108th ST SW
Lakewood, WA 98499
awoerman@motion-is-life.com

Acknowledgements

The 4th edition of this textbook could not have been published without the direct and indirect contributions of the following people:

We would first like to thank the managers and employees at The Saunders Group. Though not one of them volunteered to proofread a galley, their infallible competency and independence made it possible for us to concentrate on this project for over a year with complete confidence that the building would still be standing when we were through.

Marie Holecek, Jean Eschweiler, Katie Larkin and Dan Wolfe from Saunders Therapy Centers, and Katherine Beissner from Ithaca College asked challenging questions and provided insights that made this book better. Trevor Cmiel was a great model and was so helpful with miscellaneous requests related to this project.

Our guest authors were fantastic to work with, and weren't *too* late on their deadlines... We are very excited to have Steve Kraus and Allyn Woerman involved again in this project, as well as the new contributors— Andy Kerk, David Groom, Mike Koopmeiners, Gregg Johnson and Jim Beazell.

We would also like to thank our families for their support and encouragement. Special thanks are due to Sydney Ryan for her research assistance at the University of Minnesota's Biomedical Library, and to Audrey Fletcher-Price for the cover design.

Finally, thanks to Peter Gold from KnowHow ProServices. He finalized the layout and coached Robin on Framemaker. The final product was produced very efficiently because of his knowledge and teaching skills.

CONTENTS

INTRODUCTION

Robin Saunders Ryan, MS PT and H. Duane Saunders, MS PT

We are pleased to publish the 4th edition of *Evaluation, Treatment and Prevention of Musculoskeletal Disorders, Volume One, The Spine*. In many ways, this revision is long overdue. Many things have changed in the last 10 years, and much of it has been positive. Positive changes include progress made on the issue of direct access to physical therapy and the American Physical Therapy Association's (APTA's) support of and emphasis on evidence-based practice.[3] However, despite our positive progress, much remains to be done.

In February 2004, Ohio became the 39th state to pass direct access legislation[1], taking the physical therapy profession one step closer to its 2020 goal of consumers having direct access to physical therapy services without needing a physician's referral.[2] Reimbursement for physical therapy without a physician's referral continues to be a challenge, however.

When this textbook went to press, the Medicare Patient Access to Physical Therapist Act (HR 792 and S. 493) was still active in the United States Congress. If passed, this act will mandate Medicare payments for physical therapy services without a physician's referral. Concerns that costs would increase appear to be unfounded.[21] Still, there are opponents of this legislation.

The APTA has invested much effort on the evidence-based practice movement.[3,27] *Evidence-based practice* refers to the philosophy of choosing evaluation and treatment methods that have evidence of efficacy or effectiveness in the literature. Many articles educating physical therapists about evidence-based practice and encouraging participation in the APTA's Hooked on Evidence Database have been published.[9,11,12,14] A main driver of the push toward evidence-based practice is the skyrocketing cost of health care and the inevitable pressure on physical therapists to prove that their interventions should be paid for.

Evidence-based practice is particularly important in the specialty of back pain management. The economic impact of back pain is substantial. In one of the largest analyses of its kind, a team of Duke University Medical Center researchers found that 25.9 million adults reported back pain and approximately 26 billion dollars were spent treating it in 1998.[20] Clinicians treating back pain are under increasing pressure to show their worth, and providing research to show the effectiveness of our treatments is essential.

Unfortunately, some of the "evidence" being published is not very flattering to the physical therapy profession. Some of the methods that are in common use today by many clinicians are not shown to be effective. For example, interventions such as spinal traction, exercise for acute low back pain, the use of back supports, and patient education to prevent low back pain in industry have been criticized in recently published literature reviews or meta-analyses focusing on randomized clinical trials.[23,29,31,32,33,34]

Despite the conclusions of some literature reviews, physical therapists continue to rely on unproven interventions for a variety of reasons. The major reason cited in one study was lack of time to learn about research findings.[14] In addition, over 30% of physical therapists surveyed indicated that despite knowing about research, they felt that certain individual patients were "unique" or that certain research articles did not apply to their patient populations.[14] Some authors have acknowledged a "cultural divide" between researchers, clinicians and administrators.[13]

Research-based guidelines for treatment of low back pain have been published.[8,23,28] However, multiple studies have shown poor adherence to guidelines in actual clinical practice.[4,5,18,24] What is the reason for this dichotomy?

We believe that part of the problem is that, in some cases, few quality studies are actually being done. Most literature reviews or meta-analyses exclude studies that are not randomized clinical trials (RCTs). Then, systems are usually used to grade the RCTs on their quality. Studies not meeting the reviewers' criteria are not considered. Although it is appropriate to be selective and only consider the results from the highest quality studies, these tough criteria cause relatively few studies to be analyzed.

For example, two separate literature reviews on multidisciplinary biopsychosocial rehabilitation for subacute low back pain and neck and shoulder pain included only two articles out of 1808 references found on each subject.[15,16] In the case of neck and shoulder pain, the reviewers indicated that both articles used were considered "methodologically low-quality". In their conclusions, the reviewers stated, "there appears to be little scientific evidence for the effectiveness on neck and shoulder pain of multidisciplinary biopsychosocial rehabilitation compared with other rehabilitation methods".[15]

Our complaint is not with the tough standards used in reviews, but with the possibility of improper interpretation of conclusions when they are quoted out of context. From the evidence described in the above two reviews, we would conclude that additional research is needed, and not necessarily that multidisciplinary biopsychosocial rehabilitation is ineffective.

In some cases, published guidelines use the results of literature reviews inappropriately. For example, in the Agency for Health Care Policy and Research's (AHCPR) guidelines, *Acute Low Back Problems in Adults*, the following conclusion was published: "Spinal traction is not recommended in the treatment of patients with acute low back problems".[8] Two reviews were cited as evidence for this statement—the well-known Quebec Task Force review[28] and a 1995 review by van der Heijden G, et al.[29]

However, in the Quebec Task Force review, authors had reported a lack of evidence for lumbar traction's effectiveness but stated, "A lack of evidence supporting such interventions does not demonstrate them to be useless."[28] In van der Heijden, et al's review, the authors had reported that the studies reviewed, "…do not allow clear conclusions due to methodological flaws in their design and conduct", and they further stated, "There are no clear indications, however, that traction is ineffective therapy for neck and back pain".[29]

One can see that choice of words makes an important difference when describing the results of literature reviews. Indeed, Jules Rothstein warned in the October 2001 Physical Therapy journal's editor's note, "Keep in mind that absence of evidence is different from negative evidence".[25]

Questionable word choice is not the only difficulty encountered in reading literature reviews. Because we have found lumbar traction to be effective for some patients, we critically read the English language studies cited in the ACHPR[8], Quebec[28] and van der Heidjen[29] reviews, as well as a more recent Philadelphia Panel review.[23] A common problem found with the studies used in each of these reviews was the wide variation of methods and techniques described.

For example, some of the studies involved auto traction[17,19] and one studied bed traction.[22] Some of the studies that showed lumbar traction was ineffective were performed with forces that most clinicians would regard as insufficient[22,35,36]—they certainly used less force than we recommend in this textbook (see Chapter 12, *Spinal Traction*). Coxhead et al's study did not even report the forces or treatment times used, yet concluded that traction was of limited benefit.[10] Interestingly, this study was included in the van der Heidjen review despite these serious shortcomings, presumably because it was an RCT.[29]

Another problem with the reviewed articles was poorly defined patient selection. For example, the studies tended to group all patients with low back pain together and did not distinguish between sub-groups or by diagnosis. Recent studies have looked at traction for nonspecific low back pain and have excluded patients with herniated disc or radiculopathy—diagnoses that we consider especially appropriate for traction treatment.[6,7,30] The only two studies that looked at traction for herniated disc were done by the same primary author and did not use adequate forces.[35,36] In both articles, the authors even acknowledged that, "the treatment was carried out with a force which was in the lower end of the effective range," because they feared aggravation of symptoms if using forces recommended by other authors they cited.

One problem with studying traction and other interventions is that constraints required by good study design often require that treatment methods be studied in isolation rather than in combination with other forms of treatment. This, of course, is necessary to eliminate multiple variables that make it difficult to judge exactly which treatment helped the patient. This method has scientific merit and may be practical with certain types of research—for example, testing the effectiveness of pharmaceuticals.

However, it renders the conclusions useless if the research results were obtained in a different manner than what is actually practiced in the clinic.

For example, traction is often performed in combination with passive extension exercises for treatment of moderate to severe lumbar herniated nucleus pulposus.[26] Clinically, one would argue that it is the combination of interventions that results in success, not either technique in isolation. If either treatment was studied in isolation, results might show that neither was effective. However, when multiple treatments are studied together, it is not possible to draw conclusions about the effectiveness of the individual interventions. Such a study might be excluded from literature reviews examining a single intervention. Clearly good study design is not a straightforward task!

What is our purpose in the above critique? First, we wish to caution the reader to carefully review research articles and critique all of the methods used (such as subject selection and treatment technique), rather than assuming the study is high quality based only on its design. When reading the conclusions of literature reviews, it is important to avoid reaching sweeping conclusions based on non-homogenous studies. For example, the statement, "lumbar traction is not effective" is very different from the statement, "low force lumbar traction in a supine position has not been shown to be effective for subjects with non-specific low back pain".

Our second purpose is to justify to the reader our inclusion of "unproven" treatment techniques in this textbook. For example, we have included chapters on spinal traction and back supports—interventions that are currently out of favor in the literature. We have also recommended the use of certain types of exercise for patients with acute low back pain, despite the fact that reviewers have indicated a lack of evidence for specific exercise interventions in this population.[34] The reader will find a few instances where we recommend techniques that have not been shown to be reliable or have not been adequately researched. In each case, we have attempted to acknowledge the limitation.

On one hand, we are critical of the practice of blindly accepting conclusions reached in literature reviews. On the other hand, *we are believers* in evidence-based practice and, along with other writers, agree that there is a definite shortage of good quality, clinically relevant literature.

In the spirit of evidence-based practice, we have significantly updated the 4th edition of this textbook with the most comprehensive literature review yet. As a result, we have added new material on many subjects, including the impact fear-avoidance behaviors have on our patients' outcomes, and several other important topics. We have tried to present both positive and negative arguments for controversial tests or interventions, and we encourage the reader to follow up on our references to draw their own conclusions. We hope that we have contributed to the profession by giving the reader both "food for thought" and a practical and effective evaluation and treatment strategy.

We have added three new chapters from guest authors. To better prepare our profession for the opportunities and challenges of increased direct access, Michael Koopmeiners has contributed Chapter 3, *Medical Screening*. His chapter is an in-depth discussion of screening for non-mechanical disorders. David Groom has contributed Chapter 9, *Cervicogenic Headache*, and Andy Kerk, Gregg Johnson and Jim Beazell have collaborated on Chapter 11, *Soft Tissue Mobilization and Neuromuscular Training*. We are excited about these new subjects and are grateful for the hard work put forth by all of our guest authors.

We close this introduction by asking, "What makes a good physical therapist?" We believe the answer is a combination of passion, knowledge, solid technique, great deductive skills and intuition. Sometimes, there is a tendency to incorrectly define our patients' problems as complex, when the solutions are actually quite simple. Ironically, the more experience we obtain and the more articles we read, the more we rely on "the basics" discussed in this textbook. Therefore we have included many common-sense ideas, while attempting to provide a sound scientific basis for our rationale.

REFERENCES

1. American Physical Therapy Association's website: http://www.apta.org/news/news_releases/ohiodirectaccess
2. American Physical Therapy Association's website: http://www.apta.org/About/aptamissiongoals/visionstatement
3. American Physical Therapy Association's Website. http://www.apta.org/hookedonevidence/index.cfm
4. Armstrong MP, McDonough S and Baxter GD: Clinical Guidelines Versus Clinical Practice in the Management of Low Back Pain. Int J Clin Pract 57(1):9-13, 2003.
5. Battie MC, Cherkin DC, Dunn R, et al: Managing Low Back Pain: Attitudes and Treatment Preferences of Physical Therapists. Phys Ther 74(3):219-226, 1994.
6. Beurskens AJ, de Vet HC, Koke AJ, et al: Efficacy of Traction for Nonspecific Low Back Pain: A Randomised Clinical Trial. Lancet 346(8990):1596-1600, 1995.
7. Beurskens AJ, de Vet HC, Koke AJ, et al: Efficacy of Traction for Nonspecific Low Back Pain: 12-Week and 6-Month Results of a Randomized Clinical Trial. Spine 22(23):2756-2762, 1997.
8. Bigos S, Bowyer O, Braen G, et al. *Acute Low Back Problems in Adults.* AHCPR publication 95-0642. Rockville, Md: Agency for Health Care Policy and Research, Public Health Service, US Dept of Health and Human Services; 1994.
9. Cormack JC: Evidence-Based Practice...What is it and How Do I Do It? Joul Orthop Sports Phys Ther 32(10):484-487, 2002.
10. Coxhead CE, Inskip H, Meade TW. Multicentre Trial of Physiotherapy in the Management of Sciatica Symptoms. *Lancet* 1:1085-1088, 1981.
11. Glaros S: All Evidence is Not Created Equal: A Discussion of Levels of Evidence. PT Magazine, 11(10):42-52, 2003.
12. Guccione A: The Quest for Certainty: Goodbye to Index Cards. Phys Ther 83(11):XXXX, 2003.
13. Haines A and Jones R: Education and Debate, Implementing Findings of Research. BMJ 308:1488-1492, 1994.
14. Jette DU, Bacon K, Batty C, et al: Evidence-Based Practice: Beliefs, Attitudes, Knowledge and Behaviors of Physical Therapists. Phys Ther 83(9):786-805, 2003.
15. Karjalainen K, Malmivaara A, van Tulder M, et al: Multidisciplinary Biopsychosocial Rehabilitation for Neck and Shoulder Pain Among Working Age Adults. A Systematic Review Within the Framework of the Cochrane Collaboration Back Review Group. Spine 26(2):174-181, 2001.
16. Karjalainen K, Malmivaara A, van Tulder M, et al: Multidisciplinary Biopsychosocial Rehabilitation for Subacute Low Back Pain Among Working Age Adults.A Systematic Review Within the Framework of the Cochrane Collaboration Back Review Group. Spine 26(3):262-269, 2001.
17. Larsson U, Choler U, Lindstrom A, et al. Auto-Traction for Treatment of Lumbago-Sciatica. *Acta Orthop Scand* 51: 791-798, 1980.
18. Li LC and Bombardier C: Physical Therapy Management of Low Back Pain: An Exploratory Survey of Therapist Approaches. Phys Ther 81(4):1018-1028, 2001.
19. Ljunggren E, Weber H, Larssen S. Autotraction Versus Manual Traction in Patients with Prolapsed Lumbar Intervertebral Discs. *Scand J Rhehabil Med* 16:117-124, 1984.
20. Luo X, Pietrobon R, Sun SX, et al. Estimates and Patterns of Direct Health Care Expenditures Among Individuals With Back Pain In The United States. Spine 29(1):79-86, 2004.
21. Mitchell J and de Lisovoy G: A Comparison of Resource Use and Cost in Direct Access Versus Physician Referral Episodes of Physical Therapy. Phys Ther 77(1):10-18, 1997.
22. Pal P, Mangion P, Hossian MA, Diffey L. A Controlled Trial of Continuous Lumbar Traction in the Treatment of Back Pain and Sciatica. *Br J Rheumatol* 25:181-183, 1986.
23. Philadelphia Panel Evidence-Based Clinical Practice Guidelines on Selected Rehabilitation Interventions for Low Back Pain. Phys Ther 81(10):1641-1674, 2001.
24. Rossignol M, Abenhaim L, Bonvalot Y, et a: Should the Gap Be Filled Between Guidelines and Actual Practice for Management of Low Back Pain in Primary Care? The Quebec Experience. Spine 21(24):2893-2898, 1996.
25. Rothstein J: Autonomous Practice or Autonomous Ignorance? Editor's Note. Phys Ther 81(10):1620-1621, 2001.
26. Saal JA, Saal JS. Nonoperative Treatment of Herniated Lumbar Intervertebral Disc with Radiculopathy-An Outcome Study. *Spine* 14: 431-437, 1989.
27. Scalziti D: Happy Birthday to Hooked on Evidence. PT Magazine 11(9):56-58, 2003.
28. Scientific Approach to the Assessment and Management of Activity-Related Spinal Disorders. A Monograph For Clinicians. Report of the Quebec Task Force on Spinal Disorders. Spine 12(7 Suppl):S1-59, 1987.
29. van der Heijden G, et al: The Efficacy of Traction for Back and Neck Pain: A Systematic, Blinded Review of Randomized Clinical Trial Method. Phys Ther 75:93-104, 1995.
30. van der Heijden GJ, Beurskens AJ, Dirx MJ, et al: Efficacy of Lumbar Traction: A Randomized Clinical Trial. Physiotherapy 81:29-35, 1995.
31. van Poppel MNM, Koes BW, Smid T, et al. A Systematic Review of Controlled Clinical Trials on the Prevention of Back Pain in Industry. Occup Environ Med 54:841-847, 1997.
32. van Poppel MN, Koes BW, van der Ploeg T, et al: Lumbar Supports and Education for the Prevention of Low Back Pain in Industry: A Randomized Controlled Trial. JAMA 279(22):1789-1794, 1998.
33. van Poppel MNM, de Looze MP, Koes BW, et al: Mechanisms of Action of Lumbar Supports. A Systematic Review. Spine 25(16):2103-2113, 2000.
34. van Tulder M, Malmivaara A, Esmail R, et al: Exercise Therapy for Low Back Pain. A Systematic Review Within the Framework of the Cochrane Collaboration Back Review Group. Spine 25(21):2784-2796, 2000.
35. Weber H. Traction Therapy in Sciatica Due to Disc Prolapse. *J Oslo City Hosp* 23:167-176, 1973.
36. Weber H, Ljunggren E, Walker L. Traction Therapy in Patients With Herniated Lumbar Intervertebral Discs. *J Oslo City Hosp* 34: 61-70, 1984.

2

SPINAL BIOMECHANICS

Allyn L. Woerman, MMSc PT and Robin Saunders Ryan, MS PT

The first modern textbook on spinal biomechanics was written by Giovanni Alfonso Borelli in 1680.[40] Since then, spinal biomechanics has been explored by authors from many different disciplines. Some areas are controversial and some speculations and findings vary greatly among researchers. The complexity of the spine and its relative inaccessibility compared to the extremities has made it difficult to study. What's more, the focus of biomechanical research varies depending upon the research team's background. For example, spinal surgeons tend to focus on surgical instrumentation studies, whereas physical therapists tend to focus on studies exploring the effects of exercise.

The purpose of this chapter is not to provide the reader with an academic or detailed picture of the biomechanics or applied anatomy of the spine. Instead, this chapter will present material essential to understanding concepts presented elsewhere in this text. The reader is referred to the reference list for more complete works on spinal biomechanics and related topics.

The reader may notice a bias toward osteopathic terminology. We have found the osteopathic literature to contain excellent descriptions of normal and abnormal biomechanics and a comprehensive, common sense evaluation and treatment philosophy. Where appropriate, we have borrowed osteopathic terms and describe their usage as necessary to give the reader a clear picture of the pertinent concepts presented here.

Kapandji makes a good comparison between the vertebral column and the mast of a ship in that the spine must be able to rigidly support the trunk on the pelvis, yet provide flexibility and movement.[22] This dual role of the spine

has sometimes been referred to as "tensegrity". The spine meets these contradictory requirements through a system of muscular and ligamentous tighteners at all levels that link the shoulder girdle to the pelvis (much like the main yard and the guy ropes on a sailing ship). When these forces are in balance, the spine is straight and the pelvis and shoulders are level (rigidity). However, when the pelvis is not level, as when the body rests on one limb, the vertebral column is forced to bend (plasticity) (Fig 2-1). Since the spine is made of multiple components superimposed on one another, it will first bend in the lumbar region (convex toward the resting limb), then try to compensate by bending concavely in the thoracic region and again convexly in the cervical area. The muscular/ligamentous tighteners will actively and automatically adapt to these changes to maintain rigidity, shortening on one side and lengthening on the other. This automatic postural accommodation is under the influence of the extrapyramidal system and is geared to maintaining the eyes in the horizontal plane.

Viewed from the front or back, the spine is straight. However, viewed from the side, the spine has four curves (Fig 2-2):

1. Sacral—the fused sacrum is convex posteriorly
2. Lumbar—concave posteriorly
3. Thoracic—convex posteriorly
4. Cervical—concave posteriorly

These curves reciprocate and balance one another in such a way that in the normal spine, if a plumb line were dropped from the atlanto/occipital joint at the top of the column, it would intersect the center of motion at the lumbosacral junction at the bottom. If dropped further, the

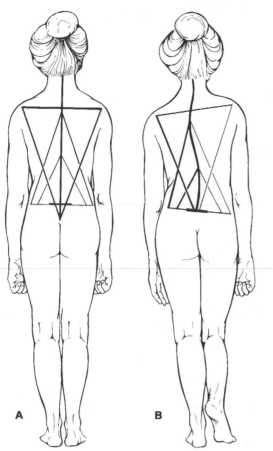

Figure 2-1: Tensegrity: A) Rigidity and B) Plasticity (adapted from Kapandji[22]).

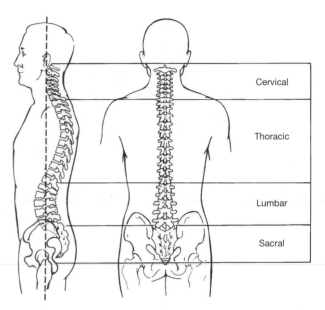

Figure 2-2: Physiological curves of the spine.

Provance's[24] texts for a more detailed explanation of the role of the muscles in biomechanical dysfunction.

Each spinal segment (i.e., two adjacent vertebræ with the intervertebral disc between) may be divided into an active portion and a passive portion. The vertebral bodies are the passive portion while the disc, intervertebral

plumb line would intersect the hip joint and the ankle. These curves not only provide balance, they provide added strength for the vertebral column to withstand axial compressive loads. Engineers have calculated that the presence of the three curves in the spine (excluding the sacrum) increases the resistance of the spine to compression ten times compared to a column with no curves at all. These curves can also be shown to influence the function of the spine as a whole. Spines with exaggerated curves tend to be more dynamic and spines with reduced or flattened curves tend to be more static[22] (Fig 2-3).

Functional Components of the Vertebral Column

In this section, the intervertebral disc and certain muscles and ligaments are discussed with some detail, while other functional components of the vertebral column are not. It is not the intent to underemphasize certain components, but to emphasize those components that have particular clinical significance to the rest of this textbook. The reader is referred to Janet Travell's[49] or Kendall, McCreary, and

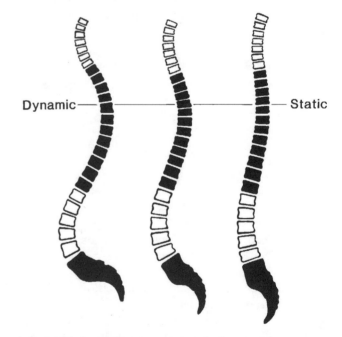

Figure 2-3: Dynamic and static spines. An increase in the normal curves tends to make the spine more flexible or dynamic. A spine with flattened curves tends to be less flexible.

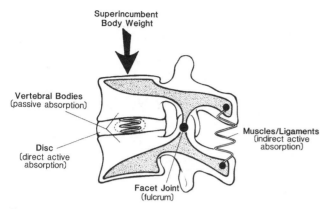

Figure 2-4: The spinal segment as a first class lever system, showing active and passive portions (adapted from Kapandji[22]).

foramen, articular processes, ligaments and muscles are the active portion.[22] Each segment, through the vertebral arches, forms a first class lever system where the articular processes (facets) are the fulcrum (Fig 2-4). Axial compressive loads are applied through the vertebral column with direct and passive absorption of some force at the disc and indirect and active absorption by the ligaments and muscles.

The Intervertebral Disc

The intervertebral disc consists of two portions: an inner gelatinous center called the nucleus pulposus, and an outer structure made up of layers of concentric fibers called the annulus fibrosis (Fig 2-5). Most published descriptions of the disc focus on the lumbar disc, but there are distinct differences in the cervical disc. The following description applies mainly to the lumbar disc, except as noted.

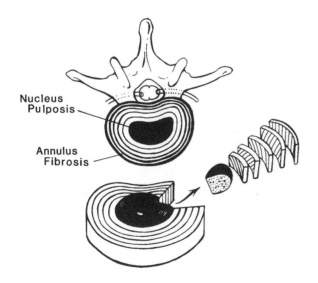

Figure 2-5: Lumbar intervertebral disc.

The nucleus, which tends to be spherical in shape, is made up of a porous-permeable, collagen-proteoglycan solid matrix that has the ability to absorb water.[6] There is a transitional area between the nucleus and the innermost of the annular rings where the gel of the nucleus is interspersed between the first few rings of the annulus. Because a blood supply is found solely in the periphery of the disc, the nutrition of disc cells is derived from diffusional and convective transport of nutrients and wastes through the porous-permeable matrix.[6] During the day, the compressional forces of the upright position cause water to be lost from the nucleus. This is why one tends to be up to one centimeter shorter at the end of the day than when first rising in the morning. During the recumbent, non-weight bearing position the nucleus imbibes water, thus increasing its height.[22] The aging process diminishes the ability of the nucleus to imbibe water.

The annulus is made up of 15 to 26 distinct layers of discontinuous concentric lamellae. The lamellae become progressively less distinct as they merge with the central nucleus pulposus.[1] The fibers of the annulus are oriented diagonally and alternate their direction between layers in a crisscross (X) fashion. The inner fibers are more obliquely oriented and the outer fibers are more vertical. This arrangement is very much like a bias-ply tire where the crisscross pattern allows for strength and flexibility. The inner fibers of the annulus are quite weak in comparison to the outer. The annular rings are firmly attached superiorly and inferiorly to adjacent vertebral bodies and the vertebral endplates and serve to maintain the nucleus under constant pressure and in a central position. In the adult, the disc is considered to be aneural except for some sensory innervation in the outermost layers of the annulus.[6]

In the adult cervical annulus, concentric lamellae with crisscross fibers are not seen. Instead, the annulus forms a crescentic mass of collagen that is thick anteriorly and tapers laterally toward the uncinate processes. The cervical annulus is deficient posterolaterally and is represented posteriorly only by a thin layer of paramedian, vertically-oriented fibers. The posterior longitudinal ligament reinforces the deficient posterior annulus with longitudinal and alar fibers.[32]

The disc is flexible, allowing motion in all directions, and serves to dissipate forces and stresses transmitted to it, especially vertical or compressive loads. The disc may thus be likened to a shock absorber. The nucleus acts predominately as a fluid under static loading conditions, generating large hydrostatic pressures.[6] Forward bending (flexion) of the spine causes compressive forces to be placed upon the anterior portion of the vertebral body and the disc, thus exerting a posterior force on the nucleus

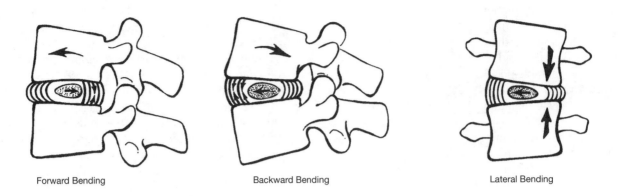

Forward Bending

Backward Bending

Lateral Bending

Figure 2-6: Effects of forward, backward and side bending on the nucleus pulposis (adapted from Kapandji[22]).

pulposus. This action is analogous to the squeezing of a water-filled balloon on one end, with the fluid moving away from the compressive force. Backward bending of the spine (extension) produces the opposite effect on the disc.[3,5,8,16,43] Side bending produces a force which is opposite to the direction of the side bend (Fig 2-6).

In the healthy disc, the annular rings tend to resist displacement of the nuclear gel, thus maintaining the nucleus in its proper shape and location. In the unhealthy disc where the annular fibers have torn, usually in a radial manner, the nuclear gel is permitted to migrate, thus setting the stage for the clinical manifestations of the herniated disc.[31] Rotation, a compressive force, causes an increase in intradiscal pressure and tends to narrow the

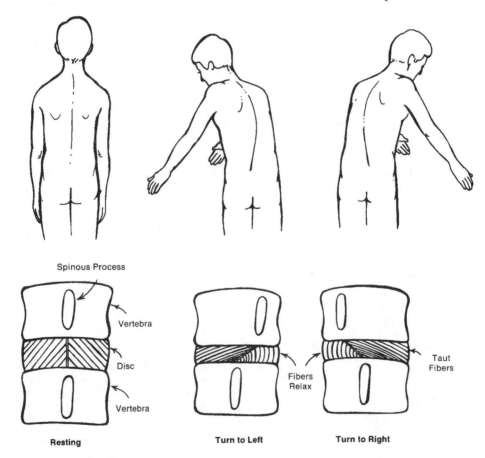

Spinous Process

Vertebra

Disc

Vertebra

Fibers Relax

Taut Fibers

Resting

Turn to Left

Turn to Right

Figure 2-7: Effects of rotation on the lumbar intervertebral disc.

joint space. When rotation occurs, the annular fibers that are oriented in the direction of the rotatory movement become taut, while the fibers that are oriented in the opposite direction tend to slacken. This situation puts the disc in a vulnerable position for injury, particularly if it is also under a load (Fig 2-7). Herniations occur most frequently posterolaterally, where the annulus is weakest.

Intradiscal pressure is greatly affected by body position and activities. Important data concerning intradiscal pressures in various body positions and under various loads is available[35,56] (Fig 2-8). Knowledge of these pressures is important to the physical therapist when designing activity and exercise programs for patients with disc problems. Note that slumped sitting and forward bending (flexion) of the spine tend to cause greater intradiscal pressures than the upright standing posture.

The mechanical properties of the disc change with age and degeneration. Aging diminishes the ability of the nucleus to imbibe fluid. Since endplate vascularity also decreases with age, disc nutrition is compromised, leading to deterioration in the structural integrity of the disc matrix.[4] The vertebral endplates become increasingly concave with age, and the presence of osteophytes increases, in men more than in women.[44]

Although it has been commonly assumed that disc height decreases with age, recent evidence shows that the disc actually thickens, and its height tends to increase with age until the seventh decade.[44] Imprecise definitions of "aging" and "degeneration" probably increase confusion, because the two terms are often used synonymously. In fact, abnormal disc degeneration should be distinguished from normal disc aging. Disc pathology involves thinning and dessication, but aging discs are not necessarily thin or desiccated. It is well-accepted that pathological disc degeneration leads to a narrowing of the disc space. However, one study examined older discs and found that 72% did not show abnormal degenerative changes.[52]

A computer modeling study has demonstrated that axial displacement, posterolateral disc bulge, and tensile stress in annular fibers all increase with increasing disc height. The authors of the study warn against concluding that "thin" discs are better than thick ones, since disc height also affects the size of the neural foramen.[26] Certainly, most clinicians tend to correlate narrowed disc spaces with greater pathology.

Muscular and Ligamentous Influences

Superficial Trunk Muscles. The superficial trunk muscles consist of the erector spinae, rectus abdominis, external obliques and internal obliques. These muscles are associated with dynamic trunk movement and control of trunk orientation and posture, whereas the deeper trunk muscles are thought to have a greater role in intersegmental stability.[41] The erector spinae consist of several individually-named muscles that extend from the sacrum to the occiput to perform neck and trunk extension. Their origins and insertions are detailed in other works[24] and will not be repeated here (Fig 2-9).

The rectus abdominis arises from the pubic crest and symphysis and inserts on the costal cartilages of the fifth,

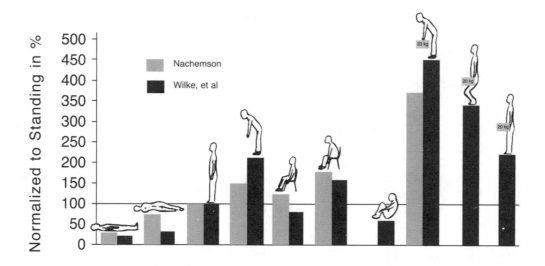

Figure 2-8: Results of research on intradiscal pressures as they relate to body positions and activities. This chart illustrates both Nachemson's and Wilke, et al's findings (adapted from Wilke, et al[56]).

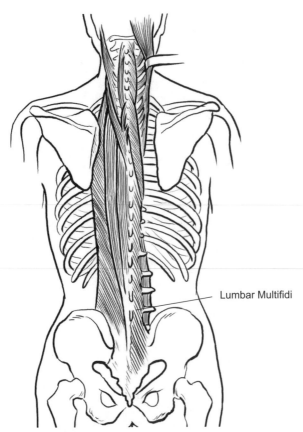

Figure 2-9: Erector spinae muscles. Note the attachment of the multifidi across the lumbosacral junction.

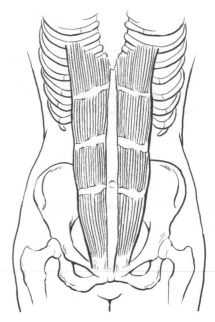

Figure 2-10: The rectus abdominis. Note the fiber direction is vertical, contributing to trunk flexion.

sixth and seventh ribs and the xyphoid process. The direction of the fibers is vertical, thus the action on the trunk is pure flexion (Fig 2-10).

The remaining abdominal muscles are illustrated in Figure 2-11. The external oblique arises from the external surfaces of ribs five through eight and inserts into the linea alba by means of a broad aponeurosis. Its fibers are oriented obliquely in an inferior and medial direction. When acting bilaterally, the external obliques flex the trunk. In unilateral action with the anterior fibers of the contralateral internal oblique, the external oblique causes trunk rotation (with the pelvis fixed) or ilium posterior rotation (with the thorax fixed).

The internal oblique originates from the lateral $2/3$ of the inquinal ligament, with a short attachment on the iliac crest near the anterior superior iliac spine. It inserts with the transversus abdominis into the linea alba and the crest of the pubis. Its fibers are oriented transversely across the lower abdomen. It, along with the transversus abdominis, compresses and supports the lower abdominal viscera.

Deep Spinal Muscles.   The deep spinal muscles are called the transversospinalis muscles and consist of the semispi-

nalis, multifidi and rotatores. The transversospinalis are named for their origins on the transverse processes and insertions on the spinous processes of vertebrae one or more levels above. The multifidi deserve special mention because of recent research supporting their important role in lumbar spine stability.

The multifidi arise from the transverse processes of L5 through C4, and span two to four vertebrae, inserting on the spinous process of a vertebra above. In the sacral region, the multifidi arise from the posterior surface of the sacrum, the medial surface of the posterior superior iliac spine, and the posterior sacral ligaments (Fig 2-9). The multifidi extend the spine, and have a minor role in rotation. They have been shown to provide up to $2/3$ the control of inter-segmental motion at L4-5,[57] and have been shown to increase lumbar spine stability significantly when co-contracting with the psoas.[41] Thus, their role in prescribed exercise programs has increased in recent years.

Other spinal muscles include the interspinales, which connect between contiguous spinous processes; intertransversarii, which connect between contiguous transverse processes; and splenius, which provide additional muscular support in the cervical and upper thoracic spine.

Transversus Abdominis.   The transversus abdominis originates from the inner surfaces of the cartilage of the lower six ribs, the thoracolumbar fascia, the anterior $3/4$ of the internal lip of the iliac crest, and the lateral $2/3$ of the

A   B   C

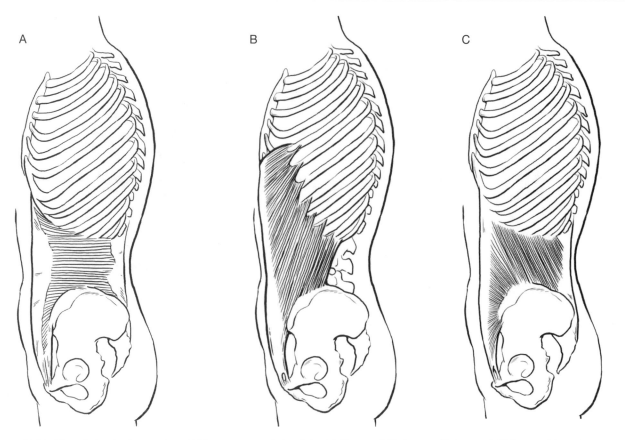

Figure 2-11: The abdominal muscles: A) Transversus abdominis; B) External Obliques; C) Internal Obliques. Note the varying orientation of their fibers, giving clues to their primary actions.

inguinal ligament. It inserts on the linea alba by means of a broad aponeurosis, pubic crest and pecten of pubis (Fig 2-11). Since its fibers are transverse, it acts like a girdle to flatten the abdominal wall and compress the abdominal viscera. There is evidence that the transversus abdominis may have a significant effect on SI joint stability, particularly when contracted independently of other abdominal muscles.[42] Prescription of specific exercise for the transversus abdominis and other transverse-oriented trunk muscles has been proposed because of the theoretical and demonstrated effect on SI joint and spinal stability. [20]

Quadratus Lumborum. The quadratus lumborum lies in the anterior compartment of the lumbar fascia. It arises from the transverse process of L5, the iliolumbar ligament and from a short length of the adjoining iliac crest. It attaches to the transverse processes of L1-L4 and to the inferior border of the 12th rib (Fig 2-12). The quadratus lumborum assists with lumbar spine extension and forced exhalation and coughing. It elevates the ilium and side bends the lumbar spine. The two quadratii, working simultaneously, can be synergistic or antagonistic in function.

An EMG study has shown that the quadratus is most active in isometric side bending. The quadratus is progres-

sively more active with increased compressive load in an upright standing posture, which emphasizes its important role in lumbar spine stability.[29]

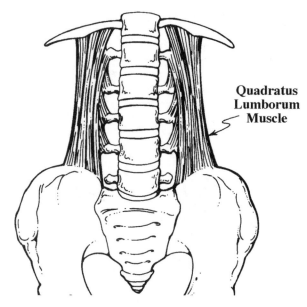

Quadratus Lumborum Muscle

Figure 2-12: The quadratus lumborum muscle.

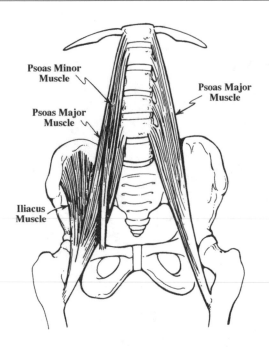

Figure 2-13: The psoas and iliacus muscles with their common insertions make up the iliopsoas.

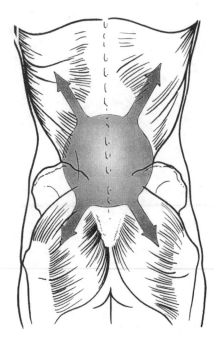

Figure 2-15: The latissimus dorsi and gluteus maximus muscles are theorized to assist lumbosacral stability via their mutual attachments through the dorsal fascia (from Porterfield and DeRosa[38]).

Iliopsoas. The iliacus and psoas major muscles share a common insertion and have similar actions. Thus, the combined mass is often called the iliopsoas. The iliacus arises from the iliac fossa, the inner lip of the iliac crest and the anterior sacroiliac ligament. The psoas major arises from the lateral and anterior portions of the lumbar vertebræ. Both muscles insert onto the lesser trochanter (Fig 2-13).

The primary functions of the iliopsoas are hip flexion and internal hip rotation, but with the hips fixed, the iliopsoas flexes the trunk. The psoas and sometimes the iliacus are active during sitting and standing. Both are active

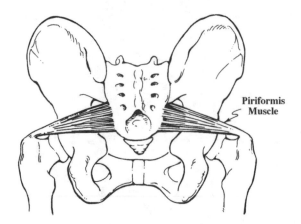

Figure 2-14: The piriformis muscle.

during ambulation. The iliacus portion is very active through the last 60° of a full sit-up. The psoas major, acting bilaterally with the insertion fixed, will increase lumbar lordosis[24] and plays a significant role in maintaining upright stance. An in vitro simulation of the psoas co-contracting with the multifidi had a significant stabilizing effect on the lumbar spine.[41] However, the psoas' role in lumbar stability remains controversial.[28]

Piriformis. The piriformis arises from the sacrum, passes laterally through the sciatic notch and attaches to the upper border of the greater trochanter (Fig 2-14). The piriformis functions as a lateral rotator of the hip when the hip is extended in non-weight bearing. It can also function as an abductor of the hip when the hip is flexed to 90°. In weight bearing, the piriformis restrains vigorous or excessive internal rotation of the hip.

Additional Muscular Support. Several other muscles directly or indirectly influence spinal stability. The latissimus dorsi and gluteus maximus are linked through the thoracolumbar fascia system. Contraction of this muscular system increases joint compression through increased tension on the fascia, and is theorized to assist in sacroiliac joint stability (Fig 2-15).[38] The biceps femoris is directly attached to the sacrotuberous ligament. Hamstring contraction during gait increases tension in the sacrotuberous ligament, which helps control the amplitude of posterior ilial

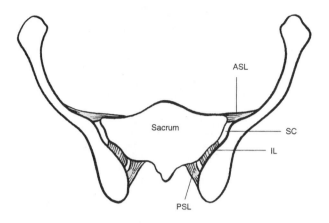

Figure 2-16: The sacroiliac joint cavity (SC) and the sacral ligaments: anterior sacroiliac ligament (ASL), posterior sacroiliac ligament (PSL), and interosseus ligament (IL) (from Porterfield and DeRosa[38]).

rotation and sacral nutation. Because of the vast muscular network potentially contributing to lumbar and sacroiliac joint stability, some authors propose general and specific muscle strengthening, rather than manual therapy techniques, to correct and control sacroiliac joint dysfunction.[38]

Spinal and Sacral Ligaments.   Spinal ligaments pass between each vertebra along the length of the spine and function to limit excessive joint motion. The ligaments include the anterior and posterior longitudinal ligaments, the ligamentum flavum, the inter- and supraspinous ligaments and the intertransverse ligaments. These ligaments run the length of the spine, except for the supraspinous ligament, which ends at L5.[1]

The sacrum is strongly supported by ligaments, including the anterior and posterior sacroiliac ligaments, the interosseus ligament, and the sacrospinous, sacrotuberous and long dorsal sacroiliac ligaments (Fig 2-16). This network of ligaments helps maintain the positional relationship of the sacrum between the ilia and prevents excessive nutation and counternutation in response to gravitational and ground forces. As mentioned above, the biceps femoris attaches to the sacrotuberous ligament, lending dynamic support during gait (Fig 2-17).[38]

The iliolumbar ligaments deserve special notice because they affect both the lumbar spine and sacrum. Movements of L4 and L5, through the pull of the iliolumbar ligaments and the action of the quadratus lumborum and iliopsoas, will affect the SI joint. Conversely, movements of the sacrum and ilium can influence the movements and position of L4 and L5.

The iliolumbar ligaments have two or three bands, depending upon naming conventions: the superior

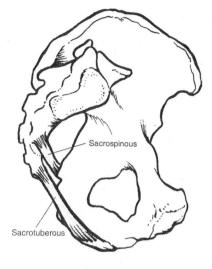

Figure 2-17: The sacrospinous and sacrotuberous ligaments (from Porterfield and DeRosa[38]).

(dorsal) band runs from the transverse process of L4 to the iliac crest; the inferior (ventral) band runs from the transverse process of L5 to the iliac crest, the anterior surface of the SI joint and the lateral sacral ala (Fig 2-18). The medial portion of the inferior band is sometimes called the sacral band, or sacroiliac portion. During side bending of the spine, these ligaments tighten contralaterally and slacken ipsilaterally. During flexion, the superior band tightens and the inferior band slackens. During extension, the reverse takes place.[22] Transection of the iliolumbar ligaments has been shown to significantly increase SI joint laxity. The inferior/ventral band is the most significant in maintaining stability.[37]

Because of the direct ligamentous influence between the L4 and L5 segments and the SI joint, these areas must be adequately examined when dysfunction exists. For example, an posteriorly rotated innominate on the left will tighten the iliolumbar ligaments ipsilaterally and tend to left side bend and left rotate L4 and L5. Thus, restriction of

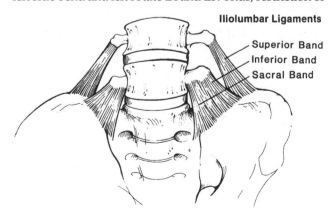

Figure 2-18: The iliolumbar ligaments.

lumbar movement into right side bending and right rotation may be observed with this dysfunction.[47]

Normal Biomechanics of the Spine and Sacroiliac Joints

Fryette, a researcher of spinal mechanics in the early 20th century, developed certain "laws" of spinal motion. Understanding these laws helps to correctly analyze spinal dysfunction and devise appropriate treatment strategies.[33]

Fryette's Law I: If the segments are in neutral (or Easy Normal) without locking of the facets (erect standing posture), rotation is in the *opposite* direction of side bending. Simply stated, if the spine is side bent to the right, rotation of the spine occurs to the left (Fig 2-19). Some osteopathic literature refers to this as Type I motion of the spine. Type I motion is considered to be the normal adaptation or physiologic movement of the spine to changes in posture.

Fryette's Law II: If the segments are in full flexion or extension with the facets engaged (or locked), rotation and side bending occur to the *same* side. Thus, if one bends forward bends (flexes) and side bends to the right, rotation of the spine will occur to the right. In the lumbar and thoracic spine, this motion is considered to be non-physiologic. In the cervical spine, however, it is considered normal physiological motion. This is sometimes referred to as Type II motion and is a non-adapting spinal response to posture or external forces. See *Adapting and Non-Adapting Spinal Dysfunction* on page 20 to see how Type I and Type II terminology is used to describe spinal dysfunction.

Fryette's Law III: If motion is introduced into a segment in any plane, available motion in the other planes is *reduced*. This means that since vertebral movements are usually coupled (concomitant), movement into one plane lessens the range of movement available in the other two planes. Motion introduced into a segment in two planes further reduces the available movement in the remaining third plane.

Normal Spinal Motion

Movement in the spine generally takes place about an axis situated slightly posterior to the center of the intervertebral disc. This axis moves slightly anterior with spinal flexion and slightly posterior with spinal extension.[22] The facet joints, sometimes referred to as zygoapophyseal or apophyseal joints, guide and limit these motions. The facet joints are diarthrodial joints complete with synovial membrane and capsule, and are highly innervated. The plane of the facet joint determines the direction and amount of movement possible between segments. These movements may generally be thought of as gliding movements. The

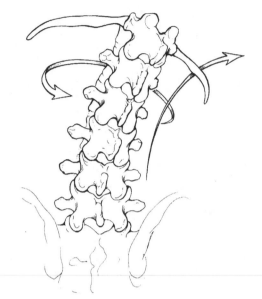

Figure 2-19: Fryette's Law I—side bending and rotation occur in opposite directions.

nucleus, due to its spherical shape, functions like a ball-bearing or a swivel.[22] This capacity facilitates the gliding of the facets. Thus, in three-dimensional space, the spinal segment has six degrees of freedom[18] (Fig 2-20). In other words, a vertebral body can move in the following six ways:

1. Along the longitudinal axis of the spine, i.e., under compression or distraction effects
2. Rotation in the transverse plane around the longitudinal axis of the spine
3. Forward and backward in the transverse plane, i.e., a degree of gliding or translation movement
4. Side bending to either side in the frontal plane around a sagittal axis
5. Lateral gliding or translation in the transverse plane
6. Forward and backward bending around the frontal axis, i.e., flexion and extension

It must be recognized that spinal movement is complex and that normal physiological movement occurs through coupling of two or more of these possible movements simultaneously.

Depending on whether the trunk movement is primarily one of side bending or of rotation, the concomitant movements will involve greater or lesser degrees of forward/backward bending versus compression/distraction of facets. For example, in the lumbar spine, if one left rotates, distraction (widening of the joint space) occurs on the left and compression (squeezing together) occurs on the

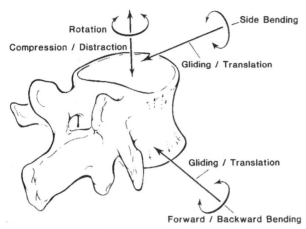

Figure 2-20: Six degrees of freedom of movement of a spinal segment (adapted from Grieve[18]).

right. If one left side bends, the left facet will glide inferiorly (close) while the right facet will glide superiorly (open). Thus, if the left facet should become restricted, the loss of motion would be most noticeable in left rotation and right side bending. Cyriax calls this the capsular pattern of motion restriction for the spine.[12]

The importance of understanding the normal physiological motions of the spine comes with the realization that one can override these movements voluntarily. One can make the spine move in ways contrary to its natural tendency for motion. This has great implication in the mechanics of injury and for subsequent treatment.

Generally speaking, spinal joints oriented in the sagittal plane and moving about a frontal axis produce the gross motions of flexion and extension; joints oriented in the horizontal plane moving about a vertical axis produce rotation; and the joints oriented in the frontal plane moving about an anterior-posterior axis produce side bending. It should be remembered that movement of the spine is described as the superior portion of the segment moving relative to the inferior portion of the segment.

Atlanto/Occipital Joint. The A/O joints, which are condyloid in nature, are oriented in the horizontal plane and move primarily about a frontal axis, producing motion in the sagittal plane. Nodding the head on the cervical spine is the most free movement with approximately 10° occurring in flexion and 25° in extension. Only small amounts of side bending and rotation take place at the A/O joints due to the concave-convex relationships of the joint surfaces. This small rotational movement is of clinical significance and can be easily palpated at the end of range.

During flexion of the head and neck all cervical vertebræ move simultaneously. The atlas may be thought of as performing a "meniscus-like" function during movements

of the head on the neck. In the normal physiological motion of flexion, where the entire cervical spine is free to move, the occipital condyles roll forward on the atlas while the atlas itself glides backward, tilting upward slightly so that the atlas and occiput approximate.[18] If the cervical spine is stabilized, either through pathological processes or by voluntary action, the occipital condyles glide backward on the atlas while the atlas moves slightly forward and cranially, moving the odontoid with it. Thus, the occiput and posterior arch of the atlas tend to move apart in this situation.

Atlanto/Axial Joint. The A/A joint (C1-2) is a plane joint whose surfaces are oriented in the horizontal plane with a vertical axis as the primary axis of movement. The presence of the odontoid process of the axis, which projects through the ring of the atlas, provides a pivot joint which further facilitates rotation at this level. Nearly one-half of the entire range of cervical rotation occurs at the A/A joint, approximately 40° to either side, with 50° or so recruited in the lower segments. There are only small amounts of motion available to the A/A joint in the sagittal (flexion-extension) and frontal (side bending) planes.

C2-C6 Segments. The facet joint planes of these segments are oriented between the horizontal and dorsal planes. These surfaces tend to separate during forward bending, approximate during backward bending and move asymmetrically in rotation and side bending. For example, in side bending to the right, the right facet joints will close and the left facet joints will open. Remembering that Fryette's Law II is true for the cervical spine, the segmental action of side bending right will occur with rotation to the right. According to Kapandji, this combined movement of side bending and rotation totals 50°. Total range of motion in flexion and extension for these segments is 100-110°. When combined with the movement of the upper cervical spine, the total range of motion is 130°.[22]

Uncovertebral Joints. The uncovertebral joints (Joints of Von Lushka) are formed by the articulations of the uncinate processes of the inferior vertebral body (superolateral plateau) and the semi-lunar facets of the superior vertebral body (inferolateral plateau). These joints are cartilaginous and encapsulated. During flexion and extension, these joints slide relative to each other, guiding the vertebral bodies into this A/P movement. During side bending and rotation, the contralateral joint tends to open while the ipsilateral joint tends to close. These joints can be of significance in cervical pathology, especially spinal stenosis and degenerative joint disease.[22]

C7-T3 Segments. These segments represent a transitional zone between the cervical lordosis and the thoracic kyphosis. Forward and backward bending are not great and all ranges are diminished (not necessarily in a graduated manner). The facet joints become somewhat more vertically oriented into the frontal plane.

T3-T10 Segments. The thoracic spine is characterized by narrow disc spaces and elongated spinous processes. These spinous processes gradually become nearly vertical in their frontal plane orientation throughout the spine. This elongation of the spinous processes limits the amount of extension possible at each segment. In forward bending, the nearly vertical facets separate superiorly, but this is somewhat restricted. Total flexion/extension motion does not exceed 5° at each segment.[1] Side bending and rotation occur in much the same manner as in the cervical spine. Both side bending and rotation are limited by the bony thorax. Side bending motions are limited to 4° or less at each segment.[1] It should be noted that all thoracic vertebræ (except T12) have three demi-facets on each side for the articulations of the ribs.

T11-L1 Segments. These segments represent a transitional zone between the thoracic kyphosis and the lumbar lordosis. While the facet joints remain vertically oriented, they begin to change from the frontal to the sagittal plane. Thus, the T12 vertebra has its superior facets in the frontal plane and its inferior facets in the sagittal plane to match those of L1. The discs also begin to increase in height. General mobility in this area is somewhat greater in comparison to the rest of the thoracic spine.

L1-L4 Segments. The lumbar facet joints are vertically oriented in the sagittal plane. Thus flexion/extension is facilitated while side bending and rotation are limited by apposition of the facets.

Lumbosacral Junction (L5-S1). The facet joints abruptly change their orientation from the sagittal plane somewhat obliquely into the frontal plane. This tight apposition of the facet surfaces limits side bending and rotation to one or two degrees but does not similarly restrict flexion/extension. Caillet[8] states that 75% of the total amount of lumbar flexion/extension takes place at the lumbosacral junction with 20% at L4-L5. The remaining 5% of motion is at the remaining segments L1-L3. Farfan, however, believes that the greatest flexion/extension range occurs at L4-L5 (10° extension and 12° flexion) with slightly less at the lumbosacral junction.[15] Yet another source reports flexion and extension motion of 9° and 5°, respectively, with rotation and side bending of 2° and 3°, respectively.[1]

Regardless of the amount of motion existing at the L5-S1 segment, the tight apposition of the facet surfaces provides the main counterbalance to the tremendous shear forces which are present at the lumbosacral junction (Fig 2-21). The normal lumbosacral angle is about 140° with a sacral inclination angle of 15-30°. The arrangement produces shear forces of 50% of the superincumbent body weight. If the sacral inclination angle increases to 40°, the shear increases to 65%. An increase to 50° produces a 75% shear force. It should also be remembered that the orientation of the auricular surfaces of the sacroiliac joint will influence this angle. Should the posterior arch become fractured (or lengthened) at the pars interarticularis, the condition of *spondylolysis* results. Should the spondylolysis be bilateral and the anterior elements begin to separate from the posterior elements, the condition of *spondylolisthesis* results. Thus, the integrity of this joint is of primary importance.

Although many non-invasive techniques to measure spinal range of motion are available, results are inconsistent and difficult to reproduce.[1] Normal ranges of spinal mobility presented in Table 2-1 are based on a variety of sources using differing methodologies, so the ranges are relatively wide.[7,9,10,14,22,23,25,30,36,50,51,53] One should keep in mind that motion will vary by age and gender.

Normal Sacroiliac Movements

The fact that the sacroiliac joints move is not a matter of conjecture. Adequate documentation exists in a variety of literature to demonstrate the certainty of their movement both in vivo and in vitro. Some sources report 1-2° rotation and about 1° translation, but studies using extreme hip positions or manual spring testing methods have demonstrated rotation of 8° and more.[27,45,46] The

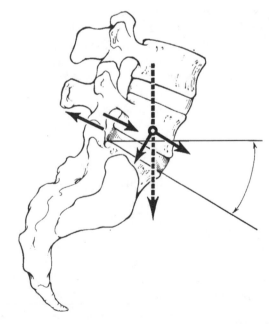

Figure 2-21: Resistance of L5-S1 facet joints to shear forces at the lumbosacral junction (adapted from Kapandji[22]).

Table 2-1: Normal Ranges of Spinal Mobility

Cervical	
Flexion	40°-70°
Extension	60°-80°
Side Bending	40°-50°
Rotation	70°-90°
Thoracic	
Flexion	20°-30°
Extension	25°-35°
Side Bending	20°-25°
Rotation	5°-10°
Lumbar	
Sacral Inclination Angle	15°-30°
Flexion	40°-75°
Extension	20°-35°
Side Bending	15°-35°
Rotation	10°-20°

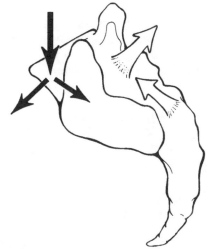

Figure 2-22: Posterior ligaments (white arrows) resist the force of the body weight on the sacroiliac joint (adapted from Kapandji[22]).

movement reported varies significantly depending upon the sample studied and the methodology of the researchers.[2,8,11,12,13,15,17,19,21,27,45,46,48,54]

In osteopathic literature, the sacroiliac joint is considered to be two joints: iliosacral (IS)—the innominates moving on the sacrum; and sacroiliac (SI)—the sacrum moving within the ilia. Functionally and from a treatment standpoint, these distinctions are meaningful, even though they are one and the same articulation.[33]

The sacrum itself is wedge shaped and fits vertically between the wings of the two iliac bones. It is suspended between the ilia by strong, dense ligaments. The wedge shape of the sacrum facilitates a self-locking mechanism of the sacrum within the ilia, with the ligaments tightening as heavier weight is imposed on it from above (Fig 2-22).[22]

With the possible exception of the piriformis, movement of the SI joint is not directly produced by muscular action. Motion of the SI joint is indirectly imposed by actions, movements, and stresses of adjacent and other body parts.[43] On the other hand, a muscular role in stability of the SI joint has been convincingly demonstrated.[20,24,38,41,42,57]

The SI joint is auricular (ear-like) in shape with corresponding parts between the sacrum and the iliac portions of the joint. The joint surfaces are irregular and characterized by peaks and valleys. Generally, there is a long crest running through the center of the iliac portion of the joint and a corresponding trough on the sacral portion.[22] According to Weisel, the cranial portion of the sacral articular facet is longer and narrower than the caudal

portion. He reports that there is a central depression at the junction of these segments and an elevation at the edge of each segment[55] (Fig 2-23). It should be recognized that natural anatomical variants of the SI joint are common. In one study, up to 19% of subjects without pathology had accessory joints in one or both SI joints. In addition, five other anatomical variants were identified.[39]

Nutation and counternutation (flexion and extension) of the sacrum occur within the ilia about a transverse axis posterior to the joint at the sacral tuberosity where the sacroiliac ligaments insert.[22] During nutation (flexion), movement of the sacral promontory is anterior and inferior (the coccyx moves posteriorly), the iliacs approximate and

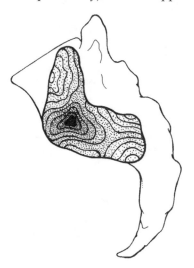

Figure 2-23: Irregular auricular surface of the sacrum, showing central depression. There is a corresponding surface on the left ilium (adapted from Kapandji[22]).

the ischial tuberosities move apart. Conversely, during counternutation (extension), the sacral promontory moves posterior and superior (the coccyx moves anteriorly), the iliacs move apart and the ischial tuberosities approximate. These movements occur naturally during forward bending and backward bending as part of the lumbopelvic rhythm.

The function of the spine is affected by the horizontal/vertical orientation of the sacrum within the ilia. A more vertical sacrum usually results in a flattened lumbar spine, which increases compression forces on it. A more horizontally oriented sacrum increases lumbar curving and also increases shear forces at the lumbosacral junction. The vertical sacrum is associated with the static spine and the horizontal sacrum with the dynamic spine previously described (Fig 2-24).

The following anatomical distinctions of the female versus the male pelvis are important to understand because they affect SI joint function and stability:[2,12,18,22]

- The lateral distance of the pelvic outlet is larger in females.
- The bone density in the female pelvis is less.
- The SI joints of females are located farther from the hip joints, creating a longer lever arm.
- Females have smaller SI joint surfaces.
- Females have flatter SI joint surfaces.
- The iliac crests are farther apart in the female.
- The vertical dimension of the pelvis is smaller in females.

Axes of Movement. Movements of the sacrum and ilia are possible about any of several axes. Mitchell, Moran, and Pruzzo[33] describe the following axes and movements (Fig 2-25):

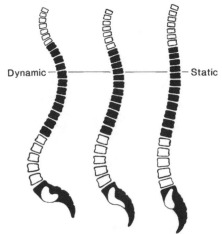

Figure 2-24: Orientation of the sacroiliac joint and its effect on the spine, producing dynamic or static types of function and posture (adapted from Kapandji[22]).

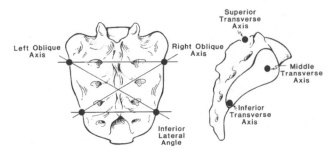

Figure 2-25: Multiple axes of the sacroiliac joint (adapted from Mitchell, Moran and Pruzzo[33]).

1. The *Superior Transverse Axis* runs through the second sacral segment horizontally. Also known as the *Respiratory Axis*, it is actually a fulcrum formed by the attachments of the posterior sacroiliac ligaments and the thoracodorsal fascia. As one inhales and exhales, the sacrum extends (counternutates) and flexes (nutates).
2. The *Middle Transverse Axis* is located at the second sacral body and is the principle axis of normal sacroiliac movement (nutation/counternutation).
3. The *Inferior Transverse Axis* runs transversely through the inferior pole of the sacral articulation and extends laterally through the PSIS. It is the principle axis of normal iliosacral motion.
4. The *Transverse Pelvic Axis* runs transversely through the symphysis pubis about which the innominates rotate, allowing movement in an anteroposterior direction during locomotion (see *Gait and Sacroiliac Joint Function* on page 19).
5. The *Right and Left Oblique Axes* run through the superior end of the articular surface of the sacrum obliquely to the opposite Inferior Lateral Angle (ILA). Each axis is named for its site of origin at the sacral base. Because iliosacral motion is conjoined with the pubis, the sacrum must make adaptive movements about these oblique axes alternately.

Multiple actions of the sacrum and ilia are possible given the number of axes of motion described. It is simplistic to think of sacroiliac joint motion only in terms of anteroposterior movements. Normal iliosacral (IS) movements are usually anteroposterior rotations of one innominate with respect to the other about the inferior transverse axis of the sacrum and the transverse pelvic axis. Other movements of the innominates on the sacrum are possible, but do not normally occur except as seen in dysfunctional states. Dysfunctional mechanics of the sacroiliac joint are described in Chapter 7, *Pelvic Girdle Dysfunction*.

Gait and Sacroiliac Joint Function

The following is a synopsis of an article by Mitchell on this topic.[34] The cycle of movement of the pelvis in walking is described in sequence as though the patient were starting to walk by advancing the right foot first:

Left thoracic trunk rotation is accompanied by left lumbar side bending, forming a convexity to the right. The body of the sacrum begins a torsional movement to the left, locking the lumbosacral junction and shifting the body weight to the left sacroiliac. This locking mechanism establishes movement of the sacrum on the left oblique axis. As the sacrum can now turn torsionally to the left, the sacral base must also move down on the right to conform to the lumbar convexity that was formed on the right.

As the right leg accelerates forward through action of the quadriceps, tension accumulates at the junction of the left oblique axis and the inferior transverse axis, and the sacroiliac joint eventually locks. As the body weight swings forward, slight anterior movement is increased by the backward thrust of the resting left leg as the right heel strikes the ground.

Tension in the right hamstrings begins with heel-strike. As the body weight moves forward and upward toward the apex of femoral support within the right acetabulum, there is a slight posterior movement of the right innominate on the inferior transverse axis. This movement is also increased by the forward thrust of the propelling leg action. This iliac rotational movement is also influenced, directed, and stabilized by the torsional movement of the pubic symphysis on this transverse axis. Also at heel-strike, the right piriformis contracts to fixate the left oblique axis at the inferior lateral angle, thus allowing for a left forward torsion of the sacrum on the left oblique axis (termed a *left-on-left forward torsion*). From the standpoint of total pelvic movement, one might consider the transverse pelvic axis as the postural axis of rotation for the entire pelvis.

As the right heel strikes the ground, trunk rotation and accommodation begin to reverse themselves. At mid-stance, as the left foot passes the right and the body weight passes over the apex of femoral support within the acetabulum, accumulating forces move to the right oblique axis, which then allows the left sacral base to move forward and torsionally to the right. The cycle of movements is then repeated in identical fashion on the left.

Lumbopelvic Rhythm

There is an interconnection of movement between the spine and the pelvis. This is especially true in the total forward bending of the spine: there is a synchronous movement in a rhythmic ratio of the lumbar spine to that of pelvic rotation about the hips.

During forward bending, the lumbar curve reverses itself from concave to flat to slightly convex. At the same time, there is a proportionate degree of pelvic rotation about the hips while the amount of movement at each lumbar level is different (more at L5-S1 and L4-5 and less at the other levels). The rhythm between levels should be so smooth and precise that at every point in the forward bending arc, there will be balance between lumbar reversal and pelvic rotation (Fig 2-26).[2] Obviously, the ability of a person to forward bend will thus be influenced by this balance or lack of it. Many factors such as facet restriction, degenerative joint disease or tight hamstring muscles can influence this balance. Thus, to achieve full, non-pathological forward bending, the lumbar spine must fully reverse itself to flat and the pelvis must rotate to its full extent. The sacrum also moves within the ilia during this action of forward bending. Initially, the sacrum nutates (flexes) but as motion in the lumbar spine is recruited and the pelvis

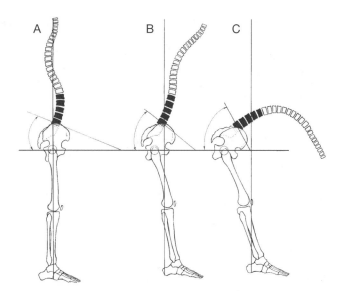

Figure 2-26: Lumbopelvic rhythm from left to right: A) Normal standing posture with lumbar concavity; body weight directly over hip joints; normal pelvic inclination angle with respect to horizontal. B) Flattening of the lumbar spine; pelvis begins to rotate anteriorly around the hips; hips and pelvis move posteriorly in the horizontal plane. C) Reversal of the lumbar lordosis to flat; pelvis rotates anteriorly to the fullest extent; hips and pelvis are posteriorly displaced in the horizontal plane.

rotates anteriorly over the hips, the sacrum begins to counternutate (extend) within the ilia. Tethering of the pelvis by the hamstrings completes the counternutation movement.

At the same time that these movements occur in the sagittal plane, there is a backward movement of the pelvis on the hips in the horizontal plane. This represents a shift in the pelvic fulcrum so that the center of gravity is maintained over the feet, otherwise the person would fall forward.

As the person returns to the standing position, just the converse occurs: the lumbar spine becomes concave, the pelvis derotates and also shifts forward. The same degree of smoothness and rhythm should be achieved with extension.

Adapting and Non-Adapting Spinal Dysfunction

The complex relationship between the pelvic joints and spine, as well as anatomic and functional asymmetries, postural problems and other biomechanical considerations, cannot be overemphasized. The spine's response to injury or biomechanical stressors can be adapting or non-adapting. It is important to understand the distinction between these responses, to determine how best to treat them.

Adapting responses are typically non-traumatic or unrelated to an injury. Functional scoliosis is an example of a normal adaptive response because it involves multiple segments, it follows Fryette's first law (side bending and rotation occuring in *opposite* directions), and is usually in response to non-traumatic factors (leg length discrepancy, pelvic obliquity, asymmetrical muscle balance, etc.)

In osteopathic terminology, adapting responses are named *Type I dysfunctions,* after Fryette's first law. Type I dysfunctions, unless of long-standing duration, are usually not treated directly with manual techniques. Instead, they are treated by addressing the cause of the adaptation. For example, functional scoliosis might be treated by correcting a leg length discrepancy or muscle imbalance.

Non-adapting responses are usually traumatic in nature, and act in accordance to Fryette's second law. For example, a lumbar spine injury caused by a slip, fall or twist often produces a single segment restriction: the vertebra will sidebend and rotate in the *same* direction. In osteopathic terminology, this abnormal response is termed a *Type II dysfunction,* after Fryette's second law, and is treated directly with muscle energy or other joint mobilization techniques. The techniques described in Chapter 10, *Joint Mobilization,* specifically address non-adapting (Type II) dysfunctions.

REFERENCES

1. Ashton-Miller J and Schultz AB: Biomechanics of the Human Spine. In Basic Orthopaedic Biomechanics, 2nd edition. VC Mow and WC Hayes, eds. Lippincott-Raven, Philadelphia 1997.
2. Beal M: The Sacroiliac Problems: Review of Anatomy, Mechanics and Diagnosis. JAOA 81(10):667-679, June 1982.
3. Beattie PF, Brooks WM, Rothstein JM, et al: Effect of Lordosis on the Position of the Nucleus Pulposus in Supine Subjects. A Study Using MRI. Spine 19(18):2096-2102, 1994.
4. Boos N, Weissback S, Rohrbach H, et al: Classification of Age-Related Changes in Lumbar Intervertebral Discs. 2002 Volvo Award in Basic Science. Spine 27(23):2631-2544, 2002.
5. Brault JS, Driscoll DM, Laakso LL, et al: Quantification of Lumbar Intradiscal Deformation During Flexion and Extension, by Mathematical Analysis of MRI Pixel Intensity Profiles. Spine 22(18):2066-2072, 1997.
6. Buckwalter J, Mow VC, Boden SD, et al: Intervertebral Disc Structure, Composition and Mechanical Function. In Orthopaedic Basic Science, Biology and Biomechanics of the Musculoskeletal System, 2nd edition. JA Buckwalter, TA Einhorn and SR Simon, eds. American Academy of Orthopaedic Surgeons, Rosemont, IL 2000.
7. Burdett R, et al: Reliability and Validity of Four Instruments for Measuring Lumbar Spine and Pelvic Positions. Phys Ther 66(5):677-684, 1986.
8. Caillet R: Low Back Pain Syndrome. 2nd edition. FA Davis, Philadelphia PA 1982.
9. Chen J, Solinger AB, Poncet JF, et al: Meta-Analysis of Normative Cervical Motion. Spine 24(15):1571-1578, 1999.
10. Cocciarella L and Andersson G, eds: Guides to the Evaluation of Permanent Impairment, 5th ed. American Medical Association Press, Chicago 2001.
11. Colachis S, Warden R, et al: Movement of the Sacroiliac Joint in the Adult Male. Arch Phys Med Rehab 44:490, 1963.
12. Cyriax J: Diagnosis of Soft Tissue Lesions. Textbook of Orthopædic Medicine, Vol 1, 8th edition. Bailliere-Tindall, London 1982.
13. DiAmbrosia R: Musculoskeletal Disorders, 258-260. JB Lippincott, Philadelphia PA 1977.
14. Dvorak J, Vajda EG, Grob D, et al: Normal Motion of the Lumbar Spine as Related to Age and Gender. Eur Spine J 4:18-23, 1995.
15. Farfan H: Mechanical Disorders of the Low Back. Lea and Febiger, Philadelphia PA 1973.
16. Fennell AJ, Jones AP and Hukins DWL: Migration of the Nucleus Pulposus within the Intervertebral Disc During Flexion and Extension of the Spine. Spine 21(23):2753-2757, 1996.
17. Frigerio N, Stowe R and Howe J: Movement of the Sacroiliac Joint. Clin Orthop and Rel Res 100:370, 1974.
18. Grieve G: Common Vertebral Joint Problems. Churchill-Livingstone, New York NY 1981.
19. Harrison DE, Harrison DD and Troyanovich SJ: The Sacroiliac Joint: A Review of Anatomy and Biomechanics

with Clinical Implications. JMPT 20(9):607-617, 1997.

20. Hodges PW: Is there a Role for Transversus Abdominis in Lumbo-Pelvic Stability? Manual Therapy 4(2):74-86, 1999.

21. Jacob HAC and Kissling RO: The Mobility of the Sacroiliac Joints in Healthy Volunteers Between 20 and 50 Years of Age. Clin Biomech 10(7):352-361, 1995.

22. Kapandji I: Spine. Vol 3 of The Physiology of the Joints, 2nd ed. Churchill Livingstone, London 1974.

23. Keeley J, et al: Quantification of Lumbar Function Part 5: Reliability of Range of Motion Measures in the Sagittal Plane and in Vivo Torso Rotation Measurement Techniques. Spine 11(1):31-35, 1986.

24. Kendall FP, McCreary EK and Provance PG: Muscles Testing and Function, 4th edition. Lippincott, Williams and Wilkins, Baltimore 1993.

25. Lantz CA, Klein G and Chen J et al: A Reassessment of Normal Cervical Range of Motion. Spine 28(12):1249-1257, 2003.

26. Lu YM, Hutton WC and Gharpuray VM: Can Variations in Intervertebral Disc Height Affect the Mechanical Function of the Disc? Spine 21(19):2208-2216, 1996.

27. Lund PJ, Krupinski EA and Brooks WJ: Ultrasound Evaluation of Sacroiliac Motion in Normal Volunteers. Acad Radiol 3:192-196, 1996.

28. McGill S: Low Back Exercises: Evidence for Improving Exercise Regimens. Phys Ther 78(7):754-765, 1998.

29. McGill S: Quantitative Intramuscular Myoelectric Activity of the Quadratus Lumborum During a Wide Variety of Tasks. Clin Biomech 11(3):170-172, 1996.

30. McGregor AH, McCarthy ID, Hughes SP: Motion Characteristics of the Lumbar Spine in the Normal Population. Spine 20(22):2421-28, 1995.

31. McKenzie R and May S: The Lumbar Spine Mechanical Diagnosis and Therapy, Vol I. Spinal Publications, Waikanae, New Zealand 2003.

32. Mercer S and Bogduk N: The Ligaments and Anulus Fibrosus of Human Adult Cervical Intervertebral Discs. Spine 24(7):619-628, 1999.

33. Mitchell F, Moran P and Pruzzo N: An Evaluation and Treatment Manual of Osteopathic Muscle Energy Procedures. Mitchell, Moran and Pruzzo Associates, Valley Park MI 1979.

34. Mitchell F: Structural Pelvic Function. AAO Yearbook II: 178, 1965.

35. Nachemson A: The Lumbar Spine, An Orthopædic Challenge. Spine 1:50-71, 1976.

36. Ng JK, Kippers V, Richardson C, et al: Range of Motion and Lordosis of the Lumbar Spine. Reliability of Measurement and Normative Values. Spine 26(1):53-60, 2001.

37. Pool-Goudzwaard A, van Dijke GH, Mulder P, et al: The Iliolumbar Ligament: Its influence on Stability of the Sacroiliac Joint. Clin Biomech 18:99-105, 2003.

38. Porterfield JA and DeRosa C: Mechanical Low Back Pain Perspectives in Functional Anatomy. WB Saunders, Philadelphia 1998.

39. Prassopoulos PK, Faflia CP, Voloudaki AE, et al: Sacroiliac Joints: Anatomical Variants on CT. Joul of Comp Asst Tomog 23(2):323-327, 1999.

40. Provencher MT and Abdu WA: Giovanni Alfonso Borelli: "Father of Spinal Biomechanics". Spine 25(1):131-136, 2000.

41. Quint U, Wilke H, Shirazi-Adl A, et al: Importance of the Intersegmental Trunk Muscles for the Stability of the Lumbar Spine. A Biomechanical Study In Vitro. Spine 23(18):1937-1945, 1998.

42. Richardson CA, Snijders CJ, Hides, JA, et al: The Relation Between the Transversus Abdominis Muscles, Sacroiliac Joint Mechanics and Low Back Pain. Spine 27(4):399-405, 2002.

43. Shah J: Structure, Morphology and Mechanics of the Lumbar Spine. In The Lumbar Spine and Low Back Pain. M Jayson, ed. Pitman Medical, London 1980.

44. Shao Z, Rompe G and Schiltenwolf M: Radiographic Changes in the Lumbar Intervertebral Discs and Lumbar Vertebrae with Age. Spine 27(3):263-268, 2002.

45. Smidt G, Wei S, McQuade K, et al: Sacroiliac Motion for Extreme Hip Positions. A Fresh Cadaver Study. Spine 22(18):2073-2082, 1997.

46. Smidt GL, McQuade K, Wei S, et al: Sacroiliac Kinematics for Reciprocal Straddle Positions. Spine 20():1047-54, 1995.

47. Stratton S: Evaluation and Treatment of the Sacroiliac Joint. Course Notes and Personal Communication. Sept 1984.

48. Sturesson B, Uden A and Vleeming A: A Radiostereometric Analysis of the Movements of the Sacroiliac Joints in the Reciprocal Straddle Position. Spine 25(2):214-217, 2000.

49. Travell J, and Simons D: Myofascial Pain and Dysfunction. Vol 2 of The Trigger Point Manual. Williams and Wilkins, Baltimore MD 1992.

50. Troke M: A New, Comprehensive Normative Database of Lumbar Spine Ranges of Motion. Clin Rehab 15:371-379, 2001.

51. Troup J, et al: The Perception of Back Pain and the Role of Psychophysical Tests of Lifting Capacity. Spine 12(7):645-657, 1987.

52. Twomey LT and Taylor JR: Age Changes in Lumbar Vertebrae and Intervertebral Discs. Clin Orthop 224:97-104, 1987.

53. Van Herp G, Rowe PJ, Salter PM: Range of Motion in the Lumbar Spine and the Effects of Age and Gender. Physiotherapy 86:42, 2000.

54. Wang M, Dumas GA: Mechanical Behavior of the Female Sacroiliac Joint and Influence of the Anterior and POsterior Sacroiliac Ligaments under Sagittal Loads. Clin Biomech 13:293-299, 1998.

55. Weisel H: Movements of the Sacro-Iliac Joint. Acta Anat 23:80-91, 1955.

56. Wilke H, Neef P Caimi M, et al: New In Vivo Measurements of Pressures in the Intervertebral Disc in Daily Life. Spine 24(8):755-762, 1999.

57. Wilke H, Wolf S, Claes LE, et al: Stability Increase of the Lumbar Spine with Different Muscle Groups. A Biomechanical In Vitro Study. Spine 20(2):192-198, 1995.

3

MEDICAL SCREENING

Michael Koopmeiners, MD

Physical therapy practice has changed dramatically in the last 10 years. While medical screening for non-musculo-skeletal conditions has always been an essential part of physical therapy practice, the changing times have placed greater emphasis on the development and implementation of well-defined screening protocols, including a description of appropriate action steps based on the outcome of the screening. Medical screening will minimally impact the majority of cases. However, the cases that will be impacted are important to identify early and to act upon.

To simplify the understanding of what medical screening entails, the process can be divided into *basic screening* and *advanced screening*, terms that will be used throughout this chapter. Basic screening is imbedded in all aspects of the patient's care including history taking, data-base analysis, physical examination and monitoring response to treatment. It simply involves being alert to findings that may indicate the patient has non-mechanical pathology.

Advanced screening involves additional inquiry or tests that are not performed during a routine musculoskel-etal examination. For example, regional organ system screening is used when the therapist suspects possible pathology in a particular organ system. The goal of both basic and advanced screening is to facilitate appropriate referral to other medical providers and to determine when special monitoring or treatment modifications will be required in the physical therapy plan of care.

Medical screening is easy to incorporate into practice. While most patients will require only basic screening, it is important that today's physical therapist be comfortable with the advanced screening skills discussed in this chapter. An appropriate response to patients who screen positive for a non-mechanical medical condition can improve patient care, efficiency, therapist satisfaction and collaboration between medical disciplines.

Historical Perspective

Medical screening has been a part of physical therapy practice for many years. The APTA guidelines mandate screening as part of the initial evaluation[6]. Physical therapy education has included course work regarding screening. In the past, screening has been somewhat cursory and has lacked clinical context. Clear instructions about what to do with a positive finding have been frequently lacking. As physical therapists expand their level of care delivery in the 21st century, it is essential to reconsider their clinical activities. In particular, there is a clear need to organize and strengthen the therapist's evaluation skills to include evaluation for co-morbid medical conditions. The ultimate driver of this change is the need to maximize quality, efficient patient care.

The historical forces driving changes in physical therapy practice started with the movement of therapy practice to an independent, non hospital-based setting. Twenty-five years ago, a hospital-based practice was the norm. The practice was mainly a prescriptive practice based on a physician's order. The physical therapist and other members of the care delivery team were in close physical proximity. Information about co-morbid conditions was readily accessible and nursing staff members were available to evaluate and treat co-morbid conditions. Today, more of physical therapy practice is done in non-hospital environments. The transition to the independent, outpatient setting means the loss of easy access to medical records and nursing personnel. Medical screening thus takes on more importance.

At the same time that physical therapy practice moved out of the hospital, hospital stays were being shortened. For example, in 1993 an average hospital stay after hip replacement was 8.9 days; in 2001 it was only 5.4 days.[7] The result is that patients are treated in the physical therapy outpatient clinic earlier in their recovery phases. A greater intensity of service is required; the patient also has a greater likelihood of developing conditions such as infection, deep vein thrombosis and worsening of previously hidden angina. The physical therapist may be the only health care professional seeing these patients regularly, and therefore needs to be competent in identifying symptoms of concern and facilitating early referrals to the appropriate provider.

Payment mechanisms also impact physical therapy practice. Fee-for-service reimbursement is less common than in previous years. More practices are being reimbursed with some expectation of demonstrating a positive outcome from the services delivered. This payment for performance is done through discounted fee-for-service with incentive models or risk sharing models such as capitation rates or case rate payment methodologies.

While the newer payment methods are frequently criticized, at least one positive change has resulted. Therapists who identify the most appropriate treatment in a timely fashion are rewarded financially. Specifically, the newer payment structures provide an incentive to identify early, and with great efficiency, those patients who may not be appropriate for therapy or who may require concurrent referral to a medical colleague. To treat a patient for three or four visits before considering the possibility of a confounding medical condition is no longer financially reasonable and does not result in optimal patient care.

The documentation of co-morbid conditions in patients receiving rehabilitative care provides justification for prolonged therapy. Physical therapists who pay attention to these facts will ensure that their patients receive more appropriate care sooner, and receive appropriate reimbursement for their services.

A new driving force in medicine is the concept of *best practice* and demonstrating value. The APTA's "hooked on evidence" project emphasizes best practice for the profession and promotes clinical decision-making based on published evidence.[1] Clinicians practicing in most areas of medicine have come to accept the concept of best practice, as evidenced by the proliferation of best practice guidelines. Best practice also drives reimbursement because payers expect the physical therapy profession to demon-

strate effectiveness. Screening is an important part of best practice.

For example, practice "A" aggressively screens their patients and identifies a subset of patients with low back pain who also have diabetes. People with diabetes with elevated blood sugars may have a prolonged recovery. If the therapists work collaboratively with these patients' treating medical providers, the patients can achieve improved control of their diabetes and minimize delayed recovery. Conversely, practice "B" does not aggressively screen for patients with diabetes and thus under-identifies these patients. Due to an increased incidence of delayed recovery, practice "B" may experience increased visit rates and poorer outcomes. This negative result has little to do with the adequacy of the therapy provider. Rather, a failure of adequate screening protocols in the practice has led to the suboptimal outcomes. An incentive model of payment would reward practice "A".

Changing demographics, especially the aging of the population, will have a significant impact on physical therapy. By 2025 over 18% of the population will be over 65 years old and 8% will be over 75 years old.[8] Degenerative processes occur with aging. Physical therapists are very familiar with one of its manifestations, degenerative joint disease (DJD). DJD leads to generalized de-conditioning, frequently resulting in joint replacement.

Other degenerative processes with which the therapist may not be as familiar include coronary artery disease, diabetes, hypertension, Parkinsonism and dementia. Besides directly impacting physical therapy, these conditions may also result in increased use of medication with adverse side effects. Screening for these and many other conditions will assume greater importance and the likelihood of positive findings will increase in the coming century.

The natural history of the degenerative process also increases the possibility that a co-morbid condition may initially manifest itself in the therapist's office. A symptom of DJD is increased pain with activity and decreased pain with rest. The increased pain caused by worsening DJD leads to decreased activity and deconditioning. Less activity also leads to less stress on the cardiac, pulmonary and nervous organ systems. Pathology of these organ systems is manifested by increased symptoms with activity and relief of symptoms with rest. Worsening disease leads to less activity. If a 66-year-old patient presents with shoulder pain with movement that is relieved with rest, is this a patient with a shoulder impingement or coronary artery disease? The physical therapist must be cognizant of the potential overlap in symptoms that these patients present.

Changing times necessitate changing behavior. The changing practice location for physical therapists, the increasing pressure on the American medical system to improve efficiency of care, the increasing role of the physical therapist in the care delivery system and the aging population all impact the day-to-day practice of physical therapy. Physical therapists must respond to these changes by becoming very efficient and effective. Screening for non–mechanical conditions plays a major role in these improvements.

Medical Conditions Impacting Physical Therapy Diagnosis

The presence of co-morbid non-musculoskeletal conditions impacts the physical therapist's diagnosis in multiple ways. Undiagnosed visceral pathology can present with primarily mechanical symptoms. Additionally, diseases may first manifest themselves due to the positive effects of therapy. Even if the patient has a known medical condition, the condition may have worsened since the patient's last physician visit. Therefore, the physical therapist must be on the alert for the signs and symptoms of visceral pathology and be prepared to react appropriately. Certain medical conditions have a significant mechanical component that needs to be treated with physical therapy. Other medical conditions and their treatments may impact the delivery of therapy services. In such cases, the physical therapist must adjust the treatment plan to appropriately address the mechanical dysfunction while making any special modifications required by the underlying medical condition.

Visceral Pathology Presenting with Musculoskeletal Symptoms

There are many examples of visceral pathology presenting with musculoskeletal symptoms. Abdominal aortic aneurysm, metastatic cancer in the lungs or lymph nodes and diverticulitis can all present with subjective and objective findings that look like mechanical dysfunction. The difficulty for the therapist is that these conditions do have some mechanical symptoms, or the onset of symptoms may sound mechanical. It is important to remember that one can find mechanical dysfunction in any patient over 20 years old. The difficulty is determining if the dysfunction is pertinent or is an incidental finding. Medical screening in the initial evaluation may sort out visceral pathology from a truly musculoskeletal condition, but it may not be until there is a lack of response to treatment that non-musculoskeletal etiology is suspected. When a patient does not respond to therapy, clinicians often begin by questioning compliance or the therapy. Instead, the clinician should first rethink the diagnosis and consider other non-mechanical causes for the symptoms.

For example, the patient with lung cancer may have posterior ribcage pain and a history of a recent fall. It is not until the patient responds poorly to therapy that a non-musculoskeletal diagnosis is considered. Advanced medical screening questions may reveal that the patient has increased pain with deep breaths and gets "winded easily" with exercise. The therapist should be suspicious of non-musculoskeletal etiology at this point.

Somatoform pain disorders are pain disorders in which psychological factors are thought to play a role. Somatoform pain disorders present a particular challenge to the physical therapist. Patients with these conditions typically have subjective complaints with poorly correlated objective findings. However, it is not uncommon to find concurrent mechanical dysfunction with a somatoform disorder, sometimes significant. This conundrum can confuse even the most senior clinician. A somatoform pain disorder should be suspected if the patient uses dramatic words to describe the symptoms and if there is discordance between the history and the physical examination. A patient reporting severe pain but having normal blood pressure and minimal functional problems may have a somatoform pain disorder. It is important to remember that these patients are ill. The therapist must efficiently rule out mechanical dysfunction and empathetically refer them to an appropriate treatment setting.

Medical Conditions with Concurrent Mechanical Dysfunction

Many disease processes present with concurrent mechanical dysfunction. The treatment of the dysfunction necessitates monitoring for the non-musculoskeletal components of the disease and close communication with other treating providers. Rheumatological diseases such as rheumatoid arthritis and the less common ankylosing spondylitis are well-known by the physical therapist. Less commonly recognized conditions are thyroid pathology, diabetes mellitus and endometriosis. Diabetes and hypothyroidism can contribute to the causation of carpal tunnel syndrome. Endometriosis leads to significant mechanical dysfunction of the pelvic floor muscles. Physical therapy plays a crucial role in helping patients with these conditions recover. However, if the underlying pathology is not treated, therapy will only relieve the patient's symptoms temporarily and will eventually become ineffectual.

Medical Conditions Arising During the Course of Therapy

Certain medical conditions may be absent during the initial evaluation but may manifest themselves during the course of therapy. Peptic ulcer disease is an example of such pathology. The patient presents with lumbar spine symptoms. The non-steroidal anti-inflammatories (NSAIDS) that are typically taken for back pain carry a significant risk of gastric irritation. As these medications help with the low back pain they also relieve the pain of the developing peptic ulcer. However, as therapy progresses and the patient uses less of the NSAID for low back pain control he begins to develop pain in the lower thoracic spine. The tendency is to consider the new thoracic spine symptoms as a mechanical consequence of therapy. To do so without considering other causes puts the patient at risk of worsening disease, e.g., gastrointestinal bleeding. Re-screening should be considered when there is a significant change in the patient's symptoms.

Similar examples are coronary artery disease (CAD) and peripheral vascular disease (PVD). With decreasing activity associated with DJD, there is progressive decrease in cardiac stress. Angina may be decreased or absent. A patient's worsening DJD may eventually lead to joint replacement surgery. Due to lack of angina, cardiac disease may not be suspected during the pre-surgical evaluation or the immediate post surgical hospital stay. It is not until the patient begins outpatient or home therapy that the patient's exertion level exceeds the threshold for angina symptoms. Therefore, the therapist may be the first medical professional to become aware of the coronary artery symptoms. Screening can not stop after the initial evaluation; it is an ongoing process during therapy, especially in high-risk individuals.

Depression is being recognized as a significant co-morbid condition in physical therapy practice. Diagnosed depression is present in 11.4% of physical therapy patients.[2] While depression is not a direct consequence of therapy, it may be noted as a problem during the course of therapy. The signs and symptoms of depression are important to recognize, and proactive planning about how to assist the patient with depressive symptoms should be a part of every therapy practice. A list of depressive symptoms is included in the review of systems questionnaire. See *Review of Systems Checklist* on page 36.

Medical Conditions Impacting Treatment

The conditions discussed so far mainly pose diagnostic dilemmas. Many diseases impact treatment choices and are just as important to recognize early in the course of treatment. Previously known disease may worsen during a course of physical therapy or may cause certain treatment techniques to be contraindicated. For example, joint manipulation and traction are contraindicated with severe osteoporosis, and exercise must be approached with cau-

tion. Additional conditions that may impact the choice of physical therapy treatment include asthma, diabetes, chronic obstructive pulmonary disease, cancer, congestive heart failure, hepatitis, aids, pregnancy and chemical dependency.

A diabetic patient requires increased attention because of the role exercise has on control of the disease. Diabetes leads to high blood sugars, which over time increases the risk of coronary artery disease, renal failure, peripheral vascular disease and neuropathy. Blood sugar levels are controlled with a combination of diet, exercise and medication. However, with injury or worsening degenerative joint disease, the activity level of the diabetic patient decreases and there must be a greater reliance on diet and medication to control blood sugars. When a diabetic patient takes part in an exercise rehabilitation program, caution and close monitoring are required. With increased activity, mild hypoglycemia leads to fatigue and sweating. If exercise is initiated too quickly, the hypoglycemia may worsen and become acute, necessitating an emergent response by the therapist. During the screening process, adequacy of control and monitoring needs to be assessed and the therapist has an obligation to warn the patient that office and home therapy may lead to hypoglycemia. During treatment, the patient needs to be monitored closely and would benefit from collaborative dialogue between the therapist and the physician. The goal would be to maximize therapy without complicating the diabetic treatment.

Another example of a medical condition impacting treatment is chemical dependency. Depending upon gender, ethnicity and age, up to 15% of the general population experiences alcohol abuse or dependence.[5] However, physical therapy studies have indicated only 4-5% of patients surveyed report drinking four or more alcoholic drinks per day.[2,3] In other words, many patients with chemical dependency concerns may not self-report during the initial evaluation. Therapists are in unique position to identify these individuals. Untreated chemical dependency results in non-compliance with treatment, poorer physical therapy outcomes and, ultimately, death.

Some screening activities are not critical for physical therapy treatment, per se, but are an important component of quality medical care. Monitoring blood pressure and referring the patient with undiagnosed hypertension is one example. Screening for skin changes consistent with skin cancer is another. Therapists have the opportunity to observe skin more than many other providers do. The screen takes minimal time and usually entails just thinking about the possibility. Skin lesions or moles that easily bleed or ulcerate, have non-distinct or irregular borders, are asymmetric in shape or larger than 6mm should raise concern.

Incidence of Co-Morbid Conditions in the Physical Therapy Patient

Boissoinault has detailed the incidence of disease, medication use, medical habits and family histories in patients being seen in physical therapy.[3] Three of his tables are reproduced here. Table 3-1 lists the type of medical conditions the patients have when they begin a course of therapy. Table 3-2 shows the varying medication that patient takes over the counter, while Table 3-3 lists prescription medication. It is clear that many patients seen in a typical outpatient physical therapy practice have multiple conditions, multiple risk factors and are on multiple medications, all of which impact physical therapy care.

The statistics in Table 3-1 were obtained from patients referred by physicians and address known conditions. With direct access, the physical therapist can expect an increased incidence of undiagnosed medical conditions. Medical screening will become even more important

Actions That May Be Required of the Physical Therapist

Basic screening should always be performed. As defined in this chapter, basic screening is simply being aware of symptoms of visceral pathology and paying attention to inconsistent findings that do not "add up." Most patients the physical therapist evaluates will have a clear history consistent with mechanical dysfunction. The past medical

Table 3-1: Incidence of patients with diagnosed illness in a physical therapy practice (n=704).[2]

Diagnosis	Number of Subjects	%
High blood pressure	108	15.3
Arthritis (other than rheumatoid)	107	15.2
Depression	80	11.4
Asthma	42	6.0
Chemical dependency	33	4.7
Anemia	30	4.3
Thyroid problems	27	3.8
Cancer	26	3.7
Diabetes	21	3.0
Rheumatoid arthritis	20	2.8
Kidney problems	9	1.3
Hepatitis	8	1.1
Heart attack	6	.9

Table 3-2: Over-the-counter medication use in physical therapy patients.[3]

Medication	Number of Subjects	%
Anti-inflammatory	1157	48
Vitamins	1140	47
Tylenol	791	32
Antacids	520	21
Aspirin	497	20
Decongestants	263	11
Antihistamines	262	11
H2 blockers	239	10
Herbal medicines	215	9
Laxatives	142	6
Sleeping pills	142	6

history and family history raise no concerns of increased risk for disease. The physical exam is consistent with the subjective exam. The patient's response to treatment is as expected. Advanced medical screening, including regional organ system screening, is not indicated for these patients, and there is no need to alter the typical therapeutic approach.

Well-controlled medical conditions will require monitoring only. The conditions will be discovered via a medical history questionnaire. The patient reports consis-

Table 3-3: Prescription medication use in physical therapy patients.[3]

Medication	Number of Subjects	%
Anti-inflammatory	984	40
Pain relievers (narcotics)	671	28
Muscle relaxants	501	21
Hypertension medications	406	17
Hormone replacement	357	15
Hyperlipidemia	325	13
Decongestants/antihistamines	306	13
Aspirin	299	12
Antidepressants	275	11
Antibiotics	172	7
Thyroid medication	163	7
Birth control	161	7
Water pills for reasons other than hypertension	121	5
Heart medications for reasons other than hypertension	114	5
Asthma medication	114	5
Stomach ulcer medication	103	4
Diabetes medication - oral	69	3

tent follow through with the physician's recommendations and successful symptom control. Examples are well-treated asthma, well-controlled hypertension and a remote history of cancer.

Certain conditions may necessitate a change in the therapeutic approach. These conditions will be discovered in the medical history questionnaire or in the physical examination. The physician is aware of these conditions and the patient is following through with the treatment plan. However, despite adequate treatment the patient may still develop symptoms that impact therapy either in the evaluation or treatment phase.

Some conditions may require a "treat and refer" approach. The physical therapist may suspect a condition that is not yet known to the referring physician, the patient may have neglected follow up for a chronic condition, there may be a change in the patient's status that has not been brought to the physician's attention, or the plan of care is clearly not having the desired effect or is not being followed. The physical therapist is well positioned to encourage appropriate follow up or inform the physician of concerns. Keep in mind that noncompliance may be due to various factors including lack of understanding by the patient, lack of financial resources or lack of desire. No matter what the reason, the physician should be informed of the patient's status.

At times, the therapist should refer the patient to a physician and place physical therapy on hold. This course of action should be followed if the potential negative health consequences are high or if physical therapy could potentially make the condition worse. Even if the musculoskeletal condition can be successfully treated with physical therapy, it may be appropriate to delay initiation of therapy while the patient is receiving evaluation for the possible medical condition. Continuing physical therapy could inadvertently cause the patient to put off an appropriate medical evaluation. An example would be the treatment of shoulder dysfunction with the presence of an enlarged, firm and irregularly shaped lymph node. Such a node is suspicious of cancer. Diagnosing and treating the potentially life-threatening disease takes priority over treatment for shoulder pain.

In very rare cases, the physical therapist will encounter a condition that is imminently dangerous and requires emergency treatment. The therapist must have a clear plan regarding these individuals. Questions that should be addressed before this situation occurs include when to call 911, when to call the physician's office and which physician to call. For example, if a patient who is referred by an orthopedic surgeon experiences unstable angina, the patient's primary care physician should be called immediately. In general these patient need urgent evaluation. The question asked of the provider is, "Where do you want the patient sent?" When in doubt have the patient sent to an emergency room or call 911 prior to calling the patient's physician. Table 3-4 lists the common emergency conditions a therapist may see.

The Evaluation Process

The goal of the evaluation process is to identify the source of the patient's symptoms, which in most cases will be a mechanical dysfunction. Additional goals are to identify the stage of healing, i.e., acute, subacute or chronic, and to define an appropriate treatment plan. This is accomplished through an organized approach to patient evaluation, which is routine for the physical therapist and discussed thoroughly in Chapter 4, *Evaluation of the Spine*. The goal of this chapter is to review the unique aspects of the evaluation that address screening for non-mechanical conditions.

Subjective History

Mechanical dysfunction has a typical presentation well known to the physical therapist. Subjective findings suggestive of a purely mechanical problem are detailed elsewhere in this text and will not be repeated here. Instead, the focus will be on those elements of the subjective history that are suspicious of non-musculoskeletal origin or a concurrent medical problem that needs to be addressed.

It is wise to approach the subjective history section of the evaluation with a healthy dose of skepticism, even if the symptoms seem straightforward. Additional historical facts will provide reassurance or cause further concern, leading the therapist to pursue the concern during subsequent parts of the evaluation.

Even when a patient presents a history that sounds purely mechanical, the therapist should be aware that additional medical factors may be involved. For example, when an injury is caused by a traumatic event, the clinician should find out what caused the event. In the elderly patient with fracture related to a fall, what caused the fall? Cardiac syncope, medication reactions, diabetes, closeted alcoholism or nutritional deficiency all are possibilities and may have ongoing impact on treatment.

Even if the cause is identified and treated the therapist must be aware of how to monitor treatment success or failure. For example, if low blood sugar contributed to the syncope, the therapist needs to be aware of this information

Table 3-4: Emergency conditions requiring immediate action.

Symptom	Possible Problem
Suicide ideation, especially with a plan	Morbid depression; imminent suicide
Severe depression symptoms	Morbid depression
Rebound abdominal tenderness	Appendicitis or peritonitis
One-sided facial pain; intractable headache	Temporal arteritis
Vaginal bleeding with acute pelvic pain	Ectopic pregnancy
Unstable angina (new onset, significant change in frequency or poor response to treatment)	Acute or impending myocardial infarction
New onset of atrial fibrillation	Atrial fibrillation causes increased risk of stroke
High blood pressure stage 3 (Systolic ≥ 180; Diastolic ≥ 110)	Poorly controlled hypertension; increased risk of stroke
Acute abdominal pain with notable abdominal bruit (swishing sound over artery)	Abdominal aortic aneurysm
New onset of pulse over 100 at rest	Atrial fibrillation; tachycardia
Melena (black tarry stool)	Gastrointestinal bleed
Bloody stools	Gastrointestinal bleed
Acute change in mentation	Stroke; aneurysm; overdose
Pelvic pain, fever and unusual vaginal discharge	Pelvic inflammatory disease
Foul odor in a non-healing wound	Gangrene; could lead to sepsis
Intractable pain any location	Needs evaluation to rule out emergency condition

and ensure the patient is monitoring blood sugars throughout the therapy session.

Most patients who come to physical therapy believe that their symptoms are appropriate for therapy. They may unintentionally present a history biased toward a mechanical cause of symptoms and may even self-diagnose. A patient reporting "shoulder tendonitis" can present more of a challenge than one who simply complains of shoulder pain. The therapist must gather all facts associated with the presenting symptoms and avoid making assumptions.

Symptoms of insidious onset are common in overuse syndromes but also raise concerns of non-mechanical pathology. For example, a gradual onset of low back pain and calf pain that is worse with walking and relieved with sitting can be either mechanical back pain with radicular symptoms or peripheral vascular disease. If the symptoms cannot be reproduced with lumbar screening tests described in Chapter 4, *Evaluation of the Spine*, the problem is not mechanical.

Even when the problem is mechanical, the therapist should be aware that visceral pathology may be involved. As previously discussed, hypothyroidism and diabetes can contribute to causation of carpal tunnel syndrome.

Several clues can help alert the therapist to the possibility of a non-mechanical problem. For example, patients with visceral pathology will often describe their symptoms using unique words. Words such as cramping, throbbing, pressure or tightness are not typical descriptors of mechanical pathology.[4]

The location of the symptoms can also warn the therapist about the potential for visceral pathology. In general, the more peripheral the symptoms, the less likely they are to be visceral. Conversely, the more central the symptoms, the more likely they are to be visceral, and the more likely regional organ system screening will be necessary. Knowing the innervation patterns of the visceral organs (Table 3-5) will direct the therapist to the organ system(s) that need to be screened. The notable exceptions to this rule are peripheral vascular disease, which should be considered with lower extremity symptoms, and the generalized conditions such as psychological, rheumatalogical, endocrine or infectious pathology.

Knowledge of symptom behavior can also help identify a potential visceral problem. The clinician should ask what activities make the symptoms worse and what relieves or abates the symptoms. When the patient reports increased symptoms with certain motions or activities, the clinician should bear in mind that non-musculoskeletal structures can be stressed with movement and can mimic musculoskeletal pathology. For example, walking stresses the hip as well as the cardiovascular system and neck range of motion stresses the thyroid gland and inflamed lymph nodes of the neck. The therapist should ask whether there is a time of day when the symptoms are better or worse.

Table 3-5: Segmental innervation of viscera and pain referral sites.

Structure	Segmental Innervation	Pain Referral Sites
Cardiopulmonary		
Heart	T1−5	Anterior cervical, upper thorax, left UE
Lungs	T5−6	Ipsilateral thoracic spine, cervical (diaphragm involved)
Gastrointestinal		
Diaphragm	C3−5	Cervical spine
Esophagus	T4−6	Substernal and upper abdominal
Stomach	T6−10	Upper abdominal, mid and lower thoracic spine
Small intestine	T7−10	Middle thoracic spine
Pancreas	T6−10	Upper abdominal, lower thoracic and upper lumbar spine
Gallbladder	T7−9	Right upper abdominal, right mid and lower thoracic spine, including caudal aspect scapula
Liver	T7−9	Right mid and lower thoracic spine
Common bile duct	T6−10	Upper abdominal, mid thoracic spine
Large intestine	T11−L1	Lower abdominal mid lumbar spine
Sigmoid colon	T11−12	Upper sacral, suprapubic, left lower abdominal quadrant
Genitourinary		
Kidney	T10−L1	Ipsilateral lumbar spine, upper and lower abdominal
Ureter	T11−L2, S2−4	Groin, upper abdominal, suprapubic, medial, proximal thigh, thoracolumbar spine
Urinary bladder	T11−L2, S2−4	Sacral apex, suprapubic, thoracolumbar
Prostate gland	T11−L1, S2−4	Sacral, testes, thoracolumbar spine
Testes	T10−11	Lower abdominal, sacral
Uterus	T10−L1, S2−4	Lumbosacral junction, thoracolumbar
Ovaries	T10−11	Lower abdominal, sacral

Night pain may be indicative of visceral pathology, but not always. It is important to look for a pattern of findings and not rely on one fact. Other questions that can help sort out visceral pathology from musculoskeletal pathology include whether symptoms are affected by food intake, defecation, urination or deep breathing. Also, female patients with pelvic pain should be asked whether the symptoms change with their menstrual cycle or during sexual activity.

During any evaluation, some parts of the history will not fit the working hypothesis of the therapist. The tendency is to gloss over these data points. However, if later questions arise about visceral pathology (e.g., if the patient responds poorly to treatment or develops additional symptoms), these previously considered pieces of extraneous data may very well provide the answer. All gathered data should be recorded.

Consideration of Demographics Data

The patient's age, gender and race should be considered. Females have a higher risk of diseases such as depression, osteoporosis and breast cancer. Males have a greater risk of chemical dependency and coronary artery disease and they have the unique risk of prostate cancer.

The patient's age can also reveal a lot about the risk of disease. Patients in their teens and twenties have a greater risk of trauma and self-destructive behaviors such as excessive drug use. Cancer is rare but if it occurs, it is more likely to be of an unusual type (e.g., young people more often have extremity tumors rather than tumors originating in the trunk). With increasing age, health problems relating to degenerative processes become more prevalent. The incidence and complications of degenerative joint disease, coronary artery disease, peripheral vascular disease and cerebral vascular disease all increase with age. Diabetes, chronic obstructive pulmonary disease, neurologic disease and cancer are more prevalent in the aging population.

Race is important to consider. For example, sickle cell anemia occurs mainly in African Americans. Hypertension has more severe consequences for African Americans than other races and prostate symptoms occur sooner than in Caucasians. Diabetes occurs more frequently in African Americans, Hispanic/Latino Americans, American Indians, and some Asian Americans and Pacific Islanders.[9]

Medical and Family History Questionnaire

Knowledge of the patient's past medical and family history may shed light on risk factors for current medical conditions. This information is obtained by asking the patient to fill out an intake form or health questionnaire that contains screening questions for current and past health issues. The goal of the medical history questions is to define the conditions for which the patient is being actively treated, and discern the type of treatments used and their results. Additionally, it is important to know what previous injuries, illnesses or surgeries have occurred and their outcomes. The physical therapist should evaluate the information, ask additional questions raised by the patient's answers, and look for any information that may possibly correlate with other parts of the subjective and physical examination.

Knowledge of past surgeries, injuries and medical conditions can be helpful in assessing the risk of non-musculoskeletal disease. Any past surgeries should be disclosed, and the therapist should understand the type of surgery performed, the reason for the surgery, its outcome and any resulting functional limitations. Most importantly, the therapist should know what the post-surgical recommendations were, and whether the patient followed the recommendations. If the surgery was for cancer, it is important to know whether subsequent monitoring studies have been done. Concerns of recurrent cancer need to be considered if the surgery was performed within the last five years, especially if there has been inadequate monitoring.

What medications are being prescribed? Will the medication impact therapy? Details of drug use including the type of medication, dosage, side effects, length of time on the medication and its effectiveness are important to document. For example, beta blockers lower pulse rate, diuretics can lower potassium levels (leading to leg cramps), and a co-enzyme A inhibitor such as Lipitor®, used to treat high cholesterol, can cause disabling muscle pain. Over-the-counter medications also have potential side effects, so the therapist should be aware of their usage. Medications like nitroglycerine and asthma inhalers are important for the patient to have immediately available during therapy. The therapist should ensure the patient brings essential medication to the appointment.

Many of today's more serious diseases are directly related to our habits. Cigarettes and other tobacco products are major risk factors for coronary artery disease, cancer and chronic pulmonary disease. Tobacco also contributes to poor wound healing. Poor diets and obesity are becoming recognized as epidemics in our society. Many patients seen in physical therapy practices use alcohol and tobacco.[2] If the behaviors the patient reports are counter productive to healthy living, the patient would benefit from the therapist making a statement to that effect. A simple statement like, "You would do better in therapy if you could cut down or cut out cigarettes. Is there anything I can do to help you stop?" can make a difference in the patient's life. If the patient denies a desire to change his behavior, at least the question was asked. If the patient shows a desire to quit, the therapist should refer the patient to his physician or the multiple Web sites or community resources that are available.

Alcohol use contributes to injuries. The patient should be questioned about alcohol use in a non-judgmental, empathetic fashion. Excessive alcohol use is perceived to be more difficult to address but the technique is the same. The therapist can state, "I am concerned about your alcohol use. It limits my ability to help you and I would encourage you to talk to your physician." At times, alcohol or drug use can be so significant that it adversely impacts the delivery of physical therapy. If the patient's safety is at risk or he is unable to follow through with a home program because of substance abuse, discharge from therapy is appropriate until the use has abated. These decisions are not easy and are best made in consultation with the referring physician.

The importance of the family history questions is that a positive response increases the risk that the patient may develop the same disease. Positive answers should be explored. The therapist should know the relative affected and the severity of the disease.

Social History Factors

Understanding the patient's social history helps to define potential support systems. The therapist should learn about the patient's living situation, including whether he lives alone or with someone who can help with therapy. Home and work responsibilities are important to ascertain. Any relevant physical or social barriers should be understood. For example, is she a single parent with several young children or is he the sole caregiver of an elder spouse with dementia? Social history has little impact on screening for medical disease, but answers to these questions can help structure the rehabilitation program.

Physical Examination

The physical examination for medical conditions consists of observation, inspection, palpation, monitoring of vital signs, auscultation, neurological testing and range of motion testing. The goal of the examination is to validate the clinical suspicions that have developed while taking the patient history. Specifically, the therapist looks for mechanical dysfunction that can contribute to the patient's symptom pattern. If the history is atypical for mechanical issues, especially if the past medical history and family history raise concerns of visceral pathology, the examination can help to clarify those concerns.

After the physical examination is performed, the therapist correlates its results with the rest of the examination performed thus far. If the history and physical examination have a high degree of concordance and minimal concerns were raised about past medical or family history, non-mechanical pathology is unlikely, and further screening is unnecessary. This should be true for well over 75% of the patients presenting for initial evaluation. Atypical histories, discordance between the history and physical examination, and atypical findings during the physical exam should lead the therapist to perform more advanced screening directed at one or more body systems.

Observation

Observation is an important and sometimes undervalued part of the examination. It is a process that is used through out the total time spent with the patient. During the history, are the patient's words and actions congruent? If the patient is reporting severe pain, does he look like he is in severe pain? Poor eye contact, sullen and withdrawn behavior and unduly negative verbiage are all signs of possible depression. Observation of gait and transitional movements can give clues to mechanical dysfunction. If the patient demonstrates a normal gait from the waiting room to the examination room but develops an antalgic gait when asked to walk during the exam, concerns about secondary gain or exaggerated symptom behavior are raised. Facial expression, arm positioning and other movements can impart significant information about the patient.

Inspection

Therapists have the opportunity to observe more skin than do most other practitioners. Skin lesions do not tend to affect physical therapy. Exceptions include metastatic skin lesions and psoriatic skin lesions associated with arthritis, which rarely occur. Nonetheless, general patient care is enhanced when the therapist recognizes a skin lesion that may be cancerous. Keep in mind that the therapist's job is not to diagnosis cancerous skin lesions, but simply to encourage the patient to have the lesion evaluated by a physician.

Scars also give the astute therapist potentially significant information. If the scars are not fully accounted for by the patient's past medical history, now is a chance to help jog the patient's memory. Some scars may be the result of trauma that the patient felt was not significant to mention, but may be important. Does the patient form keloid scars? How extensive are the scars, do they impair mobility? For

example, it may be important to know whether a hysterectomy was performed via an abdominal procedure or a laparoscopic procedure, because there are very different implications for the patient and therapist. Abdominal procedures cause substantially more scarring and potential functional limitations than the small incisions of the laparoscopic procedures. If the patient is unsure, inspection will resolve the dilemma.

Palpation

During palpation, the clinician must remember the obvious and not so obvious tissues that are being examined. Anterior shoulder palpation in a female patient may include incidental palpation of some breast tissue. If an unusual mass is found, a timely referral to a medical colleague should be initiated.

For the physical therapist, palpation of the abdomen is considered an advanced screening technique and can be performed when non-mechanical pathology is suspected. Palpation of each of the four abdominal quadrants with light pressure should be performed. The right and left upper quadrant under the anterior ribcage should be included. Progressively deeper pressure per patient tolerance will allow closer examination of particular areas of concern. The abdomen below the costal margins should be soft without any distinct firmness or mass felt.

Other significant non-mechanical palpatory findings include a pulsatile mass in the mid-abdomen, which may be associated with an aneurysm, or the presence of an enlarged liver, which may be contributing to right shoulder pain. When a therapist is palpating the iliopsoas through the abdomen, a bulge or unusual firmness could be constipation, a mass or iliopsoas spasm. In other words, the therapist needs to consider the underlying non-musculoskeletal structures during the palpation exam.

Vital Signs

Vital signs include temperature, blood pressure, pulse and respirations. The physical therapist should monitor vital signs when concerns about their stability are noted. For example, if the patient complains of chilling or has a flushed face, the therapist should take his temperature. If the patient complains of light headedness or chest pain, has clammy skin or appears lethargic or confused, all four of the vital signs should be noted. Increased respirations in an asthmatic patient (more than 30 breaths per minute at rest) may indicate poor control of the asthma.

Auscultation

Auscultation involves listening with a stethoscope over certain anatomical areas. It is usually not needed during the physical therapy examination but can be a useful advanced screening technique in certain cases. Auscultation of the abdomen should reveal 6-10 "gurgling" sounds per minute. If these are absent or slow, the patient may have constipation or a bowel obstruction.

Changes in breath sounds may point to possible lung pathology. In auscultation of the lungs, wheezing can indicate asthma, COPD or bronchial constriction caused by a severe cough or bronchitis. Rales, a "crackling" sound, can indicate fluid in the bases of the lungs. A patient with rales may have poorly-controlled congestive heart failure. Areas of absent lung sounds can indicate pneumonia or even a mass. In the asthmatic patient, auscultation or the use of a peak flow meter to confirm good lung capacity may be helpful before putting a patient on a bike.

A *bruit* is a turbulent swishing sound over an artery. Listening for bruits is indicated when poor blood flow is suspected. The presence of bruits over the carotid arteries, abdominal aorta and femoral arteries would raise concerns of an aneurysm or plaque formation. If a patient acts confused, the therapist should listen for bruits over the carotid arteries, which may indicate partial blockage.

If pain and discoloration are present in the lower leg, the therapist should listen for bruits in the femoral artery. Bruits over the abdominal aorta will change how the physical therapist approachs a tight anterior abdominal wall in a patient with back pain—deep tissue mobilization is contraindicated. Unless it is a known chronic symptom in the patient, the physician should be alerted to the presence of bruits over an artery.

Neurological Examination

In the neurological examination, the therapist should be alert for the "stocking or glove" sensation changes that may hint at diabetes. The term *stocking or glove* refers to a sensation change that encompasses the entire circumference of the limb. Rheumatologic conditions such as polymyalgia rheumatica can cause shoulder girdle and pelvic girdle weakness that may be detected during the neurological exam.

Range of Motion Testing

Specific findings during range of motion testing can give clues to non-mechanical pathology. For example, limited hip extension may be caused by diverticulitis, a colon infection. Painful rotation of the neck may be due to thyroid pathology and painful shoulder external rotation may be due to enlarged lymph nodes. Range of motion testing will stress additional non-musculoskeletal structures. The therapist must always be mindful of this fact, particularly when the patient does not respond to therapy as expected.

Advanced Screening

When the patient's evaluation findings suggest a straightforward mechanical problem, no further advanced screening is needed. However, when basic screening techniques yield suspicious findings the physical therapist should pursue a more thorough screen of the organ systems. The *Review of Systems Checklist* on page 36, is used for regional organ system screening, and includes a set of questions for the cardiovascular, pulmonary, gastrointestinal, urinary, genital/reproductive, nervous, integumentary and endocrine systems. Questions for general health and depression are also included.

Screening for general health and depression is recommended for every patient. The general health questions are screening for non-focal pathology such as cancers, infections and rheumatalogical conditions. Depression screening is performed because of its prevalence in physical therapy patients, its significant negative impact on therapy and the increased likelihood of it being missed during medical evaluations.

Using the Review of Systems Checklist

The location of symptoms will dictate what organ system to screen. Each organ system refers symptoms to predictable areas of the body (Table 3-6). For example, left upper quadrant symptoms can be associated with cardiac or pulmonary disease, whereas right upper quadrant symptoms tend to be related to pulmonary or liver pathology.

To perform screening for each organ system, the physical therapist asks the patient whether he has experienced any of the symptoms listed under the relevant organ system. See "Review of Systems Checklist" on page 36.

A positive answer to any question increases the likelihood of pathology in that organ system. Negative answers do not eliminate the possibility of visceral pathology. However, they do provide therapists with the knowledge that they have done what is possible within their scope of practice to screen for worrisome conditions.

Likewise, a positive answer does not prove visceral pathology. The greater the number of positive answers, the greater the likelihood of disease. Patients with worrisome results need to be referred back to their primary physicians for further evaluation. If the patient is found not to have the suspected pathology, this does not mean the referral was inappropriate. Fortunately, not every patient who has suspicious findings has actual disease. The more serious the potential illness, the more the therapist should err on the side of caution. Understandably, this may result in a higher

Table 3-6: Determining the organ system(s) to screen based on location of symptoms.

Location of Symptoms	Organ System to Screen
Right upper quadrant	Gastrointestinal, especially liver and gall bladder Pulmonary
Left upper quadrant	Cardiovascular Gastrointestinal
Thoracic spine	Cardiovascular Pulmonary
Lumbar spine	Gastrointestinal Genitourinary Additionally screen for PVD
Right lower quarter	Gastrointestinal Genitourinary
Left lower quarter	Gastrointestinal Genitourinary

percentage of referrals who test negative for disease. Concern about cardiac disease is a prime example of when it is better to be "safe than sorry." It is always better to err on the side of sending more rather than fewer patients for further evaluation.

Negative answers to the regional organ system screening questions are reassuring to the therapist. Documenting negative findings is just as important as documenting positive findings. Screening is an ongoing process and does not end with the initial evaluation. Re-screening every three weeks is recommended. Additionally, re-screening should be performed if there is a lack of response to therapy after three visits, a plateau in a patient otherwise making satisfactory progress and in patients who suffer recurrent symptoms.

Positive findings demand a response by the therapist, which can consist of the following:

- Emergency referral to the physician (in the clinic or, more likely, emergency room)
- Urgent referrals to the physician for less serious but still significant conditions
- Routine physician referral
- Notification of the physician during routine correspondence

Examples of symptoms that require an emergency call to the physician or even 911 were listed in Table 3-4. These symptoms possibly indicate conditions that can be immediately life or limb threatening. The patient should be kept in the physical therapy clinic until the therapist and the consultant decide on an appropriate transfer of care plan. The goal is to prevent a severe adverse outcome such as myocardial infarction, death with the rupture of an abdominal aortic aneurysm, suicide and profound infections. Concern for cancer is not in this category. While cancer is serious, it usually is not immediately deadly. Cancer and similar conditions require an urgent referral to the physician, within the next two to five days.

Urgent consultation with a medical colleague is reserved for those conditions that are not categorized as emergencies, but still require some additional evaluation because of their potential threat to life and limb. In addition to cancer, examples of such conditions include possible gallbladder disease and known atrial fibrillation with poor control of rate.

Urgent and emergency referrals necessitate an immediate phone call and a plan before the patient leaves the office. While it would be ideal to have one-on-one contact with the physician, this may not be practical at all times. The facts causing concern should be communicated. The call should end with these direct questions: "Does the patient need to be seen immediately?" and "Where would you like the patient sent?" Additional communication is best done in writing. When possible, quick notes that the patient brings along to the physician's office assist with communication and engage the patient in the process. These should be followed by a comprehensive clinic note as soon as possible after the visit.

Routine referral is reserved for those conditions that are not life or limb threatening, but are outside the scope of practice for the physical therapist. Long-standing nocturia in males or incontinence in females, patients missing medication frequently, hearing loss in the elderly and skin lesions are examples.

For very minor issues, a specific referral may not be necessary. Simple notification about the issue in routine correspondence is appreciated by the physician and results in overall better health care.

Summary

Screening for pathology other than musculoskeletal disease is an important and expected role of the physical therapist. Recent and expected future changes in physical therapy practice reinforce the need for screening being an integral part of the initial evaluation and ongoing assessment process.

Timely and directed communication with medical colleagues should lead to appropriate disposition for patients in need of additional care beyond the scope of practice of physical therapy. Desired and expected outcomes include improved patient care, improved communications between various providers of medical care and improved therapist satisfaction with practice.

REFERENCES

1. American Physical Therapy Association's "Hooked on Evidence" Website.
    http://www.apta.org/hookedonevidence/index.cfm
2. Boissonnault WG and Koopmeiners MB: Medical History Profile: Orthopaedic Physical Therapy Outpatients. J Orthop Sports Phys Ther 20(1):2-10,1994.
3. Boissonnault WG: Prevalence of Comorbid Conditions, Surgeries, and Medication Use In a Physical Therapy Outpatient Population: A Multicentered Study. J Orthop Sports Phys Ther 29(9):506-519,1999.
4. Boissonnault WG and Fabio RP: Pain Profile of Patient with Low Back Pain Referred to Physical Therapy.J Orthop Sports Phys Ther 24(4):211-222, 1996.
5. Grant B, et al: Epidemiologic Bulletin No. 35: Prevalence of DSM-IV alcohol abuse and dependence, United States 1992. Alcohol Health & Research World 18(3):243-248, 1994.
6. Guide to Physical Therapist Practice. 2nd Edition. American Physical Therapy Association, Fairfax VA, 2001.
7. HCUPnet, Healthcare Cost and Utilization Project. Agency for Healthcare Research and Quality, Rockville, MD. http://www.ahrq.gov/data/hcup/hcupnet.htm
8. United States Census Bureau, International Data Base. http://www.census.gov
9. United States Department of Health and Human Services. Centers for Disease Control and Prevention. Diabetes Public Health Resource. http://www.cdc.gov/diabetes/faqs.htm#types

ACKNOWLEDGEMENTS

The author and editor gratefully acknowledge invaluable editorial assistance and content contribution from Jackie Collins, MSN CNP.

Table 3-1 adapted from Boissonnault WG and Koopmeiners MB: Medical History Profile: Orthopaedic Physical Therapy Outpatients. J Orthop Sports Phys Ther 20(1):2-10,1994, with permission of the Orthopaedic and Sports Physical Therapy Sections of the American Physical Therapy Association.

Tables 3-2 and 3-3 adapted from Boissonnault WG: Prevalence of Comorbid Conditions, Surgeries, and Medication Use In a Physical Therapy Outpatient Population: A Multicentered Study. J Orthop Sports Phys Ther 29(9):506-519, 1999, with permission of the Orthopaedic and Sports Physical Therapy Sections of the American Physical Therapy Association.

REVIEW OF SYSTEMS CHECKLIST

I. General Health
    A. Fatigue
    B. Malaise
    C. Fever/chills sweats
    D. Nausea/vomiting
    E. Unexplained weight change
    F. Numbness/paraesthesia
    G. Weakness
    H. Mentation/cognition

II. Depression (> 5 symptoms for > 2 weeks)
    A. Depressed/irritable mood
    B. Psychomotor agitation/retardation
    C. Sleep disturbance
    D. Weight gain/loss
    E. Fatigue
    F. Feelings of worthlessness
    G. Diminished interest/apathy
    H. Diminished ability to concentrate
    I. Suicide ideation—recurrent

III. Cardiovascular
    A. Dyspnea (shortness of breath)
    B. Orthopnea (shortness of breath lying down)
    C. Palpitations
    D. Pains/sweats
    E. Syncope (layman's term please)
    F. Peripheral edema
    G. Cough

IV. Pulmonary System
    A. Dyspnea
    B. Onset of cough
    C. Change in cough
    D. Sputum
    E. Hemoptysis (coughing up blood)
    F. Clubbing of nails
    G. Stridor (upper airway constriction with breathing)
    H. Wheezing

V. Genitourinary System
    A. Urinary difficulty
        1. Frequency
        2. Urgency
        3. Incontinence
        4. Reduced caliber or force
        5. Difficulty initiating
        6. Unusual color
        7. Dysuria (difficulty or pain with urination)
    B. Male Genitalia
        1. Urethral discharge
        2. Impotence
        3. Pain with intercourse
    C. Female Genitalia
        1. Vaginal discharge
        2. Pain with intercourse
        3. Change in menstruation frequency and duration or blood flow
        4. Dysmenorrhea (menstrual period that has stopped)
        5. Date of last period
        6. Number of pregnancies
        7. Number of deliveries
        8. Menopause

VI. Gastrointestinal System
    A. Difficulty with swallowing
    B. Heartburn, indigestion
    C. Specific food intolerance
    D. Change in appetite
    E. Bowel dysfunction
        1. Color
        2. Frequency
        3. Shape/caliber
        4. Constipation/diarrhea
        5. Difficulty initiating
        6. Incontinence

VII. Nervous System
    A. Balance
    B. Gross movement patterns
    C. Mentation
    D. Tremor
    E. Asymmetric facial features
        1. Facial contour
        2. Pupil size
        3. Strabismus
    F. Muscle atrophy
    G. Muscle weakness
    H. Clonus

VIII. Integumentary System – (Unusual Lesion or Mole)
    A. Color black or multiple shades
    B. Friability/ulceration (easily bleeds)
    C. Non-distinct or irregular borders
    D. Asymmetric shape
    E. Size > 6mm diameter
    F. Mobility (decreased mobility in subcutaneous tissues)

IX. Endocrine
    A. Arthralgias
    B. Myalgias
    C. Neuropathies
    D. Cold/heat intolerance
    E. Skin/hair changes
    F. Fatigue
    G. Unexplained weight changes
    H. Bowel dysfunction
    I. Polyuria (frequent urination)

EVALUATION OF THE SPINE

H. Duane Saunders, MS PT and Robin Saunders Ryan, MS PT

Section One — The General Spinal Exam

In physical therapy, evaluation is an ongoing process. Thus, even though it may be possible to complete a full and thorough evaluation during the patient's first visit, signs and symptoms must be rechecked during the course of treatment to determine the patient's progress or lack of progress. The evaluation is the foundation upon which effective treatment rests. The evaluation findings guide the clinician to select appropriate treatments. Because many different tests, measurements and sequences can be used to collect the required data, the format chosen largely depends on individual preference. To succeed, however, the clinician must internalize a methodical and complete evaluation process.

When performing a musculoskeletal evaluation, the clinician should adhere to one method. This will allow full development of the clinician's intuitive skills. Several recognized methods of evaluation are taught in orthopedic physical therapy settings. While there are some differences in the order of questioning and emphasis, the essentials of the evaluation differ little. The emphasis, of course, should always be on thoroughness and accuracy.

The only exception to the rule of performing a complete evaluation on the initial visit is in the case of acute, severe pain or pain which is by history highly irritable. In this case, the clinician must use an abbreviated exam to determine whether the problem is likely musculoskeletal, ruling out such things as fractures or dislocations if trauma is involved. If a thorough history and brief exam does not raise the question of a possible non-musculoskeletal com-

ponent, provisional treatment to relieve pain and to expose its underlying cause is appropriate. When the severe or irritable symptoms improve sufficiently, the clinician should carry out a more thorough evaluation.

Collecting and Recording Data

The clinician must collect data that are relevant, measurable and accurate. It is important to measure and record data objectively, using tests with demonstrated reliability and validity when possible. Any subjective information also must be collected and recorded in an objective manner. For example, find out the length of time symptoms persist after a certain activity or the distance the patient can walk before the onset of symptoms. The subjective questioning protocol and objective tests a clinician uses should be individualized. Purposeful questions should be asked, but the clinician should avoid leading the patient.

Objective tests appropriate for the clinician's individual size, dexterity, physique and experience should be chosen. Physical examination findings have not been shown to be predictive of outcomes for chronic low back pain.[5] In general, this topic has not been well researched. Nonetheless, objective tests performed in the physical therapy evaluation provide comparative data that can be used to measure progress for each patient.

Certain questions and tests will have more or less meaning with individual patients. The result of one test or the answer to a question can lead to further questioning and testing. The tendency to jump to conclusions during the data collection phase must be resisted. Only thorough data collection coupled with proper interpretation will ensure correct assessment and treatment.

Sometimes, radiological examination findings can be misleading. While there are definite indications for tests such as MRI, CT scan and x-ray, clinicians in the United States tend to use them too often in routine spinal examinations. Diagnostic tests are indicated when the patient has suffered trauma or has subjective or objective findings that are suspicious of non-musculoskeletal involvement.

Radiological testing is also indicated when the patient does not respond as expected to conservative treatment. When diagnostic tests are overused, they may distract the clinician from finding the real cause of the patient's problem. For example, when diagnostic tests reveal degenerative changes, spondylolisthesis, a sacralized lumbar vertebra or a bulging disc, it is easy to implicate these findings as the cause of the patient's problem. Sources have suggested, however, that there is often little or no correlation between radiological findings and the patient's symptoms.[4,37,40,68,85]

Similarly, we must use caution when describing diagnostic findings to the patient. Using medical terminology without adequate explanation may be confusing to patients and may convince them they have no control over their problems. Terms like "degenerative arthritis", "birth defect", "slipped disc", "joint out of place", and others are particularly worrisome because they invoke frightening imagery and may make the patient less likely to take self-responsibility for the treatment plan. Even when such conditions exist, they should be described in terms of factors on which the patient can have an effect, such as stiffness, weakness or postural faults.

During an evaluation, it is important to record data in a format that other health care professionals and payers can interpret easily. A common format is the S-O-A-P note. S-O-A-P is a mnemonic for these evaluation elements: Subjective, Objective, Assessment and Plan. Evaluation reports written in the S-O-A-P format can concisely portray the patient's condition and outline a treatment plan to address deficiencies. Progress notes and the discharge summary can also follow the S-O-A-P format. In combination with the initial evaluation and treatment plan, they become the complete physical therapy record for most patients. Special tests that require an additional form, such as a complete muscle test or a nerve conduction study, can be attached to the initial evaluation.

Dictation equipment and word processors aid efficiency and clarity in record keeping, but can be relatively expensive and slow. Today's technology offers many choices in documentation. Clinic management should choose a system that is easy and time-efficient for the clinician and results in timely sharing of information. A handwritten evaluation report must be neat, easy to read, concise and complete. Physicians and other health care personnel are less likely to read an evaluation if it is more than one page in length, particularly if it is handwritten. However, thoroughness should not be sacrificed to keep the written evaluation brief. Material should always be arranged in the same order so frequent referral sources will know where to find certain information, and reference should be made to negative as well as to positive findings. To assure completeness and good organization, a worksheet should be used. One example is provided (Fig 4-1).

Table 4-1: Sequence of Spinal Evaluation, Cervical and Upper Thoracic Spine.

Standing Position	Sitting Position	Supine Position	Prone Position
Posture	Vertebral artery test	Passive cervical ROM	Upper thoracic segmental rotation
Sacral base (structural symmetry)	Posture assessment	Cervical segmental mobility tests	1st rib mobility
Aids and assistive devices	Upper thoracic segmental flex/ext	ULTT	Interscapular strength
	Active cervical ROM	Babinski's test	
	Resisted cervical muscle tests	Distraction/Compression tests	
	Resisted upper ext. muscle tests	Sensation testing	
	Clear shoulder	1st rib mobility	
	Clear elbow		
	Distraction/Compression tests		
	Palpate soft tissue and bone		
	Adson's test		
	Costoclavicular test		
	Hyperabduction test		
	Roo's test		

```
┌─────────────────────────────────────────────┐
│         PHYSICAL THERAPY WORKSHEET            │
│                                               │
│  SUBJECTIVE:                                  │
│      Complaint:                               │
│      Nature:                                  │
│      Location:                                │
│      Onset:                                   │
│      Behavior:                                │
│      Course and Duration:                     │
│      Previous Treatment:                      │
│      Occupation/Hobbies:                      │
│      Other Medical Problems:                  │
│                                               │
│  OBJECTIVE:                                   │
│      Structural:                              │
│      Mobility:                                │
│      Strength:                                │
│      Neurological:                            │
│      Palpation:                               │
│      Special Tests:                           │
│      Doctor s Report, Lab, X-ray:             │
│                                               │
│  ASSESSMENT:                                  │
│      Problem List:                            │
│      Goals:                                   │
│                                               │
│  PLAN:                                        │
│      Treatment/Education:                     │
│      Timeframes (Frequency, Duration):        │
│      Return to Work Plan:                     │
│                                               │
└─────────────────────────────────────────────┘
```

Figure 4-1: Sample evaluation worksheet for recording data.

Sequence of Evaluation

When conducting an evaluation, the clinician should follow a sequential list of tests and questions to avoid unnecessary movement of the patient (Table 4-1 and Table 4-2). The clinician should perform all tests that can be done with the patient in one position before asking the patient to change positions. This assures that tests are not overlooked and it keeps the clinician moving along in an organized, efficient manner. This sequencing should be applied to evaluation of all major musculoskeletal areas, and data gathering sheets should be developed for use as a reference to assure thoroughness in testing.

Subjective Evaluation of the Spine

This section describes the subjective evaluation in general terms. Specific questions relating to the cervical, thoracic and lumbar areas are detailed in Sections Two and Three.

Each musculoskeletal disorder presents a unique history. The clinician must possess a thorough understanding of musculoskeletal pathology and the clinical picture that each disorder presents. Even with this in mind, it is a mistake to consider treating a pathological disorder such as degenerative disc disease with a routine or "cookbook" approach. The signs and symptoms of a specific disorder in one patient may differ significantly from those in another, or signs and symptoms may alter from treatment to treatment in the same patient.

It is essential to spend time with the patient in the examination room and obtain a first hand history of the condition and events that led to the onset of symptoms. It is a mistake to accept second hand information blindly, even if it came from a physician. Because our focus is often on mechanics, posture and activities of daily living, physical therapists tend to ask an entirely different set of questions than physicians do. Often much of the information needed to make a correct assessment can be elicited from the patient during the subjective evaluation, and the information obtained helps direct and focus the objective evaluation. Knowledge

Table 4-2: Sequence of Spinal Evaluation, Lumbar, Mid and Lower Thoracic Spine.

Standing Position	Sitting Position	Supine Position	Side Lying Position
Gait	Posture	Passive flexion (knees to chest)	Segmental flexion and rotation
Posture	Sitting flexion test	Passive rotation	Palpate soft tissue and bone
Sacral base	Active rotation	Abdominal muscle testing	Tensor Fascia Latae tightness
Palpate soft tissue and bone	Segmental mobility—flexion	SLR and variations	SI tests
Correct lateral shift	Reflex testing	Hip Flexion, rotation tightness	Prone Position
Correct leg length	Resisted knee extension	SI tests	P/A segmental mobility
Standing flexion test	Clear knee	Palpate soft tissue and bone	Passive extension
Active flexion and extension	Resisted great toe extension	Sensation testing	Palpate soft tissue and bone
Active side bending	Resisted ankle dorsiflexion	Resisted hip flexion	Prone knee bend
Heel-toe raises	Clear ankle	Clear hip	Hip extension tightness
Weight shift test	Distraction test	Babinski's test	Paraspinal muscle strength
Aids and assistive devices	Slump test		

of the patient's history may influence the number of positive findings in the objective evaluation.[2]

Standardized questionnaires specifically developed for the spine can be used to obtain information about the patient's pain and functional status. The Neck Disability Index has shown sufficient reliability to detect improvement or worsening throughout the course of treatment, and is easy to administer. Several other questionnaires for neck function have been developed and reviewed in the literature.[70]

The Roland-Morris Disability Questionnaire, the SF-36 and the Oswestry Disability Questionnaire are three examples of low back function questionnaires. We have used the Oswestry with patients who have relatively severe functional limitations. It has shown sufficient reliability and responsiveness, is quick to administer and helps to objectively show pre and post treatment changes.[16]

Reliable questionnaires are essential for objectively documenting patient progress when performing research, collecting statistics and sharing treatment results with colleagues or payers. However, a questionnaire cannot replace the one-on-one questioning required to make an accurate assessment for treatment planning purposes. The following is a step-by-step description of some common areas of questioning that should be included in the subjective evaluation to obtain an adequate patient history.

Patient Complaint

When taking the history, the first question to ask is simply, "What is your complaint?" This gives the patient a chance to tell in his own words anything that he believes is important. This first question facilitates the rest of the interview by placing both the clinician and the patient at ease. It is useful to ask the patient to rate his symptoms on a 1-10 scale. It is also important to know if today is a good day, bad day or medium day, as the patient's complaints may be different from day to day.

Nature

The clinician often has to ask more detailed questions about the patient's complaint. Pain, weakness, numbness, stiffness and hypersensitivity are common symptoms. The clinician should ask for a specific description of the symptoms such as a "constant deep ache", "intermittent pain" or "sharp stab of pain", but should not lead the patient by suggesting descriptions.

It is important to differentiate carefully between "pins and needles," "tingling" and "numbness" descriptions.

The patient should be asked if there is an area of skin that can be pinched or pricked with a pin and not felt. If this is the case, nerve root impingement or peripheral nerve entrapment is a probability. "Pins and needles" and/or "tingling" are often non-specific descriptions that many patients use regardless of the disorder involved.

Weakness that is present without pain suggests a neurological deficit or disease process or may be associated with prolonged disuse. Painless weakness associated with peripheral nerve entrapment or spinal nerve root compression often follows a specific dermatomal or myotomal distribution. Weakness associated with a neurological disease or disuse will typically be more generalized. If weakness is present with pain, it is sometimes difficult to determine if the pain alone is causing the weakness or if there is also an underlying neurological deficit.

Often the patient will describe a slipping, popping or clicking sensation that is associated with certain movements. It is important to determine if this sensation occurs every time the particular movement is repeated. Many joint noises are caused by the formation of carbon dioxide gas after a sudden separation of joint surfaces results in decreased joint pressure. This type of pop cannot be repeated for a certain period of time and is completely normal. If a joint cannot be popped it is an indication that it may be hypomobile and if a joint seems to pop easily it may be an indication that it is hypermobile.

If the patient describes a joint noise that can be repeated over and over it may be an indication of: 1) an unstable joint that may be subluxing or partially subluxing with certain movements; 2) a mechanical roughness or abnormality of the joint surfaces such as a meniscus tear or osteophytosis; or 3) thickening and scarring of the soft tissue (ligament and capsule) that surrounds the joint.

Location

The patient should be asked to identify the location of the symptoms, but the clinician should remember that the location the patient describes is not necessarily a reliable indicator of the actual site of pathology.[15] Most disc syndromes cause bilateral pain in the spine. The pain will be greater on one side than the other, but it crosses the midline. On the other hand, most spinal facet joint problems are unilateral. Pain limited to one spinal segment suggests a joint or nerve root disorder, whereas pain over several spinal segments usually indicates a muscular inflammation or systemic disorder.

Interscapular pain may correspond to anterior disc pathology in the cervical spine.[12] When stimulating the

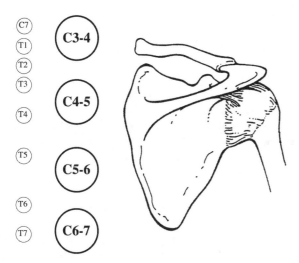

Figure 4-2: Cloward's areas. The small circles represent the spinous processes, and the large circles are Cloward's areas. Interscapular pain in the areas represented by the big circles may indicate disc pathology at the level indicated.

anterior surface of cervical discs with a needle, Ralph Cloward found that patients complained of an immediate deep, dull ache in a predictable pattern. Conversely, when the same area was injected with novocaine, the symptoms immediately disappeared. The so-called "Cloward's areas" are depicted in Figure 4-2. Cloward also found that stimulation of the posterior surface of the discs caused pain, but in a less predictable pattern. When a patient complains of interscapular symptoms, the clinician should consider cervical disc pathology as one of several possible causes. Correlating signs and symptoms for differential diagnosis is important, as many other pathological conditions can cause interscapular pain.

Pain and other symptoms are often referred distally and are rarely referred proximally. For example, cervical pain is often felt in the rhomboid muscle area, shoulder pain in the upper arm, and lower back pain in the buttocks and posterior thigh.

Pain that migrates from one joint to another suggests a systemic disease rather than a musculoskeletal disorder. Pain that spreads from the original site to the surrounding tissues is usually caused by inflammation or muscle spasm, both of which are often secondary reactions to the primary disorder.

The use of a body diagram to document the patient's complaints, their nature and location aids the clinician in two ways: First, it helps keep the clinician organized during the evaluation and decreases the likelihood that important questions will be forgotten. Second, it allows the clinician to remember details of the patient's original complaint, so

that the patient can be specifically questioned about his status during reassessments. The body diagram is kept as a part of the patient's permanent medical record (Fig 4-3).

Onset of Symptoms

The original onset of symptoms and the onset of the most recent episode should be considered. Knowing the exact mechanism of injury can be helpful. For example, sudden, unguarded movements often cause joint locking, impingement or subluxation, whereas sprains and strains involve aggravation or trauma. Inflammatory and systemic disorders present a subtler onset. Disc disorders usually have an insidious onset caused by repeated activities such as slumped sitting, forward bending and lifting, but the patient may perceive the onset as a sudden event related to one particular activity in which he was engaged when the pain was first noticed.

It is important to realize that the patient will always try to remember some incident that caused the problem. The patient also may attempt to relate present complaints to old injuries. These reports may not be reliable and it is often misleading to place too great an emphasis on the onset as described by the patient. Worker's compensation and auto insurance reporting systems tend to compound this problem, since a particular incident on a particular day must be reported for coverage to apply. Also, patients are conditioned to think that lifting or falling cause back injuries, when in reality they are caused by a multitude of lifestyle and genetic factors.

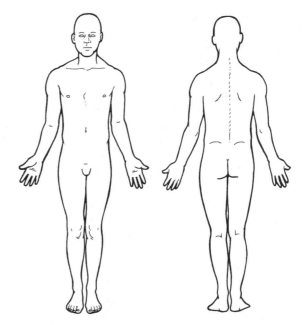

Figure 4-3: Body diagram used by the clinician to document the patient's symptoms.

Many back and neck injuries are caused by the cumulative effects of poor posture, faulty body mechanics, stressful working and living habits, loss of flexibility and strength and a general state of poor physical condition. Therefore, even when the patient reports that the pain occurred after a specific incident, it is important to obtain a detailed description of these lifestyle factors. Often the answers to both the cause and the cure of the problem are found in this area of questioning. In fact, when considering a corrective or preventive exercise program, it is usually more helpful to understand the patient's occupation, lifestyle and hobbies than it is to know about the incident that led to the current episode of symptoms.

Behavior of Symptoms

What movements, positions or activities irritate the symptoms? What movements, positions or activities ease the symptoms? Does the patient wake up with the pain in the morning? Does the weakness appear only after activity? Is there a pattern to the symptoms over a 24-hour period? The answers to these questions will help the clinician plan the objective portion of the evaluation. The effect of position can be an important clue to the cause of pain. For example, spinal pain arising from the disc is aggravated by sitting and forward bending, whereas walking tends to give relief. Pain arising from the facet joints will often be irritated by walking and relieved by sitting and forward bending. Pain associated with movement in any direction is often related to acute injury or inflammation, whereas pain that is aggravated by movement in only one or two directions is often due to joint or soft tissue dysfunction or disc pathology. Pain while resting suggests the presence of an inflammatory process. Night pain suggests a possible tumor, infection or systemic disease process, or may be indicative of an acute fracture or spondylolysis.

It is important for the clinician to identify and distinguish between an irritable and a severe condition. The information gained will help the clinician decide how vigorous and/or complete the objective part of the exam should be. If a condition is highly irritable or severe by history, the clinician's initial physical exam may have to be modified. If a position or activity causes pain, does the pain last after the position is changed or the activity is ceased? Once irritated, does the pain last for hours or days? Lingering pain indicates an *irritable* condition. If the condition is highly irritable, the clinician may choose to perform a fewer number of tests to avoid causing an increase in symptoms that may last for several hours or days after the initial evaluation. If a position causes pain, is it so intense that the patient cannot maintain the position? Inability to maintain the position indicates a *severe* condition. If the patient's symptoms are severe but not highly irritable the clinician

may be able to perform a relatively thorough evaluation by simply avoiding the end range of positions that are known by history to be problematic.

Musculoskeletal symptoms are usually irritated by certain movements and positions and are generally relieved with rest. If the symptoms do not seem related to movements or positions and are not relieved with rest, and the clinician cannot elicit a change in symptoms during the movement exam, one should suspect a systemic disease or visceral disorder and should consult with a physician.

Course and Duration of Symptoms

It is important for the clinician to consider the length of time since the onset of the symptoms to figure out whether the condition is in an acute, subacute or chronic state. The degree of acuteness or chronicity will influence treatment. The natural progression of the condition should be considered, too. Was the pain greatest when the injury first occurred, or did it worsen on subsequent days? Overall, is the condition getting worse, getting better or staying the same? Has the patient continued to work since the onset of the symptoms? Is this the patient's first back or neck injury, or have there been previous episodes? In the case of multiple episodes, how does this episode differ from previous ones?

Effect of Previous Treatment

If the patient has been to another medical practitioner, how did the treatment affect the condition? If the patient has had a previous episode any treatment that helped in the past should be considered again. Has the patient been instructed in any home treatment or exercises? Which exercises? Is the patient still doing the exercises? What medication has been prescribed? How often does the patient take the medication?

Other Related Medical Problems

The clinician should be aware of the patient's general medical history, and should be alert for possible indications of a non-musculoskeletal component to the complaint. Additionally, the clinician may need to modify evaluation or treatment techniques because of concurrent unrelated medical problems. Screening for non-mechanical conditions and the importance of coordinating care with the patient's other health care providers is discussed in Chapter 3, *Medical Screening*.

Occupation/Hobbies

The patient's occupation and hobbies are very important to note, even in a non-work related injury. For instance, a computer programmer whose hobbies are gardening and bowling has a lifestyle that involves many flexion activities. The exercises chosen for this individual may need to be extension-oriented to balance his lifestyle.

If the injury is work-related, the clinician needs to understand the current work restrictions that have been set by the physician. Additionally, the patient should describe his current routine at work and home. Often, a patient is not working at the level allowed by the physician because there is no work available at that level. For example, the post office normally handles a variety of packages that can weigh up to 70 pounds. However, a mail handler who is on a 30-pound weight restriction may be temporarily sorting letters instead of handling packages.

An astute clinician will supplement the patient's work activities and prevent deconditioning by having the patient practice lifting packages as a part of the rehabilitation. As the patient improves, the clinician will add more weight to his functional activities, and thus can give the physician input regarding appropriate changes in the patient's work restrictions.

The clinician needs to understand the patient's regular job duties to set appropriate functional goals. For example, if the above patient needs to lift 20 pounds frequently and up to 70 pounds occasionally to return to the mail handler job, the clinician will identify this as a specific goal in the initial evaluation report. The exercises and functional activities chosen for treatment will be oriented in part toward achieving this goal. For more details on functional rehabilitation, see Chapter 15, *Advanced Spinal Rehabilitation and Prevention.*

Doctor's Report, Lab and Diagnostic Tests

The patient should be asked about the results of tests performed and the physician's diagnosis. This gives the clinician information about the patient's understanding of the condition. The clinician may need to explain the diagnosis further or clarify patient misconceptions, but should avoid causing further confusion by inadvertently contradicting the patient's physician. The clinician should always confirm the patient's verbal report of the diagnosis and any tests performed with the physician's office.

Objective Evaluation of the Spine

This section describes the components of the objective evaluation, or physical examination, in general terms. Specific questions relating to the cervical, thoracic and lumbar areas are detailed in Sections Two and Three. The objective portion of the spinal evaluation consists of seven main categories:

1. Screening examination
2. Structure and posture examination
3. Mobility examination
4. Strength examination
5. Neurological examination
6. Palpation examination
7. Special tests

Screening Examination

The upper and lower quarter screening examinations consist of tests to rule out or confirm the spine as a potential cause of extremity symptoms. These exams are performed when the patient's primary complaint is extremity symptoms. If the patient's primary complaint is in the spine, the screening exams are not necessary because the clinician will perform a thorough evaluation of the spine anyway.

The neck should always be examined if the patient complains of an upper extremity symptom, since cervical spine disorders can cause arm symptoms. Similarly, the lower back should always be examined if the patient complains of lower extremity symptoms. Leg symptoms can be referred from the lumbar spine or the hip joint. As mentioned in Chapter 3, *Medical Screening*, certain visceral problems can mimic spinal disorders. The spinal screening examinations are helpful differentiation tests. If the screening examination proves negative, it should be repeated since there is the possibility that something was missed. If no spinal abnormalities are found and symptoms persist, the clinician should consult with a physician and further medical diagnostics should be pursued.

Structure and Posture Examination

Areas of specific complaint or areas that have shown some questionable signs during the screening examination should be examined in detail. The detailed objective evaluation of a specific area begins with general observation of the patient. The way the patient responds to the clinician's questions should be noted. What kind of attitude does the patient seem to have toward his condition—apprehensive, resentful or depressed? Since the behavioral attitude of the patient often has a bearing on the success of the treatment, the clinician should take time to consider this important aspect of the patient's condition.

How does the patient walk and sit? Does the patient seem to be in excruciating pain? Are there any obvious abnormalities in the way he moves about? Such observations are important for the clinician to note, as they may later tell more about the patient's progress than direct questioning does.

The structural exam involves a closer, more specific inspection of the area of complaint. Inspection involves the observation of bony, joint and muscular structures in the areas involved. It is essential that the parts to be examined are adequately free of clothing. Gym shorts and halter tops (for women) work better than patient gowns because they allow adequate observation with less awkwardness.

Postural assessment of the entire spine should be performed even if the patient's complaint concerns only one area of the spine. Any asymmetries found may be significant if correlated with other subjective and objective findings. Three types of asymmetries are discussed: Anterior/posterior, lateral and cephalocaudal.

Anterior/Posterior Symmetry. There should be a gentle continuation of anterior/posterior curves the entire length of the spine. An excessive curve in one area will usually cause an abnormal curve in an adjacent area. For example, excessive lumbar or cervical lordosis may be accompanied by increased thoracic kyphosis. It is common to see a forward head position and rounded upper thoracic spine. The forward head posture is often seen following cervical strains and can become the major cause of symptoms in the chronic stages of these injuries. Forward head posture is also often seen because of certain working positions and habits.

The lumbar and cervical spine should show a mild lordotic curve and the thoracic spine should have a mild kyphotic curve. Absence of any of the curves may indicate restriction of mobility or a disc disorder, whereas excessive lordotic curves may suggest the presence of any of a variety of structural and postural problems including joint hypermobility. A straight spine tends to be stiff and a curved spine tends to be flexible, but there are exceptions. Many pathological processes present certain predictable changes in lordosis and kyphosis and can be important clues to aid diagnosis.

It is also very important to observe the patient's sitting posture. Often the slumped lumbar flexion (flat back) posture contributes to loss of lumbar extension and to the development of a posterolateral lumbar disc protrusion. Additionally, patients with slumped lumbar sitting postures usually have forward head posture and abducted scapulae. These problems contribute to cervical and upper thoracic disorders that cannot be resolved unless the lumbar sitting posture is addressed.

Lateral Symmetry. Scoliotic curves in the spine are abnormal and are classified as functional, structural or caused by a specific pathological process. A structural scoliosis is caused by a defect in the bony structure of the spine such as wedging of the vertebral bodies. A functional scoli-

osis can be caused by a nonspinal defect such as unequal leg length, muscle imbalance or poor postural habits.

Cephalocaudal Symmetry. The clinician should observe for any cephalocaudal asymmetries, including asymmetries in the ribs or skin folds. Close attention is also paid to the sacral base during the structural evaluation, even in patients with complaints in the cervical spine. Compensatory scoliotic curves are often present in the cervical spine and may need to be treated by correcting the sacral base.

Assistive Devices and Supports. Any special assistive devices or supports used by the patient should be noted. Care should be taken to assess whether the device has been properly fitted and whether it is being used correctly.

Mobility Examination

The mobility exam consists of posture correction and active, passive and segmental mobility tests. The mobility exam helps determine what structures are involved (muscle, joint or neural tissue) and to what extent they are involved.

When performing any type of mobility test, the clinician should ask two main questions:

1. What does the test do to the patient's symptoms?
2. Is the amount of movement normal, hypermobile or hypomobile?

To perform a thorough mobility evaluation, the clinician must include all tissues from which the patient's symptoms might arise, including the joints, discs, connective tissues, neural and muscular tissues. The clinician also must determine whether any movement restrictions observed are a result of true tissue mobility restrictions or are limited by pain and muscle guarding.

Since posture often plays an important role in both the cause and treatment of many musculoskeletal disorders, an important part of the mobility exam involves observing the effects of posture correction. It is important to determine whether return to normal posture is possible and whether the patient's symptoms are altered when posture is corrected. The results of posture correction may implicate certain structures and will help determine to what extent the postural deformity is involved with the patient's current complaint.

Many spinal disorders initially present with centralized pain in the neck or lower back. As the condition worsens, pain and other symptoms begin to spread toward the periphery (arm or leg). Therefore, if spinal movements or positions cause increased arm or leg pain, this is thought to be a worse sign. Conversely, spinal movements or positions that cause increased central pain are typically less worrisome.

The tissues may be divided into two groups—non contractile and contractile. The non-contractile tissue group includes capsules, ligaments, bursae, nerves and their sheaths, cartilage, intervertebral discs and dura mater. The contractile tissue group includes muscles and tendons with their attachments. To differentiate between contractile and non-contractile tissue as the cause of the patient's symptoms, the clinician considers the results of mobility and strength testing.

Active mobility testing gives the clinician a general assessment of available range of motion and the patient's willingness to move. Pain with active movements can involve both contractile and non-contractile elements but may occur in predictable patterns that help determine the origin of the symptoms. For example, a painful recovery from forward bending often implicates a disorder of muscular origin, since the patient is using the muscles most when the pain is the greatest. Pain only at the end of range of motion in the absence of severe muscle shortening or spasm is more indicative of a non-contractile problem because the joint is the main structure being stressed. The specific joint(s) that may be hyper or hypomobile cannot be determined, but a general impression of problem areas can be gained.

Passive range of motion is tested to differentiate between contractile and non-contractile structures. These tests determine if the joint range is reduced (hypomobile), increased (hypermobile) or normal. If passive range of motion is greater than active range of motion, this implies that contractile tissue is at least in part responsible for the symptoms. If active range of motion is greater than passive range of motion, the patient is probably not able to relax well enough to allow the clinician to complete the passive range of motion testing.

The active and passive mobility tests give the clinician a general picture of the patient's joint mobility, while the *segmental* mobility tests help to find exactly where the abnormal motion is originating. Both active and passive mobility tests can be thought of as *gross* range of motion tests, in that the whole body part motion (neck or back) is being evaluated. Segmental mobility tests, on the other hand, provide information about how an *individual* joint moves.

The segmental mobility tests should be performed even when the patient has normal passive range of motion, because abnormal joint mechanics may still be present. For example, one joint may be extremely stiff, but the clinician

may not be able to detect it in the active or passive mobility exam because other joints are mobile enough to compensate for one stiff joint, giving the appearance of normal mobility. Another reason for performing segmental mobility tests is to determine whether the structure being tested (stressed) is painful, suggesting a potentially pathological process.

Segmental mobility testing is the most difficult part of the objective evaluation for many clinicians. Developing the skill of detecting subtle differences in motion from one joint to the next requires experience. In one study, even experienced manual therapists had poor interrater reliability when judging P/A stiffness of the spine.[52]

Initially, the clinician should not be concerned about detecting very subtle differences from one joint or spine to the next. Interrater reliability is important when performing research, comparing outcomes or sharing information with other clinicians. But an individual clinician can develop a "feel" that enables confident assessment and treatment, even if it cannot be precisely described or duplicated by another clinician. When an inexperienced clinician performs the segmental mobility testing procedures on every patient he encounters, he will begin to recognize that a certain segment "feels abnormal" or "is definitely stiff" when compared to the hundreds of other segments examined in the past. Eventually, that clinician will be able to detect very subtle differences. The most serious mistake the inexperienced clinician can make is to avoid testing segmental mobility for fear of not understanding the results.

A very good method to use when performing segmental mobility tests is to first find the tender segments, then perform specific mobility tests on them to detect mobility differences from right to left or from the segments above or below. Tender segments are found by palpating the soft tissues surrounding them, palpating the interspinous spaces or performing spring tests or P/A pressures on each segment. When a tender segment is found, rotation mobility testing is particularly helpful in developing a theory about the pathology. For example, if the clinician discovers that right rotation is more tender than left rotation, and right rotation is more mobile than left rotation, a possible hypermobility in right rotation exists.

Some clinicians use the following scale to grade segmental mobility:[54]

1. Ankylosed
2. Considerable restriction
3. Slight restriction
4. Normal

5. Slight increase
6. Considerable increase
7. Unstable

The use of the above scale is not universal, however, and it is usually sufficient and perhaps even more desirable to use the descriptive words rather than the numerals when describing segmental mobility in the written report.

If active and passive range of motion are full and painless in all planes, passive range of motion should be repeated with overpressures to try to reproduce symptoms. Segmental mobility testing should be performed in an attempt to find a joint that, when moved, reproduces the patient's symptoms. If none of the mobility tests and the strength tests described below reproduce the patient's symptoms, the area is considered free of musculoskeletal pathology, and the complaint is unlikely to stem from a problem that can be helped by a physical therapist.

So far, we have been discussing evaluation of joint mobility. It is also important to evaluate soft tissue mobility. These concepts are discussed in Chapter 11, *Soft Tissue Mobilization and Neuromuscular Training.*

Use of an Inclinometer in Range of Motion Testing

The AMA's Guides to the Evaluation of Permanent Impairment state that standard goniometric techniques for measuring spinal movement can be highly inaccurate and that measurement techniques using inclinometers are necessary to obtain reliable spinal mobility measurements.[13]

The reliability of visual assessment of cervical and lumbar lordosis has been shown to be fair at best.[19] For these reasons, many clinicians are using inclinometers to measure and report spinal range of motion. Inclinometers are particularly useful because changes during treatment can be measured objectively.

One issue related to inclinometer use is the lack of agreement on norms and protocols. Published normative data is device-specific and varies depending upon the protocol.[10,56] Normal ranges of spinal mobility presented in Table 4-3 are based on a variety of sources using differing methodologies, so the ranges are relatively wide.[8,10,13,18,39,41,47,59,67,82,83,84]

Even though normative data for spinal range of motion is still evolving, a properly used inclinometer with demonstrated reliability provides us with more objectivity than we have had in the past. Inclinometers can be used for the cervical, thoracic and lumbar spine. Some inclinometers have been specifically designed to measure cervical range of motion.

Table 4-3: Normal Ranges of Spinal Mobility.

Cervical	
Flexion	40°-70°
Extension	60°-80°
Side Bending	40°-50°
Rotation	70°-90°
Thoracic	
Flexion	20°-30°
Extension	25°-35°
Side Bending	20°-25°
Rotation	5°-10°
Kyphosis Posture	30°-40°
Lumbar	
Sacral Inclination Angle	15°-30°
Standing Lordosis	25°-40°
Standing Hip Flexion	45°-65°
Flexion (AMA method)	40°-75°
Extension (AMA method)	20°-35°
Flexion (curve angle method)	0°-20°
Extension (curve angle method)	60°-75°
Side Bending	15°-35°
Rotation	10°-20°

Strength Examination

The strength exam is performed to rule out muscular involvement as the source of symptoms, to decide if muscle imbalances are a source of the problem and to provide a baseline for any strengthening that will be performed as a part of the treatment. Strength tests are usually done in a comfortable neutral position within the available range of motion. The clinician attempts to elicit a strong muscle contraction with very little or no joint movement. If resisted muscular contraction of an extremity muscle produces pain, there is pathology within the muscle, tendon or its attachment.

If no pain or weakness is observed, the contractile tissues are ruled out as a source of the symptoms. Weak and painful muscle contractions do not necessarily indicate true weakness, since pain may be interfering with the patient's ability to contract. A weak and painless contraction, on the other hand, suggests neurological involvement or weakness due to inactivity (see *Neurological Examination* on page 47).

While strength tests are very helpful in differential diagnosis of the extremity joints, they are of little use in definitely implicating or ruling out muscular pathology in the lumbar and thoracic spine because of the difficulty in isolating muscle contraction without the occurrence of joint movement, especially compression, in these areas. Resisted muscle tests may be somewhat helpful in ruling out muscular involvement in the cervical spine.

Strength tests of the lumbar spine are most useful because of the relationship between trunk weakness and lumbar problems.[3,27,29,34,38,50,65] The lumbar paraspinals, lumbar stabilizers and the abdominal muscles are tested for weakness. The weakness is usually treated through exercise, because even if muscles are not the source of the patient's symptoms, weak muscles may be a part of the patient's problem.

Neurological Examination

The neurological portion of a musculoskeletal evaluation consists of a series of tests to determine if there is impingement or encroachment upon a spinal nerve root, entrapment of a peripheral nerve, tightness in the neural tissues or central nervous system involvement.

Resisted Muscle Tests. Resisted (isometric) muscle tests can help determine neurological involvement. When weakness is present with a painful contraction the clinician cannot be certain if the muscle is weak because of a neurological deficit or because of the pain itself. If pain, inactivity or immobilization have been present for a long time, the muscle also can be weak because of disuse. Specific muscular weakness that is not associated with pain or disuse is considered a positive neurological finding if it follows a nerve root distribution and correlates with other objective findings. Resisted muscle tests are done bilaterally at the same time when possible. This makes it easier to find slight differences in strength. It also makes it more difficult for the patient to exaggerate a weakness. A true weakness will be smooth and present throughout the range of motion, whereas an exaggerated weakness or weakness caused by pain will often be jerky or intermittent through the range of motion.

Muscle Stretch Reflexes. Muscle stretch reflexes are often helpful in finding neurological deficits. As a rule, hyperactive reflexes suggest upper motor nerve pathology and hypoactive reflexes suggest impingement, irritation, entrapment or injury of a spinal nerve root or peripheral nerve. Normal reflexes vary a great deal from person to person. Occasionally, reflexes appear hypoactive or hyperactive, but are symmetrical. These findings are probably normal for those patients. When a reflex appears hypo- or hyperactive when compared to the contralateral side, the finding is significant.

It is important to remember that referred pain can facilitate motor activity in the area of referral. This increased muscular activity can inhibit the antagonistic muscle group. For example, pain arising from pathology in any pain-producing structure in the lower lumbar spine can be felt as pain down the posterior aspect of the thigh. This referred pain may cause increased muscular activity in the hamstring muscles, which may inhibit the quadriceps group. This inhibitory influence on the quadriceps may cause a hypoactive muscle stretch reflex. The implication is that some muscle stretch reflex changes can be caused by referred pain rather than by spinal nerve root impingement or peripheral nerve entrapment.[64]

Sensation Testing. The patient is questioned closely during the subjective evaluation concerning sensation abnormalities. Patients will often confuse paresthesia with anesthesia. Paresthesia can suggest a certain nerve root level if it follows a given pattern but is not considered a positive neurological sign. Anesthesia, however, is a positive neurological finding. If the patient has indicated there is a sensory deficit, the clinician should confirm with pinprick testing the extent and exact location of involvement. An area of numbness that follows a dermatomal pattern or the distribution of a peripheral nerve suggests nerve root impingement or nerve entrapment or injury. If the area of numbness involves the entire circumference of an extremity (glove or stocking effect), a sensory nerve deficit due to vascular insufficiency or some other medical disorder is suspected rather than musculoskeletal pathology.

Pain that follows a dermatomal, sclerotomal or myotomal pattern does not necessarily indicate nerve root impingement or peripheral nerve entrapment. Pain may be referred from muscles, joints or other structures that are innervated by the same spinal nerve level or peripheral nerve. Pain producing structures in the spine are: 1) Paraspinal musculature; 2) Facet joints: 3) Dura mater; 4) Outer layers of the annulus fibrosis 5) Intervertebral disc; and 6) Spinal ligaments.[30,35,73,76]

Nerve root pain is often felt as a deep burning pain specific to one nerve root segment, whereas referred pain is felt as a diffuse aching pain. Since the sensory nerves supplying pain-producing structures of the spine are not specific to one level, referred pain is usually felt in more than one dermatome. Both referred pain and nerve root symptoms are usually felt first in the proximal ends of the involved dermatomes and spread toward the periphery as the symptoms intensify.

Neural Tension Tests. Physical therapy clinicians are familiar with performing neural tension tests to implicate the neural tissues for potential pathology. Examples of the most common tests performed include passive neck flexion, the straight leg raise and the prone knee bend.

More recently, however, researchers have expanded the role that adverse mechanical neural tension (AMNT) may play in a patient's symptoms or dysfunction.

Because the human nervous system is a continuous tissue tract, any peripheral limb movement will have a mechanical consequence on the peripheral and possibly central nerve tissues. For example, the ulnar nerve is stretched when the elbow is flexed, while the median and radial nerves are shortened. The human body normally provides for built-in anatomical protection of the neural tissues during movement to ensure continued chemical and electrical neural conduction. It seems appropriate, then that an evaluation of the response of the neural tissues to mechanical stresses should be included in a complete evaluation of the spine or extremities.

Symptoms related to mechanical deformation of the nervous system can result from interruption of blood supply to neural tissues, interruption of axonal transport systems or irritation of the connective tissues of the nervous system.[9] Also, there are many potential mechanical tissue interfaces where mobility of the neural tissues may be affected. These may be myofascial, bony or ligamentous. For example, the posterior interosseus branch of the radial nerve pierces the supinator muscle (myofascial), the ulnar nerve rests in the ulnar groove (bony), and the median nerve lies under the transverse carpal ligament (ligamentous). Thus, the clinician should consider these interfaces as possible causes of decreased neural tissue mobility and possibly related to symptom provocation in the peripheral limbs.

Researchers have implicated AMNT in certain disorders of the neuro musculoskeletal system and clinical studies have linked positive neural tension tests to various peripheral limb symptoms.[9,45,92] For this reason, the possibility of AMNT should be examined in any patient presenting with non-irritable symptoms where there may be a potential neural tension component. This would include any patient complaining of central or peripheral symptoms where the symptoms cannot be definitively traced to a non-AMNT source.

David S. Butler's *The Sensitive Nervous System*[9] is an excellent resource on this subject. In addition to the three traditional tests (passive neck flexion, straight leg raise and prone knee bend), the upper limb tension tests (ULTT's) and the slump test can provide information about mobility of the neural tissues. The ULTT tests are generally indicated for the upper limbs and the slump test is indicated for the lower limbs and trunk.

Neural tissue is by nature highly irritable. Therefore, neural tension testing is usually not indicated for severe, irritable, inflammatory or pathological disorders. Contraindications to neural tension testing and treatment include the following:

1. Irritable conditions
2. Inflammatory conditions
3. Spinal cord signs
4. Malignancy
5. Nerve root compression signs
6. Severe, unremitting, constant night pain
7. Neurological signs (includes true numbness, weakness or reflex changes)
8. Recent paresthesia/anesthesia
9. Active spinal motions easily provoking distal symptoms, paresthesia or anesthesia
10. Reflex sympathetic dystrophy

It should be noted that any pathological process that causes less space for neural tissue to slide freely will produce an earlier onset of symptoms with the tension tests.

Palpation Examination

The palpation portion of the evaluation procedure can impart valuable information about the condition of the skin, subcutaneous tissue, muscle, ligament and bone. Additional information about soft tissue palpation is found in Chapter 11, *Soft Tissue Mobilization and Neuromuscular Training*.

The skin is palpated and examined for tenderness, color, temperature, moisture and texture. Because pain can be referred from a proximal site, the area where the patient describes the symptoms may not be the site of the primary disorder.[15]

For example, a patient may complain of posterior thigh pain, but the pain may be coming from the lumbar spine. Tenderness to palpation can be a reliable indication about the location of the primary pathology, but prolonged muscle guarding and spasm in response to referred pain can fool the inexperienced clinician.

Temperature changes help find areas of pathology. A warm area may suggest acute inflammation or a cool area may mean chronic pathology such as soft tissue hypomobility. Dry, smooth, shiny skin indicates a chronic condition, whereas a slight rise in moisture may mean an acute condition.

The subcutaneous tissue is palpated for abnormal amounts of fat, tissue fluid, tension, localized swelling and nodules. Normally the skin can be rolled over the underlying muscle and bone freely and painlessly. If there are pathological changes at a segmental level, the subcuta-

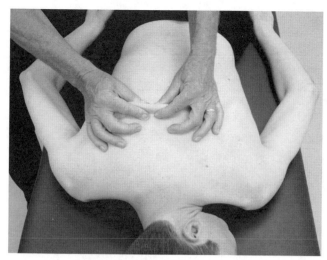

Figure 4-4: Skin rolling test.

neous tissue may be tight and painful when the skin-rolling test is done (Fig 4-4). Any moles on the skin are examined to find whether they are superficial or deep. Suspicious moles should be reported to the patient's physician (see Chapter 3, *Medical Screening*).

Muscle tenderness is examined and careful interpretation is given to any positive findings. Muscle guarding or spasm are noted. When documenting muscle changes, the clinician must take care to avoid indiscriminate use of the word "spasm." True muscle spasm is somewhat rare, especially in chronic cases. Unless the soft tissue changes found show true muscle spasm (where the muscle is in a contracted state and is unable to relax), other word choices that are more descriptive should be used.

Next, the condition of the palpable ligaments is noted. They may be tender if the joint is sprained or inflamed. They may be thickened and coarse if joint hypomobility is present.

The position of the bone is felt to rule out dislocation, subluxation or positional changes (e.g., those seen with facet joint impingement.) The clinician must not assume that all bony abnormalities are pathological. Some may be congenital and may be unrelated to the patient's present complaint.

Special Tests

The special tests section refers to specific tests performed on a particular body part or tests that do not fit into any of the other categories. The tests that are unique to the cervical spine and the lumbar spine are described in Sections Two and Three.

It is important to recognize that patients who present with musculoskeletal complaints can have a psychosocial component to their symptoms. In rare cases, patients intentionally fabricate symptoms. It is much more common for issues of secondary gain, excessive fear, depression and anxiety to accompany legitimate musculoskeletal dysfunction.

Emotional factors can significantly influence a patient's perception of pain and actually increase muscular tension. If an injury occurred at work or in an auto accident, the patient may feel a sense of entitlement to benefits and return to "normal" status that is not typically present when the injury occurs at home.

We have found that the beliefs one has about the correlation between pain and function vary drastically from one patient to the next. The patient's belief system may play a more important role in rehabilitation than the actual physical extent of the injury. It is important for the clinician to be aware of the patient's beliefs so that appropriate education and management techniques are used.

A simple questionnaire developed by Waddell, et al, sheds light on the patient's fear-avoidance beliefs, specifically with regard to work activities (Fig 4-5).[86] They found that certain fear-avoidance beliefs strongly correlated to work loss due to low back pain. Fritz and colleagues have found that fear-avoidance beliefs correlate with prolonged recovery from acute low back pain.[23,24]

We use the Fear-Avoidance Beliefs Questionnaire (FABQ) as a screening tool for all work hardening and work conditioning patients. It is also helpful to use with patients who seem to have excessive fear or anxiety about their symptoms. The patient's answers to the FABQ help create a dialogue between the clinician and patient to explore how specific beliefs can interfere with the rehabilitation process. Talking about such issues up front creates a more honest clinician-patient relationship. Specific screening tests for depression, somatic anxiety, and other psychosocial factors are also available and are essential in advanced rehabilitation programs like work hardening and work conditioning, but are outside the scope of this text.

Correlation with Other Reports and Tests

Upon completion of the evaluation, the clinician correlates his findings with other available information such as physician's reports, radiological exams, lab and other tests. So that the evaluation is done without bias, this correlation should be done at the conclusion of the evaluation instead of at the beginning. Knowledge of any severe or serious pathology is, of course, important and should be considered immediately.

Name: _____   Date: ___/___/___
                                                  mm dd yy

Here are some of the things other patients have told us about their pain. For each statement please circle the number from 0 to 6 to indicate how much physical activities such as bending, lifting, walking or driving affect or would affect your back pain.

	Completely Disagree		Unsure			Completely Agree
1. My pain was caused by physical activity.	0	1	2	3	4	5	6
2. Physical activity makes my pain worse.	0	1	2	3	4	5	6
3. Physical activity might harm my back.	0	1	2	3	4	5	6
4. I should not do physical activities which (might) make my pain worse.	0	1	2	3	4	5	6
5. I cannot do physical activities which (might) make my pain worse.	0	1	2	3	4	5	6

The following statements are about how your normal work affects or would affect your back pain.

	Completely Disagree		Unsure			Completely Agree
6. My pain was caused by my work or by an accident at work.	0	1	2	3	4	5	6
7. My work aggravated my pain.	0	1	2	3	4	5	6
8. I have a claim for compensation for my pain.	0	1	2	3	4	5	6
9. My work is too heavy for me.	0	1	2	3	4	5	6
10. My work makes or would make my pain worse.	0	1	2	3	4	5	6
11. My work might harm my back.	0	1	2	3	4	5	6
12. I should not do my regular work with my present pain.	0	1	2	3	4	5	6
13. I cannot do my normal work with my present pain.	0	1	2	3	4	5	6
14. I cannot do my normal work until my pain is treated.	0	1	2	3	4	5	6
15. I do not think that I will be back to my normal work within 3 months.	0	1	2	3	4	5	6
16. I do not think that I will ever be able to go back to that work.	0	1	2	3	4	5	6

Figure 4-5: Fear Avoidance Beliefs Questionnaire. Reprinted from Waddell G, Newton M, Henderson I, et al: Fear Avoidance Beliefs Questionnaire (FABQ) and the Role of Fear Avoidance Beliefs in Chronic Low Back Pain and Disability. Pain 52:157-168, 1993, with permission from the International Association for the Study of Pain.[86]

Section Two—The Cervical and Upper Thoracic Spine

The subjective and objective evaluation of a patient with spinal pain was discussed in Section One. Section Two takes a closer look at the objective evaluation of the cervical and upper thoracic spine. The reader should be familiar with the concepts found in Section One before proceeding.

Upper Quarter Screening Examination

The upper quarter screening examination consists of a series of mobility and neurological tests to identify problem areas in the cervical and upper thoracic spine, shoulder, elbow, wrist and hand (Table 4-4). It is most valuable when performed on a patient complaining of upper extremity symptoms and little or no neck pain. With such a patient it is important to clear the cervical spine as a source of the upper extremity symptoms. The screening evaluation is redundant if the patient is already complaining of cervical symptoms, and the clinician should skip to the rest of the objective evaluation.

A good screening evaluation performed by a skilled evaluator can make the rest of the evaluation more concise and efficient. *The purpose of the screening evaluation is to identify what anatomical areas deserve a detailed evaluation.* After the screening evaluation, the clinician will know which anatomical areas have been cleared and which ones need a closer look. The testing is done with the patient sitting in a straight-backed chair or on the edge of a treatment table.

First, a postural assessment should be made, and then the cervical spine is taken through the active ranges of motion as the clinician watches for signs of pain, muscle guarding or limited range of motion. If no signs or symptoms are observed with active range of motion, passive overpressure is performed. If no signs or symptoms are observed with passive overpressure, the joints of the cervical spine are considered clear and are not the causal structures involved.

The quadrant test is a useful screening test for cervical spine involvement. *The clinician should perform the vertebral artery test on page 53 prior to performing the quadrant test.* The quadrant test can be performed in a sitting or supine position. The cervical spine is passively taken to end range of extension, rotation and side bending in one direction. Overpressure is applied (Fig 4-6). The quadrant position places the ipsilateral facet joints in a maximally closed position and rules out or implicates the cervical spine as a source of peripheral symptoms.

Next, isometric resisted muscle tests of the cervical spine are performed in all planes of motion with the head in a neutral mid-range position. If no pain or weakness is observed, the musculature of the cervical spine is considered clear. Resisted rotation of the cervical spine is also a neurological test of spinal level C1. All other resisted muscle tests should be performed (see *Resisted Muscle Tests* on page 60).

During resisted muscle testing of the upper extremities, the clinician should look closely for asymmetries or problems with scapulohumeral rhythm. Abnormalities in scapulohumeral rhythm are clues to abnormal muscular forces in the shoulder girdle and upper back. Performing Babinski's reflex test for upper motor neuron involvement completes upper quarter screening.

Structure and Posture Examination

The evaluator should review Section One for general comments relating to structure and posture assessment, remembering that postural assessment should include the entire spine even if the patient's complaint concerns only one area of the spine. Any asymmetries found may be significant if correlated with other subjective and objective findings.

Table 4-4: Upper Quarter Screening Evaluation.

Postural assessment
Active range of motion, cervical spine
Passive over-pressures if active is symptom-free
Vertebral artery test
Quadrant test
Resisted cervical rotation (C1)
Resisted shoulder elevation (C2, 3, 4)
Resisted shoulder abduction (C5)
Active shoulder flexion and rotation
Resisted elbow flexion (C6)
Resisted elbow extension (C7)
Active range of motion, elbow
Resisted wrist flexion (C7)
Resisted wrist extension (C6)
Resisted thumb extension (C8)
Resisted finger abduction (T1)

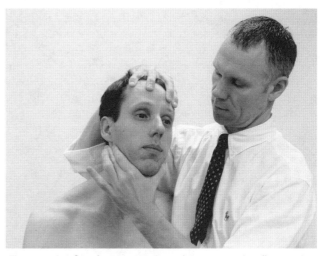

Figure 4-6: Quadrant test to rule out or implicate the cervical spine. Extension, side bending and rotation place the ipsilateral facet joint in the maximally closed packed position. Overpressure is applied.

Anterior/Posterior Symmetry

There should be a gentle continuation of anterior/posterior curves the entire length of the spine. Abnormal posturing often involves extension of the occiput and upper cervical spine, which causes a compensatory flattening (flexion) of the lower cervical and upper thoracic spine to achieve a level head position. Scapular abduction/protraction and humeral internal rotation is usually seen as well. This posture is called the forward head, rounded shoulder position (Fig 4-7). It is often caused by repetitive working positions or habits related to a sedentary lifestyle. When the patient habitually holds the occiput in extension, the suboccipital muscles adaptively shorten. This can be a source of suboccipital headaches. The flattened lower cervical lordosis that accompanies this habitual posture can lead to more serious disorders including cervical disc herniation and TMJ dysfunction.[72] The forward head posture is also often seen following acute cervical strains and can become the major cause of symptoms in the chronic stages of these injuries.

It is important to observe the patient's posture in a variety of positions. For example, patients with slumped lumbar sitting postures usually have forward head posture and protracted scapulae. These problems contribute to cervical and upper thoracic disorders that will not resolve unless the lumbar sitting posture is addressed. Indeed, sometimes the most important aid used to correct a cervical posture problem is a lumbar roll.

Lateral Symmetry

The patient should be observed closely from the front and back. Is the head slightly tipped to one side or the other? Lateral asymmetries can be the result of functional or structural abnormalities. Facet joint impingement or subluxation may cause an acute functional scoliosis in the cervical spine. This disorder involves the entrapment of soft tissue within the facet joint or facet joint subluxation, in which the patient may tip the head to the contralateral side to take the weight off the painful structure, or may tip the head toward the subluxed joint. Often, a lumbar or thoracic

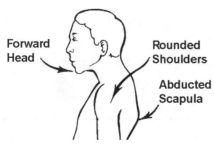

Figure 4-7: Forward head, rounded shoulder posture common in patients with spinal dysfunction.

scoliosis will cause adaptive positional changes of the head and neck. These can be thought of as functional if they are still reversible, and structural if they are long-term enough to cause permanent structural changes.

Cephalocaudal Symmetry

Cephalocaudal asymmetries can often cause lateral asymmetries. Therefore, these two conditions are closely related. When the patient is observed from the front, are the eyes and ears level? The height of the shoulders and the inferior angle of the scapulae also should be examined for levelness. The shoulder and scapula on the dominant side are often positioned lower. This is considered normal and care should be taken to avoid drawing conclusions from shoulder and scapula height asymmetries.

Asymmetrical scapulohumeral rhythm during shoulder flexion and abduction is a more significant finding. Scapulohumeral rhythm should be checked in all patients with cervical and thoracic symptoms, as asymmetries or general weakness of the interscapular musculature can contribute to problems in these areas. For example, weak interscapular musculature is often associated with protracted scapulae, forward head posturing, dysfunction of the levator scapulae and trapezius muscles and tightness of the suboccipital muscles.

The clinician should look for any asymmetries in the ribs or skin folds, sacral base and lower extremities. The sacral base should be checked closely even in patients with complaints in the cervical spine because compensatory scoliotic curves are often present in the cervical spine and may need to be treated by correcting the sacral base. The method for checking the sacral base is discussed in Section Three. Occasionally, significant abnormalities in the lower extremities (for example, unilateral genu recurvatum or subtalar pronation) also can be problematic. The clinician must use common sense and must correlate objective findings carefully when deciding if a long standing lower quarter postural defect is related to upper quarter complaints.

Assistive Devices and Supports

Any special assistive devices or supports that the patient uses, such as a cervical collar or lumbar roll, should be noted at this time. Care should be taken to assess if the device has been properly fitted and if it is being used correctly. Cervical collars are typically sold in three to five inch heights. If the patient is in acute discomfort, the taller heights are sometimes less comfortable. But if the collar is too short, it allows the patient to slump into a forward head posture. The patient must be educated about proper posture while using the collar, or it can cause more harm than good. This is especially true if the collar is used for more than a few days. Long-term use should be discouraged because of the collar's detrimental effects on the strength, range of motion and function of the cervical spine. When fitting the collar, the clinician should make sure that the collar is most comfortable when the patient is assuming proper posture. If the collar is uncomfortable when the patient slumps into undesirable posture, this is acceptable because the collar then serves as a reminder to use good posture.

Mobility Examination

When performing any type of mobility test, whether it be active, passive or segmental, the clinician should ask two main questions:

1. How does the test affect the patient's symptoms?
2. Is the amount of movement normal, hyper-mobile or hypomobile?

The findings of the mobility exam are significant if the test changes the patient's symptoms or if the amount of movement seen or felt is abnormal.

Vertebral Artery Testing

The vertebral artery test is a well-known screening procedure performed to ensure that the movements performed during cervical mobility testing or treatment will not compromise the circulation of the vertebral artery. Most clinicians are taught to perform the test during the initial evaluation. In addition, the integrity of the vertebral artery should be reassessed any time the clinician plans to perform testing or treatment that will increase cervical range of motion. For example, if a patient lacks significant extension and rotation mobility, the vertebral artery test probably will be negative initially. However, any newly gained motion could cause a circulation compromise. To emphasize its importance, the Australian Physiotherapy Association and other international associations have formalized protocols for pre-manipulative testing of the vertebral artery.[26]

The test is traditionally performed passively with the patient in a supine position. It also can be performed actively with the patient sitting. The clinician instructs the patient to keep the eyes open throughout the procedure. The patient fully extends and rotates the neck to one side, holding the position for a minimum of ten seconds (Fig 4-8). The patient should report any symptoms of tinnitus, dizziness, nausea, throbbing, confusion or unusual sensation. The clinician observes for pupillary constriction/dilation or confusion both during and a few seconds after the test. Both directions of rotation are tested. If the test is performed actively, the clinician should make sure that the

patient is fully extending and rotating the upper cervical spine. If unsure, the clinician should perform the test passively until the patient becomes familiar with the test movements.

Wendy Aspinall describes a gradual progression of vertebral artery tests.[1] When patients complain of dizziness or other symptoms that are suspicious of vertebral artery occlusion, a gradual progression may be advisable. Since vertebral artery tests themselves can compromise the artery, Aspinall's progression produces minimal stress because the least potentially provocative tests are applied first. The details of the progression are not described in this text. Clinicians desiring more information about her tests should consult the article referenced herein.

If the vertebral artery test is positive, the clinician must avoid mobilization and cervical spine movements that cause extension and rotation into the ranges of motion that produced the symptoms. The patient's physician should be alerted to the positive finding.

Posture Correction

Postural correction for the cervical and upper thoracic spine often involves the forward head, slumped sitting, abducted/protracted scapula posture that is seen in many patients who complain of a variety of musculoskeletal disorders. If correction of the poor posture can be accomplished, it should be done. If correction of posture results in some increased neck pain, it is usually acceptable. However, if posture correction causes increased pain or other symptoms in the upper extremity, attempts to correct the poor posture should be discontinued.

The *head back, chin in* position has long been a favorite of clinicians who are trying to correct their patient's posture. Yet care must be taken when prescribing it. If a patient

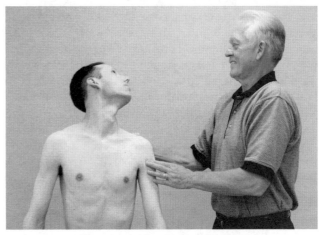

Figure 4-8: Vertebral artery test.

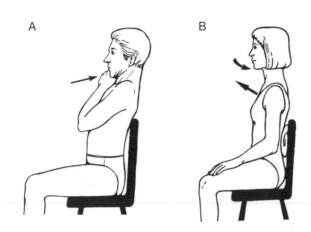

Figure 4-9: A) Overcorrection of forward head posture, which can excessively flatten the cervical spine in some patients. B) Correction technique that maintains the normal cervical lordosis. This is a better technique for most patients.

already has a flattened mid cervical lordosis, overcorrection when performing head back, chin in can make it worse (Fig 4-9). For most patients, the clinician should instruct as follows. First, the patient must be sitting upright with an adequate lumbar lordosis. The scapula should be retracted and the sternum elevated. This should not be done forcefully, but gently and naturally. Care should be taken to avoid elevating the shoulders. Often, this position alone is enough to cause an appropriate head back, chin in posture. If suboccipital muscle tightness is present, the patient should be instructed to gently nod the occiput, without flexing the cervical spine. If scapular muscle weakness or anterior shoulder tightness is present, these areas also should be addressed.

Active Mobility Testing

Atlanto/Occipital Joint

Active A/O joint mobility can be tested with the patient seated or supine by simply asking the patient to nod his head slightly. The cervical spine should be in neutral. A neutral position is most easily achieved by asking the patient to sit up straight with a normal lumbar lordosis and elevated sternum. The clinician may then use the nose and the midline of the face for reference and observe for any lateral deviations of the head during the nodding movement. Deviation to one side suggests a restriction in movement of the A/O joint on the ipsilateral side. Palpation of the suboccipital area during active motion helps the clinician to feel the quality of movement and to make sure that the movement is only taking place at the A/O joint.

Atlanto/Axial Joint

When testing active mobility of the atlanto/axial joint, one should remember that this joint is oriented in the horizontal

plane. Rotation is the main motion of the A/A joint. It has only small excursions of flexion, extension and side bending. If a rotatory restriction of the cervical spine is present, the A/A joint should be considered as a probable factor. Rotation of the A/A joint can be effectively tested actively in a sitting position by asking the patient first to fully flex the cervical spine, and then rotate. This technique isolates rotation of the A/A joint by locking the rest of the cervical spine into flexion. A passive technique in supine is shown in Figure 4-12.

Mid and Lower Cervical and Upper Thoracic Spine

Active range of motion of the mid and lower cervical and upper thoracic spine is examined with the patient sitting. From a starting position using good posture, the patient is asked to actively forward and backward bend, side bend and rotate in each direction. Any movements that are limited or that change the patient's symptoms are noted.

Next, the clinician palpates between the spinous processes while the patient performs active flexion, extension and rotation of the upper thoracic spine (Fig 4-10). This is actually a segmental mobility palpation technique, but is included in the active mobility section for simplicity because it is performed during the active mobility exam. Flexion and extension movement can be felt by placing the finger between the spinous processes as the patient forward and backward bends. Placing the thumbs on the spinous processes or pinching the spinous processes at two levels and watching and feeling the movement between the levels (the pinch test) can assess active rotation. This test also can be done with the patient lying prone, rotating the head from one side to the other. Palpating cervical segmental mobility during active motion is not as effective as in the upper thoracic spine. It is easier to palpate cervical motion using the prone and supine segmental mobility tests described later.

If all active range of motion is within normal limits and is symptom free, the movements are repeated and passive overpressures are given at the end of range of each movement. If no pain or other symptoms arise, even when overpressures are applied, the area is clear of musculoskeletal pathology.

Passive Mobility Testing

Passive range of motion is tested to differentiate between contractile and non-contractile structures. These tests determine whether the joint range is reduced (hypomobile), increased (hypermobile) or normal. In a supine position, the cervical spine is moved through each plane of motion passively by the clinician, with care being taken to ensure the patient is relaxed and not voluntarily contracting the musculature. If active range of motion is less than passive range of motion, this implies that contractile tissue is at least in part responsible for the patient's symptoms. If active range of motion is greater than passive range of motion, the patient probably cannot relax well enough to

allow the clinician to complete the passive range of motion testing. This is common in cases where the pain is severe or the patient is anxious. In such cases, the passive range of motion testing should be repeated later when the patient is more comfortable and at ease.

Segmental Mobility Testing

Atlanto/Occipital Joint

To palpate segmental mobility of the A/O joint, the clinician stands at the head of the table with the patient lying supine. The head is fully supported under the occiput by both hands while contact is made with the transverse processes of the atlas by the index or middle fingertips. This contact is indirectly made through soft tissue between the mastoid and the ramus of the mandible. The clinician can use this hand support and palpation technique for forward/backward bending, side bending and rotational movements (Fig 4-11).

Forward/Backward Bending.   The clinician passively moves the head in a nodding movement. Care should be taken to avoid flexing the entire cervical spine. The transverse processes should be felt to move symmetrically or not at all.

Side Bending.   The clinician passively side bends the head on the neck. Care should be taken to avoid side bending the entire cervical spine. The transverse process of the atlas will become more prominent on the side opposite the direction of side bending.

Rotation.   The transverse process keeps a constant relationship between the mastoid and ramus during the first few degrees of rotation. At the end of rotation range, the transverse process can be felt to approximate or even disappear behind the mastoid or the ramus depending which way the head is turned. For example, if the clinician turns the head to the left, the right transverse process will approximate/

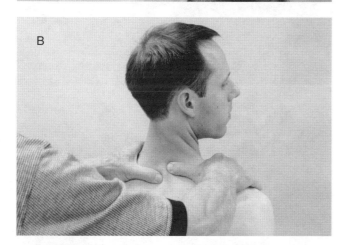

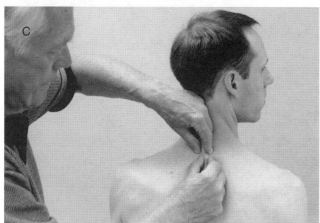

Figure 4-10: Palpating segmental mobility during active range of motion testing: A) During flexion/extension; B) During rotation; and C) Alternate method during rotation—the pinch test.

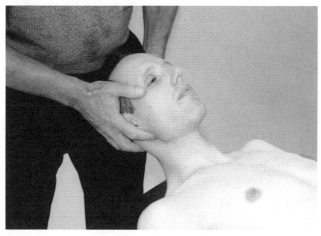

Figure 4-11: Palpating segmental mobility—A/O joint.

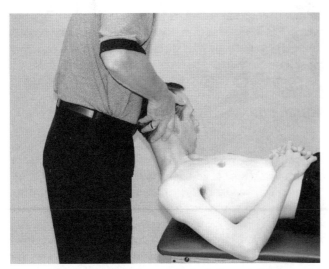

Figure 4-12: Passive upper cervical rotation—A/A joint.

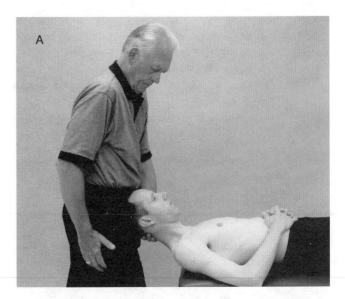

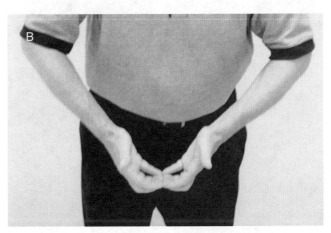

disappear behind the right mastoid. In right rotation, the opposite should occur. The two sides are compared for symmetry of movement.

Atlanto/Axial Joint

The clinician stands at the head of the table with the patient lying supine, using the same hand placement that was used in the A/O evaluation. The cervical spine is fully flexed to lock it from any other motions. The clinician then tests the A/A joint for a rotational restriction by rotating the head each direction, taking care to maintain full flexion during the movement (Fig 4-12). No other segmental mobility tests of the A/A joint are performed.

Mid and Lower Cervical and Upper Thoracic Spine

The segmental mobility tests for the mid and lower cervical spine are forward bending, backward bending, rotation, side bending and side glide. They enable the clinician to feel specific areas of hyper or hypomobility in the cervical spine.

The patient is positioned supine with the head extending over the end of the treatment plinth. It is important for the clinician to support the patient's head in such a way that the patient can relax completely, having confidence that the clinician has full control of the movements.

The treatment plinth must be adjusted to the correct height for the individual clinician. The patient's head rests against the clinician's anterior hip. The clinician must observe the neck muscles (scalenes and sternocleidomastoids) to ensure patient relaxation. The hands are cradled to hold the patient's head and neck. The index fingers support the articular pillar superior to the segment to be tested (Fig 4-13).

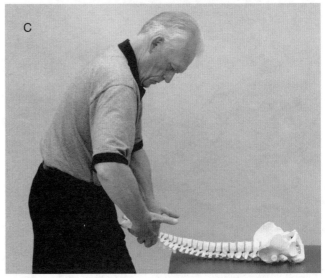

Figure 4-13: Testing cervical spine segmental mobility: A) The patient's head rests on the clinician's thigh; B) Position of the hands; C) Position of the clinician.

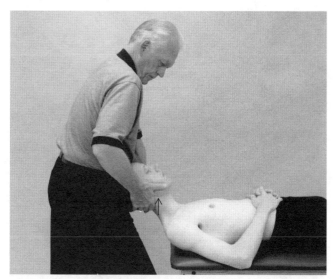

Figure 4-14: Segmental testing—cervical forward bending.

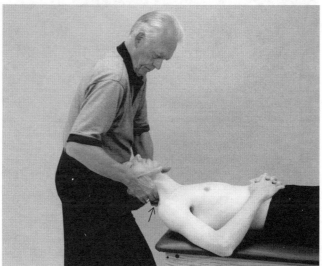

Figure 4-15: Segmental testing—cervical backward bending.

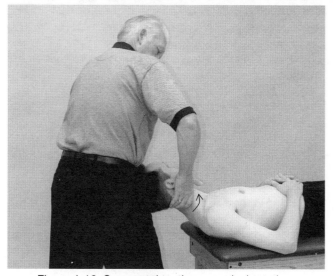

Figure 4-16: Segmental testing—cervical rotation.

Cervical Forward Bending (Forward Glide). Forward bending in the cervical spine involves superior and anterior glide of the bilateral superior articulating surfaces on the inferior articulating surfaces. The patient's head and neck are held in 30° of forward bending. This aligns the plane of the cervical facet joints perpendicular to the floor. Forward bending is performed by lifting straight upward with both hands. To start, the clinician's knees should be slightly bent. The clinician extends the knees slightly to keep the patient's head in the correct position (Fig 4-14). Most of the force is directed through the index fingers to each articular pillar, but contact is maintained with all of the neck and head so that it is carried along with the movement. The clinician should be certain that the motion occurs at the segments below the index fingers and that no segmental movement is allowed above the index fingers.

Cervical Backward Bending. Backward bending is performed in the same manner, except that the head and neck are not carried along with the movement and the test is begun with the head and neck in a neutral position. Only force through the index fingers is applied. This causes backward bending to occur at the segments adjacent to the contact point. In effect, the index fingers act as a fulcrum (Fig 4-15).

Cervical Rotation. Cervical rotation involves superior and anterior glide of the superior articulating facet on the inferior articulating facet on one side and slight inferior and posterior glide on the opposite side. Therefore, rotation is tested in the same manner as forward bending, except to only one side at a time, and it is done from the neutral position. To perform left rotation, the right hand index finger lifts upward against the articular pillar, while the left hand supports (Fig 4-16).

Cervical Side Bending. The same positioning is used for cervical side bending. Force is applied in a medial and slightly inferior direction through the base of the index finger as it contacts the lateral aspect of the neck. The point of contact on the index finger is toward the palmar surface of the metacarpophalangeal joint. This force causes the segment adjacent to the contact to side bend to the same side as the mobilizing force. In effect, the index finger acts as a fulcrum. The trunk stabilizes the spine inferiorly and the opposite hand stabilizes against the side of the head superiorly (Fig 4-17).

Cervical Side Gliding. The same basic position is used for cervical side gliding. Force is applied in a medial direction through the index finger as it contacts the lateral aspect of the neck, causing movement to occur at the segments below the contact. The point of contact on the index finger is on the palmar surface of the metacarpophalangeal joint.

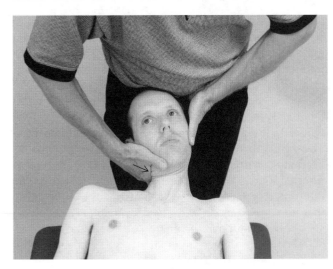

Figure 4-17: Segmental testing—cervical side bending.

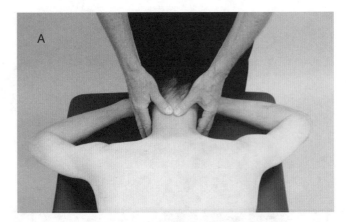

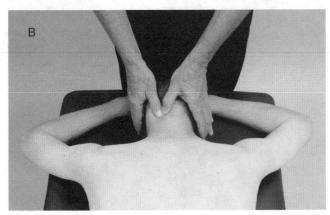

Figure 4-19: Palpating segmental P/A mobility of the cervical spine. A) Central P/A pressure on the spinous process; B) Unilateral P/A pressure on the articular pillar.

The patient's head is carried to the side with this movement. This is accomplished by the clinician shifting his hips in the direction of the movement (Fig 4-18).

Upper Thoracic Flexion, Extension and Rotation. Segmental mobility of the upper thoracic spine is palpated during active mobility testing as described earlier. The clinician palpates between the spinous processes when the patient performs active flexion, extension and rotation of the upper thoracic spine so that active and segmental mobility testing is performed simultaneously. Flexion and extension movement can be felt by placing the finger between the spinous processes as the patient forward and backward bends. Rotation can be assessed with the patient sitting or lying prone by placing the thumbs on the spinous processes or pinching the spinous processes at two levels and watching and feeling the movement between the levels as the patient rotates the head from side to side (Fig 4-10).

Posterior/Anterior Palpation Techniques for Cervical and Upper Thoracic Spine. With the patient lying prone, central P/A pressure is applied to the cervical and upper thoracic spinous processes. Unilateral P/A pressure is applied to the articular pillar. These techniques assess general mobility and symptom response and are not specific tests for flexion, extension or rotation mobility. Pain or stiffness with these P/A pressures should be correlated with other mobility tests (Fig 4-19).

Special Mobility Tests for the First Rib. The cervicothoracic junction represents the transition of cervical segments into the thoracic spine and the rib cage. It is important to assess first rib mobility because of its soft tissue attachments and its attachment to T1 (Fig 4-20).

The patient is supine on the examination table. While supporting the head under the occiput, the clinician induces passive side bending to the left. At the same time, the clinician's right thumb palpates the first rib lateral to the C7 transverse process. The clinician notes the point in side bending when the first rib starts to move cephalically into

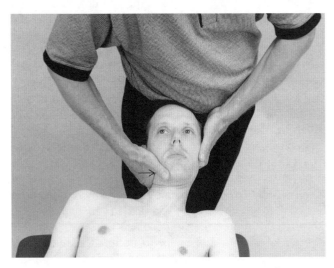

Figure 4-18: Segmental testing—cervical side gliding.

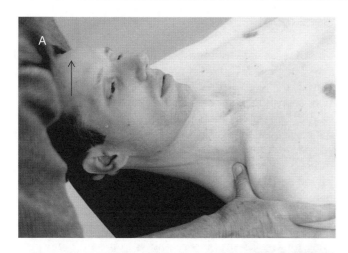

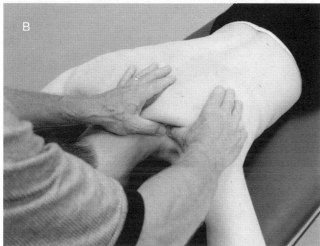

Figure 4-20: Segmental mobility tests for the first rib. A) Palpation position for detecting early rib movement; B) Caudal glide.

the palpating thumb. This is compared to the contralateral side. Asymmetries should be noted. Early first rib movement with cervical side bending may be indicative of ipsilateral scalene muscle tightness.

Joint dysfunction of the first rib can be confirmed or ruled out by testing its segmental mobility with the patient lying prone. The clinician palpates the first rib by placing the thumbs underneath (anterior to) the muscle belly of the upper trapezius just lateral to the cervical spine. A caudally directed pressure is applied. The first firm resistance felt caudally will be the first rib.

The clinician then applies pressure onto the first rib to detect differences in mobility from one side to another and to determine whether the patient's symptoms are provoked. The first rib is often tender, even in normal subjects. Therefore, tenderness is only significant if it is worse than on the uninvolved side.

Use of an Inclinometer in Cervical ROM Testing

Normative data for cervical range of motion was presented in Table 4-2. An inclinometer can be used effectively to measure cervical spine mobility. Many different inclinometer models are available, and several types have been shown to be reliable in peer-reviewed studies. The CROM is one model we like because it is easy to use (Fig 4-21). It has been shown to have good inter- and intra-tester reliability.[17,31,51] Exact instructions for measuring cervical range of motion using an inclinometer are not included here because inclinometers vary and protocols are included with the inclinometer when purchased.

Strength Examination

The middle and lower trapezius muscles are tested with the patient prone (Fig 4-22). A strong muscle contraction should be elicited with very little or no joint movement. A weak and painless contraction suggests neurological involvement or weakness due to prolonged disuse. The cervical muscles are tested with the patient sitting. The head is held well supported in a neutral, mid range position. The patient is asked to hold against resistance in each plane of motion in both directions. Shoulder elevation is also tested in sitting, and weakness implicates the upper trapezius and/or rhomboid muscles or indicates possible neurological involvement (Fig 4-23 A, B and C).

Neurological Examination

As a rule, neurological involvement of levels C4 through C7 is indicative of a cervical nerve root disorder such as a herniated disc or encroachment of the nerve root within the intervertebral foramen. The C7 nerve root is the most common root affected.[36] If neurological involvement of C8 or T1 is seen, it is often suggestive of thoracic outlet syndrome or another disorder and not cervical spine pathology.

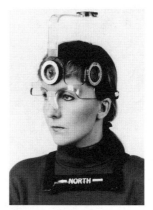

Figure 4-21: CROM cervical range of motion device (The Saunders Group, Inc.)

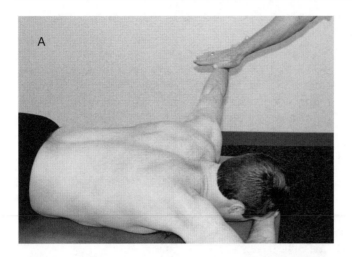

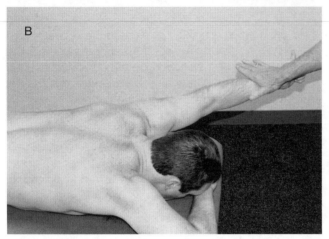

Figure 4-22: Testing trapezius muscle strength. A) Mid trapezius; and B) Lower trapezius.

Resisted Muscle Tests

As noted earlier, if resisted muscle tests are painful or painful and weak, muscular pathology may be involved. If they are painless and weak and disuse atrophy is ruled out, a neurological disorder is suggested. All resisted muscle tests for the cervical spine are done with the patient sitting.

The tests for the cervical spine involve the following motions (Fig 4-23):

- Cervical rotation (C1)
- Shoulder elevation (C2,3,4)
- Shoulder abduction (C5)
- Elbow flexion (C6)
- Elbow extension (C7)
- Wrist extension (C6)
- Wrist flexion (C7)
- Thumb extension (C8)
- Finger abduction (T1)

Sensation Testing

Specific sensation testing is carried out with the patient sitting. The clinician carefully maps out areas of numbness by using the pinprick method. The C5 neurological level supplies sensation to the lateral arm from the shoulder to the elbow. The purest patch (autonomous zone) of C5 innervation lies at the insertion of the deltoid muscle. C6 supplies sensation to the lateral forearm, the thumb, the index finger and one-half of the middle finger, with the purest patch being on the lateral portion of the web space between the thumb and index finger. C7 supplies sensation to the middle finger. Since middle finger sensation is also occasionally supplied by C6 or C8, there is no autonomous zone for C7. C8 supplies sensation to the ring and little finger of the hand and the distal half of the ulnar forearm. The ulnar side of the little finger is the purest area for C8 testing. T1 supplies sensation to the upper half of the medial forearm and the medial portion of the upper arm. T2 supplies the axilla (Fig 4-24).

Muscle Stretch Reflexes

The biceps (C5-6), brachioradialis (C6) and triceps (C7) muscle stretch reflexes are tested in the sitting position. A decreased response when compared to the contralateral limb suggests pathology at the corresponding nerve root level.

Neural Tension Tests

The upper limb tension test (ULTT) assesses pain response and tissue tension caused by passive movements of the upper limb and neck. The ULTT produces strain on the brachial plexus by a combination of movements of the upper extremity and cervical spine. The basic ULTT provides bias to the median nerve. Variations of the basic ULTT address the other nerves of the upper limb, including the radial nerve and ulnar nerve. Interested clinicians can find more information about the ULTT variations in Butler's text.[9]

Kenneally, et al have called the ULTT the "straight leg raise of the arm."[44] The basic ULTT is generally recommended for all patients presenting with non-irritable conditions of the head, cervical spine, thoracic spine and upper extremities. In situ mechanical tension measurements have demonstrated its validity for use in diagnosing nerve and plexus lesions of the upper extremity.[45] It also is a useful differentiation test for cervical radiculopathy, when used in combination with cervical range of motion, distraction and Spurling's tests.[89]

When performing the ULTT, the clinician should be mindful of contraindications discussed in Section One on page 47. Additionally, Kenneally, et al, has identified normal responses for the ULTT. They studied 400 subjects

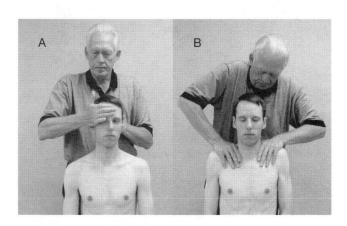

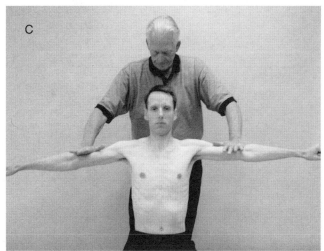

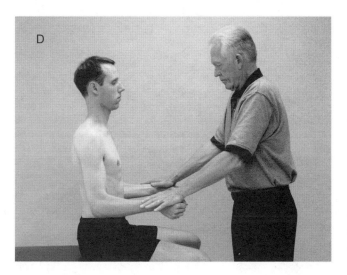

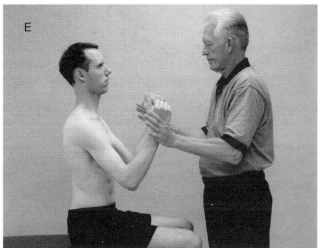

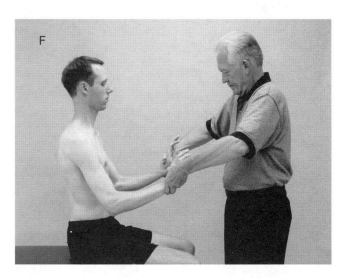

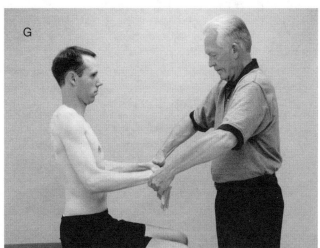

Figure 4-23: Strength testing for neurological involvement of the cervical spine. A) Cervical rotation; B) Shoulder elevation; C) Shoulder abduction; D) Elbow flexion; E) Elbow extension; F) Wrist extension; G) Wrist flexion (continued on next page).

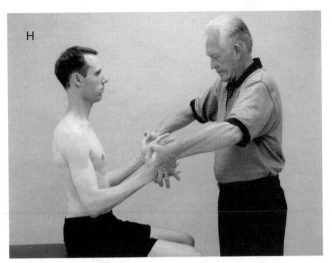
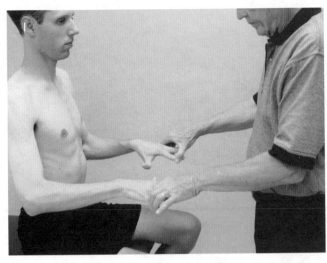

Figure 4-23 continued. Muscle strength testing for neurological involvement of the cervical spine. H) Thumb extension; I) Finger abduction.

without pathology or complaints, and described the following symptoms with the ULTT:[44]

- Deep ache or stretch in the cubital fossa (99% of subjects) extending down the anterior and radial forearm into the radial hand (80% of subjects)
- A definite tingling in the thumb and 1st three fingers
- A stretch feeling in the anterior shoulder area (small percentage of subjects)
- Increased responses with cervical side bending away from the tested side (90% of subjects)
- Decreased responses with cervical side bending toward the tested side (70% of subjects)

Therefore, the clinician must be careful when deciding whether the results of the ULTT are positive or whether they are a normal response to placing neural tissues on stretch. Any symptoms or decreased mobility found should fit with other clinical findings.

Theoretically, any pathological process that causes less space for neural tissue to slide freely will produce an earlier onset of symptoms with the ULTT.

A tension test can be considered positive in the following circumstances:

- If it reproduces the patient's symptoms
- If the test response can be altered by moving distant body parts that alter tension on neural tissues alone (e.g., when the patient is in the test position, isolated movement of the wrist or cervical spine changes the symptoms)
- If the test response differs from side to side and from a normal response described above

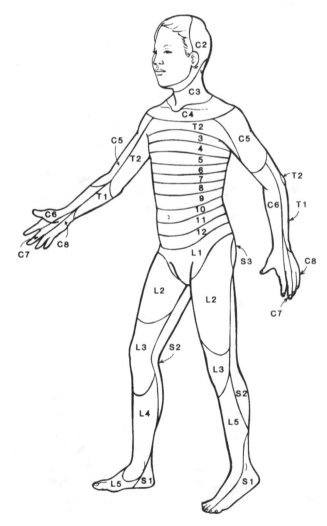

Figure 4-24: Anterolateral view of the dermatomes for sensation testing.

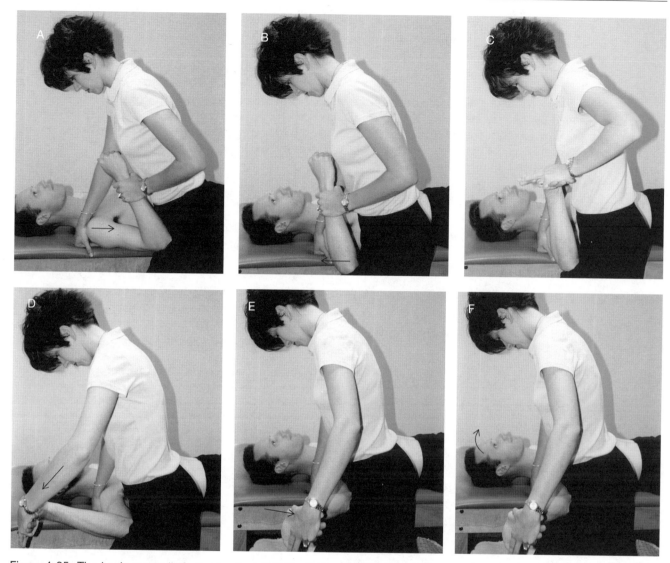

Figure 4-25: The basic upper limb tension test (ULTT). A) Shoulder depression; B) Shoulder abduction; C) Wrist and finger extension, forearm supination; D) Shoulder external rotation; E) Elbow extension; F) Cervical side bending (depicted by arrow). The clinician should carefully maintain the previous position as each new motion is added.

To perform the basic ULTT, begin with the patient lying supine on a plinth with his legs straight, feet uncrossed and opposite upper limb at his side. Then, successively perform the following steps (Fig 4-25):[9]

1. *Cervical Spine Neutral*—The patient lies in neutral, supine on the treatment table, close to the edge of the side being tested. The clinician faces the patient, one leg in front of the other, supporting the upper extremity at the wrist. Prior to the exam, the patient is instructed how to side bend the cervical spine away from and toward the upper extremity to be tested, to avoid substitution or a rotatory component in later steps.

2. *Shoulder Depression*—The clinician depresses the shoulder girdle by pressing caudally on the shoulder

as shown. This position is sustained throughout the rest of the procedure. Any change or onset in symptoms should be noted.

3. *Shoulder Abduction* – The clinician grasps the patient's wrist while supporting the upper arm with the thigh, preventing horizontal extension of the humerus. Approximately 110° of abduction should be attained.

4. *Wrist/Finger Extension, Forearm Supination* – While maintaining Step 3, the wrist and all fingers are extended, while the forearm is supinated.

5. *Shoulder External Rotation*—The clinician externally rotates the glenohumeral joint to approximately 60° while Steps 1-4 are maintained.

6. *Elbow Extension*—The clinician extends the patient's elbow to the point of symptom onset or resistance.

7. *Cervical Side Bending*—The patient is instructed to side bend the cervical spine away from the limb being examined, then toward the limb being examined. Symptom response is noted.

Each individual step must be maintained during the test, especially when the next step is added. The onset or change of symptoms or resistance should be identified and recorded after each step. Examination should include both upper limbs. In any tension testing, it is important to consider the following:

- Before beginning, carefully identify all the patient's symptoms and complaints.
- Note which symptoms are present in the starting position.
- Carefully note any change in symptoms or onset of new symptoms during each step of the test.
- Move the patient's limb in each step to the point of onset or change in symptom complaints.
- Compare the findings of the test to the contralateral limb and what is considered normal.

As with any musculoskeletal test, reassessment of the test at later intervals will help the clinician decide whether treatment is effective. To compare later findings, the clinician must document the range of motion at which the symptoms first appear, the nature and location of the symptoms and any abnormal resistance felt by the clinician during the test.

Babinski's Test

Doing a Babinski test completes the neurological exam. The test is done by quickly drawing a blunt instrument across the sole of the foot, starting at the heel, moving along the lateral aspect and crossing the ball of the foot. A positive reaction consists of great toe extension, usually associated with fanning (abduction and slight flexion) of the other toes. A positive Babinski test suggests an upper motor neuron disorder (Fig 4-26).

Thoracic Outlet Syndrome Tests

A discussion of thoracic outlet syndrome is included in this text because of its close association to the cervical spine and because differential diagnosis of cervical involvement and thoracic outlet compression is often difficult. Thoracic outlet compression syndrome involves compression or stretching of the subclavian artery, subclavian vein or the brachial plexus as they pass through the thoracic outlet. The syndrome can produce both vascular and neurological symptoms. Neurological thoracic outlet syndrome is con-

troversial and some authors believe that it is over-diagnosed.[49,74,91]

The controversy may result from the widespread use of the term to describe a variety of upper extremity symptoms that are not necessarily traced to specific anatomic origins. True neurological thoracic outlet syndrome is caused by compression of the lower trunk of the brachial plexus by the cervical ribs or fibrous band.[49]

Diagnosis for brachial plexus compression in the thoracic outlet is primarily done through ruling out other pathology in the cervical spine and upper extremities that could cause similar symptoms. Nerve compression causes various symptoms including pain, tingling or numbness that usually follow the nerve trunk. Ulnar nerve symptoms are more common than median nerve symptoms. Night pain is common.[46,63] If the tests described below reproduce neurological symptoms, and if other pathology is ruled out, thoracic outlet syndrome is a possible cause of the patient's neurological symptoms.

Arterial compression is relatively rare but is potentially very serious, particularly if arterial embolism occurs. Diagnosis of arterial compression is accomplished by the techniques described below and other objective tests not readily available to physical therapists such as arteriography and plethysmography. With arterial compression, the patient will report pain and fatigue during activity that go away with rest. Often, symptoms will start distally and proceed proximally. In later stages, cold sensitivity may be present. Any signs of possible emboli, such as cyanosis in one or more fingers, are considered serious and require immediate medical attention.[46]

Venous compression may lead to edema, skin tightness, cyanosis, pain and fatigue. After activity, venous distention may be seen in the extremity. The edema should decrease

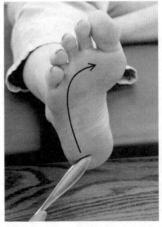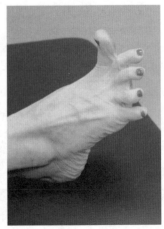

Figure 4-26: Babinski's test.

after a change in the precipitous activity. If the edema does not diminish, it is a sign of a possible venous thrombosis and requires the attention of a physician for further evaluation.

Adson's Test

Adson's test helps decide whether the neurovascular bundle is being compressed as it passes between the scalenus anticus and medius. Occasionally, a congenital defect in the scaleni may cause the bundle to pass through the muscle mass rather than between the two muscles. A review of the literature reveals that there is no clear consensus on the exact method for performing Adson's test.[28,32,63] We combine test elements described by various authors to place the neurovascular bundle and scaleni on maximum stretch.

The clinician should palpate the patient's radial pulse at the wrist as the patient takes a deep breath and holds it. The patient's arm is abducted and extended and the patient extends and rotates the cervical spine toward the arm being tested (Fig 4-27). If a marked decrease or obliteration of the radial pulse is felt and the patient's symptoms are reproduced, the test is positive. The test is repeated with cervical extension and rotation away from the arm being tested.

Costoclavicular (Military Bracing) Test

The costoclavicular test checks for the possible compression of the neurovascular bundle as it passes between the clavicle and first rib by approximating the two structures. Again, the clinician palpates the radial pulse at the wrist. The patient is asked to assume an exaggerated military position by drawing the scapulae backward and downward (Fig 4-27). The test is positive if a marked decrease or obliteration of the radial pulse is felt and the patient's symptoms are reproduced.

Hyperabduction Test

The hyperabduction test helps to determine whether the neurovascular bundle is being compressed between the pectoralis minor muscle and the ribs. The clinician palpates the radial pulse at the wrist while abducting the shoulder as far as possible (Fig 4-27). The clinician should concentrate on performing true abduction without flexion.[46] As with the other pulse palpation tests, the test is positive if a marked decrease or obliteration of the radial pulse is felt and the patient's symptoms are reproduced.

Roo's Test (EAST Test)

Roo's test involves full shoulder external rotation and abduction to 90°. It is also called the Elevated Arm Stress Test (EAST). The patient holds this position bilaterally for three minutes while repeatedly opening and closing the fists (Fig 4-27). After completing the test, the clinician quickly looks for objective changes and the patient's sub-jective response. If increased pallor, cyanosis, swelling, vein distention, tingling, numbness or pain is felt, the test is positive. The clinician should compare the affected limb to the unaffected limb.

Bilateral Brachial Blood Pressure Comparison

Cherry Koontz reported that a comparison of bilateral brachial blood pressures could give useful information about arterial compression syndromes. A difference of more than 20-30 mm Hg may be suspicious for subclavian artery stenosis.[46]

Neural Tension Tests for Thoracic Outlet Syndrome

All of the pulse palpation techniques described above are more definitive for thoracic outlet syndrome involving arterial compression. If neurological symptoms are reproduced with the tests, they are helpful at pointing toward neurological compression as well. Since neurological symptoms are present in 90-97% of all thoracic outlet syndromes,[46,80] the ULTT is very useful. In situ mechanical tension measurements have demonstrated its validity for use in diagnosing nerve and plexus lesions of the upper extremity.[45]

When performing the ULTT, the clinician looks for symptom reproduction and tissue resistance. When symptom reproduction or tissue resistance is encountered, the clinician must consider both local sources of compression (the first rib, lower cervical and upper thoracic vertebral segments and the scaleni) and remote contributing factors such as tight acromioclavicular and glenohumeral joints, or imbalanced trapezius, levator scapulae, pectoral and cervical musculature. Butler describes variations of the basic ULTT that can be more specific for the lower trunks of the brachial plexus, and his text should be consulted for further investigation of the use of neural tension testing for thoracic outlet syndrome.[9]

Palpation Examination

The palpation exam of the cervical and upper thoracic spine involves inspection of the skin and subcutaneous tissue as described in Section One. When palpating the muscles, the clinician must pay close attention to the suboccipital, upper trapezius and rhomboid muscles.

Muscle guarding and spasm in these muscles is often associated with various syndromes in the cervical spine. Painful trigger areas are often found in the levator scapulae insertion. It is often necessary to treat muscle guarding and spasm in these muscles even though they are not the primary disorders. Injury or prolonged muscle guarding of the rhomboid muscles often causes a coarseness or crepitus that can be palpated. Muscle guarding and spasm of the suboccipital muscles are often associated with headaches. Trigger points can often be palpated along the occipital

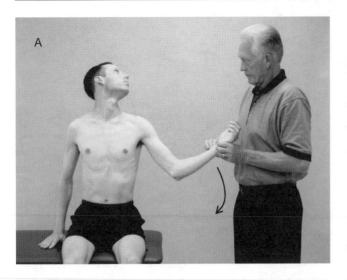
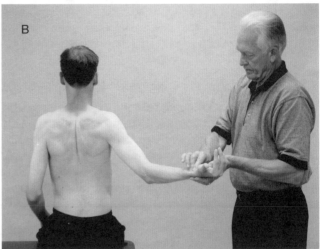
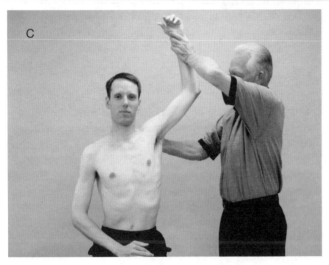
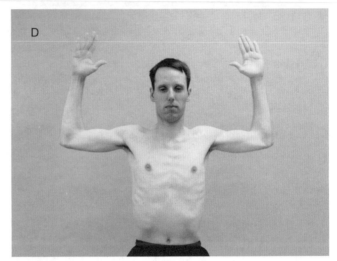

Figure 4-27: Thoracic outlet syndrome tests. A) Adson's test; B) Costoclavicular (military bracing) test; C) Hyperabduction test; D) Roo's test.

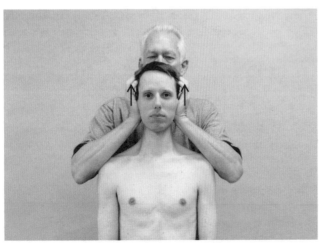
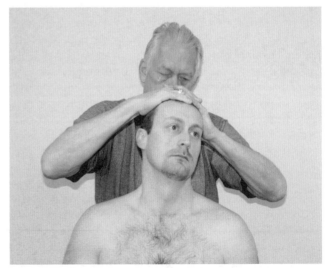

Figure 4-28: Cervical spine distraction test.

Figure 4-29: The Spurling neck compression test.

ridge and in the belly of the upper trapezius muscles. The clinician should rule out first rib involvement when a painful response to palpating the upper trapezius muscles is found, as the first rib lies directly beneath the upper trapezius and can be painful to palpation.

The supraspinous ligament and spinous processes of the lower cervical and upper thoracic spine can be palpated. In the mid and upper cervical spine, the spinous processes may be difficult to palpate. The facet joint lines of the mid-cervical spine (articular pillar) can be palpated for tenderness during segmental range of motion testing. Other important areas to palpate are described in Chapter 11, *Soft Tissue Mobilization and Neuromuscular Training*.

Special Tests

Distraction Test

The distraction test is a neurological test and a mobility test. It has been shown to be a particularly useful differentiation test for cervical radiculopathy, when used along with cervical range of motion, the basic ULTT and Spurling's tests.[89] The clinician stands behind the patient if he is seated or at the head of the patient if he is lying supine and applies long axis distraction to the cervical spine through the occiput. This maneuver opens the foramina and stretches the joint capsules. If it relieves the patient's symptoms it may show that a spinal nerve root is impinged.

It should be noted that facet joint or disc pain also may be relieved with this test. The distraction test helps determine whether traction or a cervical support to decrease

vertical loading will be beneficial during treatment (Fig 4-28).

The Neck Compression (Spurling) Test

The Spurling test involves compression with the neck side bent and extended (Fig 4-29). The Spurling test is positive if pain or tingling start in the shoulder and radiate peripherally to the elbow. Used alone, it has been shown to be sensitive but not specific for cervical radiculopathy diagnosed by EMG.[81] However, it is a useful differentiation test for cervical radiculopathy when used along with cervical range of motion, distraction and the basic ULTT tests.[89]

Valsalva Test

The patient is asked to hold his breath and bear down as if having a bowel movement. If the patient notes an increase in pain or radiation, this may suggest the presence of a space-occupying lesion such as a herniated disc or tumor.

Dynamometer Grip Strength Test

Grip strength testing is done for two reasons. First, it provides objective baseline data for cervical patients complaining of upper extremity pain or weakness. The test can be repeated during treatment to document changes in the patient's condition.

Secondly, grip strength testing has been proposed as a method of detecting submaximal effort.[78] Using the Jamar Dynamometer, the patient performs grip strength testing in all five positions (three trials at each position are aver-

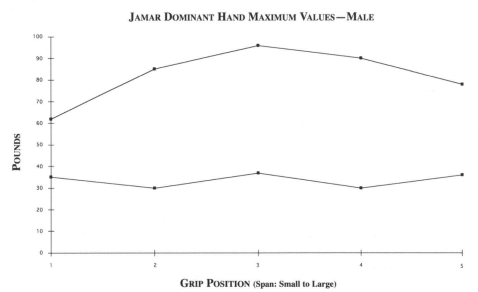

JAMAR DOMINANT HAND MAXIMUM VALUES—MALE

Figure 4-30: Sample dynamometer grip strength testing over five positions. A normal bell-shaped curve (upper) is expected. A flat or irregular curve (lower) may indicate submaximal effort.

aged). If the five values are plotted on a graph, the graph curve should be bell-shaped, with positions one and five weakest and position two or three strongest (Fig 4-30).

The bell-shaped curve should be present even with true pathology. Therefore, if a bell-shaped curve is not found, or if there is less than a five-pound variance between each value, it is possible that the patient is not exerting maximal effort.

Section Three—Mid and Lower Thoracic and Lumbar Spine

The subjective and objective evaluation of a patient with spinal pain was discussed in Section One. Section Three takes a closer look at the objective evaluation of the mid and lower thoracic and lumbar spine. The reader should be familiar with the concepts found in Section One before proceeding.

Lower Quarter Screening Examination

The lower quarter screening examination consists of a series of mobility and neurological tests to identify problem areas in the lumbar spine, sacroiliac area, hip, knee, ankle and foot (Table 4-5). It is most valuable when performed on a patient complaining of lower extremity symptoms and little or no back pain. With such a patient it is important to clear the lumbar spine as a source of the lower extremity symptoms. The screening evaluation is redundant if the patient is already complaining of lumbar symptoms, and the clinician should skip to the rest of the objective evaluation.

A good screening evaluation performed by a skilled evaluator can make the rest of the evaluation more concise and efficient. *The purpose of the screening evaluation is to identify which anatomical areas deserve a detailed evaluation.* After the screening evaluation, the clinician will know which anatomical areas have been cleared and which ones need a closer look.

The lower quarter screening evaluation begins with the patient standing so posture can be observed. Any postural abnormalities should be noted and investigated more thoroughly if they correlate with the patient's complaint or with other objective findings. The lumbar spine is then taken through active forward, backward and lateral bending as the clinician watches for signs of pain, muscle guarding or limited movement. The standing flexion test for iliosacral involvement is also performed (see Chapter 7, *Standing Flexion Test* , page 151). Heel and toe walking are completed to test for L4 and L5 (heel) and S1 (toe) nerve root involvement. Heel and toe walking also clear the ankle and foot when no pain or limitation of movement is observed. A quick technique to clear all joints of the lower extremity is to ask the patient to squat and then stand.

Table 4-5: Lower Quarter Screening Examination.

Postural assessment
Active lumbar flexion, extension and side bending
Standing flexion test/Gillet's test
Toe raises (S1)
Heel walking (L4, 5)
Sitting flexion test
Active lumbar rotation
Overpressures of lumbar motion if symptom-free
Straight leg raise (L4, 5; S1)
Resisted hip flexion (L1, 2)
Passive hip range of motion
Resisted knee extension (L3, 4)
Knee flexion, extension, internal and external rotation
Prone knee bend (femoral nerve stretch)
Babinski's reflex test (upper motor neuron test)

Next, the patient sits and the sitting flexion test for sacroiliac involvement is performed (see Chapter 7, *Pelvic Girdle Dysfunction*). Active lumbar rotation is also checked with the patient sitting. The patient is asked to extend the arms directly in front with the hands held together and then to twist to the right and left as far as possible. If no signs or symptoms are observed with active range of motion, passive overpressures are applied. If forward and backward bending, lateral bending and rotation produce no signs or symptoms even with passive overpressure, the joints and muscles of the lumbar spine are considered clear for those movements.

Resisted hip flexion, knee flexion and extension, ankle dorsiflexion and great toe extension are performed in sitting or supine (Fig 4-51 on page 83). Resisted hip flexion is also a neurological test of spinal levels L1 and L2. Resisted knee extension is a neurological test of spinal levels L3 and L4. The hip is clear if passive and resisted hip motion tests do not produce any signs or symptoms. The knee is clear if passive knee motions, including varus and valgus stresses, do not produce any signs or symptoms.

Next, the patient is positioned supine for straight leg raising, which is a neurological test of spinal levels L4 through S1. Differentiation between hamstring tightness and sciatic pain is critical. The provocative tests for sacro-iliac involvement are done in supine and side lying (see Chapter 7, *Compression-Distraction Tests*, page 154).

A femoral nerve stretch in the prone position (prone knee bend) may be indicated if the patient has described symptoms in the anterior hip, anterior thigh or groin areas.

Performing a Babinski reflex test for upper motor neuron involvement completes the lower quarter screening exam.

Structure and Posture Examination

The evaluator should review Section One for general comments relating to structure and posture assessment, remembering that postural assessment should include the entire spine even if the patient's complaint concerns only one area of the spine. Any asymmetries found may be significant if correlated with other subjective and objective findings.

Anterior/Posterior Symmetry

There should be a gentle continuation of A/P curves the entire length of the spine. Lumbar and thoracic A/P curves can be objectively measured using an inclinometer. Objective measurements are useful for patient education and documenting changes as treatment progresses.

The lumbar and cervical spine should show a mild lordotic curve and the thoracic spine should have a mild kyphotic curve. Absence of any of the curves may suggest restriction of mobility, whereas excessive lordotic curves may suggest the presence of a variety of structural and postural problems. Increased lumbar lordosis may be associated with joint hypermobility, anterior pelvic rotation, weak abdominal muscles and tight hip flexor muscles. Patients presenting with this combination of deficiencies have chronic postural strain and should be treated with a corrective exercise program. Absence or decrease of lumbar lordosis should be noted as it may be an indication of a disc disorder or may be the result of many years of living and working in sitting or forward bent postures. The patient with flat back posture often has very little lumbar extension mobility and often has tight hamstring muscles and a posteriorly rotated pelvis.

The swayback posture is often mistaken for the hyperlordotic posture, but it is actually quite different. The sway back posture is characterized by forward displacement of the hip joint, posterior rotation of the pelvis, a flat lower lumbar spine, a slight lordotic curve in the upper lumbar spine and a slightly increased thoracic kyphosis (Fig 4-31).[43]

It is also very important to observe the patient's sitting posture in the waiting room and in the examination room. Slumped lumbar flexion posture often contributes to loss of lumbar extension and possibly to development of a posterolateral lumbar disc protrusion.

Lateral Symmetry

Scoliotic curves in the spine are abnormal and are classified as either functional or structural or as caused by a specific pathological process. A structural scoliosis is caused by a defect in the bony structure of the spine such as wedging of

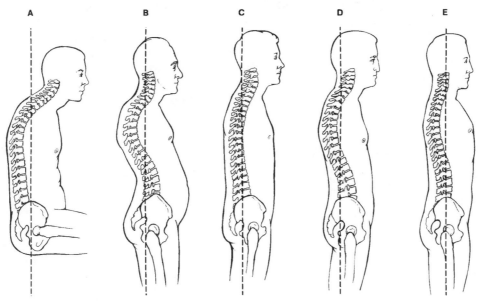

Figure 4-31: Common postural disorders. A) Forward head, rounded shoulders; B) Hyperlordosis and hyperkyphosis; C) Hypolordosis (flat back); D) Sway back; E) Ideal posture.

the vertebral bodies. A structural scoliosis does not straighten during forward bending or side bending away from the direction of the curve. Because lateral bending is accompanied by rotation, a lumbar bulge or rib hump is seen with forward bending if a structural scoliosis is present (Fig 4-32).

A functional scoliosis can be caused by a non-spinal defect such as unequal leg length, muscle imbalance or poor postural habits. Generally, a functional scoliosis will straighten during forward bending and side bending away from the direction of the curve, but this may not be true if moderate to severe muscle spasm and guarding is present or if the soft tissue structures have shortened on the concave side of the curve. The patient should be asked to hold his hands together when forward bending. This can eliminate error when trying to determine whether a rib hump represents a structural scoliosis or simply active rotation of the spine. If the patient has an uneven sacral base, it is important to level the sacral base by placing shims under the short leg before testing forward bending. This ensures that true spinal abnormalities (stiffness or structural scoliosis, for example) will be easier to identify.

Although consideration should be given to structural scoliosis, the clinician should remember that when seen in an adult, it will be a long-standing condition and may not be directly related to the patient's present complaint. Long-standing structural scoliosis may cause early degenerative joint/disc disease and may indirectly contribute to a variety of disorders. When seen in children and early adolescents, structural scoliosis has much more significance. A scoliosis specialist is required to determine whether treatment with bracing or surgery is required. Juvenile or adolescent idiopathic scoliosis cannot be treated by physical therapy alone.

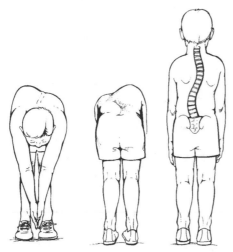

Figure 4-32: Rib hump seen with a structural scoliosis.

Facet joint impingement/subluxation may cause an acute scoliosis in any area of the spine. This disorder involves the entrapment of soft tissue within the facet joint, which may cause the patient to shift to the opposite side to take weight off the painful structure.

A more common type of lateral curve seen with acute lumbar disorders is the *lateral shift* or *protective scoliosis* (Fig 4-33). According to McKenzie, a lateral shift will often occur as the nucleus pulposus moves posterolaterally. For example, if the nucleus moves posterolaterally to the left, the patient is likely to shift his body weight anteriorly and to the right.

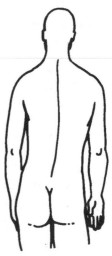

Figure 4-33: A lateral shift or protective scoliosis.

On the other hand, Finneson theorizes that a protective scoliosis is caused by the patient moving the spinal nerve root away from a disc bulge.[21] If the bulge is lateral to the nerve root it is encroaching upon, the patient will shift to the opposite side (most common). If the bulge is medial to the nerve root it is encroaching upon, the patient will shift to the same side (uncommon) (Fig 4-34).

Cephalocaudal Symmetry

The height of the shoulders and the inferior angle of the scapulae should be examined for symmetry. It is common for the shoulder and scapula on the dominant side to be positioned lower. This is considered normal and no particular conclusions can be drawn from shoulder and scapula height asymmetries, unless correlated with other findings. The clinician also should look for any asymmetries in the ribs or skin folds. Close attention is paid to the sacral base during the structural evaluation. With the patient standing upright with the feet spread shoulder width apart and weight equally distributed, the height of the iliac crests, posterior/superior iliac spines (PSIS), anterior/superior iliac spines (ASIS), trochanters, gluteal folds and fibular heads are checked (Fig 4-35). A palpation meter (PALM) can be used to measure iliac crest height differences. Good validity and interrater reliability have been demonstrated with this device.[69] The location of any asymmetries found can help pinpoint a possible dysfunction. For example, if the PSIS's are uneven and the trochanters are even, the discrepancy lies between the two structures. The sacroiliac joint, the angulation of the femoral neck or the hip joint itself are possible problem areas.

An uneven sacral base can be caused by a true leg length difference or by soft tissue or joint changes in the lower extremities or pelvis. Examples of the latter include unilateral foot pronation, genu recurvatum and ilium rotation. Asymmetries caused by soft tissue imbalances or joint impingement should be corrected via treatment when possible. Asymmetries that cannot be corrected with treatment may need to be corrected with a shoe lift. If left uncorrected, an uneven sacral base can cause lumbar scoliosis that may contribute to uneven weight distribution on the facet joints and the intervertebral discs. Theoretically, early degenerative changes or adaptive soft tissue shortening could result.

When an uneven sacral base is caused by a leg length discrepancy, its correction is somewhat controversial. Brady, et al caution against correcting a leg length inequality of less than 5 mm because of the disagreement in the literature about its clinical significance and the potential error in measurement using clinical techniques.[6]

Friberg's work, on the other hand, lends support to correcting even minor leg length differences.[22] He studied 798 subjects with low back or hip pain and 359 subjects who were symptom free. He found highly significant statistical correlation between the symptoms and leg length inequality. In 79% of the cases of low back pain with sciatica, and in 89% of the cases of hip pain, the symptoms were present on the side of the longer leg. When the LLI was corrected with a shoe lift on the short leg side, complete or nearly complete relief of symptoms occurred in the majority of cases that were followed up to six months.

Additional works suggest that leg length discrepancies are important to identify and consider for treatment purposes. For example, one study found that leg length discrepancy was associated with the side of radiating pain in patients with herniated disc. For most patients, the pain radiated into the shorter leg. This effect was statistically significant only in women.[79]

Another study found an association between a short leg and knee hyperextension and chondromalacia patellae. The authors suggested that full-sole correction of the discrepancy is advised to affect leg length during toe-off.[90]

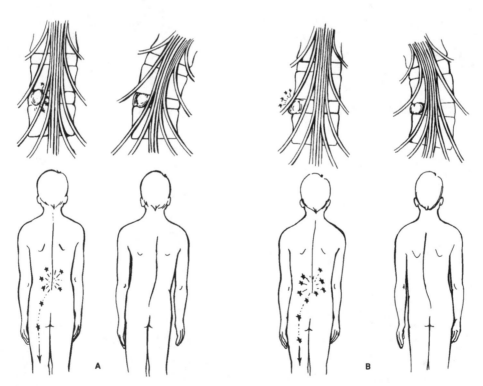

Figure 4-34: Protective scoliosis sometimes seen in patients with HNP. A) The bulge is lateral to the nerve root (most common); B) The bulge is medial to the nerve root.[21]

We believe that leveling the sacral base with a shoe lift can be very valuable, assuming that all other treatable causes for the uneven sacral base have first been addressed with joint or soft tissue mobilization, exercise or other appropriate interventions.

The height of the iliac crests also should be checked in the sitting position because it is possible for one side of the pelvis to be larger than the other. This will cause an uneven sacral base and a lumbar scoliosis while sitting. It can be corrected by using a seat cushion that is thicker on one side, after taking care that any treatable reasons for the unevenness have been thoroughly addressed.

Assistive Devices and Supports

Any special assistive devices or supports such as a lumbar corset, lumbar pillow or cane should be noted. Care should be taken to assess whether the device has been properly fitted and is being used correctly. Sometimes a patient will bring an assistive device to the appointment even though it is not regularly used. Conversely, some patients have a device that is used regularly but is not mentioned.

The use of a cane is rarely helpful with lumbar pain or radiating lower extremity pain, and it can sometimes be harmful. When a cane is used, the patient may lean on it, creating asymmetrical forces on the spine and pelvis. When true lower extremity muscle weakness exists, or if balance is a problem, a cane could conceivably be useful for helping promote a safer, more even gait pattern.

Mobility Examination

Prior to performing the mobility exam, an uneven sacral base should be corrected by placing shims under the short

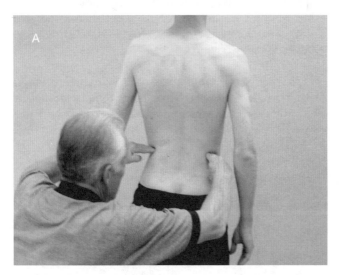
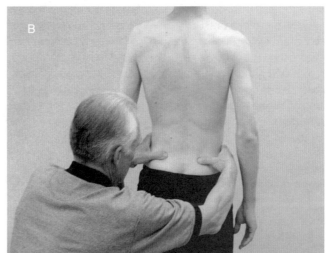
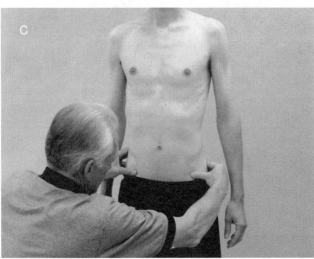
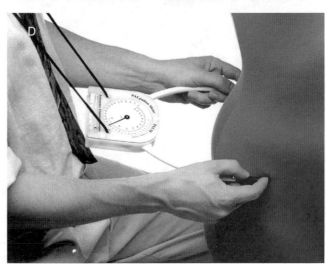

Figure 4-35: Sacral base and pelvic alignment testing. A) Iliac crest symmetry; B) PSIS symmetry; C) ASIS symmetry; and D) Using a PALM to determine iliac crest symmetry.

side. This gives the clinician a truer picture of the patient's symmetry.

Postural Correction

Postural correction in the lumbar spine involves hypolordosis, hyperlordosis or a lateral scoliosis. Hypolordosis or hyperlordosis is evaluated during active forward and backward bending testing.

When the patient has a lateral scoliosis, the clinician should first determine whether it is chronic (due to a leg length difference, uneven sacral base or structural scoliosis) or acute (a result of a lateral shift or protective scoliosis). If it is the latter, an attempt should be made to correct it (Fig 4-36). If the lateral shift is caused by a mild to moderate disc protrusion as described by McKenzie, the correction procedure will often cause centralized pain in the lumbar spine but no increase of peripheral symptoms. An exception to this would involve a large bulge in which some of the disc material is trapped outside the posterolateral edge of the vertebral bodies. In this case, attempted correction would cause increased pain or other symptoms in the lower extremity.

If the scoliosis is a protective scoliosis as described by Finneson, any attempt at correction will increase pain and other symptoms in the lower extremity.[21] At this point in the evaluation, the following rule applies: If the acute lateral lumbar scoliosis can be corrected without increasing lower extremity symptoms, it should be done. On the other hand, if attempted correction increases lower extremity symptoms, attempts to correct the shift should be ceased (see discussion in Chapter 5, *Treatment by Diagnosis*).

Active Mobility Testing

Forward Bending

To check active forward bending, the patient is asked to bend forward as the clinician assesses the general and specific mobility of the spine. If an inclinometer is used, the lumbar and thoracic curve angles at end range of motion should be measured. Does the normal lordosis in the lumbar spine flatten to neutral (normal) or does it round into considerable kyphosis (hypermobility) during forward bending? If the lordosis does not straighten completely, the spine is hypomobile. How much standing hip flexion is present? Does the thoracic spine show increased kyphosis? Is the movement smooth and is it uniform throughout the length of the spine (Fig 4-37)?

Does the patient experience pain, stiffness or any other symptoms? If so, is it central in the lower back or does it radiate into the lower extremity? Does the lower extremity pain linger after the patient returns to an upright posture? If the patient experiences increased pain when recovering

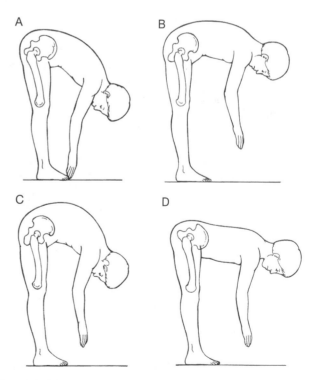

Figure 4-37: Active forward bending, checking the quality of the motion. A) Normal; B) Tight hamstrings but normal lumbar flexion; C) Tight hamstrings and excessive lumbar flexion; and D) Normal to loose hamstrings and decreased lumbar flexion.

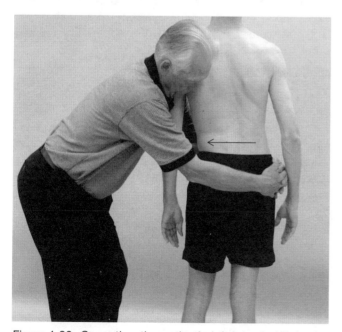

Figure 4-36: Correcting the patient's left lateral shift in the standing position.

from the forward bent position, he is said to have a torturous recovery, which suggests an active lesion in the spinal muscles.[63] The patient with a torturous recovery will often crawl the hands up the thighs to regain the standing position. Does the patient drift to the left or right instead of bending straight forward? If so, it suggests unilateral hypomobility of the soft tissue, unilateral muscular tightness or posterolateral disc protrusion. The patient should forward bend with eyes closed because it is natural for patients to fix their eyes on the floor, thus overriding any tendency to drift laterally.

Backward Bending

Active backward bending is also checked with the patient standing (Fig 4-38). Restrictions of backward bending are usually associated with disc protrusion, soft tissue hypomobility or facet joint pain. During mobility testing, it is important to note which movements cause the patient's pain to move centrally and which movements cause the pain to move peripherally.

According to McKenzie, movements that centralize symptoms are helpful; ones that cause symptoms to peripheralize are harmful.[61] If the symptoms move peripherally when testing a repeated lumbar motion in standing, it indicates the movement is making the condition worse, probably causing disc bulging. If movements centralize the pain, it is not necessarily an indication the condition is getting worse. Frequently, repeated forward bending will cause the pain to move away from the midline and into the buttock and thigh, while repeated backward bending will cause increased pain in the center of the lumbar spine. This phenomenon is suggestive of a mild disc protrusion.

Pain present at *end* of range when range is limited indicates soft tissue hypomobility. Repeated movement will typically increase motion and may decrease pain. Pain *throughout* the range of motion is characteristic of acute inflammation, strain or sprain. It is common to find hypomobility in one direction (e.g., extension) and normal or hypermobility in the other direction (e.g., flexion). Men tend to have more lumbar flexion mobility and women tend to have greater lumbar extension mobility.[83] Children and adolescents with low back pain tend to have greater restriction and more pain with extension than with flexion.[11] A feeling of slipping or a moving sensation during range of motion testing is suggestive of instability or hypermobility.

Even without a history of peripheral pain, increased central lumbar pain with backward bending must be analyzed carefully. The patient who has a flattened lumbar lordosis and who is not accustomed to backward bending will usually complain of increased lumbar pain with backward bending testing. The clinician should ask if the movement reproduces the patient's exact symptoms. The

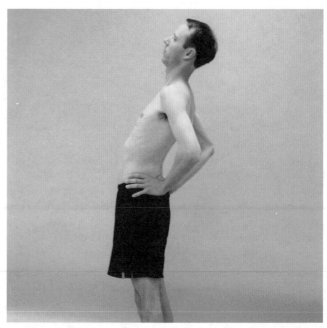

Figure 4-38: Active backward bending. Monitor for substitution of knee flexion/hip extension rather than true lumbar extension.

clinician should also ask the patient to repeat it gently several times to see if it gets better, worse or stays the same. If the increased pain is not an exact reproduction of the patient's symptoms and if it does not increase significantly with repetition, it is probably due to stiffness.

The patient with a decreased lumbar lordosis and decreased extension mobility will usually benefit from trying to increase it. To instill confidence in the corrective exercise program, the patient must be educated about the difference between soreness from stretching stiff soft tissue and a true reproduction of symptoms.

Side Bending

Active side bending is examined by first having the patient bend to one side and then the other. If the sacral base is uneven it is important to level it first with shims under the short side. Is the patient bending one way as far as the other? An easy way to assess this is to watch how far the patient's fingers reach on the side of his legs. This method is not accurate if the patient has a lateral scoliosis of any type. During side bending, one should see a gentle, smooth and continuous curve from the lumbosacral joint through the mid thoracic spine. Any straight areas suggest hypomobility and any areas of sharp bending suggest hypermobility (Fig 4-39). One must be careful to keep the patient from shifting the pelvis laterally when examining active side bending.

Rotation

Active rotation is checked with the patient sitting on the edge of a treatment plinth with the arms held straight out

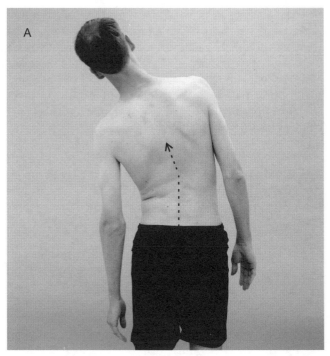

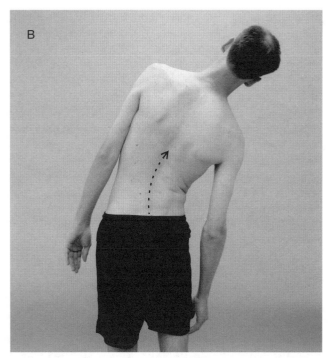

Figure 4-39: Active side bending, checking the quality of the motion. A) The left lumbar curve is rather straight in the lumbar spine, with a sharp curve above the thoracolumbar junction; and B) The right lumbar curve is smoother in the thoracic and lumbar areas.

in front and the hands together. A general assessment is made first, followed by a closer examination of the specific area of the patient's complaint. As rotation occurs in one direction, side bending will occur in the opposite direction. The spinous processes also move in the opposite direction of the rotation. The clinician should observe the position of the spinous processes during rotation, looking for smoothness and symmetry (Fig 4-40).

Findings of Active Mobility Testing

The following discussion is included in this section to guide the clinician in appropriate clinical decision making. By considering carefully the clues that the results of active mobility testing provide, the clinician can begin to formulate an idea about what potential pathological entity or treatable problems the patient may have. The clinician must remember, however, that a correct conclusion cannot be made until the entire subjective and objective evaluation is completed.

Certain pathological entities present with specific findings during the active mobility tests. Inert soft tissue restrictions (e.g., facet joint capsule and ligaments) will generally be painful at the end of range of motion and will often tend to loosen up with repeated movement. Muscular restrictions will be most painful when the involved muscle is actively contracting, as in the torturous recovery described earlier. Disc lesions tend to be irritated by certain

repeated movements, especially forward bending, and the pain often lingers after the movement is stopped.

As a rule, unilateral restrictions are more noticeable during side bending than in forward or backward bending. Conversely, bilateral restrictions will be proportionately more noticeable in forward or backward bending. A more

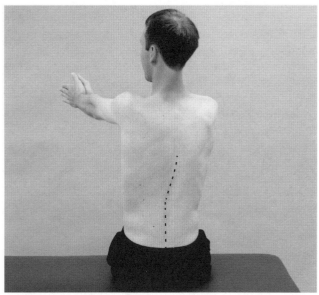

Figure 4-40: Active rotation. Both range of motion and the quality of the curve should be checked. Sharp curves or excessively straight areas may indicate hyper or hypomobilities.

detailed discussion on the objective findings of various conditions is found in Chapter 5, *Treatment by Diagnosis*.

Passive Mobility Testing

The passive mobility tests that are most useful for the lumbar spine are the knees to chest (flexion), the passive press up (extension) and rotation in supine with the knees bent. Passive overpressure in rotation is also very useful as a provocative test if no other mobility tests reproduce the patient's symptoms. Passive side bending is more difficult to perform and does not provide much additional information. Passive range of motion of the hip joint must be tested thoroughly because of the possible involvement of hip musculature, particularly the iliotibial band, the iliopsoas, the hamstrings and the piriformis.

Passive flexion is assessed in supine by having the patient hug both knees to chest (or one knee at a time). He is then asked to repeat this movement several times without letting go of the knees between repetitions. The clinician asks whether the pain increases, decreases or stays the same with repetition.

The results of passive flexion testing must be analyzed carefully. On one hand, passive flexion stretches the lumbar muscles, which may feel good to the patient. On the other hand, passive flexion compresses the disc and may be potentially harmful, causing increased peripheralization of the pain. When performing passive flexion repetitively, the patient may initially have relief of back pain but may later have increased peripheral symptoms.

Passive extension is assessed by having the patient perform a prone press up. The starting position for the hands should be directly in front of the shoulders. The clinician makes sure the patient's lumbar musculature is relaxed so that the movement is as passive as possible (Fig 4-41).[20]

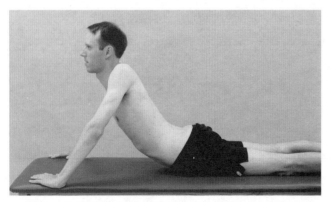

Figure 4-41: Passive extension, the press up position.

The distance of the ASIS from the table is measured (approximately 2 inches is considered within normal limits), although the quality of the curve is generally more important than the actual distance. Extreme obesity or slimness will interfere with interpretation of the measurement. One should observe flattening of the mid and lower thoracic kyphosis and an increase in lumbar lordosis, especially in the lower lumbar area.

The patient is asked to repeat the press up movement several times to determine whether a change with repetition occurs. Often, initial stiffness causes mild central pain but repeated movements become looser and the symptoms decrease.

The prone press up position is a very convenient position for testing thoracic and lumbar extension with an inclinometer. Range of motion testing using an inclinometer is discussed later in this section.

While some patients will be generally stiff throughout the lumbar spine, it is common to observe patients who have very little or no extension mobility in the lower lumbar segments and normal mobility or even hypermobility in the upper lumbar area. These two types of patients must be treated differently. The latter patient will require lower lumbar mobilization in addition to general mobility exercise.

Lumbar rotation is assessed in supine with the hips and knees bent. The legs and pelvis are passively rotated from side to side. More or less hip flexion can be used to assess the upper and lower back. If stabilization across the ribs is used, the lumbar spine is isolated (Fig 4-42).

Pain or limitation with hip motion can be a clue to involvement of the piriformis or iliopsoas muscles or can be an early indication of degenerative hip arthritis. The piriformis and iliopsoas muscles are commonly involved in the back pain patient and should not be overlooked.

Hip internal and external rotation can be tested in sitting or in supine with the hip and knee flexed to 90°. Passive hip internal rotation can be compared bilaterally in prone with the hips extended and the knees flexed to 90° by allowing the legs to rotate laterally. If passive internal rotation is more painful or restricted with the hip extended, the piriformis muscle is implicated. If passive internal rotation is more painful or restricted with the hip flexed to 90°, the hip joint capsule may be involved. Resisted external rotation with the hip and knee flexed to 90° will typically be painful if the piriformis is inflamed.

Hip extension is tested in supine with the leg hanging over the edge of the plinth (Fig 4-43). Flexion of the opposite

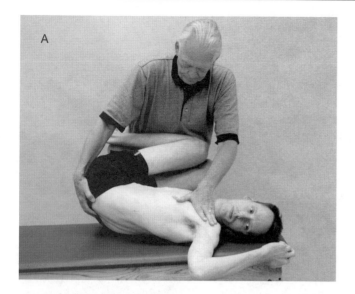

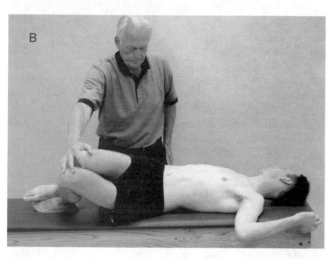

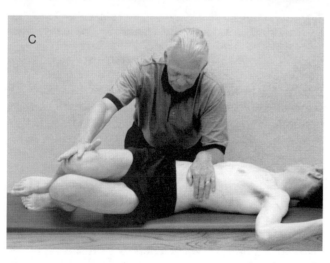

Figure 4-42: Passive rotation with varying degrees of hip flexion. A) More hip flexion involves more of the thoracic spine; B) Less hip flexion involves more of the lumbar spine; and C) Rib stabilization isolates the lumbar spine.

hip prevents lumbar hyperextension. The clinician looks for symptom provocation or any range of motion differences from one side to the other. If the hip extends fully but the knee does not flex, the rectus femoris is tight, since it crosses both the hip and the knee joint.

The length of the tensor fascia latae is assessed in side lying. The patient's uppermost hip is extended then adducted. Restriction or symptom reproduction in extension and adduction (Ober's sign) is indicative of a tight tensor fascia latae (Fig 4-43).

Segmental Mobility Testing

The segmental mobility tests for the lumbar and mid and lower thoracic spine are forward bending, backward bending and rotation. During segmental mobility testing it

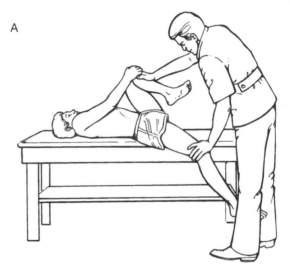

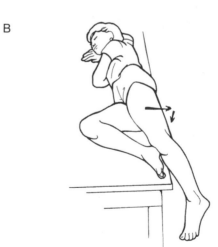

Figure 4-43: Assessing hip tightness. A) Testing rectus femoris, hip extension and contralateral hip flexion; and B) Ober's test for tensor fascia lata tightness.

is often helpful to first identify the segments that are tender to palpation. Specific segmental tenderness is often a clue to a mobility problem at that segment. The tender segments are then compared to the adjacent non-tender segments. Using this method makes it easier to detect slight but often significant differences.

During normal forward bending, the spinous processes separate slightly. Forward bending can be performed actively or passively while the clinician palpates between two spinous processes with his finger. If the clinician feels the spinous processes separate slightly and the supraspinous ligament become taut under the finger, there is movement present at that segmental level. The amount of movement felt at the involved (painful) segment is compared to other levels to determine whether it is normal, hyper or hypomobile. This test is done with the patient side lying or in the prayer position for the lumbar and lower thoracic spine, and sitting for the mid and lower thoracic spine (Fig 4-44).

During normal backward bending, the spinous processes approximate. While feeling between two spinous processes with his finger, the clinician asks the patient to perform a prone press up. If the clinician feels the spinous processes come together and the supraspinous ligament become slack under the finger, there is movement present at that segmental level. This amount of movement is compared to other levels and the clinician determines if the movement at the involved segment is normal, hyper or hypomobile.

During normal spinal rotation, each spinous process moves laterally in relation to the spinous process of the vertebra below. For example, during right rotation, each spinous process moves to the left. During left rotation, each spinous process moves to the right. The clinician, with the patient positioned in the side lying position, stabilizes the inferior vertebra and passively rotates the spine superior to the segment being tested, while feeling between two spinous processes with his finger (Fig 4-45).

If the clinician feels the superior spinous processes move laterally, as described above, there is movement at that level. This amount of movement is graded and is compared to the amount of movement at other levels and in the opposite direction. Right rotation should be tested with the patient lying on his left side, and vice versa. This technique is effective for the mid and lower thoracic and the entire lumbar spine. The clinician should begin testing superiorly and work his way inferiorly.

Segmental mobility in rotation also can be tested during the active mobility exam when the patient is sitting.

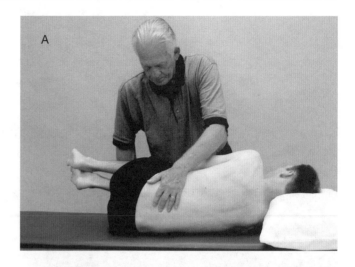

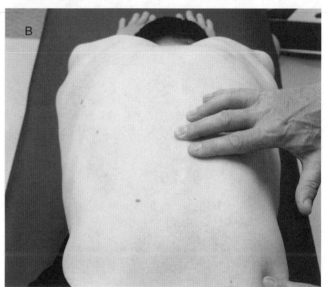

Figure 4-44: Palpating segmental thoracic and lumbar flexion. A) In side lying; and B) In the prayer position.

The clinician palpates each interspinous space in the lumbar and lower thoracic spine as the patient actively rotates. The quality and quantity of motion between each segment should be roughly the same at adjacent levels and in right and left rotation at the same level. In the mid thoracic spine, the clinician can pinch two adjacent spinous processes to check for symmetrical motion (Fig 4-10).

The anterior spring test is a special mobility test that is performed by contacting three spinous processes in a row with the thumbs. The patient is positioned prone. Downward (anterior) pressure is applied with both thumbs to the two spinous processes directly under each of the thumbs. The single spinous process between should be contacted by the tips of both thumbs, but should receive no direct pressure. If there is normal P/A movement, the two outside

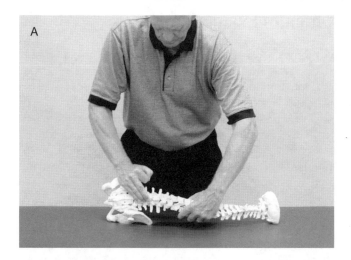

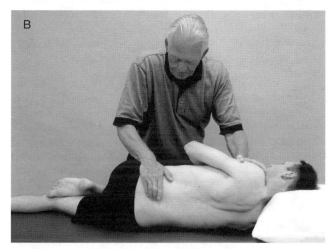

Figure 4-45: Palpating segmental thoracic and lumbar rotation. A) Showing rotation of the segments on the skeleton; and B) Palpation technique.

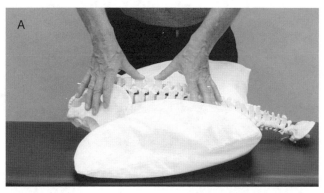

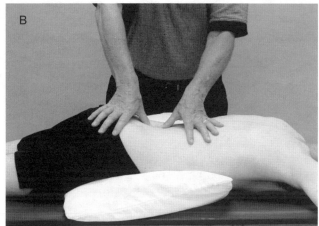

Figure 4-46: The anterior spring test. A) Showing thumb contact on three spinous processes; and B) Spring technique.

spinous processes are felt to move and the one between is felt to stay in position (Fig 4-46).

A less specific but very useful spring test is performed with the heel of the clinician's hand placed over one or two segments. The clinician repeats a gentle but firm anterior spring up and down the length of the spine. This method is useful for determining the general mobility of an entire area of the spine (mid thoracic, for example) and can sometimes be helpful for determining specific stiff or painful segments.

The coccyx should also be assessed for mobility, particularly if the patient is complaining of "tailbone" pain. Externally, the coccyx is palpated for tenderness, and P/A mobility is tested by gently springing on the dorsal surface with overlapping thumbs or the thenar eminence. The coccyx also can be palpated internally for segmental

mobility and tenderness (Fig 4-47). The clinician grasps the coccyx with the index finger in the rectum and the thumb on the coccyx externally. The position of the coccyx in neutral, flexion or extension can be felt and P/A glide can be assessed in this manner.

Because of its location, tenderness and quality of the piriformis muscle also can be palpated internally. The piriformis is assessed for tenderness or "ropiness." The internal contours of the anus should be smooth and relaxed. If ropiness or tenderness of the piriformis is found, pathology is indicated.

Use of an Inclinometer in Thoracic and Lumbar ROM Testing

Normative data for thoracic and lumbar range of motion was presented in Table 4-3 on page 46. An inclinometer can be used to measure lumbar and thoracic spine mobility. Many different inclinometer models are available and several types have been shown to be reliable in peer-reviewed studies.

More than one protocol exists for measuring spinal range of motion. Our preferred protocol for measuring

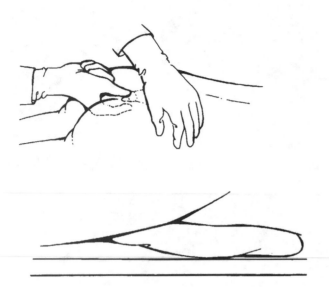

Figure 4-47: Palpating coccyx motion.

spinal flexion/extension measures the curve angle at the end of range of motion (Fig 4-48).[8,27] The AMA Guides protocol uses the standing position as the reference or zero point when measuring spinal flexion/extension.[13] The AMA Guides protocol is seriously flawed if the subject does not have normal standing posture (Fig 4-49).

Since many subjects do not have normal standing posture, we believe that the curve angle at the end of range of motion method is more useful for measuring spinal flexion and extension. Assessment of the subject's standing and sitting posture is important but must be measured separately from range of motion.

Figure 4-49 illustrates how the AMA Guides method of measuring lumbar flexion can provide misleading results. Subject B's lumbar flexion motion is less than normal when calculated using the AMA Guides method, but is within normal limits when using the curve angle at end range of motion method. If using the AMA Guides results, one might mistakenly assume the patient needs to work on flexion flexibility exercises, when in reality he probably needs to work on extension flexibility (because of the flat back posture).

Exact instructions for measuring spinal range of motion using an inclinometer are not included in this section, as inclinometers vary and protocols are usually included with the inclinometer when purchased. The clinician should make sure that the inclinometer purchased makes use of the desired protocol for measuring lumbar flexion and extension, which we believe is the curve angle at end range of motion method.

Strength Examination

Although resisted muscle tests are helpful in differential diagnosis of the extremity joints, their value in the lumbar and mid and lower thoracic spine is limited because of the difficulty of isolating a muscle contraction without at least some joint movement or compression. Torturous recovery from the forward bent position, which was described under active movements, is probably the most valid mobility test for muscular involvement in the lumbar and mid and lower thoracic spine.

Strength tests of the lumbar spine are most useful because of the well-established relationship between trunk weakness and lumbar problems.[3,27,29,34,38,48,50,65] The lumbar paraspinals and the abdominal muscles are tested for weakness or poor endurance and deficiencies are treated through exercise, whether or not the muscles are the source of the patient's symptoms.

Trunk strength can be tested with machines like the MedX® or Cybex® Back System.[14,62] Each of these back testing systems provide guidelines for interpretation of test results and the testing system can also be used for training. A major disadvantage of such systems is their cost, which can run in the thousands of dollars. The high purchase price requires high testing and rehabilitation fees to be charged to the patient or insurance company. Additionally, the validity and clinical utility of such machines has been questioned.[66]

Simple trunk strength and endurance tests that do not require machinery have been described in the literature. We recommend the use of the following tests because they are inexpensive and easy to perform. Sufficient normative data have been published to enable reasonable interpretation of results.

McIntosh, et al published norms for seven standardized tests of trunk and lower extremity endurance.[60] Subjects consisted of 548 volunteers who had not missed work due to lower back pain in the preceding six months. Isometric tests performed included a $1/4$ sit up, prone chest raise, supine bilateral straight leg raise, prone bilateral straight leg raise, and a wall squat (Fig 4-50). Isotonic tests consisted of repetitive $1/4$ sit-ups and prone chest raises. Results were analyzed by gender and categorized into age groups. Interested readers should consult the original article for details.

Ito, et al described similar tests for trunk extensor and abdominal endurance and provided normative data for both healthy subjects and people with chronic lower back pain.[33] Both Ito's and McIntosh's trunk extension tests are similar to the test described by Biering-Sorenson, which

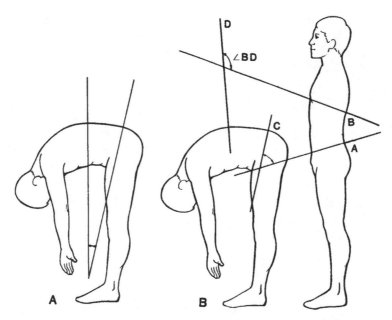

Figure 4-48: Two protocols for measuring lumbar flexion range of motion with an inclinometer. A) Measuring the curve angle at end range of motion; B) Using the AMA Guide's method. Angle AC is standing hip flexion, angle BD is gross flexion (BD-AC=lumbar flexion).

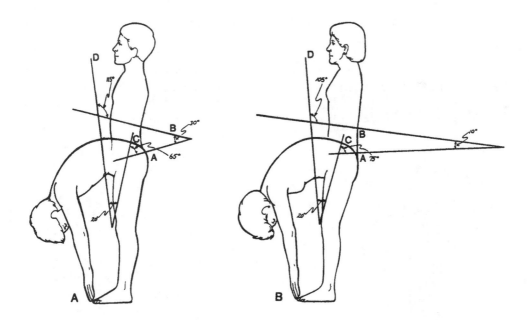

Figure 4-49: A flaw in the AMA Guide's method of measuring lumbar flexion. Subjects A and B forward bend to the same point. Using the curve angle at end range of motion method, the amount of flexion is 20° in both cases, and is considered normal. However, using the AMA Guide's method, subject A's gross flexion measures 115° and subject B's gross flexion measures 105°. The difference is because the subjects' standing postures are different (subject A=30° and subject B=10°), which affects the AMA Guide's method but not the curve angle at end range of motion method. Using the AMA Guide's formula (BD - AC = lumbar flexion), subject A has 50° lumbar flexion and subject B has 30° lumbar flexion. Normal flexion for the AMA Guide's method = 40° to 75°.

has been shown to be reliable and to correlate with risk of low back injury.[3,42,48]

Aggressive trunk strengthening and stabilization exercises are often indicated, even when the above tests

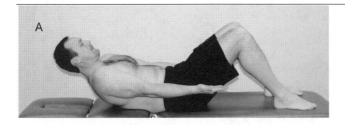

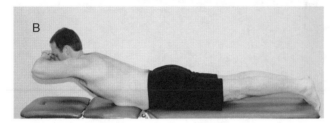

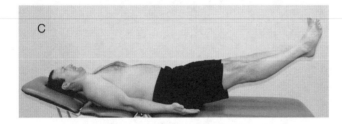

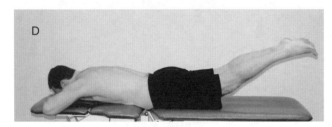

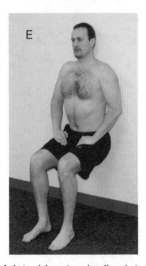

Figure 4-50: McIntosh's standardized tests of trunk and lower extremity endurance. A) ¼ sit up; B) Prone chest raise; C) Supine bilateral straight leg raise; D) Prone bilateral straight leg raise; and E) Wall squat.

show that the patient has good trunk strength. Subjects with chronic low back pain may have early extensor muscle fatigue compared to normals.[75] Extraordinary trunk strength and stability is particularly important if the patient has a high-demand job.

Additional advanced trunk exercises are described in Chapter 14, *Basic Spinal Exercise*, and the exercise positions shown can be used as tests to determine post-rehabilitation improvement.

Neurological Examination

Thoracic Spine

Spinal nerve root impingement and peripheral nerve entrapment are rare in the thoracic spine. Neurological involvement in the thoracic spine may cause weakness of the abdominal or intercostal muscles. Sensation testing of the thoracic spine involves the dermatome patterns of the thoracic spinal nerves as they pass laterally and slightly inferiorly around the torso of the body (Fig 4-24 on page 62).

Lumbar Spine

Resisted Muscle Tests

Muscle strength of the lower extremities is tested bilaterally at the same time whenever possible. This gives the clinician greater appreciation of very slight differences in strength and makes it more difficult for the patient to exaggerate weakness. Resisted muscle tests for the neurological exam of the lumbar spine involve the following muscle groups (tests are shown in Figure 4-51):

Hip flexion (L1-2) is done with the patient lying supine or sitting with the hip and knee flexed to 90°. The patient is asked to hold the position as resistance is applied. As noted earlier, increased pain with resisted muscle tests suggests muscular pathology. However, increased pain with hip flexion can also point to joint pathology in the lumbar spine or hip. The attachment of the iliopsoas muscle on the anterior lumbar vertebral bodies causes an anterior pull on the lumbar spine as the iliopsoas contracts, often causing increased pain if there is pathology in the spinal segments. Tumors or metastatic lesions should always be suspected if a true neurological deficit is found in the upper lumbar spine since spinal nerve root impingement or peripheral nerve root entrapment or injury at this level is very rare.

Knee extension (L3-4) is tested with the patient sitting with the knees slightly flexed.

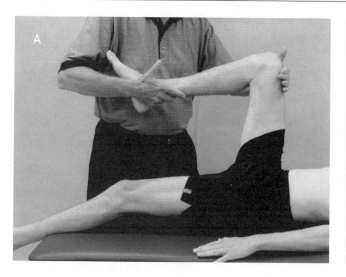 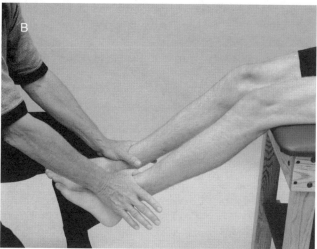

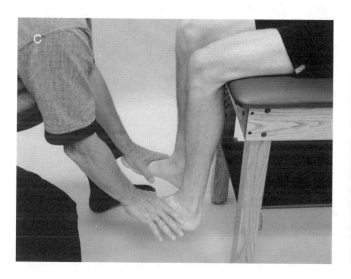 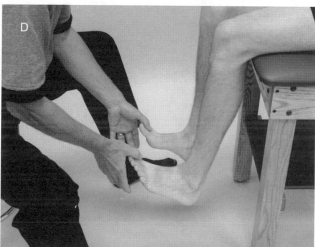

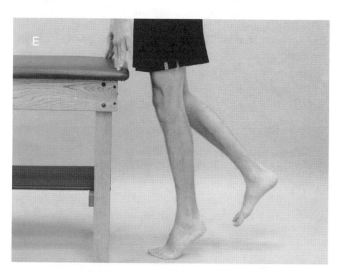 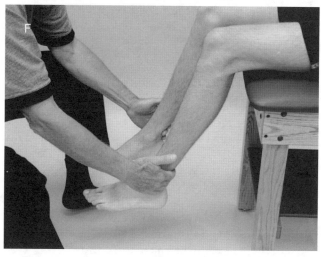

Figure 4-51: Muscle strength testing for neurological involvement of the lumbar spine. A) Hip flexion; B) Knee extension; C) Ankle dorsiflexion; D) Great toe extension; E) Ankle plantarflexion; and F) Knee flexion.

Ankle dorsiflexion (anterior tibialis muscle, L4) is tested bilaterally with the patient sitting. The patient is asked to hold the position as resistance is applied. Heel walking is another way of testing ankle dorsiflexion.

Great toe extension (L5) is tested bilaterally with the patient sitting. The patient is asked to hold the position as resistance is applied.

Ankle plantar flexion (S1) is tested with the patient standing or walking on his toes. Since the gastrocnemius and soleus muscle group is quite strong, it is often necessary to test plantar flexion by having the patient repeat 10-20 repetitions of rising on his toe, first with the uninvolved side then with the involved side, before a true comparison can be made.

Knee flexion (S1-2) is tested bilaterally with the patient lying prone or sitting.

Sensation Testing

If specific sensation testing is indicated, it is carried out with the patient standing, sitting or lying in a position that is convenient to check the specific areas involved. The pinprick tests are done to map out the areas of numbness. The exact area is measured and indicated on the body diagram (Fig 4-3 on page 41). Neurological levels L1-L3 provide sensation in oblique bands over the anterior thigh between the inguinal ligament to the knee. The L4 dermatome covers the medial side of the leg and foot.

Neurological level L5 covers the lateral leg and dorsum of the foot with the crest of the tibia being the dividing line between L4 and L5 (all that is lateral to the crest including the dorsum of the foot is L5). The S1 dermatome covers the lateral side and a portion of the plantar surface of the foot. The S2 dermatome is on the posterior lateral heel. The dermatomes around the anus are arranged in three concentric rings (S2 outermost, S3 middle and S4-5 innermost) (Fig 4-24 on page 62).[32]

Muscle Stretch Reflexes

The quadriceps (L3-4) and gastrocnemius-soleus (S1-2) muscle stretch reflexes are tested in sitting. The ankle reflex is sometimes elicited better when the patient is prone with the knees flexed. The clinician passively dorsiflexes the ankles with one hand and quickly alternates a tap on each heel cord to pick up subtle changes. The patient often tries to assist by actively dorsiflexing the foot. This can be discouraged by asking the patient to plantarflex the ankle then relax, while the clinician quickly taps the heel cord during relaxation. There is no convenient muscle stretch reflex for the L5 nerve root and the L4-5 intervertebral disc is sometimes known as the "silent disc."

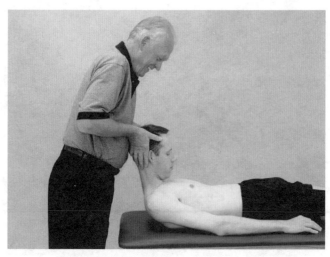

Figure 4-52: The passive neck flexion test.

Neural Tension Tests

Four neural tension tests are used in the physical examination of the lower limbs and trunk—passive neck flexion, the prone knee bend, the straight leg raise and the slump test. These tests are generally recommended for all patients presenting with non-irritable conditions of the lumbar spine and lower extremities. The clinician should be mindful of contraindications to neural tension testing already discussed. To review, a tension test can be considered positive in the following circumstances:

- If it reproduces the patient's symptoms
- If the test response can be altered by moving distant body parts that alter tension on neural tissues alone (e.g., when the patient is in the slump test position, isolated movement of the ankle or neck changes the symptoms)
- If the test response differs from side to side and from a normal response

Passive Neck Flexion. The passive neck flexion test is indicated for all spinal disorders and any headaches or extremity complaints of spinal origin. To perform the test, the patient can be supine, sitting or standing. The clinician induces neck flexion passively. Symptom response, range of motion and any resistance encountered should be noted (Fig 4-52).

Passive neck flexion should normally be painless, although a pulling sensation at the cervicothoracic junction is described occasionally. Passive neck flexion can be combined with other tension tests such as the straight leg raise to reproduce functional postures and to assess the effect of combined neural tension in provoking symptoms.

Prone Knee Bend. The prone knee bend is akin to the straight leg raise, with the prone knee bend putting selective tension on the upper lumbar segments. The prone knee bend stretches the femoral nerve and should be performed if the patient complains of pain or other symptoms in the upper lumbar spine or in the L1-4 dermatomal regions. As the femoral nerve is stretched by flexing the knee and extending the hip, the nerve roots L1, 2 and 3 are stretched across their respective intervertebral foramen. If there is reduced mobility or impingement of one of these spinal nerve roots, the patient's symptoms will increase.

The prone knee bend is performed by passively flexing the knee with the patient lying prone. Symptom response, range of motion and resistance encountered should be noted and compared to the contralateral side (Fig 4-53). One must be careful to distinguish between a painful quadriceps muscle and a true nerve root sign. If nerve root impingement is present, the symptoms may extend into the lateral aspect of the hip and into the upper lumbar spine as well as into the anterior thigh.

The normal response for the prone knee bend is not well documented. However, common clinical findings include a stretching sensation in the rectus femoris and an anterior pelvic tilt with an increase in lumbar lordosis.

Straight Leg Raise. This is the most common tension test used by clinicians. It is indicated for patients presenting with any spinal or lower limb complaints. The straight leg raise test is traditionally performed to determine if there is compromise of the nerve roots or irritation of the sciatic nerve (radiculitis). The straight leg raising test may irritate any acute, painful condition in the lumbar spine or sacroiliac joints. Tight hamstring muscles, hip joint pathology or sacroiliac joint pathology can cause a painful response to the straight leg raise. Adaptive shortening of the sciatic nerve or an adherent nerve root will cause a positive straight leg raise test. Piriformis syndrome can also be irritated by the straight leg raise test.

A systematic review of the straight leg raise test has raised questions about its reliability and predictive value in implicating particular tissue pathology (e.g., intervertebral disc herniation).[71] Therefore, careful interpretation is required, and very little can be concluded if the only evidence is a positive straight leg raise test. Additional differentiation tests can help the clinician distinguish true nerve root involvement from other musculoskeletal conditions.

The patient is positioned supine for the straight leg raise. The clinician raises the leg while making sure the knee remains straight (Fig 4-54). As the straight leg is raised, progressive tension is applied to the sciatic nerve, which in turn places tension on the nerve roots. If compromise or irritation of the nerve roots exists, symptoms will be exacerbated by this maneuver. If the test increases pain in the posterior thigh, it may not be a true neurological sign but may still be a significant clinical finding. If the straight leg raise is unilaterally limited, increases unilateral symptoms or is bilaterally limited to less than 50°, perform the following steps: raise the leg again to the onset of symptoms, lower a few degrees (to reduce pain), then successively dorsiflex the ankle, medially rotate the hip and flex the neck. Symptom reproduction by one of these tests may suggest increased root tension.[7]

The clinician should palpate the ASIS for the first sign of movement into posterior rotation. It is at this point that the hamstrings have engaged the pelvis, causing such movement to occur. By comparing both sides, the clinician can ascertain the degree of hamstring tightness. It is helpful to do hold-relax muscle stretching of the hamstring to distinguish between true nerve root signs and tight hamstrings. If the hold-relax stretching seems to increase the range of motion, the pain and restriction are probably in the hamstring. On the other hand, if the hold-relax technique does not seem to change the pain or restriction, spinal nerve root impingement or irritation may be involved. The

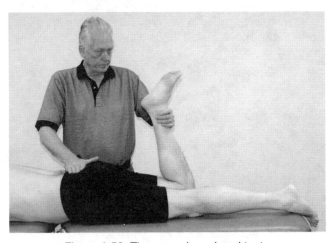

Figure 4-53: The prone knee bend test.

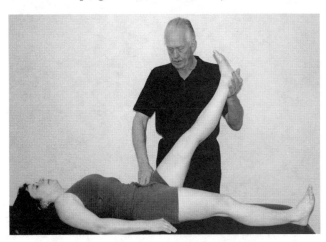

Figure 4-54: The straight leg raise test.

hold-relax technique is not advised on patients presenting with a positive straight leg raise at less than 30° hip flexion, as it may provoke an irritable condition.

The bowstring test is a useful variation of the straight leg raise test. The clinician flexes the patient's hip and knee, each to 90°. With one hand, he palpates the sciatic nerve in the popliteal fossa (Fig 4-55). When the nerve is located, the clinician extends the knee to the point of hamstring tightness and then presses on the sciatic nerve, which causes increased neural tissue tension. If pain is produced proximally, this may be a sign of nerve root irritation.

Lasegue's sign helps to further differentiate true nerve root signs. After the clinician raises the leg to the point of symptomatic response, the leg is lowered 1/2 to 1 inch. The stress to all structures, including the nerve roots, should be relieved. With the leg stationary, the foot is then dorsiflexed. This applies tension to the nerve roots without affecting the other structures (hamstring, sacroiliac joint and hip joint). Exacerbation of pain on dorsiflexion of the foot is Lasegue's sign of radiculitis.[63]

Normally, the straight leg raise test suggests more severe pathology when positive at 20° to 40° of hip flexion and less severe pathology if positive above 50°. The degree of hip flexion present when the symptoms occur should be recorded so the clinician can decide whether progress is made during a later reassessment. Occasionally, symptoms are provoked as the opposite leg is raised. This may suggest a disc herniation with protrusion medial to the nerve root. If symptoms are relieved as the opposite leg is raised a bulge lateral to the nerve root may be present. Again, careful interpretation is advised and one should not draw conclusions unless correlating evidence is found.

Slump Test. The slump test combines the sitting straight leg raise, passive neck flexion and a slump or slouch of the lumbar spine in sitting. This test was first developed and researched by Maitland in 1979.[55] The test is indicated for any patient with non-irritable low back pain or lower limb complaints.

Normal responses to the slump test are summarized below:

- When the patient initially slumps, no complaints are usually offered.
- When the neck is passively flexed, 50% of subjects report a stretch in the T8-9 area.
- When the leg is straightened, a symmetrical limitation of range when compared bilaterally and a stretch feeling in the posterior hamstring and knee is normal.
- Likewise, a symmetrical restriction of dorsiflexion is normal.
- A release of the neck flexion may increase the available range of dorsiflexion at the ankle.

The slump test is performed in the following manner (Fig 4-56):

1. The patient sits comfortably at the end of an exam table.
2. The clinician asks the patient to slump or slouch. The clinician sustains this position.
3. The patient performs neck flexion. The clinician sustains this position and asks the patient to

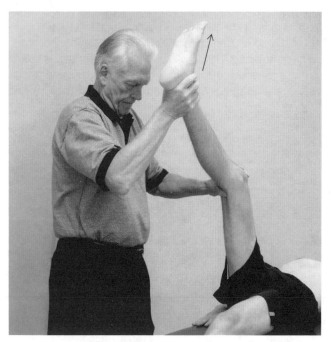

Figure 4-55: The bowstring test.

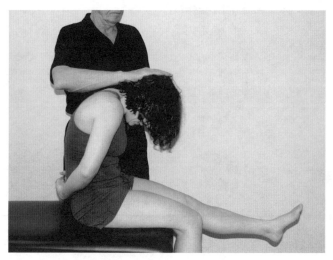

Figure 4-56: The slump test.

straighten either of his legs, while noting symptom response.

4. The clinician then asks the patient to dorsiflex the ankle, noting symptom response.
5. The neck flexion is released to neutral, and again any change in symptoms is noted.
6. The test is repeated with the opposite leg.
7. The test is repeated with both legs at once.

In any tension testing, it is important to consider the following:

- Before beginning, carefully identify all the patient's symptoms and complaints.
- Note which symptoms are present in the starting position.
- Carefully note any change in symptoms or onset of new symptoms during each step of the test.
- Move the patient's limb in each step to the point of onset or change in symptom complaints.
- Compare the findings of the test to the contralateral limb and what is considered normal.

As with any musculoskeletal test, reassessment of the test at later intervals will help the clinician decide whether treatment is effective. To compare later findings, the clinician must document the range of motion at which the symptoms first appear, the nature and location of the symptoms and any abnormal resistance felt by the clinician during the test.

Babinski's Test

The Babinski test, as described under the neurological exam of the cervical spine (Fig 4-26 on page 64), completes the neurological exam of the lumbar spine.

Palpation Examination

Palpation of the thoracic and lumbar spine is performed as described in Section One. Chronic thoracic and lumbar problems are often accompanied by changes in the soft tissue. Asymmetrical toughened or ropy areas in the paraspinal or interscapular musculature may be clues to long-standing problems.

The weight shift test is useful to detect muscle guarding or spasm in the lumbar paraspinals. With the patient standing, the clinician places his thumbs on the patient's lumbar paraspinals. The patient is then asked to shift his weight from one foot to the other (Fig 4-57). Normally, the paraspinals on the side of the stance foot will relax, but if muscle guarding or spasm are present the muscle will not relax.

The piriformis, iliopsoas and quadratus lumborum muscles receive specific attention in the palpation evaluation. The piriformis muscle is palpated at the greater sciatic notch (halfway between the ischial tuberosity and the greater trochanter) with the patient lying prone (Fig 4-58).

The iliopsoas (Fig 4-59) is palpated in three different areas with the patient lying supine: 1) Deep on the lateral border of the femoral triangle over the lesser trochanter; 2) On the inner border of the ilium behind the ASIS; and 3) Underneath the rectus abdominus (found by palpating approximately three finger-widths lateral and inferior to the umbilicus and gently pressing downward and then medially).

The quadratus lumborum (Fig 4-60) is found by positioning the patient in mild flexion and contralateral side bending to separate the 12th rib from the iliac crest. The clinician palpates deep and just lateral to the paraspinals.

Additional soft tissue palpation techniques are discussed in Chapter 11, *Soft Tissue Mobilization and Neuromuscular Training*.

When palpating the lumbar, mid and lower thoracic spinal joints (ligament and bone), the spinous processes and the supraspinous ligament are all the clinician can feel. The information gained through palpating these structures is surprisingly valuable. The supraspinous ligament is normally springy and supple. If it is thick and hardened, the segment may be hypomobile. When palpation between the spinous processes elicits pain, it may indicate the spinal segment (facet joints or intervertebral disc) is involved.

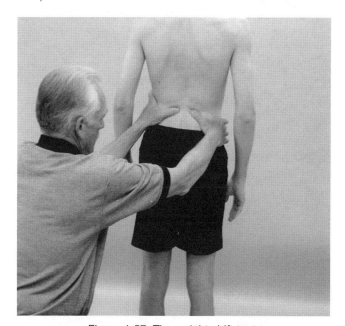

Figure 4-57: The weight shift test.

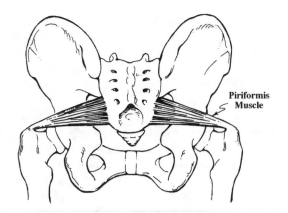

Figure 4-58: The piriformis muscle.

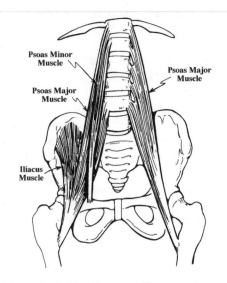

Figure 4-59: The iliopsoas (iliacus and psoas).

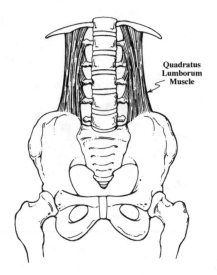

Figure 4-60: The quadratus lumborum.

The position of the spinous processes is felt to determine alignment of the spine. If one spinous process is lateral to the one below it, the segment may be locked in rotation or side bending. When the spinous processes are close together the segment may be locked in backward bending. If they are far apart the segment may be locked in forward bending or a compression fracture may be present. These *positional changes* suggest the presence of facet joint impingement or facet joint hypomobility. Positional changes are usually felt with one finger placed between two spinous processes. The pinch test also is useful in finding rotational positional changes. The pinch test was described earlier (Fig 4-10 on page 55).

Positional changes may be congenital in nature and when seen by themselves they do not necessarily mean a joint is locked or hypomobile. Mobility testing must confirm that a segment is locked or hypomobile before the final assessment is made.

The novice clinician can make the best use of the segmental mobility and palpation evaluations by successively palpating deeply at each interspinous space and spring testing at each level. When the patient complains of increased symptoms at a particular level, the clinician then examines that level more closely for signs of hypo or hypermobility, positional changes or subtle variations in soft tissue texture.

Special Tests

Distraction Test

The distraction test is a neurological test and a mobility test. If peripheral symptoms decrease when traction is applied to the spine, a possible spinal nerve root impingement is suggested. Since facet joint or disc pain can be relieved with this test also, the clinician should correlate other tests to make a proper assessment. Performing manual distraction is valuable in that it gives an indication of whether or not traction will be useful for treatment (Fig 4-61). Furthermore, if distraction relieves or centralizes the patient's symptoms, it is an indication that a back support may be helpful.

Shear Stability Test

McGill describes a useful test to detect possible instability of the lumbar joints.[58] The patient lies prone with the torso on a table and the legs hanging over the edge with the feet on the floor. Spring testing of each spinal segment is performed. When a painful segment is detected, the patient is asked to slightly raise the legs off the floor to contract the back extensors. The clinician then springs the segment again. If pain is relieved while the patient actively contracts the back extensors, the test is positive. Theoretically, the active extensors are stabilizing the painful segment to reduce the shear force, and thus relieve the pain.

Waddell's Tests

Gordon Waddell, et al have described tests for five nonorganic signs and seven nonorganic symptoms that can be used to identify abnormal illness behavior.[87,88] The original five signs have been widely used as a screening tool, sometimes inappropriately. The original article recommended that three or more signs be used to define a positive test, and cautioned against over-interpretation of isolated positive signs.[88] A subsequent article by Main and Waddell clarified that the purpose of the tests is to:

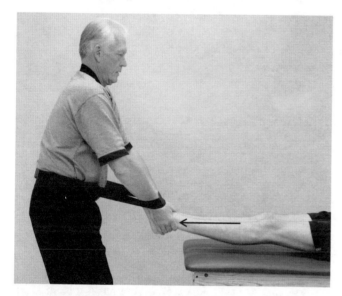

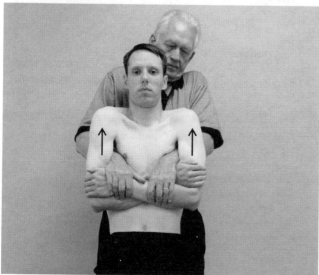

Figure 4-61: Two methods of performing manual lumbar distraction.

1. Enable the separate assessment of physical and nonorganic elements of clinical presentation and therefore clarify clinical decision-making;
2. Direct physical treatment specifically toward physical pathology;
3. Prevent the administration of inappropriate treatment; and
4. Assist in the identification of illness behavior.[53]

The authors repeated their warning to avoid over-interpretation of isolated signs and pointed out that the signs had been used inappropriately to identify "faking".[53]

Fritz, et al studied the usefulness of Waddell's signs and symptoms in predicting delayed return to work in patients with acute low back pain. For this purpose, the best definition of a positive nonorganic test was the presence of two or more signs, three or more symptoms, or three or more signs and symptoms.[25] However, the authors noted an unacceptably high level of false-negative results, which lessened the effectiveness of Waddell's signs and symptoms as screening tools. They suggest that the FABQ or other screening tools may be more valuable in predicting chronic disability.

We find Waddell's tests for nonorganic signs and symptoms useful, but agree with concerns that they be interpreted appropriately. Waddell's tests for nonorganic signs and symptoms take very little extra time because they can be easily integrated into the rest of the evaluation, and they provide useful insight about each patient's illness behavior.

Table 4-6 lists Waddell's seven symptoms. The patient is asked each of the questions. A "yes" answer is a positive test, with the exception of #5, where a "no" answer is considered positive. Table 4-7 lists Waddell's five nonorganic signs and describes a positive result for each sign.

Table 4-6: Waddell's nonorganic symptoms.

1. Do you get pain in your tailbone?
2. Do you have numbness in your entire leg (front, side, and back of the leg *at the same time*)?
3. Do you have pain in your entire leg (front, side, and back of the leg *at the same time*)?
4. Does your whole leg ever give way?
5. Have you had any time during this episode when you have had very little back pain?
6. Have you had to go to the emergency room because of back pain?
7. Has all treatment for your back made your pain worse?

We must emphasize that positive Waddell's tests do not mean that the patient is intentionally exaggerating or that he has no musculoskeletal problems at all. In fact, nonorganic signs often coexist with true physical signs.[53] However, when multiple organic signs or symptoms are present, the patient's problem is not entirely physical or musculoskeletal. Delayed recovery is probable and a more comprehensive, multidisciplinary approach to treatment may be required. The physical therapist's role is to docu- ment the existence of nonorganic signs and symptoms, without judging or over-interpreting. Additionally, the physical therapist must realize that the patient's reports of symptoms cannot be entirely relied upon, and treatment must be based on objective findings to avoid overtreating or enabling the patient.

Table 4-7: Waddell's nonorganic signs

Nonorganic Sign	Description
1. Regional disturbances	A widespread region of sensory changes or weakness that is divergent from accepted neuroanatomy.
2. Superficial/nonanatomic tenderness	Tenderness of the skin to light touch (superficial) and/or deep tenderness felt over a widespread area not localized to one structure (nonanatomic).
3. Simulation—axial loading and trunk rotation	Low back pain reported with pressure on the patient's head while standing (simulating axial loading) and/or low back pain reported when the shoulders and pelvis are rotated together in the same plane (simulating trunk rotation).
4. Distraction—straight leg raising	Inconsistent limitation of straight leg raising in the supine versus the seated position. The term "distraction" refers to the clinician distracting the patient's attention away from the purpose of the seated straight leg raise.
5. Overreaction	Disproportionate verbalization, facial expression, muscle tension, collapsing, sweating, etc., during the evaluation.

REFERENCES

1. Aspinall W: Clinical Testing for Cervical Mechanical Disorders Which Produce Ischemic Vertigo. J Orthop Sports Phys Ther 11:176-182,1989.

2. Bertilson BC, Grunnesjo M, Strender L: Reliability of Clinical Tests in the Assessment of Patients with Neck/Shoulder Problems—Impact of History. Spine 28(19):2222-2231, 2003.

3. Biering-Sorenson F: Physical Measurements as Risk Indicators for Low Back Trouble Over a One-Year Period. Spine 9(2):106-119, 1984.

4. Boos N, Rieder R, Shcade V, et al: The Diagnostic Accuracy of Magnetic Resonance Imaging, Work Perception, and Psychosocial Factors in Identifying Symptomatic Disc Herniations. Spine 20(24):2613-2625, 1995.

5. Borge JA, Leboeuf-Yde C and Lothe J: Prognostic Values of Physical Examination Findings in Patients with Chronic Low Back Pain Treated Conservatively: A Systematic Literature Review. J Manip Physiol Ther 24(4):292-295, 2001.

6. Brady RJ, Dean JB, Skinner TM et al: Limb Length Inequality: Clinical Implications for Assessment and Intervention. J Orthop Sports Phys Ther 33(5):221-234, 2003.

7. Breig A and Troup JDG: Biomechanical Considerations in the Straight Leg Raising Test. Spine 4(3):242-50, 1979.

8. Burdett R, et al: Reliability and Validity of Four Instruments for Measuring Lumbar Spine and Pelvic Positions. Phys Ther 66(5):677-684, 1986.

9. Butler D: The Sensitive Nervous System. NOI Group Publications, Adelaide Australia 2000.

10. Chen J, Solinger AB, Poncet JF, et al: Meta-Analysis of Normative Cervical Motion. Spine 24(15):1571-1578, 1999.

11. Clifford SN and Fritz JM: Children and Adolescents with Low Back Pain: A Descriptive Study of Physical Examination and Outcome Measurement. J Orthop Sports Phys Ther 33(9):513-521, 2003.

12. Cloward R: Cervical Discography: A Contribution to the Etiology and Mechanism of Neck, Shoulder and Arm Pain. Annals of Surgery 150(6): 1052-1064, 1959.

13. Cocciarella L and Andersson G, eds: Guides to the Evaluation of Permanent Impairment, 5th ed. American Medical Association Press, Chicago 2001.

14. Computer Sports Medicine, Inc. 101 Tosca Drive, Stoughton, MA 02072-1505

15. Cyriax J: Diagnosis of Soft Tissue Lesions. Textbook of Orthopædic Medicine, Vol 1, 8th ed. Bailliere-Tindall, London 1982.

16. Davidson M and Keating JL: A Comparison of Five Low Back Disability Questionnaires: Reliability and Responsiveness. Phys Ther 82(1):8-24, 2002.

17. Dhimitri K, Brodeur S, Croteau M, et al: Reliability of the Cervical Range of Motion Device in Measuring Upper Cervical Motion. J Manipulative Physiol Ther 6(1): 31-36, 1998.

18. Dvorak J, Vajda EG, Grob D, et al: Normal Motion of the Lumbar Spine as Related to Age and Gender. Eur Spine J 4:18-23, 1995.

19. Fedorak C, Ashworth N, Marshall J, et al: Reliability of the Visual Assessment of Cervical and Lumbar Lordosis: How Good Are We? Spine 28(16):1857-1859, 2003.

20. Fiebert I and Keller CD: Are "Passive" Extension Exercises Really Passive? J Orthop Sports Phys Ther 199(2):111-116, 1994.

21. Finneson B: Low Back Pain. JB Lippincott, Philadelphia 1973.

22. Friberg O: Clinical Symptoms and Biomechanics of Lumbar Spine and Hip Joint in Leg Length Inequality. Spine 8(6):643-651, 1983.

23. Fritz JM and George SZ: Identifying Psychosocial Variables in Patients with Acute Work-Related Low Back Pain: The Importance of Fear-Avoidance Beliefs. Phys Ther 82(10):973-983, 2002.

24. Fritz JM, George SZ and Delitto A: The Role of Fear-Avoidance Beliefs in Acute Low Back Pain: Relationships with Current and Future Disability and Work Status. Pain 94(1):7-15, 2001.

25. Fritz JM, Wainner RS and Hicks GE: The Use of Nonorganic Signs and Symptoms as a Screening Tool for Return-to-Work in Patients with Acute Low Back Pain. Spine 25(15):1925-1931, 2000.

26. Grant R: Vertebral Artery Testing-The Australian Physiotherapy Association Protocol after 6 Years. Man Ther 1:149-153, 1996.

27. Griffin A and Troup J: Tests of Lifting and Handling Capacity. Ergonomics 27:305-320, 1984.

28. Halbach J and Tank R: The Shoulder. In Orthopedic and Sports Physical Therapy, Vol 2. J Gould and G Davies, eds. CV Mosby, St Louis 1985.

29. Hides JA, Stokes MJ, Saide M, et al: Evidence of Lumbar Multifidus Muscle Wasting Ipsilateral to Symptoms in the Patient with Acute/Subacute Low Back Pain. Spine 19(2):165-172, 1994.

30. Hirsch C, Ingelmark B and Miller M: The Anatomical Basis for Low Back Pain. Acta Ortho Scanda 33:1-17, 1963.

31. Hole DE, Cook JM and Bolton JE: Reliability and Concurrent Validity of Two Instruments for Measuring Cervical Range of Motion: Effects of Age and Gender. Man Ther 1(1): 36-42, 2000.

32. Hoppenfeld S: Physical Examination of the Spine and Extremities. Appleton-Century-Crofts, Norwalk CT 1976.

33. Ito T, Shirado O, Suzuki H, et al: Lumbar Trunk Muscle Endurance Testing: An Inexpensive Alternative to a Machine for Evaluation. Arch Phys Med Rehabil 77:75-79, 1996.

34. Jackson D and Brown M: Is There a Role for Exercise in the Treatment of Low Back Pain Patients? Clin Orthop and Rel Res 179:39-45, 1983.

35. Jackson N, Winkelman R and Bickel W: Nerve Endings in the Lumbar Spinal Column. JBJS 48A:1272-1281, 1966.

36. Jensen G: Musculoskeletal Analysis: The Thoracic Spine. In Physical Therapy. R Scully and M Barnes, eds. Lippincott, Philadelphia 1989.

37. Jensen MC, Brant-Zawadzki MN, Obuchowski N: Magnetic Resonance Imaging of the Lumbar Spine in People without Back Pain. New Engl Joul Med 331(2):70-73, 1994.

38. Kahanovitz N, et al: Normal Trunk Muscle Strength and Endurance in Women and the Effect of Exercises and Electrical Stimulation. Part 2: Comparative Analysis of Electrical Stimulation and Exercise to Increase Trunk Muscle Strength and Endurance. Spine 12(2):112-118, 1987.

39. Kapandji I: Spine. Vol 3 of The Physiology of the Joints, 2nd ed. Churchill Livingstone, London 1974.

40. Karppinen J, Malmivaara A, Tervonen O, et al: Severity of Symptoms and Signs in Relation to Magnetic Resonance Imaging Findings Among Sciatic Patients. Spine 26(7):E149-E154, 2001.

41. Keeley J, et al: Quantification of Lumbar Function Part 5: Reliability of Range of Motion Measures in the Sagittal Plane and in Vivo Torso Rotation Measurement Techniques. Spine 11(1):31-35, 1986.

42. Keller A, Hellesnes J and Brox JI: Reliability of the Isokinetic Trunk Extensor Test, Biering-Sorenson Test, and Astrand Bicycle Test. Spine 26(7):771-777, 2001.

43. Kendall FP, McCreary EK and Provance PG: Muscles Testing and Function, 4th ed. Lippincott, Williams and Wilkins, Baltimore 1993.

44. Kenneally M, et al: The Upper Limb Tension Test: The Straight Leg Raise Test of the Arm. In Physical Therapy of the Cervical and Thoracic Spine, Vol 17 of Clinics in Physical Therapy. R Grant, ed. Churchill Livingstone, Edinburgh 1989.

45. Kleinrensink GJ, Stoeckart R, Mulder PGH, et al: Upper Limb Tension Tests as Tools in the Diagnosis of Nerve and Plexus Lesions. Anatomical and Biomechanical Aspects. Clin Biomech 15:9-14, 2000.

46. Koontz C: Thoracic Outlet Syndrome, Diagnosis and Management. Videotape in Orthopedic Physical Therapy Forum Series. AREN, Pittsburgh 1987.

47. Lantz CA, Klein G and Chen J et al: A Reassessment of Normal Cervical Range of Motion. Spine 28(12):1249-1257, 2003.

48. Latimer J, Maher CG, Refshauge K, et al: The Reliability and Validity of the Biering-Sorensen Test in Asymptomatic Subjects and Subjects Reporting Current or Previous Nonspecific Low Back Pain. Spine 24(20):2085-2090, 1999.

49. Le Forestier N, Mouton P, Maisonobe T, et al: True Neurological Thoracic Outlet Syndrome: 10 Cases. Rev Neurol 156(1):34-40, 2000.

50. Lee JH, Hoshino Y, Nakamura K, et al: Trunk Muscle Weakness as a Risk Factor for Low Back Pain. Spine 24(1):54-57, 1999.

51. Love S, Gringmuth RH, Kazemi M, et al: Interexaminer and Intraexaminer Reliability of Cervical Passive Range of Motion Using the CROM and Cybex 320 EDI. J Can Chiropr Assoc 42(4):222-228, 1998.

52. Maher C and Adams R: Is the Clinical Concept of Spinal Stiffness Multidimensional? Phys Ther 75(10):854-864, 1995.

53. Main C and Waddell G: Behavioral Responses to Examination. A Reappraisal of the Interpretation of "Nonorganic Signs". Spine 23(21):2367-2371, 1998.

54. Maitland G: Vertebral Manipulation, 5th edition. Butterworth, London 1986.

55. Maitland GD: Negative Disc Exploration: Positive Canal Signs. Australian Journal of Physiotherapy 25:129-134, 1979.

56. Mannion AF, Klein GN, Dvorak J, et al: Range of Global Motion of the Cervical Spine: Intraindividual Reliability and the Influence of Measurement Device. Eur Spine J 9(5):379-385, 2000.

57. Mayer T and Gatchel R: Functional Restoration for Spinal Disorders: The Sports Medicine Approach. Lea and Febiger, Philadelphia 1988.

58. McGill SM: Low Back Disorders. Evidence-Based Prevention and Rehabilitation. Human Kinetics, Champaign, IL 2002.

59. McGregor AH, McCarthy ID, Hughes SP: Motion Characteristics of the Lumbar Spine in the Normal Population. Spine 20(22):2421-28, 1995.

60. McIntosh G, Wilson L, Affleck M, et al: Trunk and Lower Extremity Muscle Endurance: Normative Data for Adults. J Rehabil Outcomes Meas 2(4):20-39, 1998.

61. McKenzie R and May S: The Lumbar Spine Mechanical Diagnosis and Therapy, Vol I. Spinal Publications,

Waikanae, New Zealand 2003.

62. MedX 96, Inc. 1401 NE 77th St., Ocala, FL 34479

63. Mennell J: Back Pain. Little-Brown, Boston MA 1964.

64. Mooney V and Robertson J: The Facet Syndrome. Clin Orthop and Rel Res 115:149-156, 1976.

65. Nachemson A: Exercise, Fitness and Back Pain. In Exercise, Fitness and Health: A Consensus of Current Knowledge. C Bouchard, et al, eds. Human Kinetics Books, Champaign IL 1990.

66. Newton M, Waddell G: Trunk Strength Testing with Iso-Machines. Part 1: Review of a Decade of Scientific Evidence. Spine 18(7):801-811, 1993.

67. Ng JK, Kippers V, Richardson C, et al: Range of Motion and Lordosis of the Lumbar Spine. Reliability of Measurement and Normative Values. Spine 26(1):53-60, 2001.

68. Peterson CK, Bolton J and Wood A: A Cross-Sectional Study Correlating Lumbar Spine Degeneration with Disability and Pain. Spine 25(2):218-223, 2000.

69. Petrone MR, Guinn J, Reddin A, et al:The Accuracy of the Palpation Meter (PALM) for Measuring Pelvic Crest Height Difference and Leg Length Discrepancy. J Orthop Sports Phys Ther 33(6):319-325, 2003.

70. Pietrobon R, Coeytaux RR, Carey TS, et al: Standard Scales for Measurement of Functional Outcome for Cervical Pain or Dysfunction. A Systematic Review. Spine 27(5):515-522, 2002.

71. Rebain R, Baxter GD and McDonough S: A Systematic Review of the Passive Straight Leg Raising Test as a Diagnostic Aid for Low Back Pain (1989 to 2000). Spine 27(17):E388-E395, 2002.

72. Rocabado R and Inglarsh A: Musculoskeletal Approach to Maxillofacial Pain. Lippincott, Philadelphia 1991.

73. Roofe P: Innervation of the Annulus Fibrosis and Posterior Longitudinal Ligament: Fourth and Fifth Lumbar Level. Arch Neurol Psych 44:100-103, 1940.

74. Roos DB: Thoracic Outlet Syndrome is Underdiagnosed. Muscle and Nerve 22(1):126-129, 1999.

75. Roy SH, DeLuca CJ, Casavant DA: Lumbar Muscle Fatigue and Chronic Lower Back Pain. Spine 14(9):992-1001, 1989.

76. Saal J, et al: High Levels of Inflammatory Phospholipase A_2 Activity in Lumbar Disc Herniations. Spine 15(7):674-678, 1990.

77. Shacklock M: Positive Upper Limb Tension Test in a Case of Surgically Proven Neuropathy: Analysis and Validity. Man Ther 1:154-161, 1996.

78. Stokes H: The Seriously Uninjured Hand - Weakness of Grip. Joul of Occ Med 25(9):683-684, 1983.

79. ten Brinke A, van der Aa HE, van der Palen J, et al: Is Leg Length Discrepancy Associated with the Side of Radiating Pain in Patients with a Lumbar Herniated Disc? Spine 24(7):684-686, 1999.

80. Toby EB and Koman LA: Thoracic Outlet Compression Syndrome. In Nerve Compression Syndromes. RM Szabo, ed. Slack, Thorofare, London 1989.

81. Tong HC, Haig AJ, Yamakawa K: The Spurling Test and Cervical Radiculopathy. Spine 27(2):156-159, 2002.

82. Troke M: A New, Comprehensive Normative Database of Lumbar Spine Ranges of Motion. Clin Rehab 15:371-379, 2001.

83. Troup J, et al: The Perception of Back Pain and the Role of Psychophysical Tests of Lifting Capacity. Spine 12(7):645-657, 1987.

84. Van Herp G, Rowe PJ, Salter PM: Range of Motion in the Lumbar Spine and the Effects of Age and Gender. Physiotherapy 86:42, 2000.

85. van Tulder MW, Assendelft WJ, Koes BW, et al: Spinal Radiographic Findings and Nonspecific Low Back Pain. A Systematic Review of Observational Studies. Spine 22(4):427-434, 1997.

86. Waddell G, Newton M, Henderson I, et al: Fear Avoidance Beliefs Questionnaire (FABQ) and the Role of Fear Avoidance Beliefs in Chronic Low Back Pain and Disability. Pain 52:157-168, 1993.

87. Waddell G, Main CJ, Morris EW, et al: Chronic Low Back Pain, Psychological Distress, and Illness Behavior. Spine 9:209-213, 1984.

88. Waddell G, McCulloch JA, Cummel E, et al.: Non-Organic Physical Signs in Low Back Pain. Spine 5:117-125, 1980.

89. Wainner RS, Fritz JM Irrgang JJ, et al: Reliability and Diagnostic Accuracy of the Clinical Examination and Patient Self-Report Measures for Cervical Radiculopathy. Spine 28(1):52-62, 2003.

90. Walker H and Schreck R: Relationship of Hyperextended Gait Pattern to Chondromalacia Patellae. Phys Ther 55:259-262, 1975.

91. Wilbourn AJ: Thoracic Outlet Syndrome is Overdiagnosed. Muscle and Nerve 22(1):130-138, 1999.

5

TREATMENT BY DIAGNOSIS

H. Duane Saunders, MS PT and Robin Saunders Ryan, MS PT

Chapter 4, *Evaluation of the Spine*, described the evaluative process and detailed the important subjective questions to explore and objective tests to perform during the spinal examination. In this chapter, we discuss the clinical picture one sees with common spinal conditions. The chapter is organized by diagnosis, and the major subjective and objective findings for each condition are presented. Finally, treatment considerations for each diagnosis are detailed.

Spinal assessment and treatment planning are cognitive processes. The assessment must be based on correlation of the patient's comparable signs and symptoms in a "rule out" process. This chapter is not intended to provide cookbook answers to difficult problems. Rather, it is intended to be a guide to intelligent decision making for appropriate treatment. Remember that it is not always possible to fully evaluate a patient on the first visit or to determine a specific pathological entity, in which case the therapist must assess the various problems the patient has that may be contributing to his symptoms. These problems can then be treated, often with excellent results. Chapter 6 discusses the philosophy of treating by "problem" rather than by diagnosis.

A difficulty with preparing a text of this sort is the wide difference of opinion and placement of emphasis found in the literature. All theories postulated about musculoskeletal disorders cannot possibly be discussed, but the object is to present the major schools of thought and some of the most promising trends in this area.

Many questions remain unanswered about spinal pathology. Consider the following two cases. In one instance, a disc protrusion is identified by MRI and is determined to be the cause of the patient's complaint. The disc protrusion is surgically removed but the patient's signs and symptoms remain unchanged. In the other instance, a disc protrusion is identified by CT/MRI scan, appropriate physical therapy measures or another form of treatment is applied and the patient's signs and symptoms disappear. Yet on a follow-up CT/MRI scan, the disc protrusion remains unchanged.

The point is that there is often no clear-cut cause and effect relationship between what we see, or think we see, and what may actually be causing the patient's problem. Certainly many of the things we observe, for example radiological findings, are probably unrelated to the actual problem.[3,20,41,44,45,46,88,66,88,90] What exactly is taking place when one patient with a nerve root syndrome secondary to foraminal encroachment improves with spinal traction and another patient, with presumably the same disorder, does not improve? What is really happening to the disc when a lateral shift correction maneuver is done and is followed by extension exercises? We think that the disc is reducing. Furthermore, there is some scientific evidence to support such a hypothesis. However, much of what we practice has its basis in the hypothetical realm. We must use caution when basing our treatment on our hypotheses. The same caution applies when assuming anything that shows up on the patient's radiological examination is causing the patient's complaint.

This is not to suggest or imply that just because we do not have all the answers, we should not discuss what we think may be happening. We certainly should not stop using effective treatment methods just because at this point we do not understand everything about spinal pathology. However, because specific etiologies may not be fully understood or recognized, and because much of our treatment is based in theory, we must be cautious in our approach to a patient's problem. We must work our way through the problem with each patient, individualizing treatment appropriately.

General Treatment Considerations

Generally, treatment in the acute and subacute stages of musculoskeletal dysfunction should be directed to:

1. Relieve pain
2. Restore normal anatomy and biomechanics
3. Promote healing
4. Prevent joint stiffness
5. Prevent muscle weakness
6. Prevent postural changes

Often, too much attention is focused on relief of pain (medication, rest and passive modalities and treatments) with little or no attention directed toward prevention of joint stiffness, muscle weakness and adaptive postural changes and the resulting disabilities that these disorders will ultimately produce. One should realize that pain is only a symptom of underlying pathology and that healing, in most instances, will eventually take place in spite of any treatment.

Unless otherwise indicated, the evaluation findings and treatment described for the various conditions below apply to all areas of the spine — cervical, thoracic or lumbar.

Muscle Disorders

Spinal disorders primarily of muscular origin (e.g., muscle strains) are uncommon. Muscle guarding and spasm often accompany spinal pain, regardless of the underlying cause. However, there is no neurophysiological reason for a normal muscle to spontaneously begin to spasm, nor does the concept of sudden muscle strain in the absence of traumatic injury make common sense.

Consider this scenario: Lower back pain commonly starts when a patient bends over or rises up from a bent position with no weight (e.g., the patient reports, "I just bent over to tie my shoe and my back went out!") Physical examination reveals muscle tenderness and limited range of motion. In the absence of other objective findings, a diagnosis of muscle strain is tempting. However, this would be equivalent to diagnosing biceps strain in a patient who simply bent his elbow to take a drink! We know that biceps strains do not occur in this way. Why, then, would we accept the thought that a paraspinal muscle strain can occur in such a fashion? It does not make sense that an individual who is in average physical condition would strain a back muscle during a simple bending motion. Taking this concept a step further, it does not make sense that a well-conditioned construction worker, who is used to lifting hundreds of pounds a day, would strain a back muscle while shoveling his driveway.

There are, of course, primary muscular disorders that are legitimate diagnoses. Primary muscle disorders can include strains, contusions and inflammation. In addition, trigger points can develop in muscles as a result of dysfunctional biomechanics; stressful, prolonged or repetitive positions; or in response to muscle irritation or injury. The point of the above discussion is to caution the clinician against immediately implicating the muscles as the cause of back disorders, without thoroughly considering all the subjective and objective findings and using common sense.

Muscle Guarding and Intrinsic Muscle Spasm Findings

Muscle guarding nearly always accompanies pain, regardless of the underlying cause. Muscle guarding may develop wherever pain is felt, even if it is referred from elsewhere in the body. Without a thorough evaluation, it is easy to incriminate muscle guarding and the resulting intrinsic muscle spasm as the primary cause of the patient's problem. It is unwise to make this assumption, as there is always an underlying cause of the muscle guarding. It is, however, often necessary to treat muscle guarding and intrinsic muscle spasm before treating the underlying problem.

Acute muscle spasm, or cramping, is probably the most painful feature of many back disorders. One must remember, however, that the amount of pain present is no indication of the seriousness of a problem. We have all experienced excruciating muscle cramps that were painful yet harmless. Prolonged muscle guarding or spasm, on the other hand, leads to circulatory stasis and the retention of metabolites. The muscle then may become inflamed (myositis) and a localized tenderness develops. This intrinsic muscle spasm, which is distinctly different from neurogenic muscle spasm, adds additional pain and discomfort (Fig 5-1).

Muscle guarding and intrinsic muscle spasm are detected during the palpation exam by the tension and tenderness of the muscles. A positive weight shift test indicates muscle spasm. Prolonged intrinsic muscle spasm tends to cause generalized pain along the spine and may aggravate areas of degenerative joint and disc disease.

Muscle Strains and Contusion Findings

Musculotendinous strains and contusions have a definite history of trauma such as a blow to the back, a tearing sensation while lifting or another traumatic event. Chronic strains present with a more subtle history of aggravation

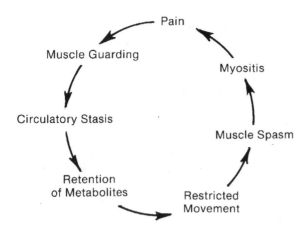

Figure 5-1: The vicious cycle that often develops with musculoskeletal disorders.

such as constant repetition of a new activity. With rest, the patient reports relief of symptoms but a sensation of "stiffening up". Initial movement usually hurts but activity will often relieve the stiffness. The patient complains of pain and a general, vague loss of active and passive movements. No particular positions or activities stand out as being especially painful. Movement is usually more painful than rest, so walking may be worse than standing or sitting.

Pain is usually referred over several spinal levels and the patient has difficulty pinpointing the location. One of the most significant objective findings is pain with muscle palpation but no pain with joint space palpation or with passive spring testing of the joint. The neurological exam is negative. Mennell describes these patients as having a torturous recovery from the forward bent position.[53] The patient may have radicular pain following the sensory distribution of the associated nerve root.[55]

Muscle Inflammation (Myositis) Findings

Muscle inflammation, or myositis, occurs in isolation only on rare occasions. The patient may describe an onset after sleeping in a draft or sitting too close to an air conditioner. Muscle inflammation more commonly follows muscle strain or contusion or develops secondary to prolonged muscle guarding or chronic stress. It essentially has the same characteristics as a muscle strain except that myositis will be of insidious onset and may show temperature and color changes over the involved musculature.

Fibromyalgia Findings

Fibromyalgia syndrome is a nonarticular rheumatologic disorder, classified with the two criteria defined by the American College of Rheumatology: 1) The presence of widespread pain of at least three months' duration; and

2) Pain upon palpation of at least 11 of 18 specific tender points.[82]

Fibromyalgia is diagnosed in women much more frequently than in men. It is considered a chronic pain syndrome and there is much disagreement in the literature about the validity of the diagnosis, with some authors opining that the diagnosis itself creates iatrogenic disability in patients.[26,91]

It is generally accepted that there is a psychological component to fibromyalgia.[22,26,82,84,91] It may be valuable to classify patients with fibromyalgia into different subgroups based on the amount of psychological distress present.[82]

Piriformis Muscle Pathology Findings

Referred pain from the piriformis may radiate to the sacroiliac region laterally across the buttock and hip to the proximal two-thirds of the posterior thigh. Piriformis symptoms may be caused by referral from trigger points within the muscle, by entrapment of the neurovascular bundle within the substance of the muscle or against the rim of the greater sciatic foramen or by sacroiliac dysfunction. Since the piriformis restrains vigorous internal and external hip rotation, piriformis strain can develop from acute overload caused by catching oneself from a fall or running.

The patient with piriformis muscle involvement will tend to squirm and shift weight frequently when seated. Pain can be referred into the posterior thigh. In the supine position, the foot of the involved side is externally rotated. Passive internal rotation of the hip will be restricted and painful and resisted external rotation will be painful. In the prone position, pelvic asymmetry may be noted. Standing examination may reveal an uneven sacral base. The piriformis muscle will be painful to palpation and painful nodules (trigger points) may be evident.

Iliopsoas Muscle Pathology Findings

Myofascial pain in the iliopsoas can result from acute overload, stress or prolonged sitting with the hips acutely flexed. Referred pain from the iliopsoas may extend along the spine from the thoracolumbar junction to the sacroiliac joint and upper gluteal region. The iliacus portion may refer symptoms into the groin and anterior thigh.[79]

The patient with iliopsoas involvement will have pain and restriction with hip extension. Resisted hip flexion will be painful. The patient will have pain with palpation or painful trigger points.

Quadratus Lumborum Muscle Pathology Findings

Myofascial pain from the quadratus lumborum is easily mistaken for radicular pain of lumbar origin. Quadratus lumborum strain often occurs as a result of simultaneously bending forward and reaching to one side to pull or lift something or as a consequence of a trauma such as a fall or motor vehicle accident.

Pain from the quadratus lumborum is usually deep and aching, although it may be sharp during movement. Referred pain will be felt along the crest of the ilium and sometimes in the lower quadrant of the abdomen and into the groin. The greater trochanter, buttock and sacroiliac joint can also be areas of referred pain. The areas of referred pain can also be tender, thus mimicking local pathology.[79]

The patient with quadratus lumborum pathology may have a functional lumbar scoliosis that is concave on the involved side. The normal lumbar lordosis may appear flattened due to the vertebral rotation that accompanies the scoliosis, even though the quadratus lumborum is a spinal extensor.[79] Lumbar flexion and extension are limited and painful, and side bending is restricted toward the pain free side (sometimes bilaterally). Rotation is usually limited and painful toward the side of involvement. In supine or prone, shortness of the muscle may distort pelvic alignment. The patient may have marked tenderness, but it is easily missed unless the examiner takes care to position the patient so that the ribs are separated from the iliac crest during palpation, and palpates deep through the lumbodorsal fascia to reach the quadratus lumborum.

Muscle Disorders Treatment

Treatment of primary muscular disorders should initially include rest with gentle activity within the pain free range. Posture support with a lumbar pillow or corset is often helpful. One may progress to mild activities and mobilization when tolerated. Gentle or vigorous stretching is indicated, depending on the irritability and chronicity of the condition. Even when in pain, the patient should be encouraged to perform mild activities that do not aggravate the condition.

Ice massage, cold packs and electrical stimulation are usually preferred in the acute stage, changing to moist heat and electrical stimulation in the subacute stage. Massage and deep tissue work is helpful for muscular disorders, especially those of the chronic strain variety. Ultrasound combined with electrical stimulation also gives the sensation of a warm massage and is helpful for many patients in the subacute or chronic stages. If definite trigger points are found (e.g., in the piriformis, iliopsoas or quadratus lumborum) they may respond to intermittent cold with stretch (spray and stretch) techniques or injection.

As symptoms decrease, the activity and mobilization treatment should also progress. Restoration of full function (strength and mobility) and normal posture should be the most important aspects of treatment. Primary muscle disorders will probably heal in spite of the care given to them, but stiffness, weakness and postural changes may take place while healing is occurring. These losses of function and adaptive postural changes can lead to more serious chronic problems and should be of primary concern to the therapist treating these disorders. It is not necessary to wait until the patient is pain free to begin active exercise. If pain with exercise is present, it is not necessarily a harmful sign. If the pain is not severe, does not last and is not progressive, exercise should be encouraged. Experience shows that more long-term harm is caused by too little activity than by too much.

Treatment for fibromyalgia can involve a short trial of modalities or manual techniques aimed at pain relief, but excessive use of passive treatments can contribute to an unhealthy focus on symptoms. Instead, active treatments geared toward decreasing fear and improving function are indicated. Patients should be weaned to independence from clinical physical therapy visits. Treatment should focus on exercise, education and cognitive behavior interventions, although the efficacy and cost-effectiveness of intense cognitive behavior therapy compared to general group education has been questioned.[22,48,84]

Joint Disorders

For classification purposes, the following structures are considered to be a part of the three-joint vertebral complex (two facet joints and the intervertebral disc): 1) Disc; 2) Cartilaginous endplate; 3) Hyaline cartilage; 4) Subchondral bone; 5) Meniscoid bodies; 6) Synovial lining; 7) Joint capsule; and 8) Ligament. Joint disorders considered in this section are impingement, sprain, inflammation and degenerative disease. Disc disorders are discussed in a separate section.

Facet Impingement Findings

Facet blockage, subluxation, fixation, locking and acute cervical torticollis are all terms sometimes used to describe facet joint impingement. Impingement is one of the disorders that has made chiropractors popular because manipulation is usually an effective treatment. The mechanism of injury is usually a sudden, unguarded movement involving backward bending, side bending and/or rotation with little or no trauma. Kraft and Levinthal describe a mechanism in which

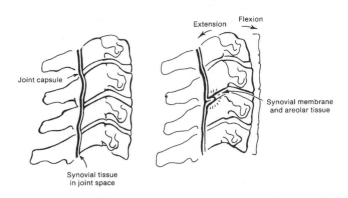

Figure 5-2: Mechanism of facet joint impingement.

the synovial and capsular tissues that line the facet joint capsule become impinged between the joint surfaces (Fig 5-2).[41] Maitland[47] and Sprague[76] have accurately described cervical joint locking, its signs and symptoms and its treatment.

The patient with a facet impingement will report that rest relieves, movement hurts and certain passive and active movements will be restricted and painful. The patient often will be "locked" into a protective posture. The protective posture will involve side bending and rotation to the same side in the cervical spine and often side bending and rotation in opposite directions in the thoracic and lumbar spine. The rotary component may not be readily observable but usually occurs according to Fryette's Laws of Spinal Motion (see Chapter 2, *Spinal Biomechanics*).

In the lumbar or thoracic spine, rotation and side bending can be limited in either the same or opposite directions, depending upon whether hyperflexion or hyperextension is present along with the rotatory and side bending components. For example, if the segment is restricted in either extension or flexion at the same time it is rotated and side bent, the rotation and side bending will be in the same direction.

Pain and restriction of movement will be present when the patient attempts movement in the direction opposite the locked position. Pain may follow the corresponding dermatomal distribution.[55] Cailliet states that pain arising from the facet joint may be felt as pain in the entire sensory distribution of the corresponding spinal nerve root.[8] For example, if a cervical segment is locked in left side bending and left rotation, the patient will have pain and restriction of movement with right side bending and right rotation. Further movement to the left is usually free and painless.

Facet joint impingement and other facet disorders should not present with the true positive neurological signs of myotomal motor weakness or dermatomal sensory loss. However, referred pain, a painful straight leg raise or depressed quadriceps muscle stretch reflex may be present (see discussion in *Radiculopathy and Other Neural Conditions* on page 116).

One of the keys to differential diagnosis of joint involvement is the palpation and segmental mobility exam as described in Chapter 4, *Evaluation of the Spine*. Spring testing or other segmental mobility tests will reveal hypomobility at a single level. When the examiner palpates between the spinous processes or along the articular pillars (cervical), the single involved segment will be tender. If the patient has had pain for more than one or two days, the muscles may also be tender from guarding and spasm alone. As previously pointed out, this reflexive guarding and spasm may sometimes be incorrectly interpreted as being the primary disorder.

Positional changes often can be felt by palpating the spinous processes (Fig 5-3). For example, if the segment is locked in rotation and side bending, the superior spinous process will not be in alignment with the adjacent inferior spinous process. If the segment is locked in forward bending, the space between the spinous processes will be wider at that level. If the segment is locked in backward bending, the space will be narrower. However, if the segment is locked in mid-range, a positional fault may not be evident upon palpation.

Lab findings and routine x-rays will be negative. Mobility x-rays, which are special techniques that show spinal motion and position, may be helpful in demonstrating a locked or immobile segment. However, such procedures seem unnecessary since the clinical exam will also demonstrate this loss of mobility or positional change.

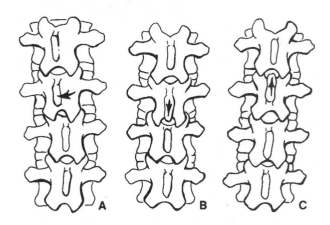

Figure 5-3: Positional changes related to facet joint impingement. A) Rotation; B) Backward bending; and C) Forward bending.

Facet Impingement Treatment

Facet joint impingements respond well to mobilization techniques and manual or mechanical traction. It is often wise to precede the mobilization or traction with ice or heat and soft tissue techniques to relieve the muscle guarding and spasm that may accompany the facet disorder. Treatment for cervical facet impingement involves manual traction and gentle rotation and side bending, first in the pain free direction. A gradual stretch into the painful direction can be achieved while the traction force is being maintained. A similar effect can be achieved in the lumbar spine if a three-dimensional mobilization table is used in combination with traction. While the traction force is being applied, the table can be moved slowly to provide a gentle mobilization force in the desired plane and direction of motion.

Facet Joint Sprain Findings

It is necessary to distinguish between facet joint impingement and facet joint sprain because the treatment for these two disorders differs. The two disorders are, of course, quite different, but their objective signs and symptoms are often hard to distinguish during the musculoskeletal examination.

The key to differential diagnosis is found in the patient's history. With facet joint sprain, the patient has a history of moderate to severe trauma, enough so that the examiner must consider the possibility of joint sprain with effusion in and around the joint. Facet joint impingement can be treated with mobilization as soon as the disorder is confirmed. Facet joint sprain, on the other hand, must be treated with a more conservative approach using physical therapy modalities, pain free movements, support and rest. The joint sprain needs time to heal.

It is possible for facet joint impingement to occur with trauma. In this case, the examiner must assume that the soft tissue around the joint has also been injured and must take a more conservative approach to treatment. Mobility tests, palpation and other signs and symptoms of joint sprain will be similar to those found with facet joint impingement, except that movement may be generally more restricted and may involve more than one specific segment. Positional faults are not as common.

Facet Joint Sprain Treatment

If the patient gradually increases activity as the joint sprain heals or if the injury is treated with mild to moderate mobilization and range of motion during the subacute stage, the joint is likely to have normal mobility by the time complete healing occurs. If the patient has been immobile during the subacute stage or there has been a great deal of muscle guarding, the joints are likely to become hypomobile (stiff) as they heal. If, on the other hand, the joint capsule or supportive ligaments are torn or over-stretched during injury, the joint may be hypermobile (unstable) when healed.

Effective treatment must guard against the development of postural changes such as forward head in a cervical sprain or slumped sitting (flat back) in a lumbar sprain. During the acute and subacute stages, it may be painful to sit or stand erect or hold the head and neck in a normal posture. Thus, the patient may tend to stand and sit slumped or develop a stooped, forward head posture. As healing occurs, the muscles and ligaments adapt to their new positions and the faulty posture is maintained. The cycle continues as the muscles weaken and a chronic postural strain develops. Short-term use of supports such as a soft cervical collar, a lumbosacral corset or a lumbar pillow often help prevent these postural changes. Modalities and medications may help relieve the pain, making normal posture possible. Above all, patient awareness that long term postural problems, stiffness and weakness can develop is imperative. Gentle exercise should be started as soon as possible and should progress to full rehabilitation as tolerated. When the patient is still experiencing acute symptoms, active range of motion exercise is preferable to passive, because pain inhibition will prevent overstretching.

Joint Inflammation Findings

Joint inflammation will have a history of insidious onset, frequently following acute joint sprain or chronic postural sprain. It will also occur secondary to aggravation or overuse in the presence of degenerative joint/disc disease. As in all joint disorders, movement will hurt. If joint inflammation is present, however, the patient may also complain of pain and stiffness at rest. The involved segments will be tender to palpation. Active and passive movement will generally be restricted. Joint inflammation often presents bilateral symptoms. The color and temperature changes characteristic of inflammation may not be noticeable because of the depth of the joints in the spine. Rheumatoid arthritis is not a consideration here since it is classified as a systemic disease and requires specialized management.

Joint Inflammation Treatment

Treatment consists of modality therapy (ice, electrical stimulation), gentle movement, support, rest and anti-inflammatory medications to promote healing. Movement exercises should be performed and can be somewhat painful. Mild pain is acceptable with exercise as long as the pain does not last or progressively worsen. Short-term support such as a lumbar pillow, cervical collar or corset may

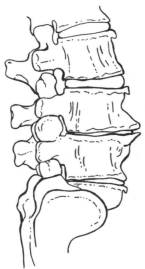

Figure 5-4: Lumbar degenerative joint/disc disease, including the narrowed intervertebral foramen seen with lateral stenosis.

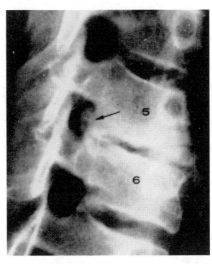

Figure 5-5: Cervical degenerative joint/disc disease (from Peterson and Kieffer).[65]

be helpful. As with other musculoskeletal disorders, passive treatments are followed by gradual reconditioning to restore strength, mobility and normal posture.

Degenerative Joint/Disc Disease Findings

Degenerative joint disease (DJD) and degenerative disc disease (DDD) are chronic and commonly progressive degenerative conditions of the facet joints and the intervertebral discs (Figures 5-4 and 5-5). There are four characteristics of DJD in synovial joints:

- Proliferation of calcific deposits in, and especially around, the periphery of the joint
- Wearing away of the hyaline cartilage
- Thickening of the synovial lining, joint capsule and other soft tissues
- Thickening of the subchondral bone

Degenerative disc disease is characterized by:

- Dehydration of the nucleus pulposus
- Narrowing of the intervertebral space
- Weakening and degeneration of the annular rings
- Approximation of the facet joints

The term *spondylosis* is used to describe various degenerative disorders of the spine, including DJD and DDD. Other conditions are closely associated with spinal degeneration. For example, degeneration that causes narrowing of the intervertebral foramen is commonly called *lateral stenosis*. *Osteophytosis* is an outgrowth of immature bony processes from the vertebrae, reflecting the presence of degenerative disease and calcification.

Although DJD and DDD are technically distinct conditions, they are usually present together and will be referred to as degenerative joint/disc disease throughout this chapter.

For evaluation and treatment purposes, lateral stenosis is considered a specific type of degenerative joint/disc disease that is significant because of its potential to impinge or irritate the spinal nerve root in the intervertebral foramen, causing radiculopathy (see *Radiculopathy Findings* on page 117).

Although degenerative joint/disc disease naturally occurs with aging and is often asymptomatic, it sometimes develops as the result of hypomobility secondary to decreased joint/disc nutrition. The intervertebral discs and the hyaline cartilage surfaces of synovial joints do not have a blood supply. The movement of body fluids is necessary for these structures to receive normal nutrition.[5,30,31,36,40] Therefore, loss of mobility contributes to early development of joint/disc degeneration. Joint hypermobility or instability also leads to early joint/disc degeneration because of the increased wear and tear to which the disc and joints are subjected.[36] When degenerative disease develops, the joint/disc is vulnerable to increased aggravation and strain, thus a progressive cycle develops as the disorder worsens.

The patient with degenerative joint/disc disease usually presents a history of joint aggravation with episodes of joint pain or stiffness. X-ray will reveal the degenerative process or a narrowing of the disc space. The patient will have tenderness at the segmental levels involved. A thickened supraspinous ligament can often be palpated.

Active and passive movements are usually restricted, but because hypermobility of the joint sometimes develops, active and passive movements are occasionally excessive. In advanced stages, pain is present with any movement. However, it should be emphasized that this disorder is asymptomatic in many cases.

The joint is more vulnerable to facet impingement, sprain and inflammation when degenerative joint disease is present. The disc can also be injured more easily.

We have seen conflicting radiological evidence in patients who seem to have degenerative joint/disc disease. Some individuals remain asymptomatic (except for hypomobility) despite radiological evidence of advanced degenerative joint/disc disease. On the other hand, physical therapists often see those patients who have no radiological evidence of disease but who have both mobility problems and pain. In such cases, it may be the soft tissue stiffness that causes symptoms, since the hyaline cartilage of the joint surfaces is aneural.

Discogenic pain related to degenerative joint/disc disease is difficult to assess clinically, but also seems to be intermittent in nature and is related to certain stressful activities. When evaluating a patient, it is often difficult to determine if the pain the patient is experiencing is coming from the disc or from the facet joints. If the pain is discogenic, it may be because of mechanical irritation or inflammation of the outer wall of the annulus. Discogenic pain may also arise because of a chemical irritation.[68] The mechanism of aggravation and analysis of the most painful positions (flexion versus extension) may give the most reliable clues. If flexion (sitting and forward bending) is more painful, the disc is probably the irritated structure. If the reverse is true and extension (standing and walking) is most aggravating, the facets are probably involved.

It must be emphasized that one cannot assume that a patient with degenerative joint/disc disease will be either hyper or hypomobile (see additional discussion in Chapter 6, *Treatment by Problem*). One could theorize that a segment with degenerative joint/disc disease would be hypermobile because of ligamentous laxity due to the narrowing of the joint and disc space. Another could argue that adaptive shortening will occur as the gradual narrowing takes place and the segment will be hypomobile. Dr. William Kirkaldy-Willis believes that the segment first goes through a hypermobile stage, and then later becomes hypomobile.[36]

At any rate, the good clinician will determine the actual mobility of the segment through segmental mobility testing or mobility x-rays rather than blindly accepting one of the above theories. Patients should not be told that they have hypermobility or hypomobility just because they have radiological evidence of degenerative joint/disc disease.

Degenerative Joint/Disc Disease Treatment

Mild to Moderate Stages

If the patient has joint hypomobility, treatment may involve ultrasound, mobilization, manual or mechanical traction and flexibility exercises. In the lumbar spine, stretching and mobilization should involve side bending away from and rotation toward the stiff side. Positional traction as described in Chapter 12, *Spinal Traction*, can be very helpful.

In the case of hypermobility, back supports are often necessary. Muscle strengthening and postural training will be important in either case, and modality therapy and medication may be necessary for relief of pain and inflammation. Usually, the patient should initially exercise in the direction opposite that of the aggravation. For example, if flexion aggravates, extension exercises are indicated. The amount of lordosis will also help determine which exercises are appropriate for each patient. If the patient is hyperlordotic, flexion exercises are indicated; if the patient is hypolordotic, extension exercises are indicated. Often, side bending and rotation exercises are better tolerated and more helpful than either flexion or extension.

Severe Stage

If the patient has joint hypomobility, it is usually beneficial to mobilize the involved segments. If this can be done without aggravating the patient's pain, mobilization is probably the treatment of choice. Traction may prove to be the most effective and least irritating way to accomplish increased general mobility. If, on the other hand, any attempt to increase mobility or activity results in increased pain or an increased inflammatory response, another approach should be considered. This approach involves bracing or support to reduce movement and vertical loading, which reduces irritation.

Bracing or support is sometimes used when the patient with degenerative joint/disc disease suffers from frequent episodes of aggravation due to activity, has a job involving heavy physical labor or participates in sports. Support may be used in all three stages (mild, moderate or severe).

Disc Disorders

Disc disorders treatable by the physical therapist usually involve some variation of herniated nucleus pulposus (HNP). Other disc disorders such as infections or congenital abnormalities are not discussed in this chapter. HNP involves displacement of the nuclear material and other disc components beyond the normal confines of the annulus. Four degrees of displacement are recognized:

l) Intra-spongy nuclear herniation; 2) Protrusion; 3) Extrusion; and 4) Sequestration.

HNP-protrusion occurs gradually over time. In the early stages, it is asymptomatic. As the protrusion progresses, the patient first experiences back pain, then back and leg pain. Finally, signs of neurological involvement accompany the back and leg pain, indicating impingement or irritation of the nerve root. We choose to classify HNP-protrusion as occurring in two stages. In the first stage (mild to moderate), the signs and symptoms are purely discogenic in nature. In the second stage (moderate to severe), the signs and symptoms also indicate involvement of the nerve root (radiculopathy). These classifications are based on treatment concepts that often change as the condition changes. It is important to note that moderate to severe HNP is only one possible cause of radiculopathy. Other conditions, such as lateral stenosis and severe disc degeneration, can also cause radiculopathy (see *Radiculopathy Findings* on page 117).

It is recommended that all other terms dealing with disc displacement such as hard disc, soft disc, disc derangement, disc prolapse, ruptured disc and slipped disc be discarded due to their imprecise meanings and because these terms do not describe a verifiable condition.

Intra-Spongy Nuclear Herniation Findings

Intra-spongy nuclear herniation refers to displacement of the nucleus into the vertebral body through the cartilaginous endplate. It is similar to a Schmorl's node except that it is a traumatic defect rather than a developmental one. Schmorl's nodes represent small invasions of the vertebral body by the nucleus protruding superiorly. According to Cyriax, they never cause any symptoms, either at the time of occurrence or later in life.[11] In fact, Schmorl's nodes are thought to stabilize the nucleus and diminish the intra-articular centrifugal force, thus rendering posterior displacement less probable. Unfortunately, they are rarely seen where they are most needed—at the fourth and fifth lumbar levels. They occur most commonly in the lower thoracic and upper lumbar spine and are purely an adolescent phenomenon since no increased frequency is observed as age advances.[9]

Similarly, traumatic intra-spongy nuclear herniation is thought to be of little clinical importance. There are few references in orthopedic literature to indicate that it is of clinical significance. However, Farfan describes a disc injury that deals with the fractured endplate of the vertebral body due to a compression injury. He maintains that these injuries can be a source of pain and that they occur in four grades:

Grade 1: Subchondral fractures in the vertebral body

Grade 2: Small cracks in the endplates

Grade 3: A crack in which a piece of bone has shifted

Grade 4: A crack in which a piece of bone has shifted and disc material is forced through the crack (intra-spongy nuclear herniation)[16]

Traumatic intra-spongy nuclear herniation usually occurs as the result of moderate to severe flexion trauma. The patient with intra-spongy nuclear herniation has pain with flexion activities, including forward bending and sitting. Actual diagnosis is by radiological examination.

Intra-Spongy Nuclear Herniation Treatment

Treatment consists of rest and avoiding compressing forces on the disc. Controlling protective muscle guarding with physical therapy modalities is important because muscle guarding contributes a compressive force. Hyperextension and mild traction may help to restore the anatomy of Grade 3 or 4 injuries. Support with a corset or brace may also be indicated.

Mild to Moderate Lumbar HNP-Protrusion (Without Spinal Nerve Root Involvement) Findings

HNP-protrusion describes the condition in which there is displacement, but not escape, of the nuclear material beyond the normal confines of the inner annulus. The protrusion produces a discrete bulge in the outer annulus. There are divergent opinions about the role of the disc in spinal pain where there is no evidence of nerve root impingement. In the past, it was thought that, except for the outermost rings of the annulus, the intervertebral disc itself was not a source of pain because of its lack of a sensory nerve supply.[27,28,29,32,33,67] Therefore, disc pain in the absence of nerve root impingement was thought to arise from mechanical deformation of the outer annulus, which is innervated by the recurrent sinuvertebral nerve. However, subsequent research has shown that disc pain can result from chemical inflammation.[68]

In the lumbar spine, 98% of herniated discs occur at the L4-L5 and L5-S1 levels.[75] HNP-protrusion is rarely associated with a single injury or incident. Rather, it is caused by the cumulative effects of months or even years of forward bending and lifting or sitting in a slumped, forward bent posture. One usually sees a generalized loss of mobility, especially spinal extension,[87] and an overall decline in general physical fitness.[7,42] Since mobility is necessary to maintain adequate nutrition to the disc, this loss of mobility leads to further weakening of the annular rings.

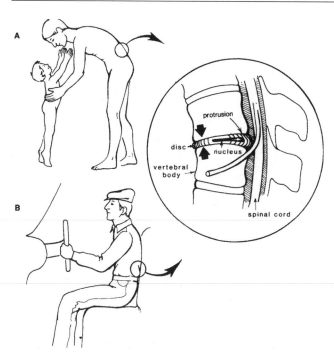

Figure 5-6: The mild to moderate herniated disc. Disc mechanics with A) Forward bending; and B) Slumped sitting. Note that the bulge is not yet touching the nerve root.

The typical patient will be 20-50 years old.[75] HNP-protrusion is uncommon in younger people—probably because the causative factors of stiffening, weakening and degeneration have not progressed enough. It is uncommon in older individuals because there is a tendency for the fluid nucleus to become more fibrous with age. Because the disc is less fluid and more fibrous it will be less likely to protrude through the small cracks in the annular rings.

In the early stages, the patient will complain of pain, usually in the lower back, but sometimes in the posterior buttock and thigh. The presence of leg pain usually indicates a larger protrusion than that of back pain alone.

Usually, the patient will not hesitate when asked, "Which hurts more—sitting, standing, walking or lying down?" The answer will be, "sitting." The patient will often report that prolonged sitting will cause the pain to move from the lower back into the leg. He will report difficulty when assuming an erect posture after sitting or lying down. However, after standing up and walking around, he usually obtains some relief of pain. When asked to locate the pain, the patient usually says that it is greater on one side of the lower back than the other, but it may be bilateral (due to a connecting branch of the sinuvertebral nerve joining its right and left portions).[17] Referred pain into the leg is usually unilateral and will correspond to the dermatomal pattern of the involved segment.

Although the patient may report a sudden onset of symptoms, usually relating to forward bending or prolonged sitting, this sudden onset is believed to be "the straw that broke the camel's back." It is much more logical to assume that the onset was insidious and related to the repetition of forward bending or sitting activities over time (Fig 5-6). The patient may not feel the gradual onset because the disc interior is not innervated.

The patient usually reports an occupation or activity that relates to a long history of a flexed lumbar posture.[13,60,75] For example, truck drivers have a higher incidence of this disorder than persons in most other occupations.[60] The patient may describe having had multiple episodes over several months or years, with episodes occurring more frequently with progressively more pain. The patient may describe a gradual worsening of symptoms with each episode, with pain spreading from the back to the buttock and then to the posterior thigh and calf.

Patients may need to be questioned closely about previous episodes of pain. They may not relate previous episodes of what may have been diagnosed as "muscle strain" to their current complaints. We believe, however, that many of these minor episodes are related, particularly when the mechanism of injury is similar. Previous diagnoses of muscle strain or mechanical low back pain actually may have represented the early stages of a disc problem. It is imperative that these patients realize this, as the importance of preventing future episodes of HNP will be more evident to them.

Figure 5-7 shows the development of the HNP-protrusion. The first drawing is of a normal disc, the second depicts the development of a slight posterolateral protrusion (this condition would be painless) and the third drawing shows a protrusion into the posterior rings of the annulus. It is at this stage that the patient begins to experience discogenic pain and symptoms. Note also that the nerve root is not involved at this stage. Therefore, it seems reasonable to assume that the patient's pain comes from the sensory innervation of the outer annulus or the surrounding soft tissues.

The objective examination will reveal a patient who sits in a slumped posture with the lumbar spine in flexion. He will often reach down to the chair seat with the hands to take the weight of the trunk off the lower back. The patient may have a lateral shift (lumbar scoliosis). Technically, there is a difference between a lateral shift as described by McKenzie[52] and a lumbar scoliosis. In a true scoliosis, there will be a more pronounced secondary curve and the patient's head and shoulders will probably be positioned directly over the pelvis. With a lateral shift, the

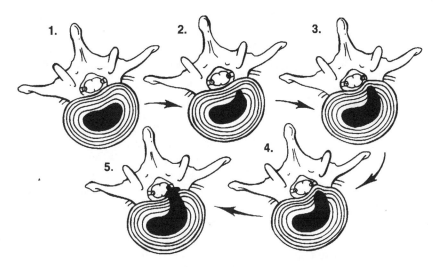

Figure 5-7: The stages of disc herniation. Stage one is normal. Stage two shows slight movement of the nuclear gel. The patient would be pain free at this stage. Stage three shows a mild to moderate protrusion. At this stage the patient may have back and leg pain but no positive neurological signs. Postural correction and extension exercises and principles are usually effective treatments at this stage. Stage four shows a protrusion that is bulging and impinging against the nerve root. The patient has back pain, leg pain and positive neurological signs. Treatment includes traction; back support and extension exercises and principles. Stage five shows disc extrusion and sequestration. In this stage, back and leg pain diminishes as neurological signs usually increase and traction becomes ineffective.

center of the patient's shoulders will be lateral to the center of the patient's pelvis.

McKenzie states that 50% of the patients with HNP-protrusion have a lateral shift because of the tendency for the nuclear gel to move posterolaterally. As the gel moves posteriorly, the patient tends to shift his weight in an anterior direction, flattening the lumbar lordosis. The patient also shifts the shoulders away from the side of nuclear movement. Therefore, the most important clinical features of this disorder are the flattening of the lordosis and the shift of the torso away from the painful side (Fig 5-8). Flattening of the thoracic kyphosis is also characteristic of the disorder.[9,52,87] There will be no positive neurological signs at this stage. The involved spinal segment will be tender to palpation and routine x-rays will usually be negative.

According to McKenzie, HNP-protrusion involves a disturbance of the normal resting position of the articular surfaces of two adjacent vertebrae as a result of a change in the position of the fluid nucleus between these surfaces. The alteration in the position of the nucleus (derangement) may also disturb the annulus.[52]

This will cause disturbance of the normal mechanics of movement. The particular pattern will depend upon the exact area where the disturbance lies. The nucleus is always under positive pressure that slightly deforms the elastic annulus. The position of the spine in flexion or extension will add to or subtract from the pressure exerted at the posterior and posterolateral borders of the annulus. The center of the nucleus is all gel and the periphery of the annulus is all collagen fiber; one merges into the other, with the fibers becoming less dense near the interior of the nucleus[52] (Fig 5-9). On extension of the spine, the intervertebral disc

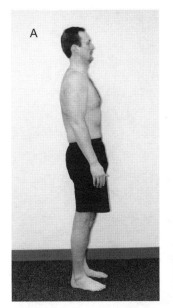
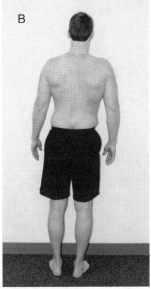

Figure 5-8: Abnormal posture commonly associated with herniated disc. A) Flattened lumbar lordosis (posterior pelvic tilt); and B) Lateral shift.

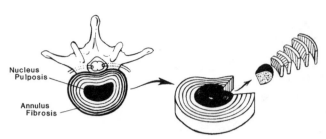

Figure 5-9: The intervertebral disc.

spaces tend to open anteriorly and close down posteriorly, thus exerting pressure on the nucleus to move it anteriorly. The converse is true with flexion.[34,52,70,72]

McKenzie theorizes that prolonged flexed lumbar posture and lifting or walking with the lumbar spine flexed will make the nucleus migrate posteriorly or posterolaterally.[52] As this condition progresses, pain sensitive structures are encountered and the patient begins to have pain in the

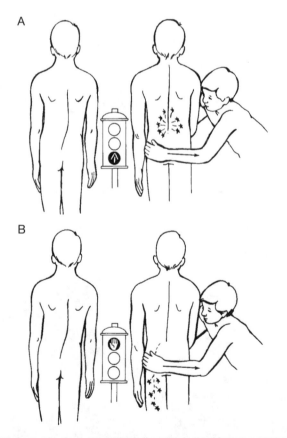

Figure 5-10: One of these two reactions is seen when an attempt to correct the lateral shift is made: A) Increased central pain, which is acceptable; or B) Increased peripheral pain, which is unacceptable.

lumbar spine (stage three of Figure 5-7). If the condition is not corrected, it may continue to progress until the patient begins to have pain in the buttock and thigh. This may eventually progress to involve nerve root impingement or irritation.

Mechanical correction of the lateral shift will usually cause increased pain. It is important to note, however, whether the increase in pain is central in the lower back or if the increase in pain is toward the periphery. If the bulge is mild or moderate, correction of the lateral shift will cause increased pain in the *central* low back. Increased central pain is acceptable. If attempts to correct the shift cause increased pain toward the periphery, they should be discontinued, at least for the present. Theoretically, if the bulge is small and the nuclear material is not displaced beyond the posterolateral edge of the vertebral body, the correction should not increase leg symptoms (Fig 5-10).

Standing forward bending is sometimes limited due to the severity of the pain and muscle guarding that may be present, but it is not uncommon for the patient to have full lumbar flexion mobility. The lumbar spine is actually often fully flattened or flexed when initially examined.

Standing flexion will cause the pain to move peripherally (Fig 5-11). This is especially true if forward flexion is repeated several times. Theoretically, repeated forward bending causes the protrusion to enlarge, producing increased pressure on the annular wall. Since this enlargement does not subside immediately, the increased pain lingers even after the movement has stopped.

If a lateral shift is present, it should be corrected before testing extension. Extension or backward bending after the lateral shift has been corrected will almost always be restricted and will cause increased pain. It is important to note whether the increase in pain centralizes or peripheralizes. If the bulge is mild to moderate (not displaced beyond the posterolateral edge of the vertebral body), extension may cause increased pain, but it will be *central* in the lower back. An increase in peripheral symptoms indicates a more severe protrusion (Fig 5-12). Occasionally, extension will dramatically relieve peripheral pain.

In summary, patients with mild to moderate HNP-protrusion usually have more pain with sitting than with walking, standing or lying down. They will also have reduced lumbar lordosis and a limitation in lumbar extension; about 50% will have a lateral shift. If the patient is asked to perform repeated flexion movements, the symptoms will worsen and *peripheralize* from the center of the spine into the leg. Once aggravated, the peripheralized pain will tend to linger for a while. On the other hand, cor-

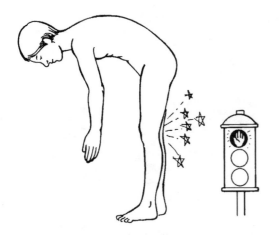

Figure 5-11: Standing flexion will cause pain to move peripherally in patients who have HNP-protrusion.

A

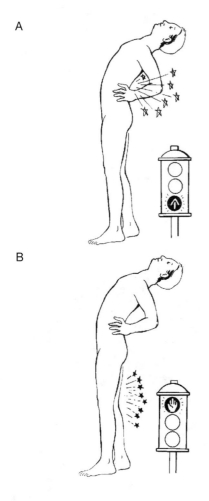

B

Figure 5-12: One of these two reactions is seen when lumbar extension is attempted with HNP: A) Increased central pain, which is acceptable; or B) Increased peripheral pain, which is unacceptable.

rection of the lateral shift and extension will tend to *centralize* the pain.

Mild to Moderate Lumbar HNP-Protrusion (Without Spinal Nerve Root Involvement) Treatment

McKenzie advocates correction of the lateral shift and passive extension exercises to move the nucleus of the disc centrally.[52] He also advocates constant maintenance of the correction to allow healing of the annular fibers to occur. The cardinal rule to always follow is: Correction of the lateral shift and passive extension may cause increased pain in the back but *must not increase the leg symptoms.* If symptoms are peripheralized by the corrective maneuvers, it indicates that either the bulge is not being reduced by the maneuver or that the nerve root is being pulled or pushed onto the bulge by the maneuver. In either case, it is wrong to proceed. Any activity that peripheralizes the pain is probably making the condition worse, whereas an activity or position that causes pain to centralize in the lower back may not be harmful and may, in fact, be the correct thing to do. If the patient has a mild to moderate bulge, correction attempts should be successful.

If attempts to correct the lateral shift in the standing position are unsuccessful, correction is attempted lying down. Sometimes elimination of the compressive force of gravity is enough to allow successful correction of the lateral shift. Several methods of correcting the lateral shift are possible, and some work better than others for individual patients. A three-dimensional mobilization table is very helpful with passive correction of a lateral shift. It can subsequently be used for passive extension (Fig 5-13).

Assume, then, that attempts to correct the lateral shift are successful, in either standing, prone or side lying. Figure 5-14 shows what is believed to be happening. One must understand that the correction is not made with one simple maneuver. Lateral shift correction may need to be performed several times before the patient can hold the correction on his own. It then becomes the patient's responsibility over the next few days to constantly keep correcting the shift until he has successfully reduced the bulge.

When the lateral shift is corrected and the back pain centralizes, the patient often feels that he is leaning or shifted to the opposite side when, in fact, he is straight. This is a temporary phenomenon resulting from improper proprioceptive feedback. One very effective way to correct a lateral shift is to stand in front of the patient and imitate his shift. Then, have the patient place a hand on his hip and push the hip inward until the spine is straight. If the patient does not feel straight, ask him to practice standing and walking while

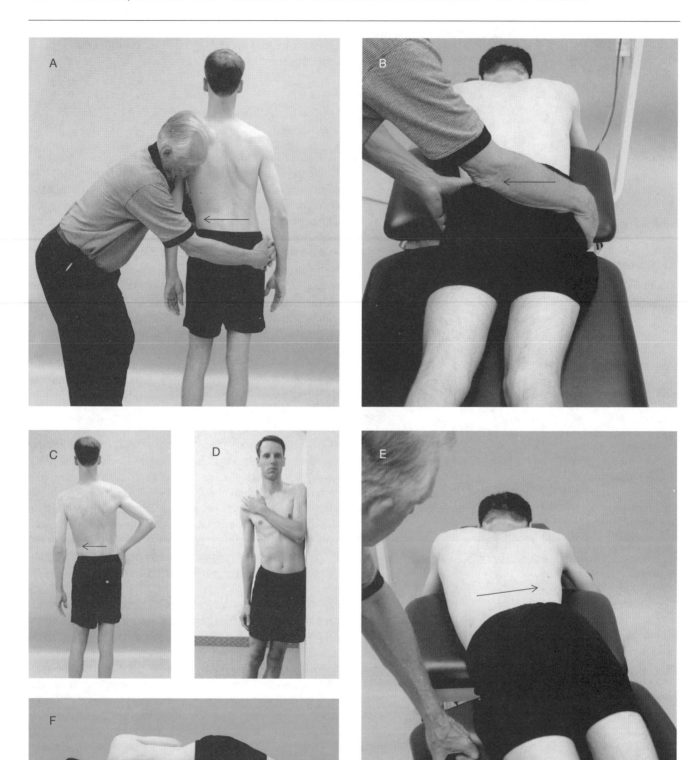

Figure 5-13: Various ways to correct a lateral shift. A, B and C) Correction of a left lateral shift; D and E) Overcorrecting a left lateral shift (patient is now in a right lateral shift); and F) Overcorrecting a right lateral shift (patient is now in a left lateral shift) Overcorrection is acceptable and often desirable, as long as the patient tolerates it without an increase in peripheral symptoms.

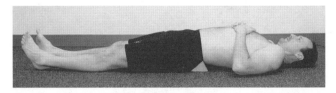

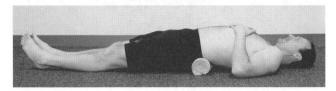

Figure 5-15: Passive extension in supine with a wedge or tightly rolled towel under the stiff segments. This is a good technique for the patient who is stiff in the lower lumbar segments but who has normal or hypermobility in the upper lumbar area.

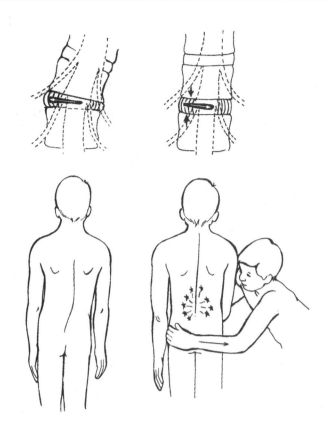

Figure 5-14: Disc mechanics with lateral shift correction (mild to moderate bulge).

keeping his hand on his hip. Working in front of a mirror also helps the patient achieve a proper correction.

When the lateral shift has been successfully corrected or if the patient does not have a lateral shift, the next step in treatment of the mild to moderate disc protrusion is passive extension exercises. Passive extension exercises are usually started in the prone position and are progressed to the standing position as tolerated. These exercises are illustrated in Chapter 14, *Basic Spinal Exercise*.

The first passive extension exercise simply consists of lying prone on a hard surface for a few minutes. This may not be necessary except for the very acute patient with a severely forward bent posture. The second passive extension exercise is the *elbow prop*, where the patient simply props on the elbows while relaxing the lower back. As described above, a three-dimensional mobilization table can be used in the clinic to achieve passive extension.

As the patient progresses with the passive extension exercises, he begins to do the passive press-ups. The stomach and back muscles must be completely relaxed as the patient pushes himself into an arched position. The patient is encouraged to do this exercise five to ten times,

several times a day. It should be noted that many patients have stiffness in the lower two lumbar segments but normal or hypermobility in the upper lumbar spine. The elbow prop and press-up exercises will not be effective with these patients. Instead, they will first require lower lumbar mobilization techniques to equalize lumbar segmental mobility. At home, they should stretch the lower lumbar spine into extension by lying supine over a wedge or tightly rolled towel placed over in the stiff area until they can properly perform prone extension (Fig 5-15). This technique ensures that the extension mobility is occurring where it is most needed — at the stiff segments.

Often, this program will cause the patient to have dramatic relief of the leg pain and it is natural for the patient to become enthusiastic about doing the program because of the success achieved. However, the patient should be cautioned to avoid overexertion because the back may become very sore. This, in turn, may cause increased muscle guarding and work against the patient's overall progress. It is better to do the exercises gently but very frequently throughout the day than to do the exercises vigorously only once or twice a day.

As soon as the patient has had success with the passive extension exercises in prone or supine, he can begin to do them in the standing position. Again, the patient is encouraged to do this exercise several times a day. It is very important to remember that if there is a lateral shift, it must be corrected before extension is done.

Figure 5-16 shows what is believed to happen when the patient can do passive extension exercises without increasing the peripheral signs. Indeed, Shah has demonstrated that the nucleus moves posteriorly with flexion and anteriorly with extension on a fresh cadaver specimen (Fig

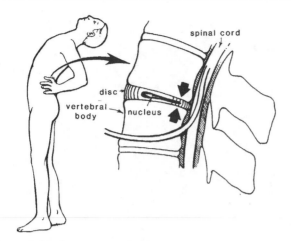

Figure 5-16: Disc mechanics with extension exercise (mild to moderate bulge).

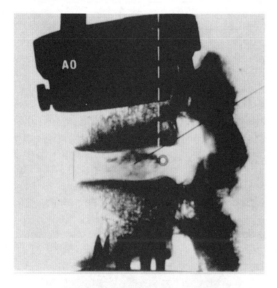

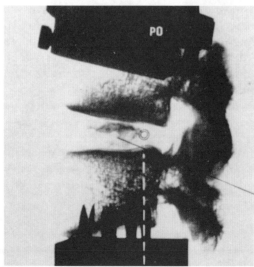

Figure 5-17: Shah's work demonstrates posterior movement of the nucleus with flexion and anterior movement with extension.[72]

5-17).[72] The patient must be given clear instructions and must be able to visualize the purpose of the corrective exercises.

To move the nucleus anteriorly, the patient must be taught to maintain the lordosis at all times and hold it there until healed. This means that sitting should generally be avoided and a lumbosacral corset or a lumbar roll must be used at all times when the patient must sit (Fig 5-18). The purpose of these external supports is to maintain and support the lordosis and to remind the patient to avoid lumbar flexion and instead bend forward at the hip joints. Many different types and densities of lumbar rolls and cushions are available. The therapist should keep several samples in the clinic to enable individualized selection for each patient.

Patient instructions for acute stages of HNP-protrusion consist of the following points:

- Maintain lordosis at all times.
- Avoid flexing the lumbar spine as it will stretch the supporting structures of the back and lead to further weakening.
- When in acute pain, sit as little as possible, and then only for short periods of time.
- While sitting, sit with a lordosis. This can be accomplished by placing a supportive roll in the small of the back.
- Bend at the hip joints, not at the back.
- Try to sit on a firm, high-backed chair if possible.
- Avoid sitting on low, soft chairs or couches.
- When rising from a sitting position, maintain lumbar lordosis.
- When in acute pain, drive as little as possible.
- When driving a car, keep the seat close enough to the steering wheel to allow maintenance of the lordosis.
- When in acute pain, avoid all bending and lifting.
- If lifting cannot be avoided, use correct lifting techniques.
- When coughing or sneezing, stand up, bend slightly backwards and increase the lordosis to lessen the strain.[52]

The patient must absolutely avoid positions and activities that increase the intradiscal pressure or that cause a posterior force on the nucleus (flexion exercises, forward bending and slumped sitting). Exercises, mobilization or activities involving rotation must be avoided initially for two reasons. First, rotation causes a narrowing of the intervertebral space and produces increased intradiscal pressure.[59] Also, as rotation of the spine occurs, there is a relaxation of $1/2$ of the oblique annular fibers while the other $1/2$ are drawn taut. This

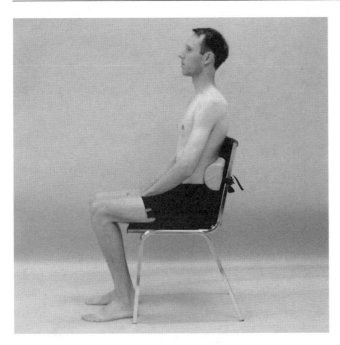

Figure 5-18: A lumbar roll encourages proper lordosis when sitting.

puts the disc in a vulnerable position for injury. When rotation exercise is initiated, the supine position should be used to eliminate the compressive force of gravity. Eventually, standing and sitting rotation exercises can be done.

There must be strict compliance with this program for two to ten weeks. The severity of the disorder and the initial success the patient has with the treatment program will determine the speed of recovery. There is evidence that healing of the disc can occur.[15,24,28,38,77] The key is to reduce the bulge and allow the disc to heal so that the scar formed will protect from further protrusion.[52] It is important to emphasize to the patient that one can recover from a disc injury and that healing can and will take place. Teaching the patient that the nucleus will become more fibrous with age and will therefore naturally tend to stabilize is important for the patient's confidence.

Additional treatment should be directed at pain relief and restoration of function and mobility. Modality therapy may relieve pain, which will reduce muscle guarding. Since spinal muscle guarding is a compressive force on the disc, it is important to control such guarding. Traction may also effectively reduce the bulge and is important to add if the patient is progressing slowly or improvement has plateaued.[11,50,61] A support or corset may allow the patient to participate in more pain free activities, aid postural correction and reduce compressive forces on the disc.[56,58]

Patients with HNP-protrusion lose range of motion because of the bulge itself but may also become restricted because of scarring and thickening of collagen tissue in and around the disc and the facet joints (joint hypomobility). Restoration of full mobility is a necessary component of treatment as soon as the protrusion is stable. Passive extension and flexion exercises, joint mobilization and traction are indicated if mobility is restricted. A particularly helpful technique is to passively extend the patient to the level of restriction using a three dimensional mobilization table and apply P/A mobilizations to the restricted segment(s). Later, the active back strengthening exercises described in Chapter 14 should be used to increase spinal strength and further promote correct posture. Finally, many of the rehabilitation techniques described in Chapter 15 should be implemented.

Mild to Moderate Cervical HNP-Protrusion (Without Spinal Nerve Root Involvement) Findings

In the cervical spine, HNP-protrusion without nerve root involvement is seen less commonly or, at least, the clinical picture is less well defined. The patient with a mild to moderate cervical HNP-protrusion will usually report increased pain with sitting and with neck flexion. Standing and walking will tend to lessen the symptoms. As the condition worsens, a progression of pain from central to peripheral (neck to shoulder to arm) is seen. Interscapular symptoms corresponding to Cloward's areas (see Chapter 4, *Evaluation of the Spine*) can help identify a particular disc level. The patient will often lack extension, but extension will cause increased central pain and decreased peripheral pain. A forward head posture is almost always present. Often, postural correction will increase central cervical pain but decrease peripheral pain (Fig 5-19).

Mild to Moderate Cervical HNP-Protrusion (Without Spinal Nerve Root Involvement) Treatment

Treatment is directed toward: 1) Returning the patient to normal posture and flexibility; and 2) Maintaining correct posture to allow the disc to heal. This is accomplished by starting with the head back, chin in exercises shown in Chapter 14, *Basic Spinal Exercise,* and progressing to cervical extension exercises. Normal cervical lordosis must be maintained. This requires a fiber or feather pillow that can be shaped to maintain the desired amount of support while sleeping. Solid foam pillows are not recommended because some muscular tension is required to maintain the head position and the solid foam does not conform adequately to the natural cervical lordosis.

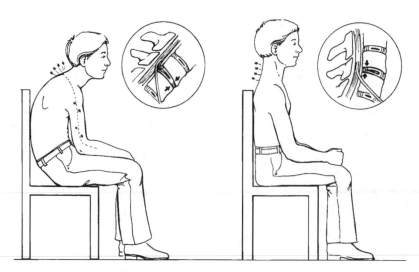

Figure 5-19: For the patient with cervical HNP-protrusion, treatment is directed toward normalizing posture. Often, posture correction increases central neck pain but decreases peripheral symptoms if the bulge is mild to moderate.

As the patient improves, full flexibility and strength must be restored. Since slumped sitting is often associated with forward head posture, a lumbar roll to improve posture and exercises to strengthen the postural muscles are often necessary.

Moderate to Severe Lumbar HNP-Protrusion (With Spinal Nerve Root Involvement) Findings

HNP-protrusion with nerve root involvement is described as a condition in which the nucleus is bulging but is still contained within the annulus or posterior longitudinal ligament. The bulge is large enough to encroach into the spinal canal or the intervertebral foramen and impinge upon or irritate the nerve root.

The patient with mild to moderate lumbar HNP-protrusion was presented earlier. This patient was a candidate for lateral shift correction and extension exercises because when these were attempted, there was no increase in *peripheral* symptoms. Now, however, the protrusion is larger and may be bulging beyond the posterior edge of the vertebral bodies. Thus, attempts to correct the lateral shift and to perform extension exercises increase the peripheral signs and symptoms. In other words, the patient has exactly the same disorder that was presented earlier, but the protrusion is simply larger and is probably pinching or irritating the nerve root (Fig 5-20). When this is the case, traction and other management techniques may be necessary before lateral shift correction and extension principles are applied.

Figure 5-21 shows the bulge in relation to the nerve roots. In nearly all cases, the bulge will encroach upon the nerve root that is descending in the spinal canal to make its exit at the segmental level *below* the bulge. An L5-S1 bulge

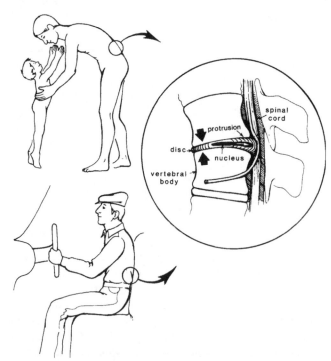

Figure 5-20: The moderate to severe herniated disc. Disc mechanics with forward bending and slumped sitting. Note that the bulge is touching the nerve root.

impinging upon the S1 nerve root is the most common example. While it is possible that the bulge can encroach upon the nerve root that is making its exit at the same level as the bulge, this is unusual. If such is the case, the bulge is usually medial and inferior to the nerve root. It is important to understand the relationship of the bulge to the nerve roots because this provides another explanation of why a patient may develop a lateral scoliosis.

Finneson theorizes that if the bulge lies lateral to the nerve root, the patient may shift to the opposite side to take the nerve root away from the bulge. When the bulge is medial to the nerve root, the patient may shift toward the side of the symptoms. Finneson calls this phenomenon *protective scoliosis*.[17] The patient with a bulge medial to the nerve root may have a painful straight leg raise on the side contralateral to the bulge. One can see that any attempt to correct the protective scoliosis will cause the nerve root to be forced back onto the bulge, which would probably increase peripheral signs and symptoms. If conventional traction with a straight pull is attempted, the spine will straighten, which will cause increased peripheral signs and symptoms. Therefore, unilateral or three-dimensional traction should be performed to preserve the protective scoliosis. See Chapter 12, *Spinal Traction*, for specific techniques.

Figure 5-22 and Figure 5-23 show what may happen when correction of a lateral shift or extension is attempted with a large protrusion. As these maneuvers are attempted, some of the disc material may be trapped instead of reduced. This is likely to cause increased pressure on the annulus as the bulge protrudes further, so peripheral signs and symptoms will increase. In any case, if lateral shift correction or extension causes increased peripheralization of signs and symptoms, further attempts to do these maneuvers should be stopped.

The patient will have all the signs and symptoms of an HNP-protrusion previously discussed, with the addition of positive neurological signs and symptoms such as strength loss, decreased muscle stretch reflexes, loss of sensation and a positive straight leg raise test. An x-ray may now show a narrowed disc space. As discussed, attempts to correct a lateral shift or to implement extension exercises may increase peripheralization of symptoms. Also, spinal flexion in the recumbent position may afford relief of some symptoms.

Occasionally, the onset is sudden with no previous history of spinal pain, but it is more common to see disc herniation with signs of nerve root involvement as a gradually worsening condition that first appears without nerve root involvement.

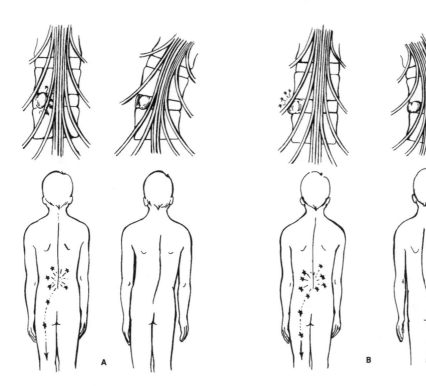

Figure 5-21: Protective scoliosis. A) The bulge is lateral to the nerve root it is encroaching upon, so the patient achieves relief by leaning away from the symptoms; B) The bulge is medial to the nerve root it is encroaching upon, so the patient achieves relief by leaning toward the symptoms.

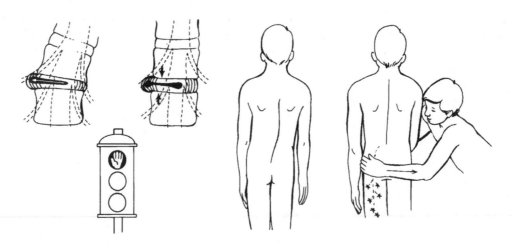

Figure 5-22: The moderate to severe herniated disc. Disc mechanics with lateral shift correction.

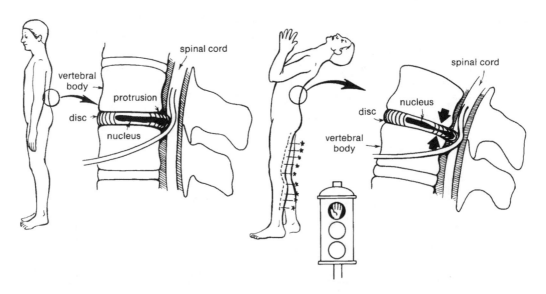

Figure 5-23: The moderate to severe herniated disc. Disc mechanics with standing lumbar extension.

Moderate to Severe Lumbar HNP-Protrusion (With Spinal Nerve Root Involvement) Treatment

In the past, conservative treatment of HNP-protrusion in the United States consisted of flexion positions, flexion exercises, bed traction and rest. It is now evident that flexion positions and exercises are potentially harmful for the patient with HNP-protrusion.[9,34,52,59,72]

However, there are some reasons why the recumbent flexed posture may give the very acute disc patient some relief. If the spine is flexed, the posterior wall of the annulus is drawn taut, which could very well take the bulge off the nerve root (Fig 5-24). This posture may afford the patient some initial relief, but it causes anterior disc compression and theoretically stops the disc from returning to its normal position. Nachemson has shown that flexed positions increase intradiscal pressure and decrease overall intradiscal space.[59]

If the patient is in an acute state of pain with muscle guarding and spasm, the flexed, recumbent posture may be necessary *initially* to allow relief. The recumbent position eliminates the compressing force of gravity when compared to sitting or standing postures, and slight flexion provides a mild stretch to the lumbar musculature. Since the patient is often medicated while undergoing this type of treatment, all of these combined factors may give the patient considerable relief.

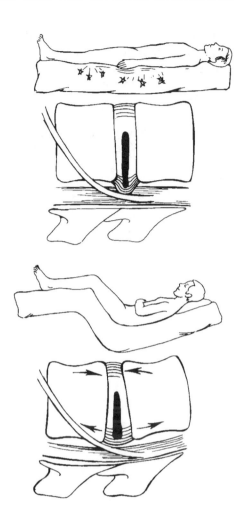

Figure 5-24: The effect of supine flexion on a disc protrusion that is touching the nerve root. Flexion draws the bulge away from the nerve root. In the long-term, however, it further stretches the posterior annulus and encourages greater disc protrusion.

Despite the potential relief it can give, the flexed position is not productive in the long run and should only be used for the very acute patient. Once some pain relief is accomplished, attempts should be made to bring the patient out of the flexed posture and to restore the normal lordosis (extension principles).

At the same time the Americans were treating HNP-protrusion with flexion, bed traction and rest, Dr. James Cyriax and other English, European and Scandinavian clinicians were using a different approach. In 1950, Cyriax reported that at St. Thomas Hospital in London the laminectomy rate for HNP patients had fallen from 1 in 40 to 1 in 200. In an article published in the British Medical Journal, he advocated sustained, prone pelvic traction of up to 300 pounds for 10-20 minutes as the treatment of choice for her-

niated disc. After the traction reduced the bulge, he stated that the patient should be locked into an exaggerated hyperlordosis with a back brace until the disc was healed.[11] Parson and Cummings advocated a similar protocol.[64]

Subsequent studies by Mathews,[49] Gupta and Ramarao[25] and Onel, et al[61] have demonstrated radiographic and clinical improvement using high forces of traction, suggesting that traction causes a suction force on the bulging nucleus. Additionally, a study by Nachemson showed that a traction load of 30 kg caused a reduction in intradiscal pressure from 30 to 10 kg in the L3 intervertebral disc.[57]

When a protective scoliosis is present, traditional traction techniques may cause the spine to straighten, forcing the nerve root onto the disc bulge. Traction may still be indicated, but the technique used must preserve the protective scoliosis. In other words, unilateral or three-dimensional traction is necessary in these cases to apply the traction force without straightening the spine.[69] Traction studies and techniques are discussed more thoroughly in Chapter 12, *Spinal Traction*.

If a protrusion is reduced with traction, it is still unstable and the patient must not aggravate the condition for a time. It must be emphasized that traction alone is usually ineffective and that a total treatment regimen must be followed or the patient will not achieve a lasting benefit. As with all the previously discussed treatments and techniques, if traction increases peripheral signs and symptoms, it must be modified or discontinued.

Total management usually involves passive extension exercises as soon as they can be done without increasing peripheral signs and symptoms. In other words, if the traction successfully reduces the extent of the bulge, the patient may then become a candidate for extension exercises and extension principles. At the very least, attempts should be made to restore the normal lordosis as the patient is able. Sometimes, passive extension principles can begin immediately after the first traction treatment. Often, however, patients are slow to return to the passive extension exercises, but they do respond well to sitting with a lumbar roll and attempting to increase their lordosis gradually when sitting or standing. Obviously, they should avoid slumped sitting and forward bending completely at this stage.

A lumbosacral corset that compresses the abdomen can decrease intradiscal pressure, causing disc unloading in both the standing and sitting positions. If the corset has steel stays, the stays should be bent into a normal or hyperlordotic position and the patient should be instructed to maintain that posture at all times. The corset is also helpful because it reminds the patient to avoid forward bending and slumped sitting and to maintain good posture.

The treatment considerations for HNP-protrusion can be summed up as follows:

1. Relieve compressive forces
2. Reduce herniation
3. Maintain correction
4. Rehabilitate

When combined with a comprehensive educational program, these principles can be effective in treating moderate to severe protrusions. Usually, one will know within a few treatments if this program will be effective for a particular patient, but it may be 6-10 weeks before the patient can return to strenuous activities, especially those involving forward bending or prolonged sitting.

For the first two or three weeks, the lumbosacral corset is used at all times when the patient is up. The patient is gradually weaned from the lumbosacral corset and may then begin using a more active back support or none at all. An active back support (see Fig 13-17 on page 337) can allow more comfortable exercise and function sooner, which ultimately benefits the patient. Back strengthening and stabilization exercises should begin as soon as the patient can perform them without increasing peripheralization of symptoms. The patient should start these exercises carefully and gradually build into a vigorous back strengthening program. Tight hamstring muscles can prevent the pelvis from flexing over the hip joint during forward bending, causing increased stress on the disc. If the patient has tight hamstrings, stretching becomes a vital part of the rehabilitation program. Eventually, overall physical fitness for the improvement of flexibility, strength and endurance should become the goal of this total program. Surgical intervention may be indicated if this management program fails and if there are signs of progressive neurological deficits or loss of bowel or bladder function. In certain cases, however, a "wait and see" attitude is justified because spontaneous regression of HNP has been documented.[15,24,28,38,77]

Moderate to Severe Cervical HNP-Protrusion (With Spinal Nerve Root Involvement) Findings

The clinical picture of cervical HNP-protrusion with nerve root involvement is usually one of gradual worsening with the symptoms starting centrally at the base of the neck, and then spreading to the shoulder and the arm as the condition worsens. Pain is also referred to the upper thoracic spine. Interscapular pain corresponding to Cloward's areas may be found. Later, positive neurological signs appear.

The slumped, forward head posture is usually seen with HNP-protrusion and attempts to correct the posture or to perform extension of the cervical spine increase the peripheral signs and symptoms because the protrusion is too large to be reduced with this maneuver and irritation or impingement of the cervical nerve root occurs (Fig 5-25).

Cervical nerve root impingement is most common at the C5-C6 segment and involves the C6 nerve root. In many cases, cervical nerve root impingement is caused by degenerative joint/disc disease rather than by disc protrusion. Often, an x-ray, CT/MRI scan or myelogram may be necessary to determine the diagnosis. The x-ray may be normal or may show very slight narrowing of the disc space. This is a clue that one is dealing with HNP-protrusion rather

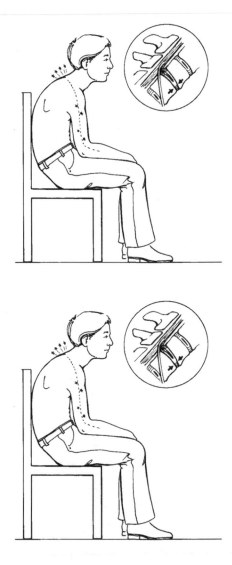

Figure 5-25: For the patient with moderate to severe cervical HNP-protrusion, attempts to normalize posture cause increased peripheral symptoms.

than degenerative joint/disc disease. Degenerative joint/disc disease significant enough to cause neurological signs will usually cause more significant changes in the radiological exam.

The following differentiation test helps distinguish nerve root irritation due to HNP-protrusion from nerve root irritation due to encroachment within the neural foramen. Cervical compression with the neck in slight flexion will reproduce symptoms if HNP-protrusion is causing the patient's symptoms. Cervical compression with the neck in slight extension will reproduce symptoms if the nerve root is being impinged in the neural foramen. Age is also a consideration, since HNP usually occurs in relatively younger people (25-45 year-olds).

Moderate to Severe Cervical HNP-Protrusion (With Spinal Nerve Root Involvement) Treatment

Treatment goals are to reduce the protrusion with traction and maintain the correction by restoring normal posture until the disc heals. Initial attempts to restore normal posture may be unsuccessful unless combined with traction. Manual traction combined with passive axial extension and/or passive backward bending exercises is often effective (see Chapter 12, *Spinal Traction*). Mechanical traction can also be used, particularly if the device allows for adjustable angles of pull and a unilateral technique.

If initial attempts at traction do not relieve the patient's peripheral pain, the therapist should try to modify the angle of pull. Sometimes, a little more flexion or a slight lateral angle may achieve the desired results. As improve-

ment is noted, the angle of pull should be reduced to regain normal posture. When the patient is able to perform posture correction and flexibility exercises without exacerbation of peripheral symptoms, he can be weaned from traction and progressed to more advanced flexibility and strengthening exercises.

HNP-Extrusion/Sequestration Findings

HNP-extrusion is defined as the disorder in which the displaced nuclear material extrudes into the spinal canal through disrupted fibers of the annulus (Fig 5-26). HNP-sequestration involves the escape of nuclear material into the spinal canal as free fragments that may migrate to other locations.

Patients with an extrusion or sequestration will have similar histories, signs and symptoms as patients with HNP-protrusion except that the peripheral signs and symptoms will probably predominate.[53] Symptoms are often unpredictable. They may change suddenly, become intermittent or follow an inexact or incomplete dermatomal pattern. The patient will often have a gradually worsening history, beginning with HNP-protrusion without nerve root signs and symptoms, progressing to HNP-protrusion with nerve root signs and symptoms, and finally to HNP-extrusion or sequestration. At this stage, there is no longer pressure on the annular wall and the pain arising from the disc bulge itself will be diminished while the signs and symptoms of nerve root irritation or impingement may be increased. In other words, at the extrusion/sequestration stage, the patient's back pain may be gone and sitting may be comfortable.

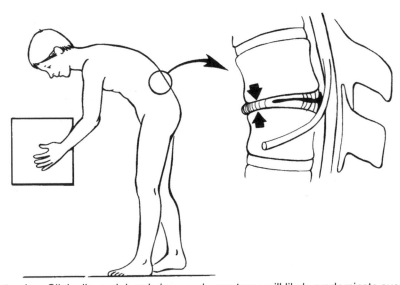

Figure 5-26: HNP-extrusion. Clinically, peripheral signs and symptoms will likely predominate over central symptoms.

HNP-Extrusion/Sequestration Treatment

No particular form of physical therapy treatment is effective at this stage except, perhaps, electrotherapy and other modalities for pain relief. Flexion exercises and the flexed recumbent position may afford relief but will not be of lasting benefit and could theoretically cause further extrusion of nuclear material. If extension causes increased *peripheral* signs and symptoms, it is contraindicated, but if extension principles can be applied without increasing the peripheral signs and symptoms, they should be cautiously implemented. Restoring and maintaining normal lordosis may close the defect in the annulus, giving the disc a better chance to heal. A lumbosacral corset should be used to help reduce intradiscal loading and to remind the patient to avoid forward bending and slumped sitting. Surgery is not always necessary because these disorders have been shown to regress spontaneously.[38] Rehabilitative exercise should be implemented as the patient's symptoms stabilize (stop worsening). After 7-10 weeks, the exercise can often get very aggressive. Even if some of the activities cause increased pain, the patient should begin to gradually work through the pain. However, if there are signs of progressive neurological involvement, a less aggressive approach or surgical intervention may be indicated.

Clinically, one occasionally sees what appears to be an extruded or sequestered disc (predominance of peripheral signs and symptoms) respond well to a combination of traction and extension principles. This causes one to conclude that the condition may have only been a protrusion and points out the importance of a trial of traction and extension principles in all such cases. In other words, one cannot be certain clinically whether a condition is a disc protrusion, extrusion or sequestration and the trial of good quality conservative care helps establish the final diagnosis.

Post-Laminectomy/Discectomy/ Chemonucleolysis

Long-term results from laminectomy/discectomy and chemonucleolysis are very often disappointing. Several follow-up studies of patients who underwent disc surgery show that 30-50% of patients had no improvement or were worse than they were before the operation.[23,43,66,66,81,85] An up to 20% reoperation rate has been reported.[35] The unimpressive results may be because little or no attention was directed toward restoring normal posture, flexibility, strength and physical fitness. Often, nothing is done to educate or motivate the post-surgical patient about proper body mechanics or other lifestyle changes that will be necessary to have a reasonably healthy back following surgery. The surgical procedure may remove or dissolve the disc herniation, but it does nothing to correct the poor

posture; faulty body mechanics; stressful living and working habits; loss of strength and flexibility; and poor physical fitness—the real causes of the problem.

There is support for comprehensive, and even aggressive, exercise rehabilitation following disc herniation surgery.[12,14,37,62] Therefore, a full rehabilitation program should be implemented for all patients who have had surgery. Gentle straight leg raise to prevent nerve root adhesions and dural tightness should be implemented quite soon in the rehabilitation process. Gentle stretching can even begin while the patient is still in the hospital. The patient should also be instructed in restoration and maintenance of normal posture (extension principles) and should eventually be instructed in a full flexibility, strengthening and fitness program, as well as a complete back care educational program.

Sometimes patients who have had previous back surgery begin to have signs and symptoms indicating that another disc disorder is developing. In such cases, the treatment protocol need not be altered because the patient has had surgery. The only exception is the patient who has had a recent (within one year) spinal fusion or a complete laminectomy. In these cases, the surgeon should be consulted about specific treatment before proceeding.

Radiculopathy and Other Neural Conditions

Radiculopathy is a disorder involving compression, impingement, irritation or inflammation of the spinal nerve root. Many terms are used to describe radiculopathy, and for the purposes of this chapter we will consider the following terms synonymous: *nerve root compression, nerve root syndrome, neuritis* and *neuropathy*. Radiculopathy is characterized by the presence of true neurological signs and symptoms.

As previously discussed, referred pain may arise from any pain-sensitive structure in the spine. It can be felt along the general distribution of the nerve roots involved. Referred pain alone is certainly not a true neurological finding. Nerve root pain tends to be felt as a deep, burning pain that is specific to one spinal nerve root sensory distribution, whereas referred pain is felt as a superficial aching pain that is somewhat more diffuse, tending to cover two or three dermatomes. For example, if one is experiencing referred pain because of a mild to moderate L5-S1 disc protrusion, the pain may be felt in the sensory distribution of both the L5 and S1 spinal nerves. This is because branches of the recurrent sinuvertebral nerve from both the L5 and S1 levels supply the L5-S1 disc. If a disc protrusion at the L5-

S1 level is impinging or irritating the S1 nerve root, the nerve root pain produced is specific to the S1 sensory distribution. Of course, in the latter example, referred pain would also be present along with the spinal nerve root pain.

Mooney and Robertson found that injection of hypertonic saline solution into a lower lumbar facet joint produced local and referred pain that radiated distally in a pattern corresponding to the dermatomal distribution of the adjacent spinal nerve roots (posterior buttock and thigh).[55] Similar pain patterns have been demonstrated by injecting irritants into spinal muscles, interspinous ligaments and the intervertebral disc.[27,28,29,32,33,67,79] Mooney and Robertson also have found increased myoelectrical activity in the hamstring muscles, painful straight leg raising and depressed quadriceps muscle stretch reflexes to be associated with the referred pain stimuli. Upon injection of a local anesthetic into the appropriate soft tissue or facet joints, these findings returned to normal. Based on their work, painful straight leg raising and quadriceps reflex changes alone do not implicate the nerve root as a source of the symptoms. Instead, specific motor weakness or specific dermatomal sensory loss is required to definitively diagnose nerve root involvement.[55]

Radiculopathy Findings

Radiculopathy is often caused by moderate to severe HNP-protrusion or advanced degenerative joint/disc disease or lateral stenosis. Other less common causes of radiculopathy include congenital anomalies, tumors and fractures. The patient with radiculopathy will have true neurological signs (numbness, weakness and reflex changes). The basic ULTT has been shown to be a useful differentiation test for cervical radiculopathy when used along with cervical range of motion, distraction and Spurling's tests.[86]

When radiculopathy is present, the clinician should attempt to determine its probable cause (e.g., HNP vs. lateral stenosis or DDD) because the treatment techniques chosen will be different.

Radiculopathy Treatment

The treatment for radiculopathy caused by moderate to severe HNP was previously described and will not be repeated here (see *Moderate to Severe Lumbar HNP-Protrusion (With Spinal Nerve Root Involvement) Treatment* on page 112).

When radiculopathy is caused by lateral stenosis or DDD, its treatment is the same as described in *Degenerative Joint/Disc Disease Treatment* on page 100, except that caution should be used with mobilization techniques and

aggressive exercises to avoid increasing nerve root irritation. If mobilization is desired, traction is likely to cause less irritation than manual mobilization techniques. If the traction force is directed specifically to the side of greatest hypomobility with a unilateral technique or three-dimensional table, traction can be even more effective.

Since many patients with radiculopathy caused by DDD are restricted in both spinal flexion and extension, exercises to increase mobility in both directions are indicated, provided they do not aggravate the nerve root. In the past, many practitioners avoided extension exercises because they believed that extension would close the foramen, further irritating the nerve. While it is true that extension does close the foramen in a normal, healthy spine, it is questionable whether the foramen closes at a spinal segment where there is already narrowing of the disc space and the facet joints are already in their maximum close packed position (full extension).

If the facet joints are indeed in maximum extension, then further extension will take place about an axis at the facet joints themselves and actual widening may occur at the intervertebral foramen and disc spaces (Fig 5-27). Therefore, both flexion and extension exercises should be attempted with this disorder and those relieving the signs and symptoms should be used. Rotation and side bending are often tolerated fairly well and are helpful for regaining general mobility. Clinical experience shows the preferred

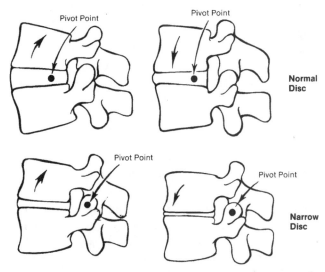

Figure 5-27: In a segment with a normal disc, flexion and extension occur about an axis slightly posterior to the nucleus. Therefore, flexion widens and extension narrows the intervertebral foramen. When a narrowed disc is present, flexion and extension may occur about an axis within the facet joint. Therefore, flexion may narrow and extension may widen the intervertebral foramen.

exercise program can only be determined by assessing each patient's individual reaction.

Nerve Root Adhesion Findings

Nerve root adhesion involves the spinal nerve root becoming entrapped by scar tissue. This disorder is also called dural adhesion or epidural fibrosis, and commonly occurs after spinal surgery. Some surgeons attempt to prevent adhesion formation by using an implantable material that acts as a resorbable barrier to adhesions. A program of passive straight leg raising starting the day after surgery and continuing until there is appreciable healing may also help preserve nerve mobility.

Nerve root adhesions may form following an episode of disc herniation. As the body attempts to heal the annular defect, collagen tissue is laid down. If the nerve root is lying close by, it may become entrapped by the scar tissue.

The patient with nerve root adhesion is likely to have had spinal surgery or a history of disc herniation or chronic spinal problems. The patient will probably retain some of the signs and symptoms of the original diagnosis, but may have had a period of complete recovery with a subsequent insidious onset of spinal or referred pain with or without positive neurological signs.

The main characteristic of nerve root adhesion is a marked restriction in standing lumbar flexion versus sitting or supine lumbar flexion, and a restricted straight leg raise or positive slump test. In other words, when the lumbar spine alone is flexed no restriction is present; the restriction is only evident when the spinal nerve is put on stretch and pulled through the intervertebral foramen. Other classical disc protrusion signs and symptoms, such as increased pain with sitting, are often absent.

Nerve Root Adhesion Treatment

Treatment for nerve root adhesion consists of gentle neural mobilization as described in the following section on treatment of adverse mechanical neural tension (AMNT) disorders. Unilateral lumbar traction is also beneficial to stretch the soft tissue around the nerve root. Prevention of adhesions via measures taken during surgery or with gentle passive straight leg raising exercises immediately post-surgery is important.

It should be noted that mobilization of the nerve root either by passive stretching or traction will cause a temporary increase in peripheral symptoms. This is an unfortunate but necessary result of the treatment itself. The symptoms should, however, subside quickly after the stretch is discontinued. If the stretch causes increased symptoms that last for more than a few seconds to minutes, indicating an *irritable* condition, it should be performed less strenuously. The patient should perform frequent, mild, prolonged stretching at home to complement the treatment performed in the clinic. Persistence is needed, as improvement is often slow. After the patient is familiar with the stretches, the majority of the treatment can be performed at home.

Adverse Mechanical Neural Tension Findings

Chapter 4, *Evaluation of the Spine*, contained a thorough discussion of AMNT theory and findings. To summarize, the therapist should test for AMNT when a patient presents with the following clinical picture:

1. Symptoms present in the spine, head or extremities
2. No neurological signs (true numbness, weakness or reflex changes)
3. No significant irritability present (the tests themselves may cause further irritation and should be approached cautiously when the patient describes a highly irritable condition)

Long-standing pins and needles in the upper or lower extremities is often a clue that AMNT may be present. The therapist should also test for AMNT in all neuromusculoskeletal patients before discharge to ensure proper neural tissue mobility. AMNT is present when a positive neural tension test is present. To review, the neural tension tests are the ULTT, the slump test, the straight leg raise, passive neck flexion and prone knee bend. An adherent nerve root is one condition that can cause AMNT, but neural tightness can result from any restriction from the spinal canal to the distal limbs.

Adverse Mechanical Neural Tension Treatment

Neural tissue is by nature highly irritable. Therefore, treatment of AMNT that causes irritability should be approached cautiously, and the treatment guidelines discussed in this section are classified according to whether the condition is irritable or non-irritable. The therapist should continually reassess the patient to determine the degree of aggressiveness with which the techniques can be applied. The therapist is cautioned to monitor and advise the patient to be aware of the possibility of latent symptom responses.

There are several other considerations that will help determine the amount and type of actual treatment. The therapist should consider and develop a clinical picture of the following:

- What are the site(s) of altered neural tissue mechanics?
- What are the specific neural tissues involved?
- What structures are juxtaposed with neural tissues along the neural tissue tract that could interfere with their normal mechanics?

Contraindications to neural tension testing and treatment include the following:

1. Irritable conditions
2. Inflammatory conditions
3. Spinal cord signs
4. Malignancy
5. Nerve root compression signs
6. Severe, unremitting, constant night pain
7. Neurological signs (includes true numbness, weakness or reflex changes)
8. Recent paresthesia/anesthesia
9. Active spinal motions easily provoke distal symptoms, paresthesia or anesthesia
10. Reflex sympathetic dystrophy

The goal of AMNT treatment is decreased symptoms and improved functional mobility of the neural structures. Butler suggests three related ways of treating neural tension problems through movement:[6]

Direct Mobilization.   Direct mobilization of the neural tissues is accomplished by reproducing the neural tension tests and their components and through joint mobilization techniques.

Related Tissue Treatment.   Related tissue treatment involves mobilization of the mechanical interfacing components of neural tension problems, which may include joints, muscles, fascia and skin interfaces. Techniques can involve soft tissue mobilization, joint mobilization, modalities and exercise.

Indirect Treatment.   This approach attempts to decrease the adverse effects of the patient's occupation and daily activities on the tissue components. Postural advice and ergonomic assessment are examples of indirect treatment approaches.

When using mobilization, successful treatment consists of many features. The therapist must develop the ability to feel or appreciate tissue resistance met during treatment, to assess the patient's symptom response and its relationship to movement, and to decide whether treatment should be strong or gentle. The therapist must continually reassess the patient and compare progress with the goals of decreased symptom response and improved functional mobility of the neural structures.

Butler states, "We can do much better than crudely stretching the nervous system."[6] Thus, it would seem appropriate that mobilization techniques traditionally used for the joints can apply to the neural tissues as well. Therefore, the graded joint mobilization and soft tissue mobilization terminology and techniques described in Chapters 10 and 11 can be adapted for mobilizing the neural tissues and their interfaces.

For example, a Grade 3 mobilization technique used in reference to a straight leg raise might involve the therapist flexing the patient's hip with the knee extended into the point where resistance is felt. A Grade 2 mobilization would stop short of the point where resistance is felt, and a Grade 4 mobilization would involve oscillation into resistance.

The treatment strategy will depend on whether or not the disorder is irritable, and to what degree it is irritable.

Irritable Problem.   The therapist may start by using a direct technique, but one that is well removed from the symptom area. For example, the therapist can use a straight leg raise or opposite limb ULTT initially to treat an acute cervical problem with right upper extremity neural tension symptoms. Initially, the techniques should be non-provoking. Suggested grades of treatment are the large amplitude, non-resistance Grade 2 mobilizations performed through range with minimal symptom provocation. It may be possible to eventually "sneak up" to resistance at a very conservative Grade 4 that gently nudges the resistance, as long as symptom responses are monitored. Gnawing, deep, constant pain should be avoided. Proper postural positioning allows the patient to be in a position of "ease" or pain relief. The patient can be taught to replicate the positioning used in the clinic for self-treatment at home.

When the problem becomes less irritable, the therapist can begin applying direct techniques to the symptom area using gentle techniques, starting with Grade 2 amplitude mobilizations. If we apply this to the previous example, the acute cervical problem with right upper extremity symptoms could be mobilized with Grade 2 right shoulder depression/elevation with the patient positioned comfortably supine. The cervical spine and distal limbs would be positioned to take the body off tension (i.e., right cervical side bending, right elbow flexion and pillows under knees). As the patient improves, tension onto the distal components of the ULTT can be progressively added (i.e., left cervical side bending, elbow extension, shoulder abduction, etc.).

Non-Irritable Problem.   Initially, techniques applied should be into the resistance, but should still stop short of symptom provocation. Grade 3 or 4 mobilizations can be used. If symptoms are provoked, they should resolve when the treatment is discontinued. Functional movements that vary from the test positions can be added. Tension onto distal components can be added, which better mimics function. For non-irritable problems, it is acceptable to provoke mild symptoms. The limiting factor is the clinician's clinical creativity. No two patients' signs and symptoms will be the same. However, some suggestions for treatment progression may be helpful for the clinician just learning to address AMNT treatment.

1. Gradually increase the number of repetitions. Oscillatory mobilizations lasting 20-30 seconds may be a good starting point.
2. Gradually increase the amplitude of the technique. This may include adding more resistance until symptoms are reproduced.
3. Symptom response should continually be monitored. Asking the patient if the symptoms are changing or building during treatment is as important as similar questioning on follow-up visits. Latency should be monitored.
4. Treatment should progress to adding more tension to the system, while taking into account the irritability of the condition.
5. Muscle energy techniques offer a careful way to add tension to interfacing components in a controlled manner.
6. Soft tissue massage techniques can be applied to nerves, where accessible, and their surrounding myofascial tissues. The techniques should be applied with all applicable tissues under tension.
7. The importance of reassessment during and after treatment application and at follow-up visits should not be underestimated.

It is usually helpful and necessary to teach patients to perform self-mobilization at home, at work and during recreation. Symptoms should be monitored carefully to avoid an unnecessary flare-up or latent symptom response. Preventive self-stretches should then be considered for maintaining neural tissue mobility.

The definitive text on the subject of AMNT is Butler's *The Sensitive Nervous System.*[6] We highly recommend it to clinicians desiring a more advanced understanding of this topic.

Thoracic Outlet Syndrome Findings

When thoracic outlet compression syndrome (TOS) causes neurological symptoms, it can actually be thought of as a type of AMNT disorder. Thus, many of the treatment principles for neurological manifestations of TOS are similar to those presented in the AMNT discussion above. However, because TOS can cause arterial or venous symptoms as well as neurological symptoms, its treatment is discussed separately.

Thoracic outlet syndrome can involve compression or stretching of the subclavian artery, subclavian vein or the brachial plexus as they pass through the thoracic outlet. Neurological symptoms account for at least 90% of thoracic outlet compression problems,[39,78] which is why the evaluation and treatment of TOS must involve neural tension testing. Mechanical tissue interfaces where compression can occur include the area between the scalenus anticus and medius, between the clavicle and the 1st rib (or a cervical rib) or between the pectoralis minor and the ribs. Diagnostic tests can help the clinician differentiate where the compression is occurring, and how best to treat it.

Subjective findings may vary depending upon whether artery, vein or brachial plexus is being compressed. With arterial compression, the patient will report pain and fatigue that occur during activity and go away with rest. Often, symptoms will start distally and proceed proximally. In later stages, cold sensitivity may be present. Any signs of possible emboli, such as cyanosis in one or more fingers, are considered serious and require immediate medical attention.[39]

Venous compression may lead to edema, skin tightness, cyanosis, pain and fatigue. After activity, venous distention may be seen in the extremity. The edema should decrease after a change in the precipitous activity. If the edema does not diminish, it is a sign of a possible venous thrombosis and requires the attention of a physician for further evaluation.

Nerve compression causes various symptoms including pain, tingling or numbness that usually follow the C8-T1 dermatome. Symptoms in the C5 through C7 dermatomes are suggestive of cervical pathology and not thoracic outlet. Ulnar nerve symptoms are more common than median nerve symptoms.[39] Night pain is common.[39,53]

When arterial compression is present, positive objective findings may include any of the following: A positive Adson's test, costoclavicular test, hyperabduction test or Roo's test. If a patient complains of symptoms with a particular position or activity, the therapist should monitor the patient's radial pulse while attempting to reproduce the position or activity. Bilateral brachial blood pressure comparison showing a difference of more than 20-30 mm Hg is suspicious for arterial stenosis. Arteriography and other objective tests not readily available to most physical therapists can also point toward arterial stenosis.

Venous compression is diagnosed objectively through plethysmography and other medical diagnostic tests not available to the physical therapist. The presence of edema, skin tightness and cyanosis or venous distention after activity may indicate venous compression. When possible, the therapist should try to reproduce the position or activity that causes the symptoms. Other possible causes of peripheral vascular symptoms should be ruled out before a definitive diagnosis is made.

Diagnosis for brachial plexus compression in the thoracic outlet is primarily done through ruling out other pathology in the cervical spine and upper extremities that could cause similar symptoms.[39] Neurological symptom reproduction with neural tension tests (the basic ULTT and variations described by Butler)[6] is suggestive of thoracic outlet syndrome. Adson's test, the costoclavicular test, the hyperabduction test and Roo's test are performed primarily to check for arterial compression, but may also cause increased neurological symptoms suggestive of brachial plexus compression.

Thoracic Outlet Syndrome Treatment

If signs of possible venous or arterial emboli are present, the patient's condition should be considered serious and immediate medical attention is required. When the patient's symptoms are not serious, careful stretching into the direction of the restriction is indicated.

For example, the patient with a positive hyperabduction test should stretch into hyperabduction. The patient with a positive costoclavicular test should stretch the shoulders and anterior chest area. The stretches should be performed often (every one to two hours) but gently throughout the day. Symptom reproduction as a result of the stretching is acceptable, but not if it lasts for more than a few minutes after the stretch is discontinued. Patience is necessary to determine the right amount of stretching for a patient whose condition is very irritable.

For patients who present with positive neural tension tests, the treatment principles presented in that section apply. It is often beneficial to stretch tight adjacent structures. For example, the patient with TOS often has a generally tight upper and mid thoracic spine. Therefore, stretching the thoracic spine into extension and rotation can be very beneficial.

Simultaneously, the patient should begin strengthening the postural muscles. Forward head, rounded shoulder posture almost always accompanies thoracic outlet compression and is often its cause. For this reason, exercises encouraging proper posture are extremely important, particularly those encouraging interscapular, lumbar and abdominal strengthening.

Mobilization techniques for tight thoracic segments or for the 1st rib are often highly beneficial. Soft tissue stretching is also beneficial but does not substitute for the patient's diligence with a home stretching program. Cervical traction is usually not beneficial and may be contraindicated.[39]

The patient must be taught early on that TOS usually takes several weeks or months to resolve. Careful, consistent attention to the patient's home exercise program is necessary for long-term resolution. In some cases, surgical resection of a cervical rib or other surgical release techniques can be successful. However, successful surgical management must include patient education and exercise to prevent factors such as poor posture, repetitive activities and poor ergonomic conditions from causing the patient's symptoms to recur.

Miscellaneous Disorders

Congenital Abnormalities

Congenital conditions can include lumbarized sacral vertebrae, sacralized lumbar vertebrae, asymmetry of the facet joints or other congenital anomalies. The clinical signs and symptoms of these conditions are quite varied and do not seem to present a clear clinical picture that can be consistently related to a definable pathological disorder. In other words, it is difficult to determine the real clinical significance of many of these congenital anomalies.

We believe that, except as these anomalies contribute to joint hypermobility or hypomobility or perhaps to degenerative joint/disc disease, they are insignificant and are often unrelated to the patient's real problem. In fact, there is a certain danger in diagnosing the patient's condition purely by radiological findings when there is no direct cause and effect relationship established during the clinical assessment, because the patient may be less likely to take responsibility for lifestyle changes or an exercise program. One should always be on guard against the temptation to use one or two isolated findings as the basis for a diagnosis.

Traumatic Fractures

X-rays need not be taken of every patient who complains of spinal pain. However, when trauma is involved, a radiological exam is necessary to determine if a fracture is present. Spinal fracture management is outside the scope of practice for a physical therapist. When a spinal fracture has healed, however, it is important to evaluate strength, mobility and posture, and to rehabilitate the patient as needed.

Compression Fractures/Osteoporosis Findings

Although osteoporosis is associated with dorsal and lumbar spinal pain, it is not likely to cause symptoms by itself. Fractured vertebra and the resulting pressure on nerve roots or sensory fibers in the periosteum probably cause the pain associated with osteoporosis. Osteoporosis has many known causes; most are classified as post-menopausal and senile. Genetic abnormalities, nutritional dysfunctions, endocrine disorders, corticosteroids, pregnancy, prolonged immobilization, inactivity and weightlessness are all known causes of osteoporosis.[1,17]

Diagnosis of compression fracture is by x-ray. The patient will often have sharp pain with or without signs of nerve root compression. In the acute state the pain will be especially sharp with movement. Flexion of the spine is usually painful, harmful and should be avoided. A single thoracic compression fracture will be characterized by the presence of a prominent spinous process and a wide interspinous space below the prominent spinous process. Multiple thoracic compression fractures are characterized by progressive increase of kyphosis, which can eventually lead to severe disability.

Compression Fractures/Osteoporosis Treatment

In most cases, only the anterior portion of the vertebral body fractures, creating a wedge. If the posterior aspect of the body has fractured, an orthopedic surgeon must direct management. Therefore, the treatment principles discussed here apply to an anterior compression fracture only, with the posterior edge of the vertebral body structurally intact.

Conservative treatment involves educating the patient about positions and activities that are beneficial or potentially harmful.[1] The rule is to encourage positions or activities that promote spinal extension and avoid positions or activities that encourage flexion. In particular, the patient should avoid using large pillows under the head and sleeping in a flexed position. The patient should be taught how to roll to the side to get up from a recumbent position. Good lumbar support when sitting will help the patient avoid flexed sitting postures. Walking and other weight bearing activities will help prevent further demineralization of the bone. Active and passive extension exercises are indicated as soon as the patient's pain has decreased to the point of tolerance. All positions and activities involving spinal flexion must be avoided. Modalities

such as moist heat and electrical stimulation may relieve some of the pain.

A spinal brace or support is often helpful to manage acute compression fractures. The function of the brace or support is to help the patient maintain extension and to prevent flexion. The type of brace or support selected will vary from a rigid three-point hyperextension brace such as the Cash™ or Jewett® brace to a semi-rigid Taylor™-type brace or a dorsolumbar corset (see Chapter 13, *Spinal Orthoses*).

An older or senile patient with an osteoporotic compression fracture will probably not tolerate a rigid hyperextension or even a Taylor brace and may only be comfortable in a dorsolumbar corset. The dorsolumbar corset, of course, does not provide as much support but may be the only reasonable solution. In contrast, a younger patient with a traumatic compression fracture probably would need more rigid support and would tolerate a hyperextension brace well.

The hyperextension brace serves only one purpose — to prevent flexion. A corset or brace that provides circumferential support, however, will reduce vertical loading on the lumbar spine. Therefore, a lumbar compression fracture may be best managed with a support or brace that provides both abdominal compression and protection from flexion. A chair back or Taylor-type brace best serves this dual purpose.

Certain patients who are strong, alert and able to carefully maintain proper extension positions and postures and avoid flexion may only need to use a brace for a very short time or may not need a brace or support at all.

Newer surgical interventions involving kyphoplasty and vertebroplasty may be helpful for severe pain and to prevent vertebral collapse.[2,21,51] Percutaneous vertebroplasty involves injection of polymethylmethacrylate cement into the collapsed vertebra for pain relief without correction of the kyphotic deformity. Kyphoplasty involves inserting a bone tamp/balloon into the vertebral body under image guidance to actually reexpand the vertebra.

Spondylolysis/Spondylolisthesis Findings

Spondylolysis is a defect involving the pars interarticularis of the neural arch of the vertebra. When the defect in the neural arch is bilateral, separation of the anterior and posterior elements at the site of these defects may occur. This displacement is called spondylolisthesis. The most common site for occurrence is L5 on S1. There is almost certainly a congenital weakness associated with this disorder, and it is thought that the defect actually occurs as a stress fracture. Many people have spondylolysis or spondylolisthesis and are symptom free.

It is important to remember that once a diagnosis of this nature is made, the diagnosis may follow the patient and be implicated as the source of all symptoms. There may, however, be another cause for the patient's complaints.

Diagnosis is by x-ray, but clinically, a "step-off" of the spinous processes can sometimes be felt. The patient will often have hyperlordosis and complain that prolonged standing increases pain, sitting relieves it and various types of vigorous physical activities aggravate the condition. The original onset of symptoms can often be traced back to athletic or other vigorous physical activities during adolescence.

If a spondylolisthesis is the true cause of a patient's symptoms, it will probably be because the segment is unstable and aggravation is due to excessive movement and stress caused by physical activity.[63] If, on the other hand, a spondylolisthesis is stable, it will probably not be the source of the patient's complaint. If the spondylolisthesis is unstable, the patient frequently will describe a slipping or movement sensation in the back when assuming certain positions or performing certain activities. A joint noise may be present. Some patients learn to self mobilize to correct this. If the spondylolisthesis is unstable, a step-off can usually be palpated when the patient is standing and side lying, but it will disappear when the patient lies prone with pillows under the lumbar spine.

Spondylolysis/Spondylolisthesis Treatment

The presence of an unstable spondylolisthesis makes the patient more vulnerable to joint sprains and muscular strains, and such a patient may need to avoid heavy labor and vigorous physical activities. General postural improvement exercises are helpful, especially those aimed at abdominal muscle strengthening and trunk stabilization.[73] It is often necessary to fit the patient with a lumbosacral support or brace to be used when performing any activities that may aggravate the condition. A lumbosacral support or brace does not actually immobilize the involved segment, but may remind the patient to limit vigorous activity. A support or brace that provides abdominal compression will also help reduce vertical loading of the spine, which may further reduce aggravation due to physical activity.[58]

In a hyperlordotic state, or in the case of obesity and weak abdominal muscles, the vertical shear forces are greatly magnified. Reduction of the hyperlordosis via abdominal strengthening or the use of a back support can reduce the shear forces. Any type of support that helps reduce a protruding abdomen has the effect of moving the center of gravity posteriorly, thus reducing the lumbar lordosis.

Teen-agers indulging in contact sports and preteen children participating in sports requiring excessive lumbar lordosis (e.g., gymnastics) are more frequently found to have spondylolysis. Traumatic spondylolysis/spondylolisthesis should be suspected and ruled out in any physically active preteen or teenage patient who has persistent back pain for more than two or three weeks. An acute spondylolysis (stress fracture) may not be evident on x-ray and a bone scan or MRI may be necessary to make the diagnosis. When a break in the pars interarticularis is found on x-ray, a bone scan may demonstrate increased metabolic activity over the pars interarticularis, which represents a stress fracture. Bracing to reduce lumbar lordosis will help heal the stress fracture.[54] In patients whose scans are not "hot," the assumption is made that nonunion has resulted. If pain is a problem in these cases, a lumbar brace or support often provides relief.[17,18] During acute episodes, rest and modality treatments are also indicated. If the displacement is great enough there may be signs of neurological impingement of the cauda equina. In such cases, Cyriax advocates traction.[10] Surgical fusion may be necessary in severe cases.

Central Spinal Stenosis Findings

First, a note about *lateral* spinal stenosis: The term *lateral stenosis* refers to narrowing of the intervertebral foramen with resulting encroachment on a spinal nerve root. Lateral stenosis is usually the result of advanced degenerative joint disease and is significant because it is a major cause of radiculopathy. For information about the findings and treatment of radiculopathy, see page 117.

Encroachment upon the cervical spinal cord resulting from a stenotic cervical spinal canal is termed *central spinal stenosis* and may cause neurological symptoms that may be confused with multiple sclerosis or other neurological diseases.[74] There are a number of ways encroachment can occur. Annular protrusions of the cervical disc, osteophytes, folding or bulging of the ligamentum flavum, subperiosteal thickening over the vertebral body and the laminal arch and congenital smallness of the spinal canal are all factors. A combination of these factors is frequently involved.[74]

Lumbar central spinal stenosis is also known as neurogenic intermittent claudication of the cauda equina.

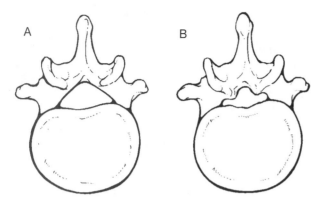

Figure 5-28: Central spinal stenosis. A) Normal spinal canal; and B) Narrowed spinal canal, i.e.,central stenosis.

Central spinal stenosis occurs much the same way in the lumbar spine as it does in the cervical spine in that it is usually associated with degenerative joint disease and a combination of factors that act together to diminish the size of the spinal canal (Fig 5-28). The ultimate mechanism producing the symptoms may be vascular insufficiency of the cauda equina nerve roots.[4]

In the cervical spine, mixed hyper and hypoactive reflexes are sometimes observed in the upper extremities, depending upon the level of encroachment. Hyperactive reflexes may be observed in the lower extremities. There may be paresthesia, pain and motor weakness in the extremities. Symptoms are aggravated by neck extension.

In the lumbar spine, the chief symptoms are pain in the lower back and one or both legs, numbness and tingling in the feet and legs, decreased muscle stretch reflexes and motor weakness in the legs. Often these symptoms are present only after walking and are relieved by rest or flexing the lumbar spine. Spinal extension decreases the volume of the lumbar spinal canal and increases nerve root bulk. Bulging of the ligamentum flavum is most pronounced in spinal extension. Therefore, it is easy to see why the symptoms are most pronounced when the patient is standing or lying flat with the lumbar spine extended.

The clinician should be aware that peripheral vascular disease (PVD) produces some of the same symptoms as lumbar central spinal stenosis. However, it does not cause back pain and is not relieved by spinal flexion. It is diagnosed by assessing peripheral circulation to the lower extremities.

Central Spinal Stenosis Treatment

Treatment centers around educating the patient to avoid aggravating or irritating the disorder. A soft collar or lumbar support is often helpful. Physical therapy modalities may provide temporary pain relief, but physical therapy interventions are not effective in correcting the causes or effects of the stenotic canal. A decompression laminectomy is indicated in severe cases.

Ankylosing Spondylitis Findings

Ankylosing spondylitis is characterized by progressive joint sclerosis and ligamentous ossification, which first appears in the sacroiliac joints and later spreads into the lumbar and thoracic spine and rib cage. In severe cases the cervical spine, hip and shoulder joints may also become involved. Complete ankylosis of the involved joints may eventually occur. Complete ankylosis eases pain, but may lead to disability depending upon the position the joints are in when they fuse. The younger the patient is at onset, the worse the prognosis; men usually do worse than women.[9]

Onset typically occurs between 20 and 35 years of age and first appears as a vague lower back pain and stiffness that is usually worse upon waking and eased by exercise. The symptoms are intermittent with episodes lasting for weeks or months at a time. The onset of each acute episode seems to be insidious, unrelated to exertion or activities.

Clinically, one sees a flattening of the lumbar lordosis and increased rounding of the thoracic and cervical spine. Since the two upper cervical joints are affected later, adaptive upper cervical hyperextension may occur. In severe cases, hip joint fusion may necessitate total hip replacement to avoid serious disability. Certain laboratory tests (e.g., elevated sedimentation rates) may be helpful in diagnosis. X-ray diagnosis may be possible only after several years, with the earliest abnormalities seen in the sacroiliac joint.[9,17]

Ankylosing Spondylitis Treatment

Patient education is of great importance. If the patient is young at onset, it is important to direct him toward a career that does not involve heavy work. It is best to tell the patient that the spine will eventually stiffen in a way that does not interfere with sedentary work, and that the pain is controllable.

A literature review supports the positive effects of physical therapy, particularly exercise.[83] Positioning and exercises to resist the gradual development of the flexed spine (and hip joints, in severe cases) play an important part. The patient must sleep on a firm mattress and should avoid lying curled up on his side or using more than one pillow when lying supine. Some prone lying is necessary and both passive and active extension exercises should be emphasized. Use of a lumbar roll (Fig 5-20) when sitting and avoidance of prolonged sitting and flexion postures is recommended. Mobilization to maintain spinal extension is also indicated and can often be taught to family members. Use of a lumbar support, medication and physical therapy modalities may be helpful during acute episodes.

Coccyx Injury Findings

Injury to the sacrococcygeal joint may occur as a sprain, subluxation or fracture. As healing occurs, the joint gradually becomes sclerosed and passive movement becomes restricted.[80] The classic patient will be one who has been to many doctors and has had very little help.

The patient will have a history of a fall directly on the coccyx or a childbirth injury. The x-ray may show a healed fracture. The patient will be unable to sit on both buttocks at the same time. The tip of the coccyx will be tender to palpate and coccyx mobility may be very limited or absent.

The normal coccyx flexes while sitting and extends when standing. When the coccyx is injured or subluxed, it may heal in the more extended position. If this happens, the soft tissue directly over the end of the coccyx develops a painful pressure point when the patient sits.

The coccyx can also be dislocated or fractured and heal in a flexed position or become fragmented or unstable in a flexed position. Palpating the position of the coccyx and testing the passive mobility of the sacrococcygeal joint can diagnose this disorder, or it may be diagnosed by radiological exam.

Coccyx Injury Treatment

Surgical removal of the coccyx may be indicated if it is hypermobile or dislocated in a *flexed* position. If the coccyx is hypomobile or subluxed and positioned in *extension*, the physical therapist can expect good results with ultrasound and passive mobilization along with other conservative management, such as a coccyx pillow.

Leg Length Inequality (LLI) Findings

Leg length inequalities are classified as either being structural (actual bony asymmetry due to fracture, growth abnormalities, coxa vara/valga, etc.) or functional (due to a pronated foot, genu valgus, tight adductor muscles, sacroiliac lesions, etc.). Leg length inequalities are included in the discussion of treatment of spinal disorders because of the frequent interrelationship between a leg length discrepancy and a functional asymmetry in the spine. One must determine the cause of the leg length discrepancy before deciding if the disorder can be treated.

The contribution of leg length inequality to low back pain and hip arthrosis remains controversial. One reason for the controversy is that LLI often escapes observation during the clinical examination. Many practitioners do not routinely check for LLI or may use inadequate assessment techniques. We feel that LLI is indeed a contributing factor in back and hip pain (see discussion and references in Chapter 4, *Evaluation of the Spine*).

A lumbar scoliosis (convexity toward the short leg) will develop secondary to an uneven leg length. This will cause unequal biomechanical stresses on the structures of the spine and can, over a long time, contribute to the development of adaptive muscle shortening, ligamentous and capsular hypomobility, degenerative joint disease and, at least theoretically, to disc protrusion. The adaptive muscle shortening and joint hypomobility will develop on the concave (long leg) side. Degenerative joint disease develops in the facets on the concave side and osteoarthritic (traction) spurring has been observed on the convex side. If a disc protrusion develops, it will probably be toward the convex (short leg) side.

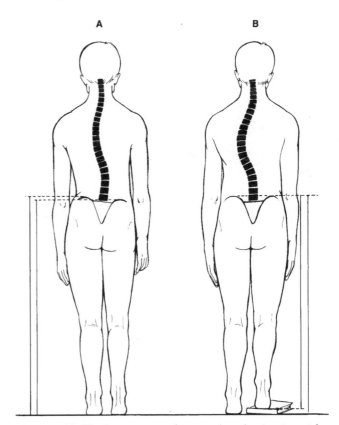

Figure 5-29: The importance of comprehensive treatment for leg length inequality. A) Long-term LLI with adaptive muscle shortening and joint stiffness on the side of the long leg (left); B) Correction of the discrepancy with a lift on the right causes the lumbar scoliosis to stay the same or worsen unless full spinal mobility is restored concurrently.

If a structural LLI exists, the iliac crests will be uneven in a standing position, but tests implicating sacroiliac joint dysfunction will be negative (see Chapter 7, *Pelvic Girdle Dysfunction*). The clinician is cautioned to beware of bony asymmetries in the iliac crests that may mimic a LLI.

Leg Length Inequality Treatment

Treatment of a *functional* LLI involves treatment of the cause. Examples include correcting sacroiliac dysfunction with mobilization and correcting strength or flexibility imbalances through exercise and soft tissue techniques. Treatment of *structural* LLI involves compensating for the leg length difference with the use of a shoe lift. Even if the leg length difference is truly structural, adaptive soft tissue shortening on the concave side of a lumbar scoliosis may be present if the problem has been long-standing (Fig 5-29). Therefore, one must be absolutely certain that balanced mobility, strength and normal posture are restored. Correcting uneven leg length in the presence of soft tissue hypomobility will not correct the lumbar scoliosis and may, in fact, increase the compensatory or secondary thoracic curve. Treatment such as ultrasound, unilateral lumbar traction, positional traction, joint mobilization and home exercises are necessary to restore full mobility in these cases.

Although full correction of the leg length discrepancy is the final goal, it may be advisable to make corrections gradually as mobility, strength and normal posture are being regained. Sometimes small corrections are made with a heel lift only. While this does correct standing leg length, it does not correct the discrepancy at toe-off during gait. Therefore, correction with a heel lift is often not adequate. Correction of more than $1/4$" discrepancy usually requires shoe modification.

The clinician should keep in mind that many factors contribute significantly to spinal pathology. Each disorder has specific subjective and objective findings, and the formulation of a unique treatment plan is necessary for each patient. Many diagnoses are related, in that one disorder may eventually progress to another more serious disorder if left untreated, or if inadequate rehabilitation takes place (Fig 5-30). Clinically, the patient often presents with more than one disorder at the same time.

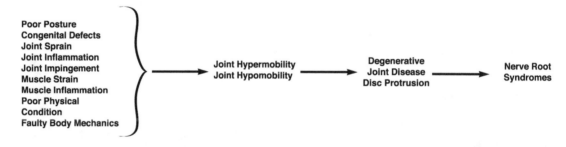

Figure 5-30: Spinal disorders often follow a natural progression, with seemingly minor disorders (left) leading to more serious disorders (right).

REFERENCES

1. Aisenbrey J: Exercise in the Prevention and Management of Osteoporosis. Physical Therapy 67:1100-1104, 1987.

2. Barr J, Barr M and Lemley T: Percutaneous Vertebroplasty for Pain Relief and Spinal Stabilization. Spine 25(8):923-928, 2000.

3. Bigos S, et al: Back Injuries in Industry: A Retrospective Study III: Employee Related Factors. Spine 11:252-256, 1986.

4. Blau J and Logue V: The Natural History of Intermittent Claudication of the Cauda Equina. Brain 101:211-222, 1978.

5. Brown J: Studies on the Permeability of the Intervertebral Disc During Skeletal Maturation. Spine 1:240-244, 1976.

6. Butler D: The Sensitive Nervous System. NOI Group Publications, Adelaide Australia 2000.

7. Cady L et al: Strength and Fitness and Subsequent Back Injuries in Firefighters. Joul of Occ Med 21:269-272, 1979.

8. Cailliet R: Low Back Pain Syndrome, 4th ed. FA Davis, Philadelphia 1988.

9. Cyriax J: Diagnosis of Soft Tissue Lesions. Textbook of Orthopædic Medicine, Vol 1, 8th ed. Bailliere-Tindall, London 1982.

10. Cyriax J: Treatment by Manipulation. Massage and Injection. Textbook of Orthopædic Medicine, Vol 2, 10th ed. Bailliere-Tindall, London 1980.

11. Cyriax J: Treatment of Lumbar Disk Lesions. Brit Med Joul 2:14-34, 1950.

12. Danielson J, Johnsen R, Kibsgaard SK, et al: Early Aggressive Exercise for Postoperative Rehabilitation After Discectomy. Spine 25(8):1015-1020, 2000.

13. Davis P: Reducing the Risk of Industrial Bad Backs. Occupational Health and Safety. May/June:45-47, 1979.

14. Dolan P, Greenfield K, Nelson R, et al: Can Exercise Therapy Improve the Outcome of Microdiscectomy? Spine 25(12):1523-1532, 2000.

15. Ellenberg M, Reina N, Ross M, et al: Regression of Herniated Nucleus Pulposus: Two Patients with Lumbar Radiculopathy. Arch Phys Med Rehabil 70:842-844, 1989.

16. Farfan H: Proceedings of the International Federation of Orthopaedic Manipulative Therapists. B Kend, ed. Vail CO 1977.

17. Finneson B: Low Back Pain 2nd ed. Lippincott, Philadelphia 1980.

18. Flemming J: Spondylolysis and Spondylolisthesis in the Athlete. In The Spine in Sports. S Hochschuler, ed. Hanley and Belfus, Philadelphia 1990.

19. Friberg O: Clinical Symptoms and Biomechanics of Lumbar Spine and Hip Joint in Leg Length Inequality. Spine 8(6):643-651, 1983.

20. Gall E: Lumbar Spine X-rays - What Can They Reveal? Occ Health and Safety 48:32-35, 1979.

21. Garfin SR, Yuan HA and Reiley, MA: Kyphoplasty and Vertebroplasty for the Treatment of Painful Osteoporotic Compression Fractures. Spine 26(14):1511-1515, 2001.

22. Goossens M, Rutten-van Molken M, Leidl RM, et al: Cognitive-Educational Treatment of Fibromyalgia: A Randomized Clinical Trial. II. Economic Evaluation. J Rheumatol 23(6):1246-54, 1996.

23. Gottlieb H, et al: Comprehensive Rehabilitation of Patients Having Chronic Low Back Pain. Arch Phys Med Rehab 58:101-108, 1977.

24. Guinto FC, Hashim H and Stumer M: CT Demonstration of Disk Regression after Conservative Therapy. AJNR 5:632-633, 1984.

25. Gupta R and Ramarao S: Epidurography in Reduction of Lumbar Disc Prolapse by Traction. Arch Phys Med Rehabil 59:322-327, 1978.

26. Hadler NM: Fibromyalgia, Chronic Fatigue, and Other Iatrogenic Dignostic Algorithms. Postgraduate Medicine 1102(2):161-177, 1997.

27. Harris R and McNab I: Structural Changes in the Lumbar Intervertebral Discs. Joul Bone Joint Surg 36B:302-322, 1954.

28. Hirsch C, Ingelmark B and Miller M: The Anatomical Basis for Low Back Pain. Acta Ortho Scanda 33:1-17, 1963.

29. Hirsch D and Schajowicz F: Studies of Structural Changes in the Lumbar Intervertebral Discs. JBJS 36B: 304-322, 1954.

30. Holm S and Nachemson A: Variations in the Nutrition of the Canine Intervertebral Disc, Induced by Motion. Spine 8:866-873, 1983.

31. Holm S and Nachemson A: Nutritional Changes in the Canine Intervertebral Disc After Spinal Fusion. Clin Orthop and Rel Res 169:243-258, 1982.

32. Jackson N, Winkelman R and Bickel W: Nerve Endings in the Lumbar Spinal Column. JBJS 48A:1272-1281, 1966.

33. Jayson M and Barks J: Structural Changes in the Intervertebral Disc. Annuls Rheum Dis 32:10-15, 1973.

34. Kapandji I: Spine. Vol 3 of The Physiology of the Joints, 2nd edition. Churchill Livingstone, London 1974.

35. Keskimaki I, Seitsalo S, Osterman H, et al: Reoperations After Lumbar Disc Surgery. A Population-Based Study of Regional and Interspecialty Variations. Spine 25(12):1500-1508, 2000.

36. Kirkaldy-Willis W: The Three Phases of the Spectrum of Degenerative Disease. In Managing Low Back Pain. WH Kirkaldy-Willis and C Burton, eds. Churchill Livingstone, New York 1992.

37. Kjellby-Wendt G and Styf J: Early Active Training After Lumbar Discectomy. A Prospective, Randomized, and Controlled Study. Spine 23(21):2345-2351, 1998.

38. Komori H, Shinomiya K, Nakai O, et al: The Natural History of Herniated Nucleus Pulposus with Radiculopathy. Spine 21(2):225-229, 1996.

39. Koontz C: Thoracic Outlet Syndrome, Diagnosis and Management. In Orthopedic Physical Therapy Forum series. Videotape. AREN, Pittsburgh, PA 1987.

40. Kornberg C and Lew P: The Effect of Stretching Neural Structures on Grade I Hamstring Injuries. J Ortho Sports Phys Ther 10(12):481-487, 1989.

41. Kraft G and Levinthal D: Facet Synovial Impingement. Surg Gynecol and Obstet 93:439-443, 1951.

42. Kramos P: New Rules to Fight Back Injuries. Health and Safety 44:42-44, 1975.

43. Loupasis G, Konstadinos S, Katonis P, et al: Seven- to 20-Year Outcome of Lumbar Discectomy. Spine 24(22):2313-2317, 1999.

44. Magora A and Schwartz A: Relation Between Low Back Pain and X-ray Changes IV: Lysis and Olisthesis. Scand J Rehabil Med 12:47-52, 1980.

45. Magora A and Schwartz A: Relation Between the Low Back Pain Syndrome and X-ray Findings I: Degenerative

Findings. Scand J Rehabil Med 8:115-126, 1976.

46. Magora A and Schwartz A: Relation Between the Low Back Pain and X-ray Findings II: Transitional Vertebra (Mainly Sacralization). Scand J Rehabil Med 10:135-145, 1978.

47. Maitland, G: Palpation Examination of the Posterior Cervical Spine: The Ideal, Average and Abnormal. Aust J Physiother 28:3-12, 1982.

48. Mannerkorpi K and Iversen MD: Physical Exercise in Fibromyalgia and Related Syndromes. Best Pract Res Clin Rheum 17(4):629-647, 2003.

49. Mathews J: Dynamic Discography; A Study of Lumbar Traction. Ann Phy Med 9:275-279, 1968.

50. Mathews J: The Effects of Spinal Traction. Physiotherapy 58:64-66, 1972.

51. Mathis JM, Eckel TS, Belkoff SM, et al: Percutaneous Vertebroplasty: A Therapeutic Option for Pain Associated with Vertebral Compression Fracture, Joul Back and Musculo Rehabil 13(1):11-17, 1999.

52. McKenzie R and May S: The Lumbar Spine Mechanical Diagnosis and Therapy, Vol I. Spinal Publications, Waikanae, New Zealand 2003.

53. Mennell J: Differential Diagnosis of Visceral From Somatic Back Pain. Joul of Occ Med 8:477-80, 1966.

54. Micheli L: Back Injuries in Gymnasts. Clin Sports Med 4(1):85-93, 1985.

55. Mooney V and Robertson J: The Facet Syndrome. Clin Orthop and Rel Res 115:149-156, 1976.

56. Morris J, Lucas D and Bresler M: Role of the Trunk in Stability of the Spine. J Bone and Joint Surg 43A:327-351, 1961.

57. Nachemson A and Elfstrom G: Intradiscal Dynamic Pressure Measurements in Lumbar Discs. Scand J Rehabil Med (Suppl)1:1-40, 1970.

58. Nachemson A and Morris J: In Vivo Measurements of Intradiscal Pressure. J Bone Joint Surg 46A: 1077-1092, 1964.

59. Nachemson A: The Lumbar Spine, An Orthopaedic Challenge. Spine 1:50-71, 1976.

60. Nordby E: Epidemiology and Diagnosis in Low Back Injury. Occupational Health and Safety 50:38-42, 1981.

61. Onel D, et al: Computed Tomographic Investigation of the Effect of Traction on Lumbar Disc Herniations. Spine 14(1):82-90, 1989.

62. Ostelo R, de Vet HC, Waddell G, et al: Rehabilitation Following First-Time Lumbar Disc Surgery. A Systematic Review Within the Framework of the Cochrane Collaboration. Spine 28(3):209-218, 2003.

63. O'Sullivan PB, Twomey LTand Allison GT: Evaluation of Specific Stabilizing Exercise in the Treatment of Chronic Low Back Pain with Radiologic Diagnosis of Spondylolysis or Spondylolisthesis. Spine 22(24):2959-2967, 1997.

64. Parson W and Cummings J: Mechanical Traction in the Lumbar Disc Syndrome. Can Med Assoc Joul 77:7-11, 1957.

65. Peterson H and Kieffer S: Introduction to Neuroradiology. Harper and Row, Philadelphia 1972.

66. Quinet R and Hadler H: Diagnosis and Treatment of Backache. Sem in Arth and Rheu 8:261-287, 1979.

67. Roofe P: Innervation of the Annulus Fibrosis and Posterior Longitudinal Ligament: Fourth and Fifth Lumbar Level. Arch Neurol Psych 44:100-103, 1940.

68. Saal J, et al: High Levels of Inflammatory Phospholipase A2 Activity in Lumbar Disc Herniations. Spine 15(7):674-678, 1990.

69. Saunders H: Unilateral Lumbar Traction. Phys Ther 61:221-225, 1981.

70. Schnebel B, et al: A Digitizing Technique for the Study of Movement of Intradiscal Dye in Response to Flexion and Extension of the Lumbar Spine. Spine 13(3):309-312, 1988.

71. Scientific Approach to the Assessment and Management of Activity-Related Spinal Disorders. A Monograph For Clinicians. Report of the Quebec Task Force on Spinal Disorders. Spine 12(7 Suppl):S1-59, 1987.

72. Shah J: Shift of Nuclear Material With Flexion and Extension of the Spine. In The Lumbar Spine and Low Back Pain. M Jayson, ed. Pitman Medical, London 1980.

73. Sinaki M, et al: Lumbar Spondylolisthesis. Archives of Phy Med 70:594-598, 1989.

74. Smith B: Cervical Spondylosis and Its Neurological Complications. Thomas, Springfield IL 1968.

75. Spangfort EV: The Lumbar Disc Herniation. Acta Orthop Scand (Suppl 142):5-95, 1972.

76. Sprague R: The Acute Cervical Joint Lock. Phys Ther 63:1439-1444, 1983.

77. Teplick J and Haskin M: Spontaneous Regression of Herniated Nucleus Pulposis. AJNR 6:331-335, 1985.

78. Toby EB and Koman LA: Thoracic Outlet Compression Syndrome. In Nerve Compression Syndromes. RM Szabo, ed. Slack, Thorofare, London 1989.

79. Travell J and Simons D: Myofascial Pain and Dysfunction - The Trigger Point Manual. Vol 2. Williams and Wilkins, Baltimore 1992.

80. Turck S: Orthopædics. 2nd edition. Lippincott, Philadelphia 1967.

81. Turk D and Flor H: Etiological Theories and Treatments for Chronic Back Pain II: Psychological Models and Interventions. Pain 19:209-233, 1984.

82. Turk DC, Okifuji A, Sinclair JD, et al: Pain, Disability and Physical Functioning in Subgroups of Patients with Fibromyalgia. J Rheumatol 23(7):1255-1262, 1996.

83. van der Linden S, van Tubergen A and Hidding A: PHysiotherapy in Ankylosing Spondylitis: What is the Evidence? Clin and Exp Rheumatol 20 (Suppl 28):S60-S64, 2002.

84. Vlaeyen J, Teeken-Gruben N, Goossens M, et al: Cognitive-Educational Treatment of Fibromyalgia: A Randomized Clinical Trial. I. Clinical Effects. J Rheumatol 23(6):1237-1245, 1996.

85. Waddell G, et al: Failed Lumbar Disc Surgery and Repeat Surgery Following Industrial Injury. JBJS 61A(2):201-207, March 1979.

86. Wainner RS, Fritz JM Irrgang JJ, et al: Reliability and Diagnostic Accuracy of the Clinical Examination and Patient Self-Report Measures for Cervical Radiculopathy. Spine 28(1):52-62, 2003.

87. Waitz E: The Lateral Bending Sign. Spine 6:388-397, 1981.

88. Weisel S et al: A Study of Computer-Assisted Tomography - The Incidence of Positive CAT Scans in an Asymptomatic Group of Patients. Spine 9(6):549-551, 1984.

89. White A and Gordon S: Idiopathic Low Back Pain. Spine 7:141-149, 1982.

90. Witt I, et al: A Comparative Analysis of X-ray Findings of the Lumbar Spine in Patients With and Without Lumbar Pain. Spine 9:298-299, 1984.

91. Wolfe F: The Fibromyalgia Problem. J Rheumatol 24(7):1247-1249, 1997.

6

TREATMENT BY PROBLEM

H. Duane Saunders, MS PT and Robin Saunders Ryan, MS PT

In Chapter 5, treatment of the spine by diagnosis was discussed. That treatment philosophy was based on the assumption that all spinal signs and symptoms can be traced to distinct pathological processes. A diagnosis is made and the pathological entity is treated with a plan designed to resolve the pathology. The approach of treating the spine by diagnosis is ideal and often works well; however, clinical experience has shown there are situations in which this approach is not successful or well understood.

First of all, there is poor agreement among clinicians concerning an accurate diagnosis. Differences of opinion exist between disciplines, with one clinician calling a *facet syndrome* what another clinician would call a *disc bulge*. Often, the diagnosis depends on which university or postgraduate courses one attended, rather than a clear consensus supported by the literature.

Even when the diagnosis is less controversial, every clinician has been confronted with those patients who simply don't respond to a treatment plan that *should* work, based on the literature and clinical experience with other patients. Also a clinician sometimes finds a patient who presents with signs and symptoms that do not fit any particular diagnosis. If the clinician's only approach was to treat by diagnosis, he often would be frustrated and many patients would not be helped.

Many patients who do not present with a clear pathological entity do present with easily identifiable problems such as pain, decreased soft tissue or joint mobility, abnormal posture and muscle weakness. When treatment is directed toward resolution of these problems, the signs and symptoms often disappear. In retrospect, one could conclude that the pathology (whatever it was) was properly treated by addressing the problems. This chapter is devoted to discussing some of these problems and how to treat them.

When the particular musculoskeletal pathology cannot be clearly diagnosed, the clinician must at least make sure the patient's signs and symptoms are musculoskeletal in nature before embarking on a treatment plan. Warning signs that the patient's problem may not be musculoskeletal were discussed in *Chapter 3, Medical Screening*.

In this chapter, eleven specific problems, a summary of their findings and their suggested treatments will be discussed:

- Pain, Inflammation, Guarding and Spasm
- Soft Tissue Hypomobility
- Joint Hypermobility
- Segmental Instability
- Muscle Weakness
- Poor Posture
- Poor Body Mechanics
- Poor Ergonomic Conditions
- Poor Physical Condition and Health Habits
- Psychosocial Involvement
- Abnormal Function

Even in cases when the diagnosis is clear, additional treatment for identifiable problems is often required. For example, a diagnosis of moderate to severe herniated disc typically requires traction and extension exercise treatment. However, in addition to the patient's *diagnosis* of herniated disc, he may have the *problems* of soft tissue stiffness and poor posture. Therefore, principles from both Chapters 5 and 6 will be applied for full rehabilitation of this patient. In fact, this scenario tends to be the rule rather than the exception. Most patients seen in the physical therapy clinic have one or more treatable problems that should be addressed. One of the most important roles of the physical therapist is that of educator/motivator. The clinician should make sure that patients understand the multiple goals of treatment and continue to work on improving musculoskeletal problems long after they have been discharged from physical therapy care.

Pain, Inflammation and Spasm

Mechanical irritation and soft tissue inflammatory processes often cause pain, muscle guarding, muscle spasm and other symptoms. Regardless of their underlying cause, treatment of these symptoms may be necessary to promote healing. As discussed previously, a complete evaluation may not be possible the first day the clinician examines the patient. The pain and muscle guarding may be severe enough to interfere with a thorough evaluation. It is quite acceptable for the clinician to begin treating the symptoms before the underlying pathology is determined, as long as the clinician reassesses the patient's condition as soon as the initial symptoms are under control.

Sometimes, the patient's symptoms are relieved entirely before the clinician ever finds the true source of the symptoms. This is acceptable as well. It is not always necessary for the clinician to know whether the pain is coming from the joint capsule, ligaments, disc or muscle, as long as the patient improves and normal posture, mobility, strength and function are restored.

Findings for Pain, Inflammation and Spasm

The patient's main complaint will be of pain, sometimes of an incapacitating nature. A positive weight shift test is indicative of spasm or guarding. Palpable tension or nodules in the paraspinals or interscapular muscles are often seen. Inflammation will sometimes cause the skin to be warm to the touch. Cold, clammy skin is sometimes seen when the patient is experiencing acute symptoms. A unilateral difference in tissue tension and temperature is often palpated.

Treatment for Pain, Inflammation and Spasm

Immobilization and rest for short periods may be necessary to help the patient avoid activities that injure healing tissue, aggravate the symptoms or inhibit the healing process. Immobilization and rest may take the form of bed rest, activity restrictions, positions of comfort and the use of supportive braces, corsets or cervical collars.

Attitudes have changed considerably about the benefits and dangers of bedrest and immobilization in the last two decades. We no longer require prolonged bedrest after childbirth, heart attack or surgery. Nor do we recommend

strict immobilization for several weeks with certain fractures. We now realize that excessive bedrest and immobilization delay healing while promoting depression, weakness, and deconditioning. Conversely, exercise and activity generally promote healing, strength and a positive mental outlook. Only in the past several years have practitioners begun to see these benefits for their back patients; many still have that lesson to learn. The change in attitude is encouraging. Many respected sources are now advocating the use of bedrest only in cases of severe symptoms, and then for no more than two days at a time without reassessment.[4,14,22,66] Even when bedrest is prescribed, most patients should get out of bed and move about frequently (every two to four hours).

Modality therapies and medications have long been used for relief of pain and muscle spasm. The various forms of heat and cold are usually effective. Ice should be used initially in the case of acute trauma. Electrotherapy and massage are often useful to promote healing and relieve pain. Modalities reducing edema, promoting circulation and stimulating cellular activity all speed the healing of irritated tissue and promote relaxation of muscle guarding and spasm.

When the possibility of tissue irritation is no longer an issue, joint or soft tissue mobilization often relieves pain effectively. The techniques employed usually consist of gentle traction or graded movements in the pain free range.

Soft tissue techniques used can consist of myofascial release, muscle energy techniques, or other soft tissue mobilization or stretching techniques. Techniques involving the active participation of the patient and incorporating functional movements are preferred to those that are entirely passive.[10,76,77]

It should be noted that most of the passive modalities have not been shown to be effective in the literature. However, clinical experience shows that they are helpful on an individual basis. Therefore, we recommend their use, but caution clinicians to avoid the excessive use of passive modalities when the patient is not experiencing a clear benefit or showing objective signs of current inflammation, muscle guarding or spasm. Within a few visits, most patients should show functional improvement and should progress to more active therapies. Passive modalities have been overutilized in years past.

Soft Tissue Hypomobility

Adaptive Muscle Shortening

Any skeletal muscle has a given number of sarcomeres at its normal resting length. The muscle can adaptively add or subtract sarcomeres at the musculotendinous junction, thus increasing or decreasing length according to the stresses placed on it. This is a normal, non-pathological response that begins shortly after the new position is introduced. For example, the biceps will adaptively shorten when the elbow is casted in flexion (sarcomere subtraction). Additionally, within one to two weeks, the collagen fibers of the connective tissue will adaptively shorten and thicken. Following cast removal, the biceps must lengthen (add sarcomeres) and the collagen fibers must be stretched for the biceps to regain normal resting length.[77]

Similarly, postural and structural changes that can lead to adaptive changes in the muscle often occur in response to injury, working positions or habits. For example, one usually sees the forward head, slumped posture develop secondary to cervical injuries or with an occupation requiring prolonged sitting. The muscles in the upper back, chest and neck soon adapt to the new posture. Another example is adaptive shortening of the lumbar spinal muscles secondary to hyperlordosis or sway back. Adaptive shortening of muscles may also occur if normal range of joint mobility is lost. Thus, the clinician must always take into account the possibility of adaptive muscle shortening when treating patients with postural changes or restricted joint motion.

Adaptive Changes of the Intervertebral Joint Complex Related to Joint Hypomobility

When many clinicians speak of joint hypomobility, they tend to forget the entire joint complex is involved. Hypomobility involves adaptive changes in muscular, ligamentous, joint and intervertebral disc tissue.[10,34,76,77] For this reason, adaptive muscular or soft tissue changes and joint hypomobility should really be thought of as the same condition or a continuation of a progressive condition.

Joint hypomobility is a disorder generally involving the entire spinal segment and is the result of prolonged immobilization, usually secondary to injury, poor posture or inactivity. The facet joint capsule, the disc, the supporting ligaments or any combination of the above may be the primary site of restriction. Joint hypomobility may be due to molecular binding of the collagen fibers within the joint capsule, adhesions or scarring of the surrounding soft tissue following injury (Fig 6-1). It may result following acute sprain if normal mobility and posture are not restored as healing occurs. Hypomobility may occur during and following episodes of disc herniation when certain movements are restricted or when scar tissue is laid down to repair the annular defect, or may simply be the result of prolonged poor posture, faulty working positions and general inactivity.

When joint hypomobility occurs over time as the result of habitual activities and postures, the joints may be normal or hypermobile in one or more directions, but hypomobile in another direction. A classic example would be a person whose occupation involves standing stooped at a bench all day. The person's thoracic spine may flex quite well, because he is used to rounding the shoulders and flexing the spine at work. Over time, however, the thoracic joints may lose their ability to extend, especially if the person is relatively sedentary at home. Joint hypomobility can lead to early degenerative change or predispose the patient to further injury.

William Kirkaldy-Willis[34] describes degenerative changes that occur in the entire intervertebral joint complex, including the muscle, synovium, articular cartilage, capsule and disc. Posterior joint changes produce a reaction on the disc and vice versa. For example, synovitis and a minor facet joint sprain may result in protective guarding, which leads to hypomobility, which in turn produces degenerative changes in the annulus of the disc. As the dysfunction becomes more severe, radial tears in the annulus may form, and a disc herniation can occur. Of course, the adaptive muscular changes described above also occur.

Findings for Soft Tissue Hypomobility

As discussed above, muscular length and strength imbalances are often seen in combination with joint hypomobility. For example, in the case of cervical joint hypomobility, interscapular muscles may be stretched and weak, while suboccipital muscles, scalenes and pectoralis muscles are tight. Palpable muscle changes such as areas of ropiness or trigger points may be felt. Mobility tests will reveal a limitation of active and passive movement at the involved segments.

Joint hypomobility may be specific to one or two segments, or may be general throughout an entire spinal area. The involved levels will be tender to palpate. The tenderness may involve only the interspinous space and facet

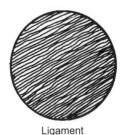
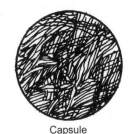

Ligament   Capsule

Figure 6-1: Collagen fibers are arranged in parallel in ligaments and irregularly in joint capsules. The irregular arrangement allows greater mobility. However, collagen fibers can bind together easily with immobilization.

joints, or it may involve the surrounding soft tissue as well. Pain may be referred and is usually unilateral. As with all joint problems, pain is associated with movement and is noticed especially at the end of available range. Lab findings and routine x-rays will initially be normal. Prolonged segmental hypomobility may lead to degeneration of both the disc and the facets, with pathology becoming evident on x-ray.[34] As with other soft tissue problems, there will be no true neurological signs.

Treatment for Soft Tissue Hypomobility

Treatment of adaptive changes of the intervertebral joint complex should be directed specifically to the tissues that have undergone the adaptive changes. As discussed above, these changes can involve the muscle tissue, non-contractile tissue or both.

Treatment of adaptive muscle length changes is most effectively accomplished by emphasizing normal physiological function (active exercises) rather than passive stretching or other techniques.[10,76,77] Some of the soft tissue mobilization techniques, such as myofascial release, can be useful. However, such techniques should be considered adjunctive to more active forms of therapy.

When treating adaptive muscle shortening, one should concurrently treat the joint hypomobility and any structural or postural changes that may be present. It is important to get the patient on an active exercise program as soon as possible in the treatment program. Emphasis on return to activities of daily living such as walking, work and general fitness exercise is very important. Active exercises can be done in short arcs of motion or isometrically if the patient's primary disorder is aggravated by exercising through the entire range of motion. At any rate, muscles need to be exercised functionally as soon as the condition of the primary disorder allows.

When joint hypomobility is present, joint mobilization should be used. The earlier mobilization is begun, the more beneficial it can be—provided it is done without aggravating any concomitant soft tissue injury. Mobilization can take many forms. When one thinks of mobilization, the manual therapist, osteopath or chiropractor comes to mind; however exercise, traction and posture correction are also forms of mobilization. Mobilization techniques may be uncomfortable, and the patient should be told that some soreness can be expected when using techniques that increase mobility. Ultrasound reduces soft tissue tightness and can be beneficial when used in combination with mobilization. Ice is often helpful following mobilization to prevent mild inflammation or soreness caused by the mobilization. Ultrasound or other modalities alone are not beneficial, but when combined with exercise and mobilization they can be effective adjuncts to treatment. Modalities can be overdone, and caution should be used in applying multiple modalities for pain relief, especially after the first few sessions. The patient must be educated that hypomobility is the main cause of the problem, and restoration of mobility must be the treatment focus.

Methods used to restore mobility can be general or specific. Exercise and traction tend to be more general, whereas some of the mobilization techniques discussed in Chapter 10, *Joint Mobilization* can be more specific. The key to successful treatment is a thorough evaluation, as the clinician must apply specific mobilization techniques and exercise protocols appropriate for the identifiable problems.

Joint Hypermobility

Joint hypermobility is defined as excessive range of motion. Joint hypermobility usually involves the entire spinal segment and can be the result of a variety of situations. For example, hypermobility may be caused by postural problems, congenital defects, injury caused by trauma such as whiplash, overtreatment by manipulation, excessive stretching related to sports like gymnastics and dancing or conditions such as hypermobility syndrome[67,68] or Ehlers-Danlos syndrome. In addition, sacroiliac hypermobility often develops with pregnancy and spondylolisthesis is sometimes hypermobile.

Sometimes increased motion develops at the spinal segment above or below a hypomobile or fused joint, particularly in the cervical spine.[15] Although some manual therapists teach that a stiff joint is always accompanied by a hypermobile joint, in our experience the tendency for this to happen is overstated. Joint hypermobility adjacent to a stiff or fused joint only occurs when the patient resumes a relatively active lifestyle that would normally cause significant movement in the stiff area. In such a case, the stiff joint does not move normally as it should. Because the patient is very active, the adjacent joints move more to compensate for the stiff joint's lack of movement. However, many patients who have experienced significant spinal injury or surgery naturally self-limit their activities, so the above phenomenon does not occur. In fact, such patients usually suffer more from general stiffness and muscle weakness because of the tendency toward a more sedentary occupation or lifestyle.

Compensatory joint hypermobility is more likely to occur in the cervical spine than in the thoracic and lumbar spine because even sedentary patients tend to achieve functional motion of the cervical spine after injury. For example, a patient may have a stiff upper and mid thoracic spine yet develop hypermobility of the cervical spine because it is necessary to regain full rotation mobility to drive a car comfortably. On the other hand, a sedentary patient with a stiff lower lumbar spine may not notice the stiffness because he is not challenged with activities of daily living requiring full lumbar mobility. The latter patient will not develop a compensatory hypermobility.

Joint hypermobility can lead to early degenerative change or predispose the patient to further injury. It also can be inherently painful because of the chronic stress placed on the joint capsule and soft tissues when the joint is at end range for prolonged periods.

Findings for Joint Hypermobility

Patients with joint hypermobility complain of general soreness in the spine with or without referred pain down one or both extremities. They generally cannot maintain positions for more than a few minutes without pain and they feel a need to change positions frequently. Pain usually worsens following increased physical activity.

If joint hypermobility is present, the mobility exam will reveal increased active and passive movement at the involved levels in one or more directions. It should be noted that hypomobility may be present in one direction (e.g., extension) while hypermobility may be present in another direction (e.g., flexion). The patient will not have any true neurological signs unless the condition is so severe that the bony structure is impinging on a nerve root. There is evidence that joint hypermobility can lead to joint/disc degeneration due to changes in biomechanical stresses and the increased stress and wear and tear placed on the joint during activity.[11,34,73]

Treatment for Joint Hypermobility

Patient education and exercise are the keys to treatment of the patient with joint hypermobility. Strengthening exercises for the muscles around a hypermobile joint can give support to the joint. The patient must learn corrective posture, and should be taught to avoid positions or activities that place the joints at extreme ranges of motion.

Spinal orthoses are helpful, especially in an acute phase of discomfort and when performing stressful activities such as heavy work or sports. Patient compliance with the long term use of corsets or supports is often poor. Furthermore, back supports promoting inactivity should be discouraged because strengthening and stabilization should be emphasized. A more active back support is more practical for prolonged use, and since it encourages activity, is not contraindicated (see Chapter 13, *Spinal Orthoses*). The patient must be taught that using a back support does not replace proper exercise and

posture principles. However, it is our experience that most patients do not tend to become dependent on a support. Instead, they learn to use it when performing activities that have a history of causing aggravation. For non-aggravating activities, most patients will choose to go without the back support.

In extreme situations of hypermobility, surgery may be indicated.

Segmental Instability

Instability is defined as a loss of control or excessive motion in a spinal segment's neutral zone.[59] Frymoyer and Selby further define segmental instability as, "loss of motion segment stiffness such that force application to that motion segment will produce greater displacement than would occur in a normal structure."[19] It is easy to confuse spinal instability with hypermobility, but they are two different problems. Discussing movement of the shoulder joint provides an analogy that helps clarify the distinction (Fig 6-2).

The rotator cuff muscles stabilize the shoulder. One can have normal shoulder range of motion or even hypomobility and at the same time have shoulder instability caused by rotator cuff muscle weakness. The same is true of the spine. When we evaluate range of motion in most chronic patients, we find joint and soft tissue hypomobility. At the same time, these patients often have joint instability because of weakness of the stabilizing muscles (e.g., multifidi and rotatores).

Some authors report that mild to moderate degenerative joint/disc disease causes hypomobility, but that severe degenerative joint/disc disease is accompanied by instability.[34] Severe disc degeneration may cause ligamentous laxity, and therefore segmental hypermobility, due to the narrowed disc space. However, it is also possible that the opposite occurs—ligaments may adaptively shorten in response to the narrowed disc space, causing joint and soft tissue hypomobility. The results of degenerative joint/disc disease probably vary from patient to patient.

Regardless of the joint status (hyper or hypomobile), it makes sense that the patient can have segmental instability *in either case*, if the stabilizing muscles are deconditioned. Exercise to improve segmental stability cannot harm the situation and will probably help.

Findings for Segmental Instability

Patients with lumbar instability will tend to have a painful arc of motion with trunk flexion or on return from trunk flexion. A reversal of lumbopelvic rhythm is often seen

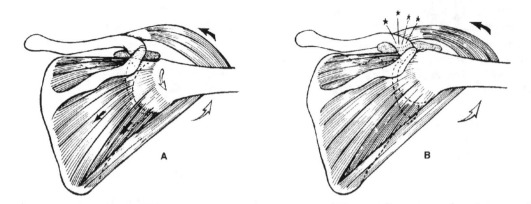

Figure 6-2: The rotator cuff muscles as stabilizers of the shoulder joint. A) Strong cuff muscles stabilize the glenohumeral joint during shoulder abduction. Inferior glide of the humeral head prevents pinching of the subacromial structures, including the bursa and supraspinatus tendon insertion; B) With weak cuff muscles or poor neuromuscular control, insufficient inferior glide allows impingement of the subacromial structures. This can be equated to "instability".

during return from flexion (i.e., the trunk extends first followed by hip and pelvis extension). The patient may use the hands on the thighs to obtain upright posture (e.g, from sit to stand or upon return from forward bending).[12] All of these behaviors represent a painful response to segmental motion or an attempt of the patient to stabilize himself to prevent pain. The shear stability test described in *Chapter 4, Evaluation of the Spine*, page 88, is useful for detecting lumbar joint instability.

When instability is accompanied by joint hypermobility, motion testing may reveal a catch or "clunk" when moving through an arc of motion. This sensation may be reported by the patient or may be palpated by the clinician. Mobility x-rays also may help reveal an unstable joint.

Treatment for Segmental Instability

Treatment for segmental instability involves specific muscle stabilization exercises, general strengthening and education in postural control and body mechanics. A back support may be necessary to provide pain relief during an acute episode and helps provide additional support during vigorous activity. In severe cases, surgical fusion of the segment may be necessary.

Muscle Weakness

In this category, we consider both muscle strength and endurance issues, as well as poor motor control. As discussed, muscle weakness and poor endurance is related to spinal instability. It is also related to other problems discussed in this chapter, such as poor posture and poor body mechanics. Weak muscles are less able to support the trunk in the positions of strength needed to prevent injury. Lumbar

muscle fatigue impairs the ability to sense a change in lumbar position.[78] Additionally, improper muscle recruitment[27,29,61,86] and slowed reaction time[42,43,44,62] experienced by patients with chronic low back pain may cause abnormal stress to tissues and contribute to a high incidence of reinjury.

There is growing evidence that loss of strength and endurance is a common finding in patients with chronic back problems or intermittent episodes of back pain. Trunk muscle strength is poor in patients post-HNP surgery compared to normals.[23] Altered muscle recruitment patterns have been demonstrated in patients with sacroiliac joint pain.[30] Radiographic evidence of paraspinal and psoas muscle wasting has been seen in patients with chronic low back pain.[10]

Much attention in the recent literature has focused on the lumbar multifidi. Significant weakness of the lumbar multifidi has been demonstrated in patients with back pain. Further, post-injury multifidi weakness does not spontaneously recover when the patient becomes pain free.[24] The deficit is most notable on the ipsilateral side of pain.[25] The weakness leaves the patient vulnerable to further injury once normal activities are resumed. Importantly, Hides and colleagues demonstrated that targeted rehabilitation of the multifidi resulted in less recurrence of low back pain compared to a control group.[26]

In addition to the multifidi, the transversarii, the abdominal muscles (particularly transversus abdominis) and quadratus lumborum have been shown to have important roles.[20,28,29,36,39,50,52,58,65,69,79,84] These muscles co-contract during activity to stabilize the spine, in much the same way as the rotator cuff muscles act to stabilize the shoulder during upper extremity activity.

There is controversy about which muscle groups are most important in trunk stabilization and injury prevention. However, one recurring theme in the literature is that patients who have a history of multiple back pain episodes, or even one significant episode, will have poor muscle strength and endurance unless rehabilitated post-injury. All of the trunk muscles play an important role in spinal stability, including the abdominal muscles, the lumbar paraspinals, the quadratus lumborum and latissimus dorsi.

Findings for Muscle Weakness

Once patients have passed the acute stage of an injury, their muscle strength and endurance should be tested by performing pertinent exercises shown in Chapter 14, *Basic Spinal Exercise*. If the patient cannot attain or maintain the exercise positions shown, weakness is present and should be addressed. Alternately, tests described by McIntosh, et al can be used and results compared to normative data (see Fig 4-50 on page 82).[53] Patients who have advanced functional demands (heavy work or sports) will require more strength and endurance. Muscle testing should be adjusted accordingly by requiring more advanced positions, more repetitions, a greater hold period or more exertion against resistance.

Treatment for Muscle Weakness

Proper spinal rehabilitation after injury is the key to preventing the post-injury weakness cycle described. The question of what "proper rehabilitation" is remains somewhat controversial. On one hand, Richardson et al, promote an intensive rehabilitation program that places emphasis on a step-wise progression through successively more difficult stabilization activities. The focus is on the lumbar multifidi and the transversus abdominis. The recommended program can require up to 10 weeks of supervised physical therapy visits. It may be difficult to teach, in that several subjects in one study took as long as 4 or 5 weeks of specific training before an accurate pattern of co-contraction could be achieved.[58] While such programs may be effective, they may not be practical.

Additionally, McGill cautions against focusing excessively on one muscle group for stabilization training. He reports that virtually all trunk muscles play a role in ensuring stability, but their importance at any point in time is determined by the unique combination of functional demands. Therefore, he recommends a series of exercises that improve the strength and endurance of all the trunk muscles and impose a relatively low load on the spine.[51]

The use of "high-tech" machines to test and strengthen back and neck musculature have become popular in recent years. The MedX® and Cybex® systems are two such machines.[9,55] Studies of lumbar extensor muscle strengthening[40,57] and neck muscle strengthening[16] using the MedX machines have shown good results. Good results have also been shown with the DBC110, a Finnish high-tech back strengthening machine.[32] However, no studies have convincingly shown the MedX or the DBC110 to have an advantage over "low-tech" exercise. One study showed that treatments incorporating either MedX or low-tech exercise consisting of regular weights and pulleys were equally effective in treating chronic neck pain.[16] Another study showed that for chronic low back pain patients, low-tech exercise compared favorably to using a Cybex isokinetic back strengthening machine and was considerably less costly. Since a major disadvantage of the high-tech systems is their expense, it is hard to justify their use without more compelling evidence of their superiority.

Indeed, many different types of exercise programs have yielded good results, but studies directly comparing the various ways of exercising are sparse. Manniche, et al, showed favorable results using aggressive back extension and latissimus dorsi strengthening with chronic low back pain patients. The back extension exercises did not require special equipment.[45,46] Positive effects have been shown for both strength and endurance of the back extensors using a relatively inexpensive variable-angle Roman chair device.[83] Additional studies have shown good results using low-tech, high intensity back extension exercises.[66,73,75,80]

Some authors have demonstrated positive results with general exercise that doesn't directly focus on back musculature. For example, one randomized trial showed that the results of low impact aerobics classes compared favorably to specific trunk strengthening exercises for chronic low back pain treatment. The aerobics classes were more cost-effective than clinician-supervised exercise sessions.[47,48]

Lindstrom, et al, showed that a focus on general fitness and education, combined with an operant-conditioning approach to improve confidence, allowed patients with sub-acute low back pain to return to work significantly earlier than a control group. The fitness exercises consisted of back-stroke swimming, general weight lifting, general cardiovascular exercise, prone lumbar extension against gravity and trunk curls for abdominal muscle strengthening.[41]

We should note that comparisons between the above studies should be made with caution, since several studies had methodological flaws, and the populations studied and exercise methods used were not homogenous.

In light of the conflicting evidence in the literature, how should clinicians choose the best exercise programs for their patients? In their review, VanTulder et al, said, "There is strong evidence that exercise therapy is effective for chronic low back pain, and there is no evidence in favor of one of these exercises".[82] Still, we don't advise clinicians to blindly choose from among the various exercise options.

As we've repeated throughout this text, the clinician must perform a thorough evaluation of the patient, consider the evidence available in the literature and decide upon a treatment strategy using sound clinical judgment. Part of the evaluation process involves determining factors that might make certain patients more challenging to treat or more prone to future reinjury. For example, patients who have had frequent recurrences or lengthy episodes in the past may require more subtle stabilization training with greater supervision. On the other hand, patients whose job or sport requires intense physical effort may need a wider variety of general strengthening and more intense paraspinal endurance training. There are many variations, and what works for one patient may not for another. We use common-sense and develop the program by considering each patient's functional goals. Many of the exercises we recommend are illustrated in Chapter 14, *Basic Spinal Exercise.*

To summarize, we tend to use exercises that are easy to teach yet provide sufficient challenge for an advanced exercise progression. For most patients, we focus on exercises that can be done at home but require occasional recheck visits to update the program. The cost-benefit of a professionally supervised program versus a home program has not been thoroughly analyzed, but researchers have provided some evidence that professional supervision results in a better outcome.[17,81] Each patient's need for supervision should be determined on a case-by-case basis.

In general, we like exercises that require minimal or easily-accessible equipment. Patients are more likely to continue such exercises long-term (or at least resume them if a future episode "reminds" them to take self-responsibility for their spinal fitness). Exceptions are cases where intensive, supervised exercises or work simulation techniques are justified to counter excessive fear-avoidance behavior or meet advanced functional goals (see Chapter 15, *Advanced Spinal Rehabilitation and Prevention*).

Poor Posture

Poor posture contributes to many types of spinal disorders. Therefore, postural correction is often a primary treatment consideration.

True postural strain syndromes fall into three categories:

- Lumbar flexion syndrome
- Lumbar extension syndrome
- Forward head syndrome

Lumbar Flexion Syndrome

Findings for Lumbar Flexion Syndrome

The lumbar flexion syndrome (flat back) is characterized by the patient who slumps with a flattened lumbar spine while sitting or standing. Working postures often contribute to this disorder. Consider, for example, the secretary who slumps over the desk or the assembly worker who stands slightly bent forward at his bench. Tight hamstring muscles may also contribute to this syndrome by preventing full pelvic mobility.

Pain is intermittent and only comes on after being in a flexed position for some time. Sitting usually hurts more than standing. Coming to the standing position after prolonged sitting is especially painful and difficult. Changing posture or position usually brings relief. Ligaments maintained under prolonged tension will adaptively lengthen. Thus, the ligaments stabilizing the spine in flexion (posterior longitudinal ligament, supraspinous and interspinous ligaments) are all subject to stretch. Overstretching these ligaments decreases support for the facet joints and disc. Pain arising from the ligaments or posterior annulus is often bilateral and may refer symptoms to the extremities. Patients with lumbar flexion syndrome are usually pain free after resting at night. Bilateral backache is the chief complaint but leg ache may also be present. Initially, full mobility is present but prolonged maintenance of these postures will eventually lead to a loss of lumbar extension. This situation may lead to disc herniation because of increased intradiscal pressure resulting from the flexed posture and the tendency for flexion to displace the nucleus posteriorly.[33,54,70]

Treatment for Lumbar Flexion Syndrome

Treatment consists of avoiding prolonged sitting and standing unless maintaining a lumbar lordosis. A lumbar pillow or roll placed against the lumbar spine will help maintain the lumbar lordosis while sitting. Hamstring stretching and lumbar stretching and strengthening exercises are often necessary to maintain full extension range of motion and to strengthen the back muscles. If the poor posture is work related, it may be necessary to raise the work area so that patients can stand or sit with a normal lordosis at work. Since one cannot always eliminate all stressful postural positions from daily routines, it is essential the stressful positions be interrupted or changed frequently when they are a necessary part of the patient's daily activities.

Lumbar Extension Syndrome

Findings for Lumbar Extension Syndrome

The lumbar extension syndrome (hyperlordosis) is characterized by a complaint of dull backache that comes on after prolonged standing. Standing usually hurts more than sitting. The pain often covers a large non-specific area. There is often a leg ache in one or both legs. The patient actually slumps into lumbar extension while standing by "hanging" on the anterior hip ligaments (Fig 6-3). He often will have tight hip flexor muscles and weak abdominal muscles. A large, protruding abdomen, as with obesity or pregnancy, adds to the strain. In cases of prolonged excessive lordosis, adaptive shortening of the posterior spinal musculature and ligaments occurs and flexion may become restricted. As with other postural problems, the patient will obtain relief by changing positions. Rest and recumbency will relieve symptoms and the patient is usually asymptomatic in the morning with a gradual return of symptoms during the day. The patient with lumbar extension syndrome is often younger and hypermobile. The level of physical fitness may vary from very athletic to very sedentary. The pregnant woman often suffers from this syndrome.

Treatment for Lumbar Extension Syndrome

Treatment consists of postural correction, abdominal muscle strengthening and exercises to stretch the hip flexor muscles and the posterior spinal segment. Weight loss may be important. Severe cases may require a corrective support. If prolonged standing is necessary, resting one foot on a small stool may be helpful. Frequently changing the stressful position is essential when it cannot be eliminated from the patient's daily activities.

In either the flexion or extension syndrome, it is the extreme, often prolonged posture that creates difficulty. It is a sad fact that many medical practitioners have prescribed the routine use of generic exercises to treat specific postural syndromes. To avoid this cookbook approach, it is essential that the problem be assessed properly and specific principles be applied knowledgeably.

Forward Head Syndrome

It is often difficult to determine the exact pathological process involved when treating a patient with spinal pain. This is especially true with cervical and upper thoracic problems. Postural change is often the only objective evidence we see. Clinical experience teaches that almost every neck pain patient has some degree of forward head posture syndrome. When poor posture is corrected with patient education and exercise, the patient often has symptom relief. In this case, the treatment is correct and the patient gets well, yet the clinician may never know the exact nature of the pathology. There is nothing wrong with this approach to treatment. In fact, it may be the only reasonable approach available in some cases.

Findings for Forward Head Syndrome

In the forward head postural syndrome, the upper cervical spine is extended while the lower cervical and upper thoracic spine is relatively flexed. Additionally, forward head posture is usually accompanied by rounded shoulders, slumped sitting, upper back muscle weakness, anterior chest and upper cervical muscle tightness and scapular abduction (Fig 6-4).

When the head is held in the forward position, there is considerably more weight and tension exerted at the cervi-

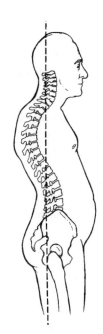

Figure 6-3: Lumbar extension syndrome (hyperlordosis).

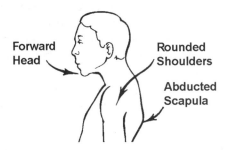

Figure 6-4: Forward head posture.

cothoracic junction. Normally, the bony structures of the neck should act as a weight bearing column and simply transfer the weight of the head to the trunk. In the forward head posture, however, the neck acts as a lever arm, causing a torque force at the base of the cervical spine.

Treatment for Forward Head Syndrome

Treatment of forward head postural syndrome depends on its cause. When forward head posture results as a secondary or concurrent response to lumbar postural problems, treatment of the primary lumbar problem, appropriate spinal strengthening and general physical fitness exercises are all indicated. For example, it is nearly impossible to correctly treat forward head posture when the lumbar spine is excessively flat or hyperlordotic.

The forward head posture may result from the development of joint or muscular tightness in the upper cervical spine due to muscular tension or poor ergonomic factors. Because of muscular tension or awkward positions, the upper cervical spine tilts more and more into extension. As this occurs, the lower cervical and upper thoracic spine is flexed to keep the eyes level. Squinting and shoulder elevation often accompany this scenario.

Treatment in this case consists of mobilization and stretching (traction) of the upper cervical spine and postural training. Relaxation and biofeedback training may be necessary, as many patients do not realize they are tensing up and inadvertently causing suboccipital muscle tightness. If awkward working positions are contributing to the muscular tension, the ergonomic or body mechanics factors need to be addressed as well.

The forward head posture may result from weakness of the lower cervical, upper thoracic and interscapular stabilizing muscles, and tightness of the anterior chest/suboccipital muscles. In this case, treatment consists of spinal and interscapular muscle strengthening exercises, anterior chest/suboccipital muscle relaxation and stretching exercises and postural training.

Finally, forward head posture may result from a chronic problem secondary to a previous cervical sprain or strain. Pain in the acute and sub-acute stages of cervical sprain or strain causes the patient to assume a slumped posture. In time, the cervical extensors and stabilizers become weak and the joints of the lower cervical spine lose extension mobility. At the same time, the upper cervical spine extends to keep the head and eyes level. By the time the precipitating injury has healed, the patient is fixed in the new posture.

Chronic forward head posture causes a strain on the ligaments and muscles in the posterior lower cervical and upper thoracic spine. This syndrome is characterized by generalized, non-specific pain in the neck and upper back, headaches and occasional referred pain into the upper extremities. The upper trapezius, levator scapulae and rhomboid major muscles are most often involved. A constant state of muscle guarding, spasm, ligamentous stress and generalized inflammation will often cause the patient to believe the original injury has never healed even though many months or years have passed.

Treatment in this case must be directed toward: 1) restoring any loss of flexion mobility in the upper cervical spine and extension mobility in the lower cervical and upper thoracic spine; 2) strengthening the muscles of the posterior cervical, upper thoracic and interscapular areas; 3) stretching the anterior shoulder and chest muscles if they have become adaptively shortened due to the postural changes; and 4) making the patient aware of the correct posture he must achieve if treatment is to be successful.

Exercises used to treat forward head syndrome are described and pictured in Chapter 14, *Basic Spinal Exercise*.

Poor Body Mechanics

Poor use of body mechanics directly affects other problems a patient may have. For example, constantly bending at the waist when performing functional activities can overstretch spinal ligaments and muscles and contribute to abnormal muscle recruitment and abnormal disc mechanics. Theoretically, this would predispose one to injury. After an episode of back or neck pain, use of improper body mechanics inhibits the normal healing process and can contribute to the development of abnormal posture syndromes and joint hyper or hypomobility. These facts are true whether or not the patient has a labor intensive occupation. For this reason, teaching proper body mechanics cannot be overlooked with any spinal patient.

There is controversy over the definition of proper body mechanics. For lifting, some clinicians promote an anteriorly tilted pelvis with a lordotic lumbar position, while others teach a posterior pelvic tilt. Most clinicians are now teaching a neutral lumbar position and generally agree that body mechanics training should be individualized, since what is considered optimal in a normal individual may change in the presence of pathology.

We believe that it is unrealistic for most people to lock the spine in a true lordosis, even though a slightly lordotic lifting position would be theoretically ideal. When the hips and knees are flexed in a partial squat, ligamentous and muscular tightness will usually prevent a true lumbar lordosis. The important principle for lifting is to "lock" the

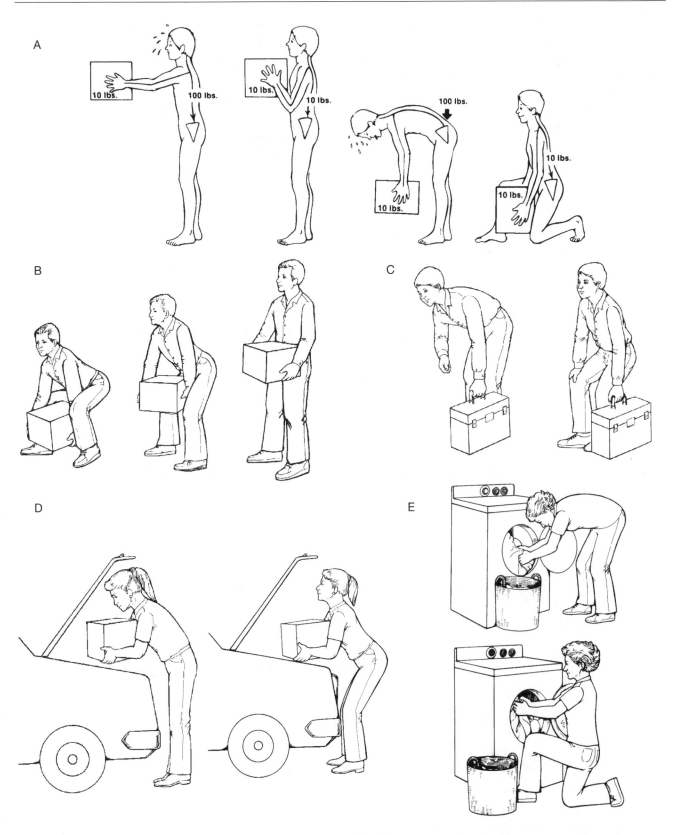

Figure 6-5: Examples of good and bad body mechanics. All of the "good" examples involve maintaining the spine in the "power" position—head up, spine stabilized and weight held close to the body. Note that bending occurs at the hip joints, not in the lumbar spine.

spine, so that segmental movement is minimized. In other words, the lumbar segments should not flex, extend, rotate or side bend for the duration of the lift. Instead, the patient should keep the head up, the weight should be held as close as possible, and the hips and knees should provide the concentric muscular effort with the spine muscles holding isometrically. We call this position the "power position" and teach patients to strive for a lordotic lumbar position, while realizing the best most can probably achieve is spinal neutral (Fig 6-5).

When considering whether the use of good body mechanics comes naturally, one only needs to look to children for the answer. The toddler who is just discovering how his body moves uses good body mechanics quite easily. His spinal range of motion is equal and fluid in flexion, extension, rotation and side bending. Hip mobility is excellent. All muscles work in harmony to keep him from toppling over. The child bends naturally from the hips rather than the low back, and uses good posture when sitting (Fig 6-6).

The child does not begin to break these good habits until later, when he develops a more sedentary or specialized lifestyle. When the child begins to attend school, the spine begins to flex more than it extends. The child's legs do not get as much exercise, so he begins to bend over because bending expends less energy than squatting. When the child reaches adulthood, he may choose an occupation and hobbies that do not promote spinal balance. When consid-

ering all of these factors, it is no wonder many humans learn to use their bodies incorrectly. It can easily be argued that, at least initially, good body mechanics do come naturally!

Treatment for Poor Body Mechanics

The physical therapist must be skilled at evaluating each patient's individual circumstances. An individual body mechanics training program must be designed. Techniques for lifting, bending and reaching should be taught to all patients, since nearly everyone must perform these activities to some extent during an average day. The patient should be quizzed about other significant activities. Often, a patient will not realize a simple activity that does not cause pain can be problematic. For example, a patient may think lifting is the main issue when repetitive and prolonged bending is just as important (Fig 6-7). Body mechanics training should begin the first day of treatment, as any treatment performed in the clinic can be counteracted by the harmful effects of poor body mechanics at home.

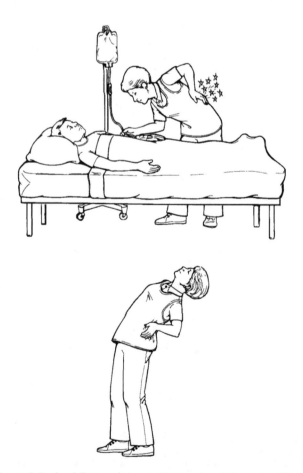

Figure 6-7: Avoiding or interrupting prolonged or repetitive positions is as important as using proper lifting techniques.

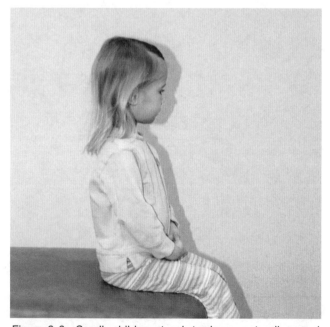

Figure 6-6: Small children tend to have naturally good posture.

Poor Ergonomic Conditions

The significant injury recurrence rates experienced by patients returning to work show that ergonomic factors cannot be ignored. Worker behaviors and work station or job design problems often need to be addressed to completely resolve the patient's musculoskeletal problems. As discussed in Chapter 4, *Evaluation of the Spine*, the physical therapist's initial evaluation must include a detailed discussion of the patient's work and home activities, both of which can be direct or indirect causes of the patient's problem.

The clinician should teach patients basic ergonomic principles so they can conduct their own "common sense" ergonomic evaluations. We find it helpful to have patients watch a video about the most important ergonomic principles, and follow this with a detailed discussion about applying the general principles in their specific work environments. Watching a video alone or reading about ergonomics is not enough. Detailed discussion and problem-solving is essential.

In some cases, the physical therapist should perform a job site evaluation to help patients and their employers develop a solution. The clinician should suggest ideas, but should be careful to avoid inadvertently putting patients at odds with their employers by suggesting unrealistic changes in the workplace. There are often many simple, inexpensive changes that can drastically improve the work environment. Complex changes in work flow or capital equipment purchases are not realistic unless the clinician has been hired as a consultant for overall ergonomic advice.

Employer cooperation varies with individual circumstances. Sometimes, the clinician must be very tactful when approaching a change. Likewise, the clinician should be sensitive to the fact that the employer may not be able to make a change because of logistic or economic considerations. The employer is sometimes more motivated to make a positive change when the injury involves a workers' compensation claim, because lost days from work represent a significant insurance expense. Employers also may be motivated to make changes in non-workers' compensation cases because of the 1992 Americans with Disabilities Act (ADA). The ADA mandates certain requirements for larger employers to accommodate disabled individuals in the workplace.

Poor Physical Condition and Health Habits

Sometimes it is difficult to find objective problems in the person complaining of spinal pain. This is particularly true of patients complaining of intermittent, non-severe episodes of pain. The patient's joints may move fairly symmetrically, and no particular muscle group seems to be involved. However, the patient is generally in poor physical condition and leads a fairly sedentary lifestyle. The patient initially may have had a significant injury, after which the pre-injury physical condition was not restored. With such a patient, improvement of general physical fitness is the key. More and more evidence is linking general physical fitness to neck and back fitness. For example, a study by Cady, et al, found firefighters who were fit had significantly fewer episodes of back pain than those who were unfit.[6] Additional studies with similar findings can be found in the literature.[1,2,3,5,13,71] Lack of fitness is often seen in conjunction with poor posture, joint hypomobility and poor use of body mechanics. All of these factors should be addressed, but simply improving general physical fitness may simultaneously improve the other problems.

General fitness is not the only lifestyle issue that influences back pain. Deyo and Bass demonstrated a significant relationship between body weight and smoking and the occurrence of low back pain.[13] Other authors have demonstrated correlations between smoking and low back pain[21,31,37] or poor results from low back pain treatment.[49,74] Obesity and low back pain are correlated.[31,38] We know general health habits such as diet and rest have considerable effect on illness, specifically on healing disease and injury.[13,18,33,56]

Although definitive causal relationships with spinal pain have not been established, one can conclude from the evidence that practicing healthy lifestyle habits is an important factor in prevention and treatment of back pain.

Treatment for Poor Physical Condition

One of the bigger challenges the clinician faces is encouraging patients to change their lifestyles. If patients smoke or are overweight, they should be informed of the affect these factors can have on spinal health. Patients usually are aware that smoking and obesity negatively affect their overall health, but dealing with back pain may give them one more reason to make a good change.

Education is very important to help patients understand that progress will be slow. Lifestyle improvements are expected to cause long-term benefit—immediate pain relief is not the goal. Progress should be measured in months, not weeks.

For exercise programs it may be helpful to initially begin in the clinic two to three times per week. A positive, supportive environment may help motivate the slow starter. Ultimately, however, the patient must take responsibility for self-management of his condition. While verbally encouraging self-responsibility, the clinician must avoid inadvertently giving the patient a mixed message.

The clinician should avoid the following:

Overusing passive treatments for pain relief. The clinician absolutely must convince patients that the exercise, posture and lifestyle changes are helping—not the ultrasound and mobilization!

Underexplaining the role of physical fitness The clinician must be a cheerleader. Quoting statistics and studies about exercise, such as the firefighter study above, can be helpful.

Giving patients too many exercises to perform. The clinician should become skilled at determining how much each patient is willing to participate in his own recovery. If a patient is only willing to invest five minutes per day, it will not help to give him a 20-minute exercise program. The clinician should choose the most essential exercises and seek the patient's commitment to doing them.

Giving patients pre-printed exercise sheets. When patients are given a standard handout of exercises titled, "Back Pain Exercises", they do not feel the exercises are individualized. Many of these handouts end up in the patient's garbage can. Standard exercise diagrams can be used, but the combination of exercises chosen should clearly show each patient that the clinician designed a special exercise program for him.

Using special equipment not available to patients elsewhere. Most patients should not require specialized equipment to rehabilitate a spinal problem. Equipment such as free weights, balls, mats and elastic tubing should be used. Aerobic activities that can be performed at home or in a health club the patient already attends should be prescribed. Persistence, not high technology, is the key.

Psychosocial Involvement

The role of mental fitness and its effect on back injuries cannot be ignored. Stress, emotional problems, chemical dependency and lack of job satisfaction are just a few of the many factors that can influence a patient's response to symptoms and treatment.[4,60] Diagnosing and treating psychosocial issues is not within the scope of a physical therapist's training. However, the therapist must be aware that the existence of adverse psychosocial factors will influence the effects of treatment. Some physical therapists make the mistake of continuing to treat patients with concurrent psychosocial issues as though they have only a physical problem. Such treatment is not helpful to the patient and can be harmful because it prevents the patient from addressing important issues.

Findings/Treatment for Psychosocial Issues

Findings for depression were outlined in Chapter 3, *Medical Screening*. Excessive fear-avoidance behavior can be detected with the FABQ, described in Chapter 4, *Evaluation of the Spine*. Additionally, inconsistencies in presentation, excessive anxiety or somatic focus are often noticed in evaluation or treatment sessions.

As physical therapists, our role is to treat physical problems and educate the patient about his role in recovery. Improving the patient's symptoms and general physical condition can relieve stress. Teaching self-management techniques can restore a feeling of confidence and control. A cognitive behavior approach designed to decrease fear and emphasize activity is very important (see Chapter 15, *Advanced Spinal Rehabilitation and Prevention*). In fact, the results of one study suggest that decreasing fear may be more important than decreasing pain in increasing physical capacity for work.[85] When we have done all we can from a physical and educational perspective, we should refer the patient to appropriate sources or to his primary physician for additional care.

Abnormal Function

Treatment to restore active function is the most important part of practicing orthopedic physical therapy. All other treatment goals, such as relieving pain or restoring normal mobility, are important because they will help normalize function. Treatment principles already discussed often improve function naturally, because as the patient feels and moves better, his function normalizes. In some cases, however, physical therapists and other medical practitioners are unable to relieve pain and restore normal mechanics. Every experienced clinician has met patients whose pain cannot be relieved with current medical techniques. The goal of treatment for these patients is restoration of function. Regardless of the patient's level of pain or disability, function can almost always be improved.

Treatment for Abnormal Function

Patient education is the key to restoring function. The patient must understand and accept the goals of treatment, even when they fall short of the patient's initial expectations. It is often difficult for a patient to accept that functional improvement, not pain relief, is the only realistic goal.

Exercise is also essential. Exercises chosen for the patient should be directly related to restoration of function. Some of the exercise and functional restoration techniques go beyond the scope of this text. Work hardening and chronic pain programs are often necessary because they address more factors than a physical therapist alone can address. These factors often include psychosocial issues, vocational issues and family issues. Functional restoration is discussed in greater detail in (see Chapter 15, *Advanced Spinal Rehabilitation and Prevention*).

To summarize this chapter, the philosophy of treating a patient's identifiable problems can be very successful, even if a particular pathological entity is never identified. Even when a definitive diagnosis is made, not all patients respond the same to treatments that usually work. The clinician should never hesitate to use a common sense approach when treating a patient's musculoskeletal disorder. An overly analytical cookbook approach is never superior to sound thinking and good clinical decision making.

REFERENCES

1. Anderson C: Physical Ability Testing as a Means to Reduce Injuries in Grocery Warehouses. International Joul of Retail and Distribution Management 19(7):33-35, 1991.
2. Anderson C: Preplacement Screening: Survival of the Fittest. Risk Management 44-46, Nov 1987.
3. Biering-Sorenson F: Physical Measurements as Risk Indicators for Low Back Trouble Over a One-Year Period. Spine 9:106-119, 1984.
4. Bigos S, et al: Back Injuries in Industry: A Retrospective Study III: Employee Related Factors. Spine 11:252-256, 1986.
5. Boyer M and Vaccaro B: The Benefits of Physically Active Workforce: An Organizational Perspective. Occupational Medicine 5:691-706, 1990.
6. Cady L et al: Strength and Fitness and Subsequent Back Injuries in Firefighters. Joul of Occ Med 21:269-272, 1979.
7. Callaghan JP, Gunning JL and McGill SM: The Relationship Between Lumbar Spine Load and Muscle Activity During Extensor Exercises. Phys Ther 78:8-18, 1998.
8. Callaghan MJ: Evaluation of a Back Rehabilitation Group for Chronic Low Back Pain in an Out-patient Setting. Physiotherapy 80(10):677-681, 1994.
9. Computer Sports Medicine, Inc. 101 Tosca Drive, Stoughton, MA 02072-1505.
10. Cooper RG, St. Clair Forbes W and Jayson MIV: Radiographic Demonstration of Paraspinal Muscle Wasting in Patients with Chronic Low Back Pain. British Joul Rheum 31:389-394, 1992.
11. Cyriax J: Diagnosis of Soft Tissue Lesions. In Textbook of Orthopædic Medicine, Vol 1, 8th edition. Bailliere-Tindall, London 1982.
12. Delitto A, Erhard RE and Bowling RW: A Treatment-Based Classification Approach to Low Back Syndrome: Identifying and Staging Patients for Conservative Treatment. Phys Ther 75:470-489, 1995.
13. Deyo R and Bass J: Lifestyle and Low Back Pain: The Influence of Smoking and Obesity. Spine 14:501-506, 1989.
14. Deyo R, Diehl A and Rosenthal M: How Many Days Of Bed Rest For Acute Low Back Pain? N Engl J Med 315:1064-1070, 1986.
15. Eck JC, Humphreys C, Lim T-H, et al: Biomechanical Study on the Effect of Cervical Spine Fusion on Adjacent-Level Intradiscal Pressure and Segmental Motion. Spine 27(22):2431-2434, 2002.
16. Evans R, Bronfort G, Nelson BW, et al: Two-Year Follow-up of a Randomized Clinical Trial of Spinal Manipulation and Two Types of Exercise for Patients with Chronic Neck Pain.

Spine 27(21):2383-2389, 2002.
17. Frost H, Klaber-Moffett JA, Moser JS, et al: Randomised Controlled Trial for Evaluation of Fitness Programme for Patients with Chronic Low Back Pain. BMJ 319:151-154, 1995.
18. Frymoyer J and Cats-Baril W: Predictors of Low Back Pain Disability. Clin Orthop and Rel Res 221:89-98, 1987.
19. Frymoyer JW and Selby DK: Segmental Instability: Rationale for Treatment. Spine 10:280-286, 1985.
20. Gardner-Morse MG and Stokes IAF: The Effects of Abdominal Muscle Coactivation on Lumbar Spine Stability. Spine 23(1):86-90, 1998.
21. Goldberg M, Scott S and Mayo N: A Review of the Association Between Cigarette Smoking and the Development of Nonspecific Back Pain and Related Outcomes. Spine 25(8):995-1014, 2000.
22. Hagen KB, Hilde G, Jamtvedt G, et al: The Cochrane Review of Bed Rest for Acute Low Back Pain and Sciatica. Spine 25(22):2932-2939, 2000.
23. Hakkinen A, Kuukkanen T, Tarvainen U, et al: Trunk Muscle Strength in Flexion, Extension and Axial Rotation in Patients Managed with Lumbar Disc Herniation Surgery and in Healthy Control Subjects. Spine 28(10):1068-1073, 2003.
24. Hides JA, Richardson CA and Jull GA: Multifidus Muscle Recovery is Not Automatic After Resolution of Acute, First Episode Low Back Pain. Spine 21(23):2763-2769, 1996.
25. Hides JA, Stokes MJ, Saide M, et al: Evidence of Lumbar Multifidus Muscle Wasting Ipsilateral to Symptoms in Patients with Acute/Subacute Low Back Pain. Spine 19(2):165-172, 1994.
26. Hides JA, Jull GA and Richardson CA: Long-Term Effects of Specific Stabilizing Exercises for First-Episode Low Back Pain. Spine 26:e243-248, 2001.
27. Hodges PW and Richardson CA: Altered Trunk Muscle Recruitment in People with Low Back Pain with Upper Limb Movement at Different Speeds. Arch Phys Med Rehabil 80:1005-1012, 1999.
28. Hodges PW and Richardson CA: Contraction of the Abdominal Muscles Associated with Movement of the Lower Limb. Phys Ther 77:132-144, 1997.
29. Hodges PW and Richardson CA: Inefficient Muscular Stabilization of the Lumbar Spine Associated with Low Back Pain: A Motor Control Evaluation of Transverse Abdominus. Spine 21(22):2640-2650, 1996.
30. Hungerford B, Gilleard W, and Hodges P: Evidence of

Altered Lumbopelvic Muscle Recruitment in the Presence of Sacroiliac Joint Pain. Spine 28(14):1593-1600, 2003.

31. Kaila-Kangas L, Leino-Arjas P, Riihimaki H, et al: Smoking and Overweight as Predictors of Hospitalization for Back Disorders. Spine 28(16): 1860-1868, 2003.

32. Kankaanpää M, Taimela S, Airaksinen O, et al: The Efficacy of Active Rehabilitation in Chronic Low Back Pain. Effect on Pain Intensity, Self-Experienced Disability, and Lumbar Fatigability. Spine 24(10):1034-1042, 1999.

33. Kelsey J: An Epidemiological Study of Acute Herniated Lumbar Intervertebral Discs. Rheumatol Rehabil 14:144, 1975.

34. Kirkaldy-Willis W: The Three Phases of the Spectrum of Degenerative Disease. In Managing Low Back Pain. WH Kirkaldy-Willis and C Burton, eds. Churchill Livingston, New York NY 1992.

35. Klaber Moffett J, Torgerson D, Bell-Syer S, et al: Randomised Controlled Trial of Exercise for Low Back Pain: Clinical Outcomes, Costs and Preferences. BMJ 319:279-283, 1999.

36. Lam KS and Mehdian H: The Importance of an Intact Abdominal Musculature Mechanism in Maintaining Spinal Sagittal Balance. Spine 24(7):719-722, 1999.

37. Leboeuf-Yde C, Hyvik K, Bruun N, et al: Low Back Pain and Lifestyle. Part I-Smoking. Information from a Population-Based Sample of 29,424 Twin Subjects. Spine 23(20):2207-2213, 1998.

38. Leboeuf-Yde C, Hyvik K, Bruun N, et al: Low Back Pain and Lifestyle. Part II-Obesity. Information from a Population-Based Sample of 29,424 Twin Subjects. Spine 24(8):779, 1999.

39. Lee JH, Hoshino Y, Nakamura K, et al: Trunk Muscle Weakness as a Risk Factor for Low Back Pain. Spine 24(1):54-57, 1999.

40. Leggett S, Mooney V, Matheson LN, et al: Restorative Exercise for Clinical Low Back Pain. Spine 24(9):889-898, 1999.

41. Lindstrom I, Ohlund C, Eek C et al: The Effect of Graded Activity on Patients with Subacute Low Back Pain: A Randomized Prospective Clinical Study with an Operant-Conditioning Behavioral Approach. Phys Ther 72:279-293, 1992.

42. Luoto S, Aalto H, Taimela S, et al: One-Footed and Externally Disturbed Two-Footed Postural Control in Patients with Chronic Low Back Pain and Healthy Control Subjects. A Controlled Study with Follow-Up. Spine 23(19):2081-2089, 1998.

43. Luoto S, Hurri H and Alaranta H: Reaction Times in Patients with Chronic Low-Back Pain. Eur J Phys Med Rehabil 5:47-50, 1995.

44. Luoto S, Taimela S, Hurri H, et al: Psychomotor Speed and Postural Control in Chronic Low Back Pain Patients; A Controlled Follow-Up Study. Spine 21(22):2621-2627, 1996.

45. Manniche C, Lundberg E, Christensen I, et al: Intensive Dynamic Back Exercises for Chronic Low Back Pain: A Clinical Trial. Pain 47:53-63, 1991.

46. Manniche C, Hesselsoe G, Bentzen L, et al: Clinical Trial of Intensive Muscle Training for Chronic Low Back Pain. The Lancet 31:1473-1476, 1988.

47. Mannion AF, Muntener M, Taimela S, et al: A Randomized Clinical Trial of Three Active Therapies for Chronic Low Back Pain. Spine 24(3):2435-2448, 1999.

48. Mannion AF, Taimela S, Muntener M, et al: Active Therapy for Chronic Low Back Pain. Spine 26(8):897-908, 2001.

49. McFadden J: Cigarette Smoking May Adversely Affect Chemonucleolysis. Orthopædic News 8(2):Mar/Apr 1986.

50. McGill SM, Juker D and Kropf: Quantitative Intramuscular Myoelectric Activity of Quadratus Lumborum During a Wide Variety of Tasks. Clin Biomech 11:170-172, 1996.

51. McGill SM: Low Back Disorders. Evidence-Based Prevention and Rehabilitation. Human Kinetics, Champaign, IL 2002.

52. McGill SM: Low Back Exercises: Evidence for Improving Exercise Regimens. Phys Ther 77:132-144, 1997.

53. McIntosh G, Wilson L, Affleck M, et al: Trunk and Lower Extremity Muscle Endurance: Normative Data for Adults. J Rehabil Outcomes Meas 2(4):20-39, 1998.

54. McKenzie R and May S: The Lumbar Spine Mechanical Diagnosis and Therapy, Vol I. Spinal Publications, Waikanae, New Zealand 2003.

55. MedX 96, Inc., 1401 NE 77th St., Ocala, FL 34479.

56. Nachemson A: Exercise, Fitness and Back Pain. In Exercise, Fitness and Health: A Consensus of Current Knowledge. C Bouchard, et al, eds. Human Kinetics Books, Champaign IL 1990.

57. Nelson BW, O'Reilly E, Miller M, et al: The Clinical Effects of Intensive, Specific Exercise on Chronic Low Back Pain: A Controlled Study of 895 Consecutive Patients with 1-Year Follow-Up. Ortho 18:971-981, 1998.

58. O'Sullivan PB, Twomey LT and Allison GT: Evaluation of Specific Stabilizing Exercise in the Treatment of Chronic Low Back Pain with Radiologic Diagnosis of Spondylolysis or Spondylolisthesis. Spine 22(24):2959-2967, 1997.

59. Panjabi MM: The Stabilizing System of the Spine, Part II: Neutral Zone and Instability Hypothesis. J Spinal Disord 5:390-396, 1992.

60. Quazi M: Body and Spirit. Occupational Health and Safety 34-38, 52 and 57, July 1992.

61. Radebold A, Cholewicki J, Panjabi MM, et al: Muscle Response Pattern to Sudden Trunk Loading in Healthy Individuals and in Patients with Chronic Low Back Pain. Spine 25(8):947-954, 2000.

62. Radebold A, Cholewicki J, Polzhofer GK, et al: Impaired Postural Control of the Lumbar Spine is Associated with Delayed Muscle Response Times in Patients with Chronic Idiopathic Low Back Pain. Spine 26(7):724-730, 2001.

63. Richardson CA, Jull G. Muscle Control-Pain Control. What Exercises Would You Prescribe? Man Ther 1:2-10, 1995.

64. Richardson CA, Jull GA, Toppenberg RMK, et al: Techniques for Active Lumbar Stabilization for Spinal Protection: A Pilot Study. Aust J Physiother 38(2):105-112, 1992.

65. Richardson R, Jull G, Hodges P, et al: Therapeutic Exercise for Spinal Segmental Stabilization in Low Back Pain. Churchill Livingstone, Philadelphia 1999.

66. Rissanen A, Heliovaara M, Alaranta H, et al: Does Good Trunk Extensor Performance Protect Against Back-Related Work Disability? J Rehabil Med 34:62-66, 2002.

67. Russek LN: Examination and Treatment of a Patient with Hypermobility Syndrome. Phys Ther 80(4):386-398, 2000.

68. Russek LN: Hypermobility Syndrome. Phys Ther 79(6):591-599, 1999.

69. Saal JA: Dynamic Muscular Stabilization in the Nonoperative Treatment of Lumbar Pain Syndromes.

Orthop Rev 19:691-700, 1990.

70. Schnebel B, et al: A Digitizing Technique for the Study of Movement of Intradiscal Dye in Response to Flexion and Extension of the Lumbar Spine. Spine 13(3):309-312, 1988.

71. Schonfeld B, et al: An Occupational Performance Test Validation Program for Fire Fighters at the Kennedy Space Center. Joul of Occ Med 32:638-643, 1988.

72. Scientific Approach to the Assessment and Management of Activity-Related Spinal Disorders. A Monograph For Clinicians. Report of the Quebec Task Force on Spinal Disorders. Spine 12(7 Suppl):S1-59, 1987.

73. Sheon R, et al: The Hypermobility Syndrome. Postgrad Med 71:199-209, 1982.

74. Silcox DH, Daftari T, Boden SD, et al: The Effect of Nicotine on Spinal Fusion. Spine 14:1549-1553, 1995.

75. Sinaki M and Grubbs N: Back Strengthening Exercises: Quantitative Evaluation of Their Efficacy for Women Aged 40 to 65 Years. Arch Phys Med Rehabil 70:16-20, 1989.

76. Tabary J, et al: Experimental Rapid Sarcomere Loss in Concomittant Hypoextensibility. Muscle Nerve 4:198-203, 1981.

77. Tabary J, et al: Physiological and Structure Changes in the Cat's Soleus Muscle Due to Immobilization by Plaster Casts. Joul Physiol 224:231-244, 1972.

78. Taimela S, Kankaanpaa M, Luoto S: The Effect of Lumbar Fatigue on the Ability to Sense a Change in Lumbar Position: A Controlled Study. Spine 24(13):1322, 1999.

79. Taylor JR and O'Sullivan PB: Lumbar Segmental Instability: Pathology Diagnosis and Conservative Management. In: Physical Therapy of the Low Back, 3rd edition. LT Twomey and JR Taylor, eds. Churchill Livingstone, Philadelphia 2000.

80. Timm K: A Randomized-Control Study of Active and Passive Treatments for Chronic Low Back Pain Following L5 Laminectomy. J Orthop Sports Phys Ther 20(6):276-286, 1994.

81. Torstensen TA, Ljunggren AE, Meen HD, et al: Efficiency and Costs of Medical Exercise Therapy, Conventional Physiotherapy and Self-Exercise in Patients with Chronic Low Back Pain. Spine 23(23):2616-2624, 1998.

82. VanTulder MW, Koes BW and Bouter LM: Conservative Treatment of Acute and Chronic Nonspecific Low Back Pain. Spine 22(18):2128-2156, 1997.

83. Verna JL, Mayer JM, Mooney V, et al: Back Extension Endurance and Strength. The Effect of Variable-Angle Roman Chair Exercise Training. Spine 27(16):1772-1777, 2003.

84. Vleeming A, Pool-Goudzwaard AL, Stoeckart R, et al: The Posterior Layer of the Thoracolumbar Fascia: Its Function in Load Transfer from Spine to Legs. Spine 20:753-758, 1995.

85. Vowles KE and Gross RT: Work-Related Beliefs About Injury and Physical Capability for Work in Individuals with Chronic Pain. Pain 101:291-298, 2003.

86. Wilder DG, Aleksiev AR, Magnusson ML, et al: Muscular Response to Sudden Load; A Tool to Evaluate Fatigue and Rehabilitation. Spine 21(22):2628-2639, 1996.

7

PELVIC GIRDLE DYSFUNCTION

Allyn L. Woerman, MMSc PT

This chapter describes dysfunctional mechanics of the sacroiliac joint and introduces evaluation and treatment techniques for the most common pelvic girdle dysfunctions. The reader should refer to Chapter 2, *Spinal Biomechanics*, for prerequisite understanding of basic biomechanical principles, normal sacroiliac joint mechanics and terminology.

To evaluate pelvic girdle dysfunctions properly, the hip joint and the lumbar spine, especially the L5 and L4 segments, must also be assessed. Dysfunction in any of these joints may lead to dysfunction in the others. The influence of the entire kinetic chain on the function of these joints should not be underestimated. Biomechanical problems such as a pronated foot, genu varus/valgus knees, anteverted/retroverted hips and others will influence the entire chain.

The treatment techniques described in this chapter are primarily osteopathic in nature and use muscle energy techniques popularized by Fred Mitchell, Sr., DO[25] and Phillip Greenman, DO.[16] A muscle energy technique (MET) is a manipulative treatment procedure that uses a voluntary contraction of the patient's muscle against a distinctly controlled counterforce. The contraction is performed from a precise position and in a specific direction. METs are considered to be active techniques. They require direct positioning (where the motion restriction barrier is engaged but not stressed). METs may be used to lengthen shortened muscles, strengthen weakened muscles, reduce localized edema and mobilize restricted joints.[14,25,31,34]

Evaluation of the sacroiliac joints and pelvic complex by the osteopathic system of positional assessment uses a common sense approach that correlates comparable signs.

This means that a given dysfunctional lesion will reflect a fairly consistent pattern of findings. When considered together, these findings yield an assessment of the affected segment in three-dimensional space and in relation to adjoining segments. The clinician simply collects the raw data using palpatory and observational skills, correlates the data to a set of signs and symptoms, and formulates an assessment. The clinician then applies a specific technique to the affected segment based on that assessment. It should be kept in mind that each test viewed by itself does not make an assessment. It is only when all the data are collected and correlated that the clinician can make the correct assessment.

Signs of Pelvic Girdle Dysfunctions

Symptoms of pelvic girdle dysfunctions vary.[17,20,25,31,32,34] The pain may be sharp or dull, aching or throbbing, and so forth. The pain is often unilateral and local to the sacroiliac joint (sulcus) itself, but may be referred distally (usually posterolaterally and not below the knee) possibly due to multiple levels of innervation.[30] There are no associated neurological signs with pelvic girdle dysfunction. A straight leg raise test may be positive but only for pain in the joint or the gluteal region and usually in the higher arc above 60°. The pain is usually aggravated by walking and stair climbing and the patient may limp (with Trendelenburg or similar gait pattern). Pain intensity usually does not increase with prolonged sitting; however, when the condition is acute, the patient may sit shifted onto the opposite ischium. The patient often maintains lumbar lordosis or a flat back posture in forward bending, recruiting motion around the acetabula, and may complain of lumbar pain with forward bending. Ipsilateral tension over the erector spinæ muscles may be noted. The clinician may see a slight swelling over the dorsal aspect of the sacrum. Pain may often be present on the non-blocked side (i.e., the dysfunctional side may be non-painful but cause the opposite side to become hypermobile and painful). Finally, sacroiliac pain is more common in females than in the general population.[7]

Differentiation of Structural Asymmetry

Structural asymmetry is very common, particularly in the lumbosacral spine. If the relative position of comparable anatomic parts (right and left PSIS's, inferior lateral angles of the sacrum, etc.) remains constant through the full flexion-extension range of motion, then the asymmetry is probably due to *structural variation* of the anatomic part and may not be treatable. However, if the relative position of comparable anatomic parts changes in the full flexion-extension range of motion, then the perceived asymmetry is probably due to *functional alteration* of the parts. These are the treatable pelvic dysfunctions.

The clinician must be able to palpate various anatomical landmarks accurately and consistently and be able to relate their relative positions to one another in three-dimensional space. Only then is the clinician able to assess the patient and to test, re-test and evaluate the effects of treatment. The following landmarks are the keys to accurate assessment: iliac crests, anterior superior iliac spines (ASIS), posterior superior iliac spines (PSIS), ischial tuberosities, greater trochanters, medial malleoli, pubic tubercles, sacral inferior lateral angles (ILA), sacral sulci, sacrotuberous and sacrospinous ligaments, piriformis and tensor fascia latæ.

Dysfunctional Mechanics of the Sacroiliac Joint

The following discussion describes a model for sacroiliac dysfunction as taught by osteopathic practitioners.[25] The symptoms associated with a variety of sacroiliac joint dysfunctions are similar; certain disease processes or mechanical problems will manifest themselves in localized sacroiliac pain. Diseases such as ankylosing spondylitis, Paget's disease, or tuberculosis all may give rise to sacroiliac pain as an initial complaint.[12] Therefore, differential diagnosis of the various sacroiliac joint problems depends upon a thorough understanding of sacroiliac joint biomechanics.

Normal and dysfunctional motion about the principle sacroiliac joint axes is discussed in this section. Dysfunctional motion about the axes forms a basis for evaluation and a rationale for treatment. For simplicity, motion about each one of the axes is described individually. It must be remembered, however, that very few motions in the human body occur in a single plane about a single axis. So it is with the sacroiliac joint.

In the general population, acute strains with joint involvement are actually rare. This may not be true in certain populations such as athletes and the military.[33] Far more common in terms of mechanical dysfunction are structural and muscular imbalances and joint hypermobilities/hypomobilities which give rise to sacroiliac complaints.

The osteopathic model of dysfunction considers the sacroiliac joint to be mechanically two joints: the *iliosacral* and the *sacroiliac*. The term *iliosacral* implies the innominates moving on a fixed sacrum. The term *sacroiliac* implies the sacrum moving within fixed innominates. The common iliosacral dysfunctions are anterior and posterior innominate rotations, pubic shears, innominate upslips and downslips, and innominate inflares and outflares. The common sacroiliac dysfunctions are forward and backward sacral torsions, and unilateral sacral flexions and extensions.

Iliosacral Dysfunctions

Innominate Rotations. There are two principle rotatory dysfunctions of the innominates: anterior (forward) and posterior (backward) rotations. The axes through which these rotations occur are the Transverse Pelvic Axis and the Inferior Transverse Axis of the sacrum (refer to Chapter 2, *Spinal Biomechanics*, for a review of the sacral axes). Innominates found to be in dysfunction are described either as anterior or posterior according to the side of involvement (e.g., left posterior, right anterior innominate). By far the most common of these dysfunctional rotations is the left posterior innominate with the right anterior being second most common.[25] These two dysfunctions make up the vast majority of sacroiliac joint dysfunctions.[25]

Pubic Shears. Pubic shears are, as the name implies, a sliding of one joint surface in relation to the other in a superior or an inferior direction. Pubic shears are probably the most commonly overlooked pelvic dysfunction, however, their recognition and proper treatment are mandatory for treating pelvic and sacroiliac dysfunctions successfully. Pubic shears are associated with innominate rotations and upslips/downslips.

Superior Innominate Shears (Upslips). Innominate shears, particularly the superior, were once thought of as rather rare. However, Greenman[15] has indicated that their occurrence is much more common than previously thought. As the name suggests, a dysfunction here is a sliding of one entire innominate superiorly in relation to the other. These shears are usually traumatic in nature and result from a fall onto an ischial tuberosity or as an unexpected vertical thrust onto an extended leg.

Sacroiliac Dysfunctions

Sacral Torsions. Sacral torsions are perhaps the hardest dysfunctions to conceptualize. They occur as fixations on either of the oblique axes, usually during the gait cycle, and are held dysfunctionally by the piriformis muscle (right piriformis restricts the left oblique axis). Torsions do not occur purely on one of the two oblique axes but have a side bending component as well as a flexion/extension component. Torsions are defined by the direction in which the face of the sacrum has turned and by the axis on which this motion has occurred. It must be remembered that anatomic referencing takes place from the standard anatomic model but clinically, patients with back problems are viewed from the posterior aspect. Confusion can arise if this is forgotten.

To help visualize the concept of sacral torsion, the reader is invited to take a matchbook cover to represent the sacrum in three-dimensional space. Hold the top left corner and the bottom right corner between the thumb and long finger. The diagonal axis between the fingers represents the left oblique axis. Push forward on the top right corner of the matchbook and allow the "sacrum" to rotate between the fingers. This action approximates that of a sacral torsion to the left occurring on the left oblique axis. Thus, this torsion is labeled a Left Forward Sacral Torsion on the Left Oblique Axis or a Left-on-Left Forward Torsion (L-on-L).

By simply changing the finger holds on the matchbook to the opposite diagonal corners and pushing forward on the top left corner, the reader has now approximated a Right Forward Torsion on the Right Oblique Axis or a Right-on-Right Forward Torsion (R or R). *Note that forward torsions are only right-on-right or left-on-left.*

Backward sacral torsions positionally in space appear to be identical to forward torsions. They are, however, quite different. To visualize this concept, again take the matchbook and hold it on the left oblique axis (top left and bottom right corners). Now pull back on the top right corner. This approximates a Right Backward Torsion on the Left Oblique Axis or a Right-on-Left Backward Torsion (R-on-L). Grasping the opposite diagonal corners (top right and bottom left) and pulling the top left corner backward approximates a Left Backward Torsion on the Right Oblique Axis or a Left-on-Right Backward Torsion (L-on-R). *Note that backward torsions are only left-on-right or right-on-left.*

Unilateral Sacral Flexions. This dysfunction begins with the sacrum being fully nutated about the middle transverse axis. At this point, usually secondary to trauma, the sacrum is forced down the long arm of the joint where it becomes restricted. Thus, there is a large side bending component in this dysfunction as well as a flexion component. Because of this, the sacrum is unable to counternutate on that side.

Again using the matchbook cover, hold it about one-third the way down on each side. This simulates the middle transverse axis. Turning the cover forward between the fingertips simulates nutation. Now, by turning forward with one hand and turning backward with the other and adding a downward tilt to the side turning backward, the sacral flexion lesion is approximated.

Subjective Evaluation of the Pelvis

The reader is referred to the Subjective Evaluation section in Chapter 4, *Evaluation of the Spine*, for a thorough discussion of important questions to ask the patient with back and leg pain. Additional questions that have particular significance for a suspected pelvic girdle problem are:

Have you had a sudden sharp jolt to the leg, e.g., after unexpectedly stepping off a curb? (This is a very common mechanism for innominate rotations, shears, and upslips.)

Have you recently fallen directly onto your buttocks? (This is a very common mechanism for innominate rotations, shears, and sacral flexion lesions.)

How is the pain affected by sitting, standing, walking, or maintaining a sustained posture? (If pain increases with sitting, then a discogenic etiology is more suspect, especially with radicular pain; if pain increases with standing, then the sacroiliac joint may be implicated, especially if the patient stands unilaterally a great deal. If the pain increases with walking, then the sacroiliac joint is very much implicated, and a sacral torsion is quite likely.)

Have you recently experienced a sudden trunk flexion with rotation, e.g., chopping wood or shoveling snow? (This is a common mechanism for sacroiliac joint strain.)

Certain mechanisms of injury are particularly common with innominate rotations. Posterior innominate dysfunctions occur most frequently from repeated unilateral standing; a fall onto an ischial tuberosity; a vertical thrust onto an extended leg; lifting in a forward bent position with the knees locked; or, with females, intercourse positions involving hyperflexion and abduction of the hips. Anterior innominate dysfunctions occur most frequently following a golf or baseball swing; a horizontal thrust of the knee (dashboard injury); or any forceful movement on a diagonal (ventral) PNF pattern such as chopping wood.

Objective Evaluation of the Pelvis

Evaluation of the sacroiliac joint and pelvis begins the moment the patient enters the office. Observation of gait, and the patient's ability to sit down, stand and bend will give valuable clues about whether the patient's problem is primarily lumbar in nature or from the pelvic girdle.

In addition to simple observation, several evaluative procedures are recommended. Each procedure is performed to either provoke (or sometimes relieve) pain (thus implicating the SI joint as a potential source of symptoms), or to determine the relative positions of palpatory landmarks (to determine the type of SI joint dysfunction). Although pain provocation tests have been shown to be valid, several articles have called into question the reliability or validity of palpatory and other sacroiliac evaluative techniques.[10,18,23,35,36] Most studies showing poor reliability of SI joint tests were done on asymptomatic subjects. One study has shown the reliability of using four tests together to detect sacroiliac joint dysfunction (positive standing flexion test, uneven PSIS's in sitting, a positive supine long sitting test and a positive prone knee flexion test).[4]

The reader is encouraged to learn, practice and use the tests described in this chapter, even if their reliability has not been proven. To avoid a palpatory evaluation of the pelvis until proof of reliability exists would deprive the clinician of valuable information that can be correlated with other tests and the subjective evaluation. Certainly, caution should be used to avoid over-interpretation of any one test. A key to making an accurate diagnosis of SI joint dysfunction is to make sure all tests uniformly agree.[6] It is important to recognize that the MET treatment procedures recommended are non-invasive, gentle, and reversible. If, in the worst case, poor reliability of a test leads to inaccurate assessment of the type of dysfunction, the likelihood of harm occurring from the resulting treatment is negligible. Responsible clinicians practice to improve their personal evaluative skills, interpret all tests carefully with regard to reliability and validity concerns, and choose treatment techniques that have low risk commensurate with the certainty of the assessment.

The following clinical testing procedures and their meanings are categorized according to patient position to minimize patient position changes. The assumption is that the reader is performing a comprehensive spinal evaluation. The components of the objective evaluation as listed

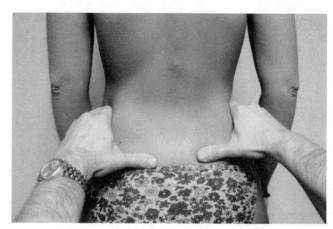

Figure 7-1: Checking the iliac crest height.

here are adjunctive to the evaluation described in Chapter 4, *Evaluation of the Spine*.

Standing Position

Posture. Make sure the feet are hip width apart and the knees are fully extended. Observe the patient from the anterior, posterior and lateral aspects for the general postural conditions (i.e., scoliosis, kyphosis, lordosis, protracted shoulders, forward head, slope of waist distances of arms from sides).

Iliac Crest Height. Iliac crest height is best observed by using the radial borders of the index fingers and the web spaces of the hands to push the soft tissue up and medially out of the way, and then pushing down on each crest with equal pressure (Fig 7-1). The clinician's eyes must be in the same plane as his hands to assess whether or one side is more caudad or cephalad than the other. This method quite accurately and precisely detects leg length discrepancies.[2] If an asymmetry is found, a lift of appropriate dimension should be placed under the short side before any of the other standing position motion tests are executed. The lift can provide pelvic balance and muscle tone symmetry before testing motion. Placing a lift under the foot is appropriate whether the asymmetry is due to a structural or functional leg length discrepancy.

Posterior Superior Iliac Spine Position. In the standing position, localization of the PSIS's is very important. An assessment should be made about the relative superoinferior and mediolateral relationships. This may be done with the ulnar borders of the thumbs or the tips of the index fingers by hooking them under the inferior aspect to the posterior spine. The clinician must be at eye level with the PSIS's to make an accurate assessment (Fig 7-2).

Anterior Superior Iliac Spine Position. As with the PSIS's, the relative superoinferior and mediolateral relationships of

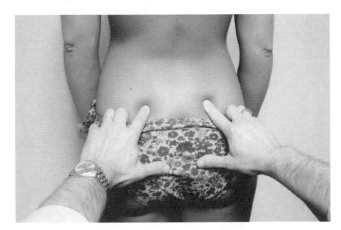

Figure 7-2: Checking PSIS position.

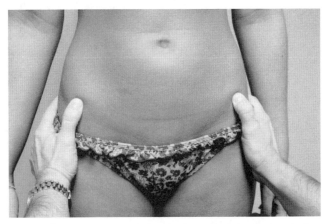

Figure 7-4: Checking ASIS position from in front of the patient.

the ASIS's must be assessed. This may be done from behind the patient with the clinician's arms extended (Fig 7-3) or from the front by visual inspection and palpation with the thumb (Fig 7-4).

Trochanteric Levels. Trochanteric levels are palpated using the same method as for the iliac crests, with the radial borders of the index fingers and the web spaces resting on the tops of the greater trochanters (Fig 7-5). Levelness here and unlevelness at the iliacs indicate pelvic dysfunctions producing an apparent leg length discrepancy. Unlevelness here only indicates a structural leg length discrepancy below the femoral neck level.

Gait. Observe the patient's gait pattern. Frequently, a pelvic girdle dysfunction produces a Trendelenburg gait or a gluteus maximus gait. The patient may side bend the trunk away from the affected side, walk with difficulty or may limp.

Standing Flexion Test . The standing flexion test of iliosacral motion is used to help the clinician determine the type of dysfunction and the side of involvement. For example, if

the standing flexion test is positive on the left, it tells the clinician that a left-sided iliosacral problem may be present (see further discussion under Sitting Flexion Test).

The standing flexion test is accomplished by localizing the PSIS's and noting their relative positions. The patient is asked to bend forward as if to touch the toes. The head and neck should be flexed and the arms should hang loose from the shoulders. As the patient bends forward, the examiner should note the cranial movement of the PSIS's (Fig 7-6). If asymmetrical motion exists, the side that moves first and/or the farthest cranially is the blocked (positive) side. The standing flexion test may be thought of as iliosacral motion recruited from the top down.

Gillet's Test (Sacral Fixation Test). Like the standing flexion test, Gillet's test is also a test of iliosacral motion, but recruitment is from the bottom up. The PSIS's are localized again. The patient is asked to stand first on one leg and then on the other while pulling the opposite knee toward the chest (Fig 7-7). If asymmetry is found, the PSIS on the unblocked side will move farther inferiorly. The blocked side will move

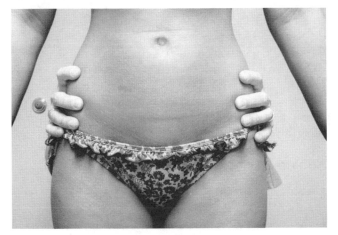

Figure 7-3: Checking ASIS position from behind the patient.

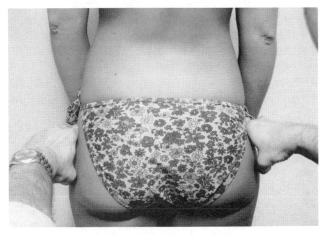

Figure 7-5: Checking greater trochanter height.

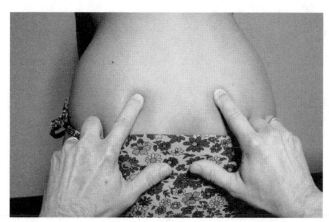

Figure 7-6: The standing flexion test of iliosacral motion. The side that moves superiorly first or farthest is the positive (blocked) side.

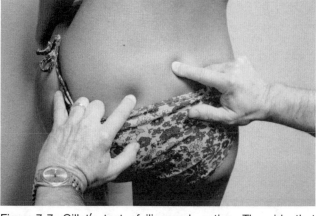

Figure 7-7: Gillet's test of iliosacral motion. The side that moves farthest inferiorly is the negative (unblocked) side.

very little. An alternate method of assessment uses the S2 spinous process as a fixed reference point for the relative PSIS movement as the patient alternately pulls the knees to the chest. Hip flexion must reach at least 90°.[20,22] The reliability of Gillet's test has been challenged.[10,23] However, performing Gillet's test may be useful to confirm the results of the standing flexion test or when patients cannot forward bend for the standing flexion test.

Active Lumbar Movements. Since lumbar lesions often occur along with iliosacral and sacroiliac dysfunctions, restrictions of lumbar movements must be assessed as well. When a pelvic girdle dysfunction exists, side bending the lumbar spine toward the affected side will often exacerbate pain. Pain on backward bending may indicate a pelvic girdle lesion as well.

Sitting Position

The sitting position fixes the innominates to a chair or table and eliminates the influence of the hamstrings on the pelvis. This allows for sacral movement within the innominates when testing motion. Additionally, active trunk rotation can best be tested since hip and pelvic motions are stabilized. The clinician should also note the posture of the patient in this position; the patient with sacroiliac joint dysfunction often tends to sit on the unaffected buttock. The sitting position also facilitates the neurological evaluation.

Iliac Crest Height. Iliac crest height is observed in the sitting position to eliminate the influence of the lower extremities on symmetry. If crest height is uneven in the sitting position, structural variation in the innominate bones is a likely cause. Other possible causes of uneven crest height in the sitting position may be shortening or spasm of the quadratus lumborum or a structural scoliosis. If asymmetry is present, a lift of appropriate size should be placed

under the ischial tuberosity of the short side before performing the sitting flexion test.

Neurological Evaluation. The clinician performs resisted muscle tests, lower extremity sensation and muscle stretch reflexes, as described in Chapter 4, *Evaluation of the Spine*.

Sitting Flexion Test. The sitting flexion test of sacroiliac motion is used to help the clinician determine the type of dysfunction and the side of involvement. For example, if the sitting flexion test is positive on the left, it tells the clinician that a left-sided *sacroiliac* problem may be present.

The clinician must again localize the PSIS's. The patient is asked to cross the arms across the chest and pass the elbows between the knees as if to touch the floor. The patient's feet should be in contact with the floor, or resting on a stool if seated on the edge of an examination table (Fig 7-8). The PSIS on the involved side will move first and/or farther cranially (i.e., the blocked joint moves solidly as one, while the sacrum on the unblocked side is free to move through its small range of motion with the lumbar spine).

If a blockage is detected in this test, and it is more positive (greater) than a restriction noted in the standing flexion test, then a sacroiliac dysfunction is implied. If the two PSIS's move symmetrically in the seated test position, yet a positive standing flexion test or Gillet's test was noted, then an iliosacral dysfunction is implied. If the standing flexion test and the sitting flexion test are both equally positive, then a soft tissue lesion is suspected.

Supine Position

Straight Leg Raising. The straight leg raising test is a common clinical test used to evaluate low back pain. It is perhaps one of the more commonly misinterpreted clinical tests as well.[26] The test applies stress to the sacroiliac joint

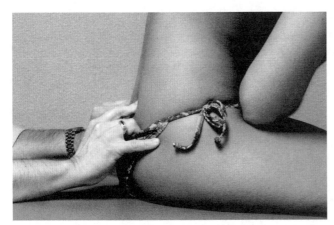

Figure 7-8: The sitting flexion test of sacroiliac motion. The side that moves superiorly first or farthest is the positive (blocked) side.

in the higher ranges of the arc and can indicate the presence of a unilateral dysfunction of the joint. It could also indicate a coexisting lumbar problem. The guidelines in Table 7-1 can help interpret the results of the straight leg raising test:

Table 7-1: Straight leg raising test results.

Range	Probable dysfunction
0 – 30°	Hip pathology or severely inflamed nerve root
30° – 50°	Sciatic nerve involvement
50° – 70°	Probable hamstring involvement
70° – 90°	Sacroiliac joint is stressed

The patient is supine on the examining table. The clinician lifts one of the patient's legs by supporting the heel while palpating the opposite ASIS (Fig 7-9). The leg is raised until the clinician can detect pelvic motion under the fingertips of the palpating hand. This determines the hamstring length in the leg being raised.[19] The other side is then tested similarly.

An active straight leg raise test has been proposed by some authors to implicate the SI joint as a potential cause of symptoms.[24,27] The patient is asked to raise one straight leg five centimeters. The test is then repeated while a manual compressive force is applied through the ilia (Fig 7-12) or with a sacroiliac belt applying circumferential pressure around the pelvis to improve SI joint stability. A positive test is denoted by improved ability to raise the leg.

Long Sitting Leg Length Test. A positive long sitting leg length test indicates an abnormal mechanical relationship of the innominates moving on the sacrum (an iliosacral dysfunction) and helps determine the presence of either an anterior innominate or a posterior innominate by a change in the relative length of the legs during the test.

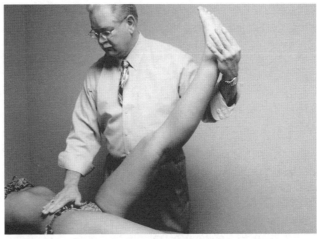

Figure 7-9: The straight leg raise test. Palpation of the opposite ASIS is done to detect pelvic motion when the hamstrings are maximally stretched.

Malleolar levelness is initially assessed in supine. The patient is then asked to perform a sit-up (with the clinician's assistance), keeping the legs straight. The clinician observes any change between the malleoli (Fig 7-10). The presence of a posterior innominate will make the leg in

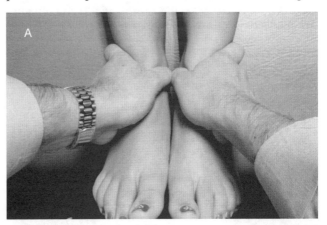

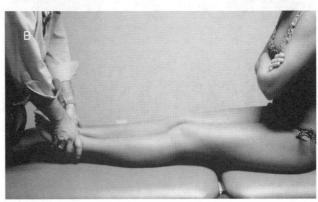

Figure 7-10: A) Assessing malleoli levelness with the patient lying supine; B) Reassessing the malleoli position after the patient assumes the long sitting position.

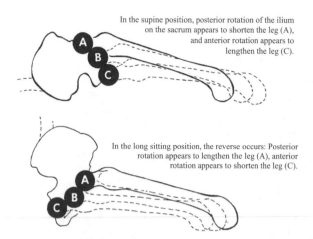

In the supine position, posterior rotation of the ilium on the sacrum appears to shorten the leg (A), and anterior rotation appears to lengthen the leg (C).

In the long sitting position, the reverse occurs: Posterior rotation appears to lengthen the leg (A), anterior rotation appears to shorten the leg (C).

Figure 7-11: Interpreting the results of the long sitting leg length test.

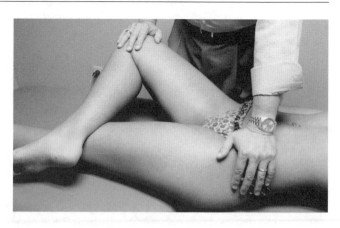

Figure 7-13: FABER (Patrick's) test. The clinician presses down on the patient's knee while stabilizing the opposite ASIS.

question (same side as the positive standing flexion test) appear to lengthen from a position of relative shortness. This occurs because, in the supine position, the posterior rotation of the innominate moves the acetabulum and the leg in a superior direction and carries the leg along with it. Thus, the leg appears shortened.

Just the opposite occurs in the anterior innominate. When the long sitting leg length test is performed, the leg

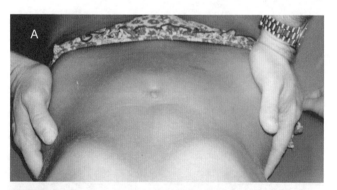

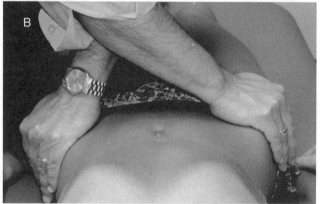

Figure 7-12: Sacroiliac joint compression-distraction test. A) Compression; and B) Distraction. The compression test can be performed in side lying if more force is required.

in question will appear to shorten from a position of relative elongation (Fig 7-11).[1]

Pelvic Rocking. The pelvic rocking test simply involves assessing the end-feel for the relative ease or resistance to passive overpressure for each innominate. The clinician places his hand on the ASIS's and gently springs the innominates alternately several times to assess the end-feel to this motion. A harder end-feel indicates a probable movement restriction on that side.

Compression-Distraction Tests. Compression-distraction tests are provocative tests performed to determine the presence of joint irritability, hypermobility, or serious disease such as ankylosing spondylitis, Paget's disease or infection. For compression, the clinician performs a quick compressive maneuver to the iliac wings laterally. In doing so, the clinician compresses the anterior and distracts the posterior sacroiliac joints. For distraction, the hands are crossed on opposite ASIS's. Downward pressure is applied to take up any slack, then a sudden, sharp spring is given to the ASIS's. This action compresses the posterior and gaps the anterior sacroiliac joints. Pain as a result of either of these maneuvers is a positive sign. Both compression and distraction have adequate inter-tester reliability (Fig 7-12).[21]

FABER (Patrick's) Test. The FABER test can be used to differentiate between hip and sacroiliac joint pain. Reliability of this test for hip range of motion has been established.[29] The hip is **F**lexed, **AB**ducted, and **E**xternally **R**otated, and the lateral malleolus is allowed to rest upon the opposite thigh above the knee. The opposite ASIS is stabilized, and pressure is applied to the other externally rotated leg at the knee (Fig 7-13). Pain located in the groin or anterior thigh is more indicative of hip joint pathology. Pain over the trochanteric region indicates hip capsular problems. Pain in the sacroiliac joint indicates sacroiliac joint involvement.

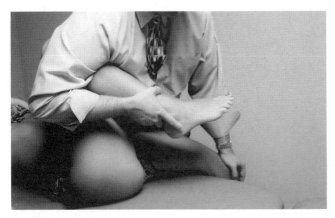

Figure 7-14: Gaenslen's test. Overpressure is applied to stress the sacroiliac joint. A painful response implicates the sacroiliac joint.

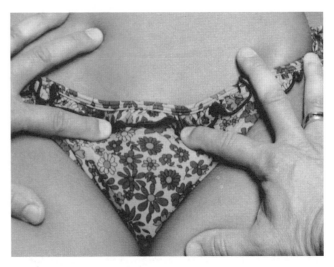

Figure 7-16: Assessing pubic tubercle height with the fingertips.

Gaenslen's Test. Gaenslen's test is a provocative test involving pelvic torsion, performed to implicate the sacroiliac joint as a source of symptoms. The patient lies supine as the contralateral hip is flexed and the ipsilateral hip is extended. Overpressure is applied to force the sacroiliac joint to its end range. Pain indicates a positive test. Gaenslen's test has been shown to have good reliability (Fig 7-14).[21]

Piriformis Tightness. Piriformis muscle tightness is easily checked by flexing the hip and knee to 90° and then passively rotating the hip into internal rotation through the lower leg (Fig 7-15). Relative end-feel and range of motion can be assessed.

Pubic Tubercle Position. The pubic tubercles are assessed for their relative superior-inferior and anteroposterior relationships. If they are unlevel, the positive side is correlated

to the side of the positive standing flexion or Gillet's test. To avoid embarrassment and unnecessary probing in this region, it is recommended that the clinician slide the heel of his hand down the abdomen until contact is made with the pubic bone. The tubercles may then be easily located with the fingertips (Fig 7-16). In most men and some women, because of the strength of the abdominal muscles, it sometimes helps to ask the patient to flex the knees a little to relax the muscles. Palpation is further facilitated by asking the patient to take a breath; upon exhalation, the clinician slides his fingers over the top and presses down upon the tubercles.

Anterior Superior Iliac Spine Position. The ASIS's must be assessed for any change from the standing position. To assess the superoinferior and mediolateral relationships, the clinician places his thumbs under the lip of the ASIS and observes the patient. To determine the anteroposterior relationship of the ASIS's, the clinician places the fingertips

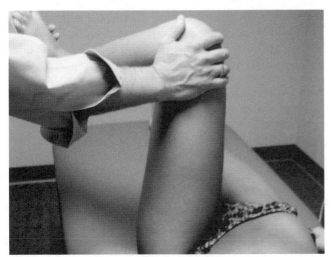

Figure 7-15: Checking for piriformis tightness in the supine position.

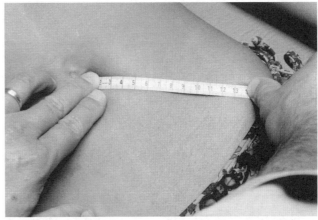

Figure 7-17: Measuring the distance from the umbilicus to the ASIS to check for inflare or outflare.

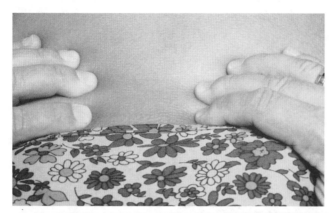

Figure 7-18: Assessing the depth of the sacral sulci.

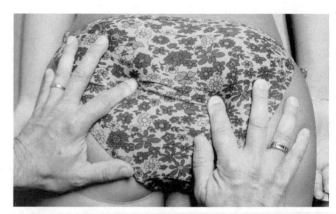

Figure 7-20: Assessing the position of the sacral ILA's.

on the tips of the ASIS's and sights along the plane of the abdomen. The umbilicus also becomes a reference point for mediolateral positioning. A tape measure may be used from the umbilicus to the inside border of the ASIS to determine the presence of an iliac inflare or outflare (Fig 7-17).

Prone Position

Depth and Tenderness of Sacral Sulci (Medial PSIS). The depths of the sacral sulci are best determined if the clinician uses the tips of the long fingers while curling his fingers around the posterior aspects of the iliac crests (Fig 7-18). The clinician assesses not only the relative depth of each sulcus but the quality of the ligaments, by palpating for tightness, tenderness and swelling. If a sacroiliac joint problem exists, tenderness in the sulcus can be quite localized. If one side is found to be deeper than the other, this could indicate a sacral torsion or an innominate rotation.

The depth of the sacral sulci is then reassessed with the patient in the Sphinx position (prone on elbows) or press-up position (Fig 7-19). The clinician notes whether any difference found in sulci depth becomes more pronounced or less pronounced in the Sphinx position. This distinction

helps determine whether a possible sacral torsion is backward or forward.

Inferior Lateral Angles. The ILA's are compared as to their relative caudad/cephalad and anteroposterior positions (Fig 7-20). If one side is found to be more caudad or posterior, then a sacroiliac lesion is implicated. If the ILA's are level but a deep sacral sulcus was found, the lesion may be in one of the innominates.

The position of the ILA's is reassessed with the patient in the Sphinx position. The clinician notes whether any differences found in ILA position become more pronounced or less pronounced in the Sphinx position. If a sacral torsion is present, this distinction will determine whether the sacral torsion is backward or forward.

Sacrotuberous and Sacrospinous Ligament Symmetry. These ligaments must be palpated through the gluteal mass (Fig 7-21). The clinician must assess changes in tension and springiness from one side to the other. If such changes are noted, they are due to positional changes of the ilium.

Piriformis Tightness. The piriformis was tested in the supine position while on stretch. It is now tested while not on stretch by having the patient flex the knees to 90° and internally rotate the hips (Fig 7-22). This position also tests the short rotators of the hip.

Ischial Tuberosities. The clinician checks for the relative anteroposterior and cephalad/caudad relationships of the ischial tuberosities by using the thumbs to push soft tissue out of the way (Fig 7-23). A change in the anteroposterior relationship may indicate an innominate rotation. A change in the cephalad/caudad relationship may indicate an ilium upslip or downslip.

Rotation of L4 and L5. To test for rotation of L4 and L5, the clinician uses the thumbs to palpate the transverse processes bilaterally at each level and compares their relative levelness (Fig 7-24). The test is repeated with the patient's lumbar spine in both flexion and extension. This is easily

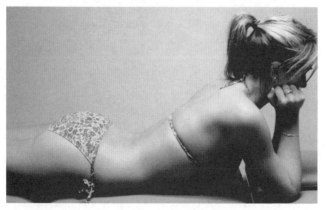

Figure 7-19: The Sphinx (prone on elbows) position.

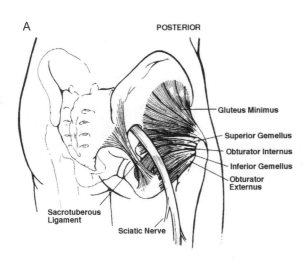

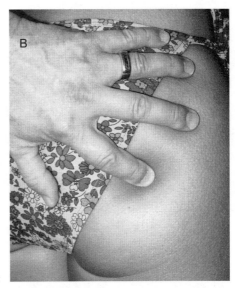

Figure 7-21: Locating the sacrotuberous ligament. A) Drawing showing anatomy; B) Palpation location.

accomplished by the patient assuming the sphinx position for testing extension or assuming the prayer position for testing flexion (Fig 7-25). If unlevelness is seen, the segment is rotated in the direction of the most posterior transverse process. Rotation of the lower lumbar segments may indicate a compensated curve or non-compensated problem in response to a pelvic girdle dysfunction.

Sacral Mobility Test. To test the passive mobility of the sacrum within the innominates, the clinician palpates the sacral sulci while applying posteroanterior pressure on the sacrum (Fig 7-26). Hypermobility or hypomobility can be assessed by the relative amount of movement between the PSIS and the dorsal aspect of the sacrum.

Lumbar Spring Test . The standard spring test is applied to the lumbar spine to help rule out the possibility of a lumbar lesion (Fig 7-27).

Prone Leg Length Test. The clinician stands at the foot of the examination table and holds the patient's feet in a symmetrical position with thumbs placed transversely across the soles of the feet just forward of the heel pad. Sighting through the plane of the heel with eyes perpendicular to the malleoli, the clinician assesses the relative length of the legs in the prone position (the short side may not be the same as in the supine or standing position). If one leg appears short, it is the positive side. The knees are then simultaneously flexed to 90° (Fig 7-28). Care must be taken to maintain the feet in the neutral position and to bring the feet up in the midline. Deviation to either side will cause a false impression. If the leg still appears short, an anterior innominate is suspected. If the leg that seemed short now appears longer, a posterior innominate should be suspected.

Hip Rotation Range of Motion. Asymmetrical hip range of motion has been shown to correlate with sacroiliac dysfunction. Cibulka, et al showed that patients who had evidence of a posterior innominate had greater external rotation than internal rotation on the side of the posterior innominate. In patients with low back pain without evidence of sacroiliac involvement, hip internal and external rotation were more symmetric between sides, although external rotation exceeded internal rotation.[5] Hip range of motion is measured in prone in neutral abduction/adduction and with the knee flexed to 90°.

Sacral Provocation Tests. Sacral provocation tests should be done only when the above series of tests has not provided a clear picture of the dysfunction. These tests should not be performed if the previous tests have demonstrated a hypermobility. They are performed in a manner similar to the sacral mobility test (Fig 7-26). In chronic sacroiliac joint pain, provocation should increase symptoms due to adaptive shortening of the soft tissues. Sacral provocation tests include:

- Anteroposterior pressure on the sacrum at its base (this encourages sacral flexion)

- Anteroposterior pressure on the sacrum at its apex (this encourages sacral extension)

- Anteroposterior pressure on each side of the sacrum just medially to the PSIS's (this encourages motion about the vertical axis)

- Cephalad pressure on the sacrum applied near the apex (note pain or movement abnormalities)

- Cephalad pressure on the sacrum applied near the base (note pain or movement abnormalities)

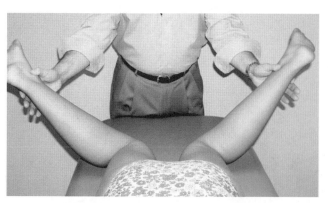

Figure 7-22: Checking for piriformis tightness in the prone position.

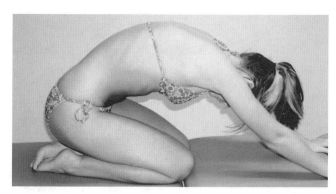

Figure 7-25: The prayer position.

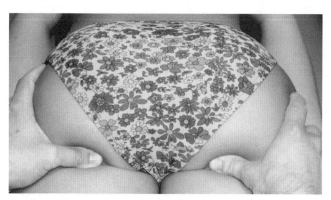

Figure 7-23: Checking the positions of the ischial tuberosities.

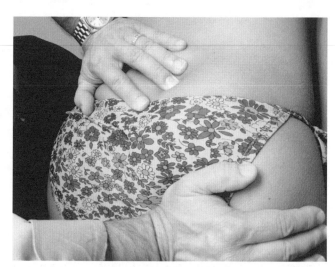

Figure 7-26: A sacral mobility test. The clinician palpates the sacral sulcus while pressing downward on the inferior sacrum. This test can also be performed for provocation of symptoms.

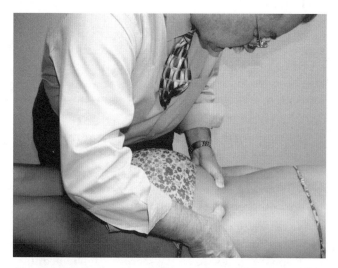

Figure 7-24: Testing for rotation of L4 and L5 in prone. This can also be done in standing.

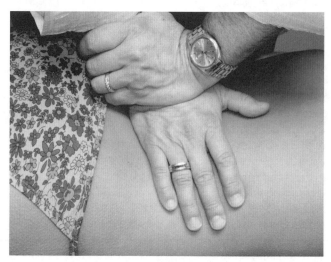

Figure 7-27: The lumbar spring test.

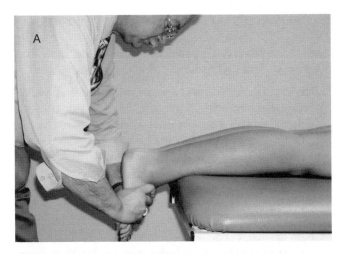

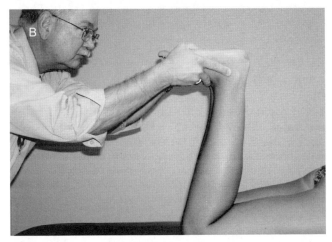

Figure 7-28: Assessing leg length in prone. A) Starting position; B) Rechecking leg length after the knees are bent to 90°.

If a sulcus is found to be deep, pressure is applied on the opposite ILA to see if the sulcus becomes more shallow (this encourages torsional movement about the oblique axis).

Side Lying Position

Tensor Fascia Latæ. Length of the tensor fascia latæ is assessed in side lying. The patient's uppermost hip is extended then adducted (Fig 7-29). The clinician should stabilize the pelvis to prevent side bending of the lumbar spine, thus producing a false-negative result. Restriction or symptom reproduction in extension and adduction (Ober's sign) indicates a tight tensor fascia latæ.

Physical Findings and Assessment of Pelvic Girdle Dysfunctions

Physical findings for the major pelvic girdle dysfunctions are summarized in diagram form (Fig 7-30). The physical

findings are correlated to the results of the standing and sitting flexion tests. The standing and sitting flexion tests are important because they help determine whether the dysfunction is iliosacral or sacroiliac. In the following paragraphs, Gillet's test can be used to confirm the results of the standing flexion test or instead of the standing flexion test if the patient does not have adequate forward bending mobility:

- If the standing flexion test is positive, an *iliosacral* lesion is implicated.
- If the sitting flexion test is positive, a *sacroiliac* lesion is implicated.
- If both the standing and sitting flexion tests are positive, the patient likely has a combination lesion (multiple lesions) or soft tissue restriction.
- In both the standing and sitting flexion tests, the side that moves first and/or farthest is the restricted side.

Using the diagrams in Figure 7-30 is simple, once the nomenclature and thought process is understood. First, choose either diagram A or B, depending on whether the standing flexion or the sitting flexion test is positive. Then, perform each additional test listed at the left of the applicable diagram, and use the results on the right to classify the dysfunction. "SS" refers to the same side as the positive standing flexion or sitting flexion test, and "OS" refers to the opposite side.

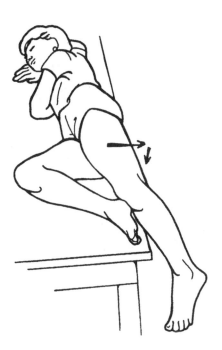

Figure 7-29: Testing for tensor fascia latæ tightness.

Note that combination or multiple lesions are more common than simple isolated lesions. For simplicity, the findings for each lesion in the following section are presented as though they occur singularly without another dysfunction present. In reality, the patient often presents with findings that do not clearly fit with any of the diagnostic entities.

In the case where two or more findings conflict, the clinician should place more emphasis on the tests that were the *most* positive, and/or correlate more readily with other objective and subjective findings (i.e., if the standing flexion test is more positive than the sitting flexion test, the restriction is more likely to be iliosacral, and vice versa).

Iliosacral Lesions (Positive Standing Flexion)

Iliosacral lesions can involve the following: 1) Posterior innominates; 2) Anterior innominates; 3) Pubic shears; and 4) Iliac subluxations (upslips).

Posterior Innominate. The posterior innominate is a unilateral iliosacral dysfunction. It is by far the most common pelvic dysfunction, particularly on the left.[33] The main findings for a left posterior innominate are summarized in Figure 7-30. In addition, the clinician may note tenseness of the sacroiliac ligament, decreased lumbar lordosis, and sacral sulcus or unilateral buttock pain.

Anterior Innominate. The anterior innominate is also a unilateral iliosacral dysfunction. It is essentially the reverse of the posterior innominate and occurs more commonly on the right. The main findings for an anterior innominate are summarized in Figure 7-30. The clinician may also note a possibly increased lumbar lordosis and concurrent cervical and lumbar symptoms.

Pubic Shear. Dysfunctions of the pubic symphysis are probably the most commonly overlooked lesions of the pelvis. The lesions that usually occur at this joint are shear lesions in a superior or an inferior direction. Anterior and posterior shears are rare and are usually the result of trauma. The main findings for a superior pubis are summarized in Figure 7-30. Almost every pubic shear lesion occurs simultaneously with a posterior innominate or upslip.[15]

Innominate Shear (Upslip). Once considered uncommon, vertical shear lesions of an entire innominate have been shown to occur more frequently than originally thought.[15] The main findings for a superior shear are summarized in Figure 7-30.

Sacroiliac Lesions (Positive Sitting Flexion)

Sacroiliac lesions can involve the following: 1) Sacral Torsions, and 2) Sacral Flexions.

Sacral Torsion. Assessment and terminology of sacral torsions can be confusing. First, the clinician must decide whether a sacral torsion is present. Then he must determine whether the torsion is a forward torsion or a backward torsion. This is done by retesting the position of the sacral sulci with the patient in an extended (Sphinx) position as described previously. Finally, the torsion must be named. Forward torsions are always *right on a right* oblique axis or *left on a left* oblique axis. Backward torsions are always *right on a left* oblique axis or *left on a right* oblique axis. The axis of involvement is the same as the side of the shallow sacral sulcus. Most sacral torsions occur around the left oblique axis. The findings for a sacral torsion are summarized in Figure 7-30.

Sacral Flexion. Unilateral sacral flexion occurs primarily around the middle transverse axis of the sacroiliac joint. It might be thought of as failure of one side of the sacrum to counternutate from a fully nutated position. When this occurs, a side bending component is present, driving the sacrum down the long arm of the joint. Findings for a unilateral sacral flexion are summarized in Figure 7-30.

Treatment of Pelvic Girdle Dysfunctions

If the clinician finds multiple lesions, they should all be treated, but in this suggested order:

1. Pubic lesions
2. Nonadapting lumbar compensations
3. Sacroiliac lesions
4. Iliosacral lesions

This treatment order takes advantage of the axes of motion, so that unlocking a restriction in one area helps unlock the restriction in another. A very common combination of lumbopelvic dysfunctions consists of left superior pubic shear, left-on-left forward sacral torsion, and left posterior innominate. The lumbar spine is usually adaptive in response to these dysfunctions and does not need correction. If the lumbar spine dysfunction is non-adaptive, it should be treated using the muscle energy or joint mobilization techniques discussed in Chapter 10, *Joint Mobilization.*

Muscle Energy Techniques

As discussed previously, a muscle energy technique (MET) is any manipulative treatment that uses a voluntary contraction of the patient's muscles against a distinctly

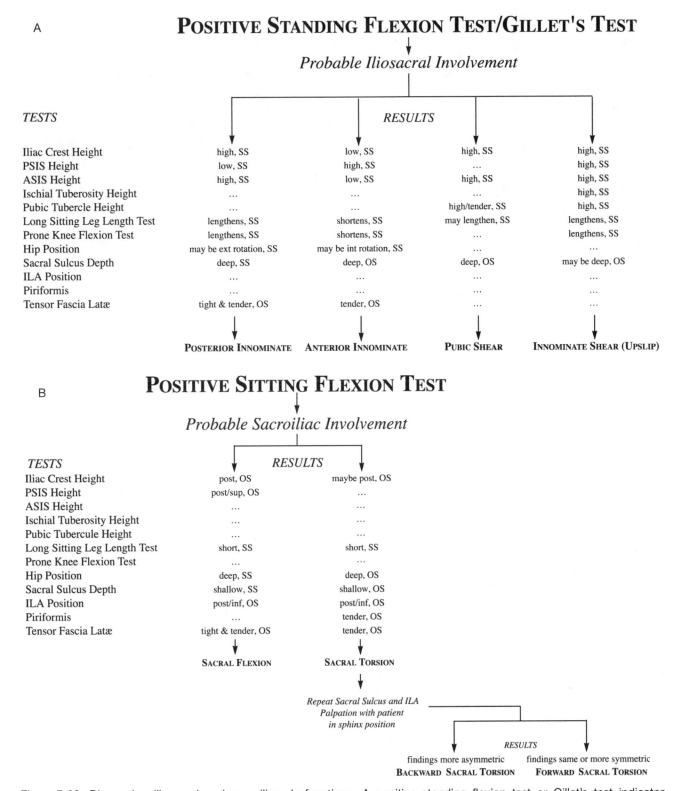

A

POSITIVE STANDING FLEXION TEST/GILLET'S TEST

Probable Iliosacral Involvement

TESTS	RESULTS			
Iliac Crest Height	high, SS	low, SS	high, SS	high, SS
PSIS Height	low, SS	high, SS	...	high, SS
ASIS Height	high, SS	low, SS	high, SS	high, SS
Ischial Tuberosity Height	...	...	...	high, SS
Pubic Tubercle Height	...	...	high/tender, SS	high, SS
Long Sitting Leg Length Test	lengthens, SS	shortens, SS	may lengthen, SS	lengthens, SS
Prone Knee Flexion Test	lengthens, SS	shortens, SS	...	lengthens, SS
Hip Position	may be ext rotation, SS	may be int rotation, SS	...	...
Sacral Sulcus Depth	deep, SS	deep, OS	deep, OS	may be deep, OS
ILA Position	...	...	...	...
Piriformis	...	...	...	...
Tensor Fascia Latæ	tight & tender, OS	tender, OS	...	...
	POSTERIOR INNOMINATE	**ANTERIOR INNOMINATE**	**PUBIC SHEAR**	**INNOMINATE SHEAR (UPSLIP)**

B

POSITIVE SITTING FLEXION TEST

Probable Sacroiliac Involvement

TESTS	RESULTS	
Iliac Crest Height	post, OS	maybe post, OS
PSIS Height	post/sup, OS	...
ASIS Height	...	...
Ischial Tuberosity Height	...	...
Pubic Tubercule Height	...	...
Long Sitting Leg Length Test	short, SS	short, SS
Prone Knee Flexion Test	...	...
Hip Position	deep, SS	deep, OS
Sacral Sulcus Depth	shallow, SS	shallow, OS
ILA Position	post/inf, OS	post/inf, OS
Piriformis	...	tender, OS
Tensor Fascia Latæ	tight & tender, OS	tender, OS
	SACRAL FLEXION	**SACRAL TORSION**

Repeat Sacral Sulcus and ILA Palpation with patient in sphinx position

RESULTS

findings more asymmetric   findings same or more symmetric
BACKWARD SACRAL TORSION   **FORWARD SACRAL TORSION**

Figure 7-30: Diagnosing iliosacral and sacroiliac dysfunctions. A positive standing flexion test or Gillet's test indicates probable *iliosacral* involvement. A positive sitting flexion test indicates probable *sacroiliac* involvement. The clinician consults either diagram A or B to interpret the results of additional tests to determine the type of dysfunction. SS=same side and OS=opposite side of the applicable test (standing flexion/Gillet's or sitting flexion). Refer to the text for more assistance in interpreting these diagrams.

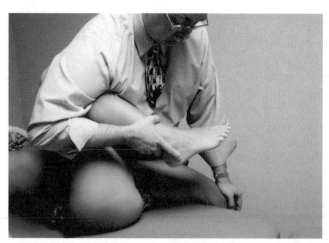

Figure 7-31: Position for treatment of a left posterior innominate with muscle energy technique.

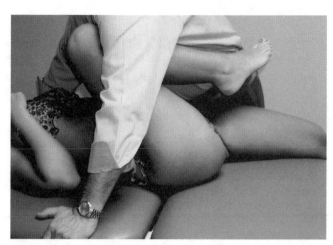

Figure 7-32: Position for treatment of a right anterior innominate with muscle energy technique.

controlled counterforce from a precise position and in a specific direction. METs may be used to lengthen shortened muscles, strengthen weakened muscles, reduce localized edema, and mobilize restricted joints.[14,25,31,34] The focus of this section will be on the use of METs to mobilize joint restrictions.

Posterior Innominate (Fig 7-31). The main features of a posterior innominate were summarized in Figure 7-30. Muscular correction of this positional fault uses muscles that can rotate the innominate in an anterior direction. In this case, the rectus femoris is the major mover:

1. The patient is supine with the involved leg hanging freely over the edge of the treatment table as pictured. The hip is extended and the knee is flexed.

2. The opposite hip and knee are flexed up toward the patient's chest until the freely hanging leg begins to come up. The patient is instructed to hold the flexed knee and hip in that position with his hands. The clinician may assist with a hand, arm or shoulder.

3. The clinician places the other hand on the anterior supracondylar area of the freely hanging knee and gently pushes down to take up the slack.

4. The patient is then instructed to push the freely hanging leg up against the clinician's hand with a submaximal force, holding it constant for 7-10 seconds while breathing in a relaxed, smooth manner. It is important for the clinician to give unyielding resistance to the contraction.

5. As the patient relaxes the contraction, the clinician takes up the slack by pushing down on the freely hanging leg and helps the patient pull the flexed hip and knee up to the new barrier. The contraction is then again executed in the new position. This procedure is repeated three or four times.

6. The patient is now re-examined for any changes produced by these efforts, usually by the long sitting leg length test. Treatment is repeated if necessary.

This technique can be used at home by hanging the uninvolved leg from the edge of a bed or other raised surface and bringing the opposite hip and knee to the chest. The patient should then hold that position for 2-3 minutes and perform slow, relaxed breathing, taking up any slack occurring from the stretch.

The breathing techniques used for both the anterior and the posterior innominate procedures take advantage of rotatory motion of the innominate around the superior transverse (respiratory) axis of the sacroiliac joints.

Anterior Innominate (Fig 7-32). The main features of an anterior innominate were summarized in Figure 7-30. Muscular correction of this positional fault uses muscles that can rotate the innominate in a posterior direction. The major mover is the gluteus maximus.

1. The patient is supine with the opposite leg hanging freely from the edge of the treatment table, supported at approximately the level of the ischium.

2. The hip and knee are flexed on the involved side until the freely hanging leg begins to come up.

3. The clinician may then stabilize the flexed knee with his shoulder or instruct the patient to hold the leg in that fixed position with his hands.

4. The patient is then instructed push the knee on the involved side against his hands or the clinician's shoulder with a submaximal sustained contraction

(isometric). Note that the hip is not allowed to move into extension at any time, only flexion.

5. As with other METs, the forces generated are submaximal, the contraction is held for 7-10 seconds, the slack is taken up to the new barrier, and the technique is repeated three or four times until all slack is taken up.

6. The patient is now re-examined for any change, usually by the long sitting leg length test or the standing flexion test. The treatment is repeated if necessary.

The patient can perform this treatment as a home program two to three times per day for the next several days. It should be noted that this technique is a powerful rotator for the innominate and can be easily overdone unless specific guidelines are given.

Superior Pubic Shear (Fig 7-33). The main features of a superior pubic shear were summarized in Figure 7-30. Muscular correction of this very common pelvic dysfunction uses the combined forces of the rectus femoris and the hip adductor group to effect the mobilization:

1. The patient is supine with the leg on the involved side hanging freely from the edge of the table. The clinician stands on the same side as the lesion.

2. The lower portion of the freely hanging leg is passively extended at the knee and is held in this position, supported between the legs of the clinician.

3. The clinician then reaches across the patient and places one hand on the ASIS opposite the side of involvement to stabilize it.

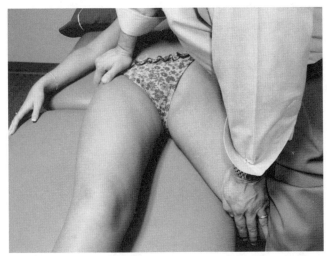

Figure 7-33: Position for treatment of a left superior pubic shear by muscle energy technique. The clinician's left leg is maintaining the position of the patient's left leg in passive extension and abduction.

4. With the other hand, the clinician gently presses down on the supracondylar areas of the freely hanging leg and takes up the available slack at the hip. The clinician does this maintaining the position of the knee in passive extension between her own legs.

5. The patient is then instructed, "Squeeze your thigh toward the table and push your leg up against my hand." The clinician offers unyielding resistance to the upward contraction, and the table offers unyielding resistance to adduction. The knee must be maintained in passive extension as the patient tries to raise the leg.

6. As with other METs, the forces generated are submaximal, the contraction is held for 7-10 seconds, the slack is taken up to the new barrier, and the technique is repeated three or four times until all slack is taken up. Stabilization of the opposite ASIS is particularly important during this test.

The patient is reexamined and treatment is repeated as needed.

Combined Treatment for Superior and Inferior Pubic Shear (Fig 7-34). This technique is a powerful mover of the pubic symphysis. It first employs the hip abductors to "gap" the joint and then the hip adductors to "reset" the joint in its normal position.

1. The patient is supine with her knees flexed and together. The clinician stands at either side of the table.

2. The clinician places his hands on the outsides of the patient's knees and instructs the patient, "Push your legs apart," (abduct the knees). This is done with maximal force, and the clinician resists this effort by pushing against the lateral aspects of the patient's knees. This isometric contraction is held for 7-10 seconds. The patient is then instructed to relax.

3. The patient is then instructed to allow her legs to "fall apart" (abduct the knees). The clinician guides this action so that the feet are held together and the legs abduct 30-45°. Step 3 is repeated in this new position, with the patient giving a maximal contraction into abduction while the clinician resists this effort.

4. As the patient relaxes the contraction, the clinician quickly places his forearm between the patient's knees (the clinician's hand and elbow make contact with the medial aspects of the patient's knees), and the patient is instructed, "Squeeze your knees together against my hand" (adduct the knees). This is also done with a maximal contraction.

5. The contraction is held for a few seconds and then relaxed. It may need to be repeated once or twice

more before repositioning the patient on the table to retest. Treatment may be repeated if necessary. Many times an audible "pop" is heard during this treatment. This represents a separation of the pubic symphysis, allowing it to "reset" itself. This technique can be used separately or in combination with the specific pubic subluxation technique previous described.

Superior Innominate Shear (Upslip) (Fig 7-35). The main features of an iliac upslip were summarized in Figure 7-30. This technique is a direct action thrust technique but applies principles of "close-packed" versus "loose-packed" joint mechanics to effect the mobilization.

1. The patient lies prone, and the clinician stands at the foot of the treatment table on the side of the lesion.

2. The clinician grasps the patient's distal lower leg above the ankle and raises the entire leg into approximately 30° of hip and lumbar extension, 30° of hip abduction, and hip internal rotation. This approximates the closed-packed position of the hip as much as possible.

3. The clinician then instructs the patient to grasp the top table edge with his hands. The clinician proceeds to take up the slack by distracting the leg along its long axis until tightness is perceived along the kinetic chain.

4. The clinician now instructs the patient, "Take a deep breath and cough." Timing is important. As the patient coughs, the clinician gives a quick, caudad tug on the leg.

5. The patient is then retested and treatment is repeated if necessary.

By employing the closed-packed position of the hip, the effect of the distraction is applied to the innominate instead of the hip. Mobilization of the hip is done supine in the loose-packed position.

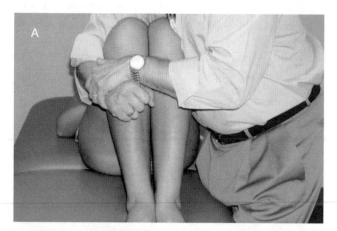

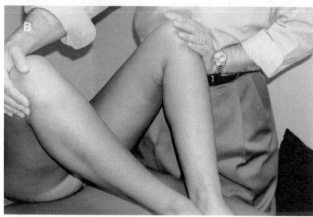

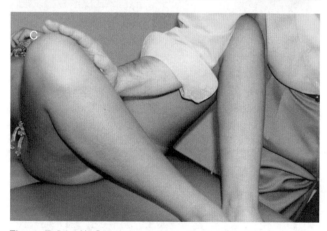

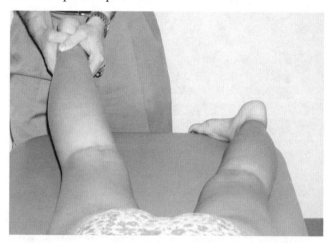

Figure 7-34: A) Starting position for treatment of a pubic shear by muscle energy technique. The patient tries to abduct the hips as the clinician holds her knees together. B) The clinician repositions the hips into more abduction, and the patient repeats resisted abduction. C) Final position for treatment of a pubic shear. The clinician quickly places his forearm between the patient's knees and asks her to squeeze the knees together.

Figure 7-35: Position for treatment of a right superior iliac subluxation (upslip) by direct action thrust technique. The leg is extended 30°, abducted 30° and internally rotated to approximate the close packed position of the hip.

Forward Sacral Torsion (Left-on-Left or Right-on-Right) (Fig 7-36).   The main features of a forward sacral torsion were summarized in Figure 7-30. Muscular correction of forward sacral torsion uses the piriformis muscles to move the sacrum on one of its oblique axes. In a *left-on-left forward torsion*, the right piriformis is holding the sacrum so that it cannot move normally on its left oblique axis. The right oblique axis is free to move. In the following description of treatment for a left-on-left forward torsion, the right internal rotators contract, causing reciprocal inhibition of the right piriformis. This allows the sacrum to move on the left oblique axis. At the same time, the left piriformis contracts, which moves the sacrum into its correct position.

1. The patient lies on the side corresponding to the axis of involvement. Therefore, a patient with a left-on-left torsion would lie on the left side. The clinician stands at the side of the table, facing the patient.

2. The patient should be as close to the edge of the table as possible. The downside arm should rest behind the trunk (the hand may be used to stabilize the patient by gripping the edge of the treatment table behind the patient). The topside arm hangs over the edge of the table closest to the clinician as the trunk of the patient is rotated forward and the chest approximates the table.

3. The clinician's cephalad hand palpates the lumbosacral junction while the caudad hand flexes the patient's knees and hips approximately 70-90° or until the clinician can appreciate motion occurring at the lumbosacral junction. This is best achieved by grasping both legs together at the ankles and moving the hips passively into flexion. The patient's knees should be resting in the hollow of the clinician's hip as the clinician translates his body laterally toward the patient's head to flex the patient's hips.

4. The clinician now moves his hand from the lumbosacral junction and places it on the patient's shoulder near the edge of the treatment table. The patient is instructed, "Take a deep breath," and as she exhales, "Reach toward the floor." As the patient does this, the clinician assists by pressing down on the patient's shoulder to take up the slack. This is repeated two or three times until all the slack is gone.

5. The clinician now returns that hand to the lumbosacral junction and, using the hand holding the ankles, lowers the ankles toward the floor until resistance is met and/or motion is felt at the lumbosacral junction.

6. The clinician now instructs the patient, "Lift both ankles toward the ceiling." This causes contraction of the right internal rotators and the left piriformis. This is a submaximal contraction, and the clinician must

be sure to give unyielding resistance (hold-relax contraction) to the patient's effort. The contraction is held for 7-10 seconds and is then relaxed.

7. As the contraction is relaxed, the clinician takes up the slack by translating his body cephalad (to increase flexion) and lowers the ankles toward the floor until resistance is met or motion felt at the lumbosacral junction (to increase side bending), and the patient reaches toward the floor with the hanging arm (to increase rotation).

Steps 6 and 7 are repeated two or three times. Then the patient is retested to check for changes in sacral position. The treatment is repeated if necessary.

In some instances, the edges of the treatment table are uncomfortable to the patient's downside thigh during the contractions in step 6. The clinician must some times support the patient's knees with his own thigh or may sit on the treatment table and perform the technique from that position.

Backward Sacral Torsion (Left-on-Right or Right-on-Left) (Fig 7-37).   The main features of a backward sacral torsion were summarized in Figure 7-30. Muscular correction of backward sacral torsion uses muscles that will cause the sacrum to move forward on an oblique axis. The technique described uses the gluteus medius, tensor fascia latæ and the gluteus maximus:

1. The patient lies on the side corresponding to the axis of involvement. This means that a patient with a left-on-right torsion would lie on the right side. The patient lies as close to the edge of the table as possible, and the clinician stands at the same edge facing the patient.

2. The clinician grasps the patient's downside arm (usually above the elbow) and pulls it out from under the patient. The patient's trunk is now rotated so that the back approximates the table surface. The clinician now somewhat flexes the patient's topmost leg at the hip and knee. The downside leg is allowed to remain straight for the moment.

3. The clinician now palpates the patient's lumbosacral junction with the cephalad hand. With the other hand, the clinician reaches behind the patient's topside flexed knee and passively extends the patient's bottom hip by pushing the leg posteriorly. The clinician does this until motion is perceived at the lumbosacral junction.

4. The clinician now repositions his hands so that the caudal hand now palpates the lumbosacral junction.

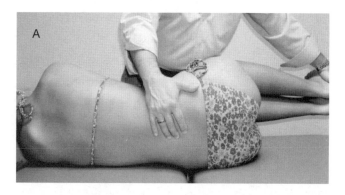

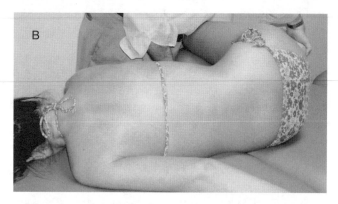

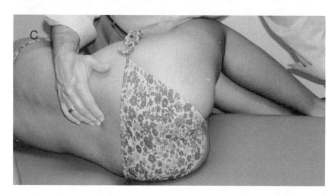

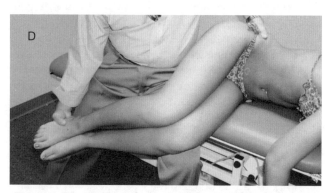

Figure 7-36: Treatment of a left-on-left forward sacral torsion by MET. A) Starting position; B) After flexion and rotation of the patient's spine; C) Lowering the ankles to left side bend the lumbar spine until movement is felt at the lumbosacral junction; D) Alternate position.

5. The clinician now uses the forearm of his caudad arm to stabilize the pelvis and instructs the patient, "Take a deep breath." As the patient exhales, the clinician presses downward on the shoulder, causing greater trunk rotation and further approximating the trunk to the table surface. This maneuver is repeated two or three times to take up all the slack. The clinician must be careful not to allow the pelvis to move and change its alignment.

6. Maintaining trunk rotation and pelvic alignment, the clinician instructs the patient, "Straighten the topside knee and allow the leg to hang freely from the table." Being careful not to change pelvic alignment, the clinician slides the caudad hand down the thigh to the lateral supracondylar area of the patient's knee.

7. The patient is then instructed, "Lift the knee toward the ceiling," while the clinician provides unyielding resistance to the effort. The contraction is held for 7-10 seconds and is then relaxed.

8. The clinician takes up slack by moving the downside leg back a little (to increase extension), rotating the trunk a little (to increase rotation), and pushing down on the hanging leg until resistance is met (to increase side bending).

Steps 7 and 8 are repeated two or three times, and the patient is then retested to check for positional changes of the sacrum. Treatment is repeated if necessary.

Unilateral Sacral Flexion (Fig 7-38). The main features of a unilateral sacral flexion were summarized in Figure 7-30. Muscular correction of this sacral positional fault takes advantage of the normal nutation-counternutation movement of the sacrum during respiration. By accentuating the breathing pattern and applying direct pressure, the sacrum can be made to move up the long arm of the joint axis to its normal resting position:

1. The patient lies prone. The clinician stands on the same side as the lesion.

2. With a finger, the clinician palpates the sacral sulcus on the side of the lesion and abducts the patient's hip on the involved side approximately 15°, then internally rotates that hip. This hip position is maintained throughout the procedure.

3. Using a straight arm force, the clinician places a constant downward pressure on the ILA on the side of the lesion with the heel of the hand in the direction of the navel.

4. Maintaining pressure on the sacrum, the clinician instructs the patient to take in his breath in "small sips" (as through a soda straw) until she can hold no

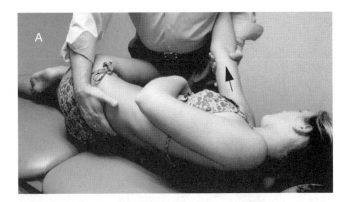

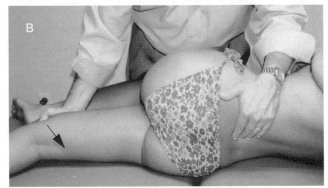

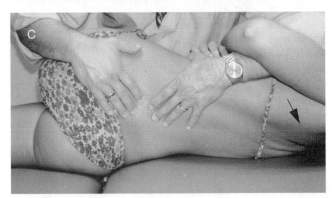

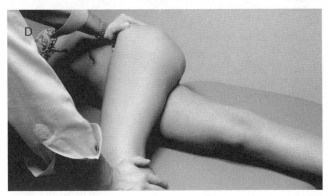

Figure 7-37: Treatment of a left-on-right backward sacral torsion by muscle energy technique. A) Trunk rotation; B) Extending the patient's lumbar spine until movement is felt at the lumbosacral junction; C) Localizing lumbar rotation; D) Stabilizing the final position as the patient attempts to raise her top leg toward the ceiling.

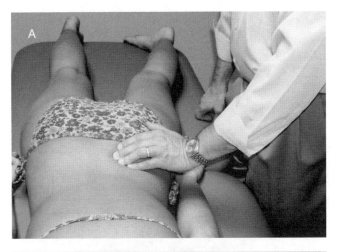

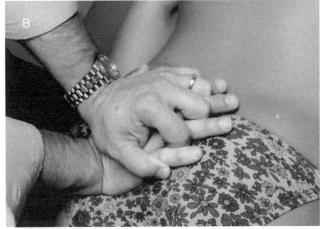

Figure 7-38: Treatment of a left unilateral sacral flexion. A) Palpation of the sacral sulcus with abduction and internal rotation of the hip; B) Exerting downward pressure on the left ILA.

more air, then hold this breath with lungs maximally filled.

5. After several seconds, the clinician instructs the patient to release this air while the clinician maintains the constant downward pressure on the ILA.

Steps 4 and 5 are repeated three or four times, and then the patient is retested for positional changes of the sacrum. Treatment is repeated if necessary.

Self-Treatment Techniques

Posterior Innominate. Self-treatment for a posterior innominate is done by hanging the involved extremity off the edge of a bed or table, while holding the contralateral knee to the chest (Fig 7-39). Ankle weights can be added. The patient should be encouraged to relax completely. An alternate technique involves the patient half-kneeling on the involved extremity (Fig 7-40).

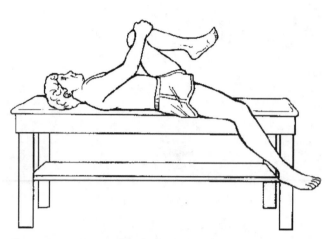

Figure 7-39: Self-treatment using the supine position for right posterior innominate.

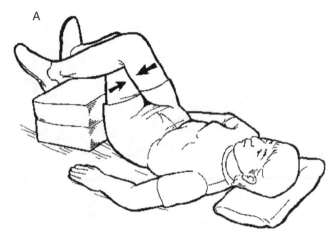

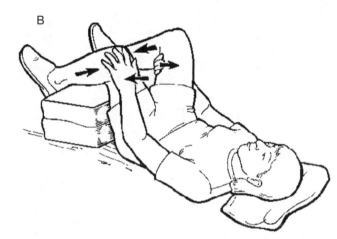

Figure 7-41: A) Self-treatment for a right anterior and left posterior innominate; B) Alternate technique.

Anterior or Posterior Innominate. Self-treatment for an innominate rotation can consist of contract-relax techniques that are less specific than the muscle energy techniques described earlier. For a right anterior or left posterior innominate, the patient lies supine and places the right hand behind the right knee and the left hand on the right anterior thigh. The patient performs an isometric contraction of the right hip extenders and the left hip flexors as shown (Fig 7-41).

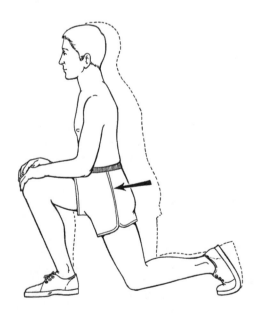

Figure 7-40: Self-treatment using the half-kneel position for a left posterior innominate.

Unilateral Sacral Flexion. To self-treat a unilateral sacral flexion, the patient is instructed to sit in a chair with the legs abducted. He takes a deep breath, holds it, and flexes the trunk between his spread knees, passing the elbows between the knees (Fig 7-42). After several seconds, the patient releases the air and straightens the trunk.

Manipulation Techniques

The focus of the techniques presented has been on the "patient-active" muscle energy techniques. A variety of high-velocity thrust mobilizations for the sacroiliac joint exist. They primarily produce rotatory forces on the innominates and are thus more appropriate for the iliosacral lesions. Two particularly effective thrust techniques for an anterior innominate are included for completeness. The first technique is performed with the patient supine (Fig 7-43):

1. The patient is supine with hands locked behind the head (fingers interlaced).

2. The clinician stands opposite the affected side and makes hand contact with the patient's ASIS on the affected side using the caudad hand.

3. With the cephalad hand, the clinician reaches through the crook of the patient's elbow on the affected side from behind and allows the dorsum of her hand to contact the patient's chest.

4. Using the dorsum of the hands as a fulcrum against the patient's chest, the clinician rolls the patient's torso toward her. The clinician instructs the patient, "Relax, hang on to your head, and let me turn you."

5. The clinician takes up the slack through the pelvis using a stiff arm, applying force down and away.

6. The clinician instructs the patient, "Take in a deep breath and let it out." As the patient does so, the clinician takes up the remainder of the slack through the torso and pelvis and gives a quick thrust to the pelvis through the ASIS.

The above technique has been shown to be effective for runners with hip pain who show signs of sacroiliac joint dysfunction.[3] Flynn, et al have described a clinical prediction rule to help determine when this technique will be most effective for low back pain. In their study, five predictive factors were identified: 1) Duration of symptoms greater than 16 days; 2) Fear Avoidance Beliefs Questionnaire (FABQ) work subscale score greater than 19; 3) At least one hip with greater than 35° internal rotation; 4)

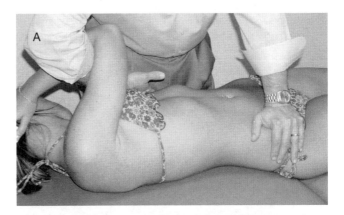

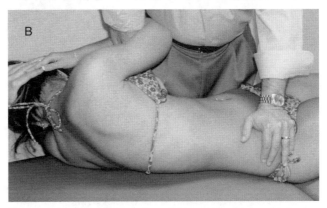

Figure 7-43: Treatment of a right anterior innominate by direct action thrust technique. A) Starting position; B) Trunk rotation positioning in preparation for the thrust.

Hypomobility of the lumbar spine; and 5) No symptoms distal to the knee. The presence of four of five variables increased the likelihood of success with this manipulation from 45% to 95%.[11]

In a subsequent study by some of the same authors, six variables were identified as being related to *inability* to improve with this manipulative technique: 1) Longer symptom duration; 2) Symptoms distal to the low back; 3) Lack of hypomobility in the lumbar spine; 4) Reduced hip rotation range of motion; 5) Little discrepancy in hip internal rotation from side to side; and 6) Negative pain provocation using Gaenslen's test. They suggest that if a patient exhibits several of these signs during the evaluation, the likelihood of improvement with this technique is minimal.[13]

The second thrust technique for an anterior innominate is performed with the patient side lying with the involved side up. Graded passive movements and stretches can also be used with this technique (Fig 7-44):

1. One hand is place on the ASIS and the other is on the ischial tuberosity. The anterior rim of the ilium is

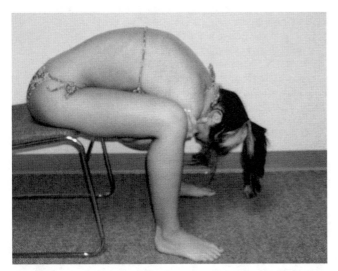

Figure 7-42: Self-treatment for a unilateral sacral flexion lesion.

pushed posteriorly while the ischial tuberosity is pushed anteriorly, producing a force couple.

2. When slack is completely taken up, the clinician gives a quick thrust in the direction of posterior ilium rotation.

3. Additional force may be added by stabilizing the bottom hip in extension and flexing the top hip.

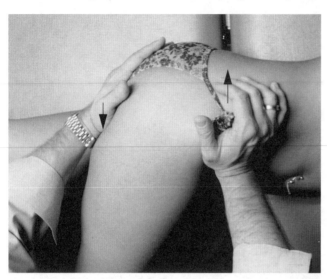

Figure 7-44: Posterior rotation of the ilium on the sacrum.

Even more force can be imparted by extending the top knee and allowing it to hang over the edge of the treatment table. This tethers the hamstring muscles and helps pull the innominate posteriorly.

Transversus Abdominis Strengthening

It has been shown that contraction of the transversus abdominis significantly decreases sacroiliac joint laxity in subjects without low back pain.[28] Theoretically, these exercises can be helpful in the treatment of sacroiliac hypermobility, but clinical trials have not been performed to test this theory.

Sacroiliac Supports

The use of a pelvic belt strapped firmly around the pelvis just below the ASIS has been shown to decrease SI joint laxity.[9] Using a sacroiliac support theoretically increases stability via compression, and can be helpful if symptoms are persistent or recur after treatment for dysfunction. This method of treatment may be particularly effective postpartum with patients who had SI joint pain during pregnancy, since continued SI joint laxity may contribute to lingering symptoms after delivery.[8] Supports are also available for use during pregnancy. Sacroiliac supports are discussed in more detail in Chapter 13, *Spinal Orthoses*.

REFERENCES

1. Bemis T and Daniel M: Validation of the Long Sit Test on Subjects with Iliosacral Dysfunction. J Orthop Sports Phys Ther 8(7):336, 1987.

2. Binder-MacLeod S and Woerman AL: Leg Length Discrepancy Assessment: Accuracy and Precision in Five Clinical Methods of Evaluation. J Orthop Sports Phys Ther 5:230, 1984.

3. Cibulka MT and Delitto A: A Comparison of Two Different Methods to Treat Hip Pain in Runners. J Orthop Sports Phys Ther 17(4):172-176, 1993.

4. Cibulka MT, Delitto A and Koldekoff RM: Changes in Innominate Tilt after Manipulation of the Sacroiliac Joint in Patients with Low Back Pain, an Experimental Study. Phys Ther 68:1359-1363, 1988.

5. Cibulka MT, Sinacore DR, Cromer GS, et al: Unilateral Hip Rotation Range of Motion Asymmetry in Patients with Sacroiliac Joint Regional Pain. Spine 23(9):1009-1015, 1998.

6. Cibulka MT: Understanding Sacroiliac Joint Movement as a Guide to the Management of a Patient with Unilateral Low Back Pain. Manual Therapy 7(4):215-221, 2002.

7. Cyriax J: Diagnosis of Soft Tissue Lesions. *Textbook of Orthopædic Medicine*, Vol 1, 7th edition. Bailliere-Tindall, London 1978.

8. Damen L, Buyruk HM, Guler-Uysal F, et al: The Prognostic Value of Asymmetric Laxity of the Sacroiliac Joints in Pregnancy-Related Pelvic Pain. Spine 27(24):2820-2824, 2002.

9. Damen L, Spoor CW, Snijders CJ, et al: Does a Pelvic Belt Influence Sacroiliac Joint Laxity? Clin Biomech 17:495-498, 2002.

10. Dreyfuss P, Michaelsen M, Pauza K, et al: The Value of Medical History and Physical Examination in Diagnosing Sacroiliac Joint Pain. Spine 21(22):2594-2602, 1996.

11. Flynn T, Fritz J, Whitman J, et al: A Clinical Prediction Rule for Classifying Patients with Low Back Pain Who Demonstrate Short-Term Improvement with Spinal Manipulation. Spine 27(24):2835-28-43, 2002.

12. Frigerio N, Stowe R and Howe J: Movement of the Sacroiliac Joint. Clin Orthop and Rel Res 100:370, 1974.

13. Fritz JM, Whitman JM, Flynn TW, et al: Factors Related to the Inability of Individuals with Low Back Pain to Improve with Spinal Manipulation. Phys Ther 84(2):173-190, 2004.

14. Goodridge JP: Muscle Energy Technique: Definition, Explanation, Methods of Procedure. J Am Osteopath Assoc 82(4):249, 1981.

15. Greenman P: Innominate Shear Dysfunction in the Sacroiliac Syndrome. Manual Med 2:114, 1986.

16. Greenman, P: Principles of Manual Medicine, 3rd ed. Lippincott Williams & Wilkins, Baltimore 2003.

17. Grieve G: *Common Vertebral Joint Problems*. Churchill-Livingstone, New York 1981.

18. Harrison DE, Harrison DD and Troyanovich SJ: The Sacroiliac Joint: A Review of Anatomy and Biomechanics with Clinical Implications. J Manipulative Physiol Ther 20(9):607-617, 1997.

19. Kendall F, McCreary E and Provance P: *Muscles: Testing and*

Function. 4th ed. Lippincott, Williams and Wilkins, Baltimore 1993.

20. Kirkaldy-Willis W: *Managing Low Back Pain*, 2nd edition. Churchill Livingstone, New York 1988.

21. Laslett M and Williams M: The Reliability of Selected Pain Provocation Tests for Sacroiliac Joint Pathology. Spine 19(11):1243-1249, 1994.

22. Liekens M, Gillets HL: *Belgian Chiropractic Research Notes*. 10th ed. Brussels 1973.

23. Meijne W, van Neerbos K, Aufdemkampe G, et al: Intraexaminer and Interexaminer Reliability of the Gillet Test. J Manipulative Physiol Ther 22(1):4-9, 1999.

24. Mens JM, Vleeming A, Snijders CJ, et al. The Active Straight-leg-raising Test and Mobility of the Pelvic Joints. Eur Spine J 8:468-74, 1999.

25. Mitchell FL Jr, Moran PS, Pruzzo NA: *An Evaluation and Treatment Manual of Osteopathic Muscle Energy Procedures*. Mitchell, Moran and Pruzzo Associates, Valley Park MO 1979.

26. Mooney V and Robertson J: The Facet Syndrome. Clin Orthop and Rel Res 115:149-156, 1976.

27. O'Sullivan PB, Beales DJ, Beetham JA, et al: Altered Motor Control Strategies in Subjects with Sacroiliac Joint Pain During the Active Straight-Leg-Raise Test. Spine 27:E1-E8, 2002.

28. Richardson CA, Snijders CJ, Hides JA, et al: The Relation Between the Trasversus Abdominis Muscles, Sacroiliac Joint Mechanics, and Low Back Pain. Spine 27(4):399-405, 2002.

29. Ross MD, Nordeen MH and Barido M: Test-Retest Reliability of Patrick's Hip Range of Motion Test in Healthy College-Aged Men. J Strength Cond Res 17(1):156-161, 2003.

30. Solonen K: The Sacroiliac Joint in the Light of Anatomical, Roentgenological and Clinical Studies. Acta Orthop Scand (Suppl 27):1-115, 1957.

31. *Somatic Dysfunction: Principles of Manipulative Treatment and Procedures*. PE Kimberly, ed. Kirksville College of Osteopathic Medicine, Kirksville MO 1980.

32. Stoddard A: *Manual of Osteopathic Technique*. Hutchinson, London 1978.

33. Stratton S: Evaluation and Treatment of the Sacroiliac Joint. Course Notes and Personal Communication. Sept 1984.

34. Tutorial on Level I Muscle Energy Techniques. Michigan State University College of Osteopathic Medicine, East Lansing MI 1986. Course Notes.

35. van der Wurff P, Meyne W and Hagmeijer RHM: Clinical Tests of the Sacroiliac Joint. A Systematic Methodological Review. Part 2: Validity. Manual Therapy 5(2):89-96, 2000.

36. Vincent-Smith B and Gibbons P: Inter-examiner and Intra-examiner Reliability of the Standing Flexion Test. Manual Therapy 4(2):87-93, 1999.

8

TEMPOROMANDIBULAR DISORDERS

Steven L. Kraus PT OCS MTC

Section One—Introduction, Anatomy and Kinematics

Clinicians are faced with challenges in the management of patients with head and neck pain. Head and neck pain can originate from dental, neurologic, otolaryngologic, vascular, metaplastic, infectious disease or musculoskeletal conditions.[117] *Temporomandibular disorder* (TMD) is a collective term embracing a number of clinical problems that involve the temporomandibular joints (TMJ), muscles of mastication and associated structures.[132] Epidemiological studies indicate 3% to 6% of the population would benefit from treatment of TMD. This figure represents up to 17,000,000 patients.[47] Since physical therapists are skilled in treating non-disease musculoskeletal structures, they have a significant role to play in the management of TMD. The physical therapist's primary role in TMD management involves the evaluation and treatment of the temporomandibular joints, muscles of mastication and cervical spine tissues. Not all patients with signs of TMD will require modalities, exercises or manual procedures. However, all patients will require education to decrease fear and anxiety and correct misperceptions about their TMD conditions.

Voluminous textbooks, journal articles and continuing education courses address TMD. Unfortunately, discussion about the etiology, terminology, evaluation and management of TMD is often clouded by confusion and controversy. Despite all the scientific evidence supporting a particular evaluative and treatment procedure, an equal volume of contradictory material exists. This leaves both novice and seasoned clinicians in the physical therapy, dental and medical professions confused about TMD management.

This chapter focuses on the subclassifications of TMD that fall within the domain of physical therapists. Essential background such as anatomy, kinematics and terminology is presented, and the reader is exposed to a comprehensive classification, evaluation and treatment scheme.

Ideal management of patients with head and neck pain involves a team approach. For maximum patient benefit, each member of the dental, medical and physical therapy teams needs to understand what the other can offer in the management of TMD.

Osseous Structures

Temporal Bone

The temporal bone forms the roof of the TMJ. Pertinent bony landmarks are the postglenoid spine, mandibular fossa, articular eminence, articular crest, and articular tubercle (Fig 8-1).

The *postglenoid spine* or process is a downward extension of the squamosal portion of the temporal bone.[53] The postglenoid spine forms the posterior aspect of the *mandibular fossa* and is positioned anterior to the external auditory meatus. The postglenoid spine does not extend all the way laterally. Inserting a finger partially into the external auditory meatus provides reasonable access to tissues located posterior and lateral to the head of the condyle. This is one of several examination procedures used to identify possible inflammation of the TMJ.

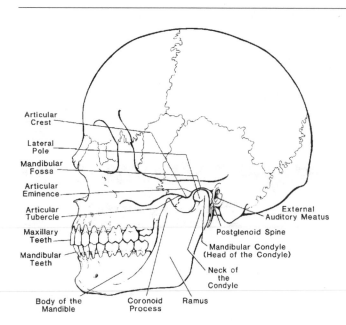

Figure 8-1: Skeletal Anatomy

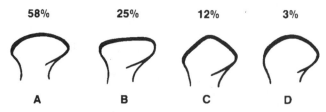

Figure 8-2: Various shapes of the mandibular condyle viewed in the frontal plane: A) Convex; B) Flat; C) Angular; D) Rounded

is referred to as the *long axis of the condyle*. Extending the long axis of each condyle medially forms an obtuse angle varying from 145° to 160° (Fig 8-3).[10]

Only the lateral pole can be palpated. The lateral pole is located directly in front of the tragus of the ear (Fig 8-1). Inflammation of the tissues that attach to or extend over the lateral pole can occur with TMD. Inferior to the head of the condyle is the neck of the condyle. Between the neck and the ramus (angle of the mandible) is the projection of the coronoid process for the attachment of the temporalis muscle (Fig 8-1). The ramus continues anterior to become the body of the mandible, which contains the lower arch of teeth.

The postglenoid spine offers attachments for the capsule and posterior attachment.[118] The concave mandibular fossa is occupied by the posterior band of the disc. The mandibular fossa is a non-articular portion of the TMJ.

The *articular eminence* is convex in the anteroposterior direction and concave mediolaterally. The articular eminence has a slope ranging from 40° to 60°.[10] Anteriorly, the articular eminence is separated from the *articular tubercle* by a bony landmark referred to as the *articular crest*. The articular tubercle is the most anterior portion of the roof of the TMJ. The articular tubercle area is concave in the mediolateral direction. During mandibular opening, the condyle translates along the articular eminence. With full mouth opening, if the head of the condyle translates onto the articular tubercle, TMJ hypermobility is present.[44]

Condyle

The condyle forms the floor of the TMJ (Fig 8-1). The condyle has an elliptical shape measuring approximately 20 mm mediolaterally and 10 mm anteroposteriorly.[190] The condyle is convex both anteroposteriorly and mediolaterally. Variation in the size and shape of the condyle is common, both from person to person and from one side to the other (Fig 8-2).[190]

The lateral pole of the condyle lies anterior to the transverse axis of the condyle and the medial pole lies posterior to the transverse axis of the condyle (Fig 8-3). A line running between the medial and lateral poles of each condyle

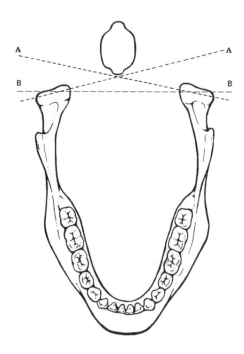

Figure 8-3: A) The long axis of the condyle is represented by a line drawn from the lateral to the medial pole. If the long axes of each condyle are extended, they intersect anterior to the foramen magnum. B) The lateral pole of the condyle lies anterior to the transverse axis of the condyle and the medial pole lies posterior to the transverse axis of the condyle.

The Occlusion

Unlike any other joint, the TMJ has teeth at one end of its lever arm (the mandible). The maxillary teeth are contained in the maxillary bone (Fig 8-1). Dawson defines centric occlusion or maximum intercuspation as the "relationship of the mandible to the maxilla when the teeth are in maximum occlusal contact, irrespective of the position or alignment of the condyle-disc assemblies".[36] Centric occlusion is the rigid end point of mandibular closure.

Malocclusion is any deviation or irregularity in the position, form or relation of teeth.[2] There are varying opinions as to the contribution of a malocclusion in the development and treatment of TMD. Clinicians who believe that malocclusion contributes to TMD would treat TMD by any one or a combination of occlusal adjustments, prosthetic rehabilitation, orthodontics and orthognathic surgery.[106] However, the literature suggests that malocclusion does not significantly contribute to TMD.[30,92,108,155,168] No reliable criteria exists to identify patients whose malocclusion is contributing to their TMD. McNamara and colleagues suggests that "the dental profession should be encouraged to manage TMD symptoms with reversible therapies, only considering permanent alterations of the occlusion in patients with very unique circumstances."[108] Nonetheless, clinicians should have a basic understanding of occlusal factors that have a potential association with TMD. A thorough discussion of occlusal factors is beyond the scope of this text, but patients with TMD who have malocclusion and have not responded to physical therapy should be referred to a dentist knowledgeable in TMD management.

TMJ—A Load Bearing Joint

The TMJ is a load bearing joint.[17,112] Joint loading occurs at the articulating surfaces on the temporal bone and head of the condyle.[10] The articulating surface on the temporal bone is located on the articular eminence, articular crest and articular tubercle areas. On the head of the condyle, the articulating surface is located on the anterior/anterosuperior portion (Fig 8-1).[118]

The articulating surfaces of the TMJ are covered by fibrocartilage that is avascular and aneural. Fibrocartilage has the same general properties found in hyaline cartilage but tends to be less dense,[81] has greater potential to remodel and is less likely to breakdown over time.[133]

In the TMJ, degenerative joint disease occurs first laterally, because TMJ loading occurs more laterally than medially. Lateral loading also might explain why the lat-

eral collateral ligament of the TMJ loses its integrity with a subsequent affect on disc position.

The articular surfaces of the TMJ have been shown to be remarkably adaptable.[34] However, the adaptive capacity of the TMJ is not infinite, and some joints adapt better than others. Degenerative changes in the TMJ are the result of maladaptation to increased joint loading.[111] The articular disc affords some protection against excessive loading. Disc displacements may contribute to degenerative joint disease by increasing functional demands on the articular surfaces of the TMJ. The notion that disc displacement leads to degenerative joint disease has encouraged both surgical and nonsurgical approaches to "reposition" the displaced disc. Successful long-term repositioning of the disc is believed to stop the progression of advanced degenerative joint disease.[111] On the other hand, successful long term repositioning of the disc is sometimes problematic (see *Treatment for Disc Displacements – All Stages* on page 199). Some histological models suggest that degenerative joint disease may actually precede disc displacements. Therefore, disc displacement may be a sign of degenerative joint disease and not its cause.[41]

Intracapsular Structure

Articular Disc

The TMJ disc is a biconcave fibrocartilage structure lying between the head of the condyle and the temporal bone (Fig 8-4).[118] The disc consists of dense bundles of collagen fibers.[112,114] A firm yet flexible structure, the disc accommodates to the incongruities in the shape of the articulating surfaces. Knowledge of the disc's anatomy and attachments is essential to understand disc displacements and gain a realistic perspective on treatment.

The disc divides the joint into superior and inferior compartments or joint spaces. The upper joint space is larger than the lower joint space, extending further anterior

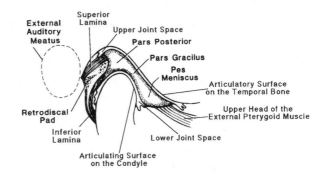

Figure 8-4: A sagittal view of the intracapsular structures of the right temporomandibular joint.

in the sagittal plane and overlapping the lower joint space in the coronal plane (Fig 8-5). The volumes of the upper and lower joint space are 1.2 ml and 0.9 ml respectively.[13]

Rees divides the disc into three bands according to thickness: anterior (pes meniscus), intermediate (pars gracilis) and posterior (pars posterior) (Fig 8-4).[141] The posterior band is thicker than the anterior band and the intermediate band is the thinnest. In centric occlusion, the posterior band of the disc is positioned superior on the condyle and in the mandibular fossae (Fig 8-4).[174] The intermediate band is positioned over the anterosuperior part of the condyle and along the articular eminence. The anterior band lies anterior to the condyle and anterior on the articular eminence.

The intermediate band of the disc is avascular and aneural.[189] In contrast, the disc's peripheral non-load bearing areas are vascularized and innervated. During mandibular function, the intermediate band maintains its position between the temporal bone and head of the condyle where load-bearing occurs.[174]

The thin intermediate band connecting the thicker posterior and anterior bands creates a biconcave shape. This anatomical feature creates a "self-seating" relationship of the disc to the condyle.[103,133] The self-seating feature, along with tight medial and lateral collateral ligaments, allows the disc to rotate anterior and posterior on the condyle[10,133] without displacing anterior to the condyle.[103]

Disc Attachments

Anterior Attachment. The disc attaches anteriorly to the capsule and to the upper head of the lateral pterygoid muscle (Fig 8-4).[12] The upper head of the lateral pterygoid muscle influences disc movement.

Medial and Lateral Attachments. The medial and lateral collateral ligaments attach the disc firmly to the medial and lateral poles of the condyle.[174] The lateral collateral ligament is relatively thin compared to the medial collateral ligament.

Posterior Attachment. The disc is contiguous with the posterior attachment (Fig 8-4).[133] The posterior attachment consists of the superior lamina or stratum and the inferior lamina or stratum with the retrodiscal pad lying between the two laminae.[151,152]

The posterosuperior disc attaches to the superior lamina. The superior lamina travels posteriorly to attach in the area of the postglenoid spine. The superior lamina contains a branching meshwork of elastic fibers.[151] The extensibility of the superior lamina ranges from 7 to 10 mm in the fresh cadaver specimen.[141]

The posteroinferior disc attaches to the inferior lamina. The inferior lamina courses posteriorly around the back of the condyle to attach to the posterior aspect of the neck of the condyle.[151] The inferior lamina is composed mainly of collagenous fibers with little elastic tissue.

The retrodiscal pad is a part of the posterior attachment.[151,152] The retrodiscal pad contains small-caliber, loosely associated collagen fibers, a branching system of elastic fibers, fat deposits, a specialized arterial supply, a large venous plexus, lymphatics, a profuse nerve supply and many large blood-filled endothelium-lined spaces.[151,152] When the condyle translates forward, the volume of the retrodiscal tissue expands due to venous distention, filling the mandibular fossa.[152,174] During closure, the retrodiscal pad returns to its smaller size and shape.

Intracapsular inflammation of the TMJ can result from inflammation of the posterior attachment. Inflammation of the posterior attachment should be suspected if the patient complains of pain during jaw movement and the patient's symptoms are reproduced or increased with palpation via the external auditory meatus.

Periarticular Tissues

Capsule

The capsule is composed of fibrous connective tissue.[74] Superiorly, the capsule is attached to the temporal bone. Inferiorly, the capsule tapers to attach to the neck of the condyle. The capsule blends medially and laterally with the medial and lateral collateral ligaments only at the medial and lateral poles in the lower joint space (Fig 8-5).[74]

In the superior joint space, the capsule has no medial and lateral attachments to the disc.[74] Further laterally, the capsule thickens to become the TMJ ligament. The close anatomical relationship between the capsule and TMJ ligament makes it difficult to distinguish between the two.[53] Anteriorly, the capsule blends with the upper and lower head of the external pterygoid muscle and anterior disc.[12] Posteriorly, the capsule attaches to the postglenoid spine.[74]

The capsule is lined by a highly vascular, synovial fluid-producing membrane that supplies nutrients to the avascular intracapsular tissues. The capsule is richly innervated with sensory receptors and nociceptors.[125,171]

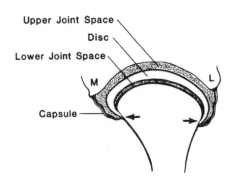

Figure 8-5: A frontal view of the left TMJ. Arrows depict attachments of the collateral ligaments and capsule to the medial and lateral poles.

The capsule contains articular mechanoreceptors that initiate reflexes possibly involved in jaw control and kinesthetic and perceptional awareness of the mandible.[125] The capsule contains four types of receptor nerve endings that are differentiated based on morphological and functional characteristics.[33,171] TMJ receptors are located in the fibrous joint capsule, the TMJ and lateral collateral ligaments and the posterior attachment, but are absent from the central disc and synovial tissues. Terminating on the receptors are the deep temporal, masseteric and auriculotemporal nerves which originate from the mandibular division of Cranial V.[86]

Injection of a local anesthetic into the capsule of healthy subjects causes decreased jaw control and significant deterioration in perception of mandibular position.[85] Fibrous adhesions of the capsule or joint inflammation causing joint effusion may contribute to a patient's lack of awareness of jaw movement and position.

Temporomandibular (TMJ) Ligament

The temporomandibular (TMJ) ligament is often referred to as the lateral ligament because it is continuous with the capsule and reinforces the capsule laterally (Fig 8-6).[21] The TMJ ligament is composed of two parts: a superficial oblique portion running laterally from the zygomatic portion of the temporal bone to the neck of the condyle, and a deeper more horizontal part from the same origin to the lateral pole.[149]

The inner (horizontal) portion of this ligament limits posterior movement of the condyle, protecting the posterior attachment from trauma.[120] Some authors state that the arrangement of the outer (oblique) fibers prevents separation of the condyle, disc and temporal fossa and restrains condylar movement on maximum mandibular opening,

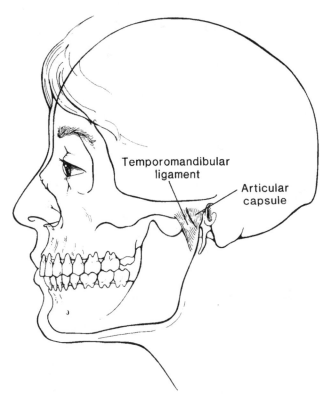

Figure 8-6: A lateral view of the temporomandibular joint showing the outer oblique TMJ ligament and capsule.

protrusion and lateral excursion.[69,120,133] The TMJ ligament is also believed to assist in the transition from condylar rotation to condylar translation.[69,70]

Stylomandibular and Sphenomandibular Ligaments

The stylomandibular and sphenomandibular ligaments are extracapsular ligaments (Fig 8-7).[21] The stylomandibular ligament extends from the styloid process of the temporal bone to the angle of the mandible. The sphenomandibular ligament has partial attachment superiorly to the sphenoid spine of the sphenoid bone; the remaining attachment is continuous with the medial capsule. In the medial capsule, a portion of the sphenomandibular ligament enters the petrotympanic fissure merging with the anterior malleolar ligament. Inferiorly, the sphenomandibular ligament attaches medially to the mandible.[149]

The role of the stylomandibular and sphenomandibular ligaments during mandibular dynamics is uncertain. Their role may be to protect the joint during wide excursive movements.

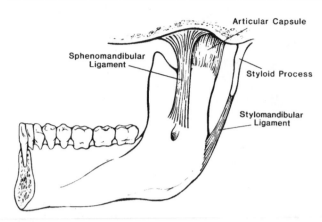

Figure 8-7: A medial view of the right temporomandibular joint showing the spenomandibular and stylomandibular ligaments and capsule.

Anterior Malleolar Ligament

The anterior malleolar ligament is a connection of fibrous tissue between the TMJ and the middle ear.[5,139] The anterior malleolar ligament, along with the sphenomandibular ligament, originates from the sphenoid bone and the medial capsule. It passes through the petrotympanic fissure to insert on the malleus. When tension is applied to the sphenomandibular ligament or the medial capsule of cadavers, movement of the chain of ossicles and the tympanic membrane is observed.[139] The functional importance of the anterior malleolar ligament has been debated.[5,149] It is speculated that ear symptoms may result from tension of the anterior malleolar ligament. Anterior malleolar ligament tension may be caused by tension of the sphenomandibular ligament occurring at end range jaw movements. Anterior malleolar ligament tension may also occur from disc displacement placing tension on the medial capsule.

Innervation

The TMJ is primarily innervated by the auriculotemporal nerve.[170] The auriculotemporal nerve is a branch of the posterior trunk of the mandibular nerve, a division of the trigeminal nerve. The auriculotemporal nerve innervates the posterior attachment and the posterior and lateral joint capsule. The anterior and medial joint is innervated by the masseteric and posterior deep temporal nerves, which come from the anterior trunk of the mandibular nerve.

Anesthetic block of the auriculotemporal nerve can help determine whether the patient's pain is arthrogeneous in origin.[10] If the patient's symptoms are myogenous or referred from other adjacent areas (e.g., cervical spine),

symptoms are not affected by an anesthetic block. Clinicians should be aware of the placebo effect, which may result in a false positive response to this procedure.

Muscles Associated with the TMJ

The many skeletal muscles involved with mandibular movement are called the muscles of mastication. Muscles that attach directly to the mandible have the greatest influence on jaw function. Muscles in the neck provide secondary support during jaw function and should not be ignored. Eggleton and Langton provide a more detailed description of the origin and insertion of each muscle.[53]

Controversy exists over the number of heads of the lateral pterygoid muscle, but most sources agree there are two heads—a superior and an inferior.[12] Therefore, the following discussion assumes two heads.

Primary Muscles for Mandibular Closure

Temporalis. The temporalis is a large fan-shaped muscle originating from the temporal fossa. The temporalis inserts primarily along the coronoid process and extends to the anterior border of the ramus just posterior to the third molar.

Masseter. The masseter is a quadrilateral muscle originating from the anterior two thirds of the lower border of the zygomatic arch. The fibers run down and back to insert on the lateral aspect of the ramus.

Medial (Internal) Pterygoid. The medial pterygoid is a quadrilateral muscle originating from the pterygoid plate and palatine bone. The insertion is along the medial angle of the mandible.

Primary Muscles for Mandibular Opening

Inferior Head of the Lateral (External) Pterygoid. The lateral pterygoid muscle originates from the lateral surface of the lateral pterygoid plate. The insertion is into the medial half of the neck of the condyle. This muscle opens the mouth and protrudes the mandible. It cannot be palpated extraorally or intraorally.

Masticatory muscle involvement often causes a limitation in mandibular opening. However, if the inferior head of the lateral pterygoid is in spasm, patients are unable to bring their back teeth together on the side of the lateral pterygoid spasm. In theory, spasm of the lateral pterygoid muscle is caused by a quick stretch. Examples include a blow to the chin or an abrupt change in the patient's centric occlusion.

Other Muscles of Mastication

Superior Head of the Lateral Pterygoid. The origin of the superior head is on the greater wing of the sphenoid bone. Approximately 1/3 of the superior head inserts on the anterior and medial disc and capsule.[12] The remaining portion of the superior head attaches to the medial 1/3 of the neck of the condyle.[12,133] The superior head stabilizes the disc during function.

Hyoid Muscles. The hyoid muscles facilitate mandibular opening. The infrahyoid muscles stabilize the hyoid bone while the suprahyoid muscles open the mouth. The origin and insertions of the suprahyoid and infrahyoid muscles are not detailed here.[53]

Osteokinematics

The TMJ is a synovial ginglymoarthrodial joint. The TMJ is ginglymoid in that it provides a hinging movement and arthrodial in that it provides for a freely movable gliding motion.[118] The disc moves independently of both the condyle and temporal bone during active movements of the mandible.

Osteokinematics pertains to the overall movement of bones with little reference to their related joints.[100,101] Osteokinematics of the mandible are depression, protrusion and lateral excursion. These movements are often measured in millimeters during the physical examination.

Reported ranges for normal mandibular movements are rather arbitrary.[167] Clinically, it is more important to base treatment decisions on the patient's perception of what is functional. If measurements are used, age and gender should be taken into account, because wide variation exists. Baseline measurements can be useful to assess the patient's response to treatment. "Normal" ranges for osteokinematic movements of the mandible should be used as guidelines only and not as rigid goals in treatment.

Deviation and deflection are also assessed during mandibular opening and protrusion. *Deviation* is movement of the mandible away from midline and back to midline. Deviation is a "S" curve movement of the mandible. *Deflection* is movement of the mandible away from midline that does not return to midline. Deflection is a "C" curve movement of the mandible.

Clinicians like to see symmetry with jaw dynamics. However, when deviations and deflections are observed, it is important to remember that midline opening can be affected by deviations in anatomy caused by adaptive remolding of the joint surfaces and normal anatomical vari-

ations in the size and shapes of the condyle heads, the slope of the articular eminence, the long axes of the condyle heads and their relationship to the necks of the condyles, and differences in the distance between the condyles and rami.[157,176] Asymmetry is the rule rather than the exception. Treatments goals should be directed toward pain reduction and functional improvement, and not necessarily toward symmetrical mandibular dynamics. As a general rule, deviations and deflections associated with functional opening and protrusion are not significant. Deflection associated with limited mandibular movement is significant, and may indicate limited condylar translation on the side the deflection occurred toward. Deviation is rarely associated with limited mandibular function.

In addition to providing a baseline, measuring osteokinematic movements may help to differentially diagnosis TMD arthrogenous involvement from TMD myogeneous involvement. A patient who has limited opening but has normal protrusion and lateral excursion likely has myogeneous dysfunction. On the other hand, if the patient has limited opening, limited protrusion and limited lateral excursion, the dysfunction is likely arthrogenous.

Depression

Mandibular depression is mouth opening. Maximum opening of normal subjects ranges from 33 to 72 mm, depending on gender and age.[71,167] *Functional mandibular depression* is roughly 40 mm.[167] Mandibular depression is measured with a millimeter ruler between the tip of the right or left maxillary and mandibular central incisors (Fig 8-8).

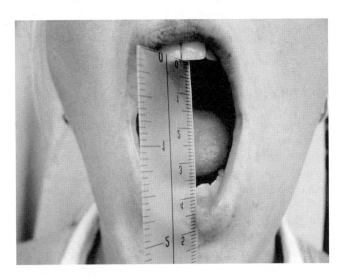

Figure 8-8: Mandibular depression measured with a millimeter ruler. Functional mandibular depression is roughly 40 millimeters.

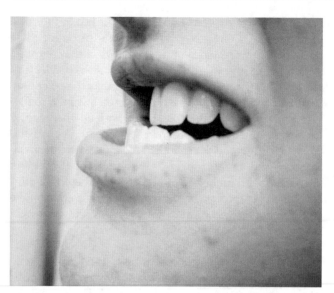

Figure 8-9: Functional protrusion with the bottom central incisors moving past the tip of the upper central incisors.

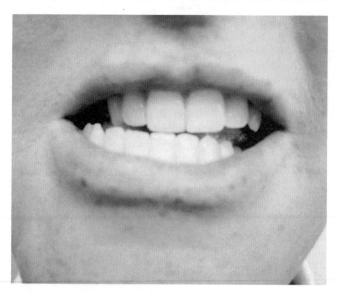

Figure 8-10: Functional lateral excursion to the right with the bottom canine moving past the tip of the upper canine.

Protrusion

Protrusion is anterior movement of the mandible in the horizontal plane. Normal protrusion ranges from 5 to 7 mm.[167] Though a ruler can be used to measure protrusion, it is easier to assess by visually inspecting the relationship between the patient's central incisors.

Functional mandibular protrusion is the ability to actively protrude the mandible to at least an end to end position between the maxillary and mandibular central incisors. Ideally, the mandibular central incisors should move past the maxillary central incisors by 1 to 2 mm (Fig 8-9). This amount of protrusion will allow patients to pronounce words such as "hiss", "house", "church", "judge", and "steeples", and to bite into an apple.

Lateral Excursion

Lateral excursion involves moving the mandible laterally in the horizontal plane. Normal lateral excursion is 5 to 7 mm to each side.[167] Though a ruler can be used to measure lateral excursion, it is easier to assess by visually inspecting the relationship between the patient's canines.

Functional lateral excursion is the ability to actively move the mandible laterally to at least an end to end position between the mandibular and maxillary canines. Ideally, the mandibular canine should move past the maxillary canine by 1 to 2 mm bilaterally (Fig 8-10). This range of lateral excursion will allow patients to chew food, since chewing involves lateral movements.

Arthrokinematics

Arthrokinematics pertains to active and passive accessory movements between two joint surfaces. Arthrokinematic movements permit full, pain-free movements in diarthrodial joints.[101]

Active accessory movements occur in response to muscle contraction. The active accessory movements of the TMJ are compression, rotation, translation, and spin. Compression occurs during all mandibular movements since the TMJ is a load bearing joint.

Passive accessory movements of the condyle are distraction and lateral glide. Passive accessory movements are the result of an external force, not muscular contraction. Passive accessory movement is also referred to as *joint play*. Joint play is the inherent quality of the joint to "give" and is minute.[110] An example of joint play is rotation of the metacarpophalangeal (MCP) joint. Although one cannot actively rotate the MCP joint, MCP rotation occurs when grasping a baseball. The external force causing MCP rotation is the baseball. Similarly, chewing food causes ipsilateral condylar distraction and lateral glide.[70,73,78,140] The bolus of food is the outside force causing these joint play movements.

Accessory Movement During Mandibular Depression

Condylar rotation and translation occur during mandibular opening and closing.[59] Contraction of the supra and infrahyoid muscles initiates mandibular opening.

Condylar rotation occurs during the first 10 mm of opening. After 10 mm, contraction of the lower head of the lateral pterygoid translates the head of the condyle anteriorly. After 10 mm, rotation and translation occur together until functional opening has been achieved.

During opening, the TMJ ligament is thought to assist the muscles in the transition from condylar rotation to translation. As the condyle rotates, the neck of the condyle moves posteriorly. This tightens the oblique portion of the TMJ ligament (Fig 8-11). TMJ ligament tightening occurs at approximately 10 mm of opening. Additional opening occurs only if the condyle translates anteriorly, thereby decreasing tension in the TMJ ligament.[69,70]

Clinically, tightness of the TMJ ligament may cause limited translation of the condyle. A tight TMJ ligament can occur from trauma or joint immobility, the same events that cause fibrous adhesions (See *Fibrous Adhesions* on page 203.)

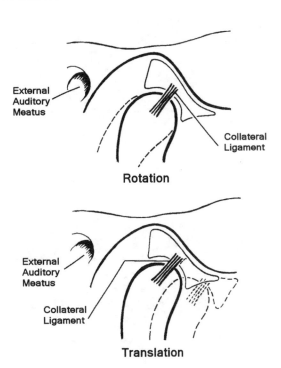

Rotation

Translation

Figure 8-12: Rotation occurs in the lower joint space between the condyle and the inferior surface of the disc. Translation occurs in the upper joint space between the superior surface of the disc and temporal bone.

Condylar translation is a result of ipsilateral contraction of the lower head of the lateral pterygoid.

Disc Movement with Mandibular Opening

Though the disc is firmly attached to the head of the condyle by collateral ligaments, the disc and condyle can still rotate independently from one another. During active mandibular opening, rotation occurs in the lower joint space between the condyle and the inferior disc surface.[10,133] Translation occurs in the upper joint space between the superior disc and the temporal bone (Fig 8-12).

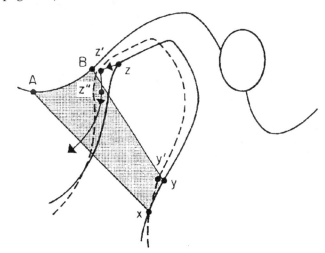

Figure 8-11: Upper (A and B) and lower (x and y) attachments of the temporomandibular ligament. During opening, rotation of the condyle moves points x and y posteriorly, thereby tightening the ligament. Functional opening occurs when the condyle translates forward.

Accessory Movement During Mandibular Protrusion

Condylar translation occurs during mandibular protrusion, and is a result of contraction of the lower head of the lateral pterygoid muscle.

Accessory Movement During Mandibular Lateral Excursion

Mandibular lateral excursion is accompanied by condylar translation contralaterally and condylar spin ipsilaterally.

For the first 10 mm of mandibular opening, the condyle rotates below a relatively stationary disc. After 10 mm of opening the condyle translates anteriorly. The disc also translates anteriorly with the condyle because it is firmly attached to the condyle by the collateral ligaments.[133] As the disc and condyle both translate anteriorly, the disc rotates posteriorly in relationship to the condyle. Posterior rotation of the disc on the condyle occurs because of the "self-seating" disc to condyle relationship and from tension developing in the posterior attachment (superior lamina).[10,103,137] At the end of mandibular opening, both the disc and condyle have translated anterior in relationship to the temporal bone as the disc rotated posteriorly on the condyle (Fig 8-13).

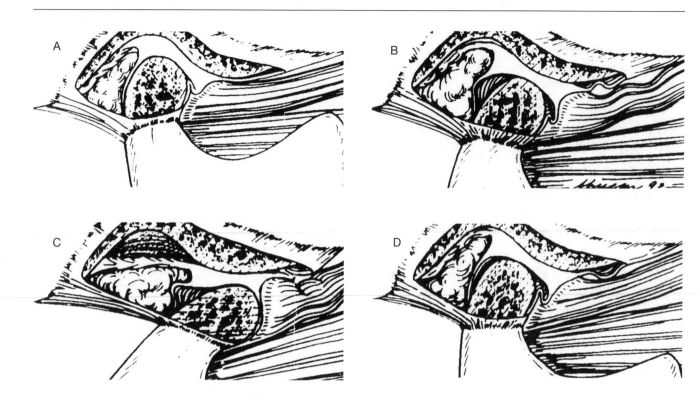

Figure 8-13: Normal disc movement during mandibular opening and closing. A) Position of disc with back teeth together; B) After 10 mm of mouth opening, condylar rotation and anterior translation occur as the disc rotates posterior in relationship to the condyle; C) At full opening, the disc is rotated posterior in relationship to the condyle and translated anterior in relationship to the temporal bone; D) During closing, condylar rotation and posterior translation occur in relationship to the temporal bone as the disc rotates anterior in relationship to the condyle (adapted from Okeson).[133]

Disc Movement with Mandibular Closing

During closing, both the disc and condyle translate posteriorly in relationship to the temporal bone. However, the disc rotates anteriorly on the condyle (Fig 8-13). Anterior rotation of the disc occurs because of the "self-seating" disc to condyle relationship and from tension developing in the superior head of the lateral pterygoid muscle.[102,118,137]

Electromyographic (EMG) studies have demonstrated that the superior head of the lateral pterygoid muscle is active on mouth closure.[102,107] The superior head of the lateral pterygoid "pulls" or rotates the disc in an anteromedial direction in relation to the condyle. The disc's behavior during opening and closing allows its thin avascular and aneural intermediate portion to stay between the condyle and temporal bone. MRI, CT, arthrotomy and arthroscopy inspections confirm this behavior.[174]

Comments on Arthrokinematic Movements

Fibrous adhesions of the capsule, TMJ ligament or disc can limit both active and passive accessory movements, including translation, distraction and lateral glide. A restriction in translation appears to be the most significant factor limiting functional mandibular dynamics. Three classic osteokinematic restrictions are observed when translation is limited (Fig 8-14). Condylar rotation and spin are rarely limited with arthrogeneous conditions except with the uncommon condition of bony ankylosis.

Even with restricted condylar translation, mandibular opening of 20 to 25 mm can be achieved.[133] Patients with less than 20 mm opening may have muscle pain or joint inflammation limiting their opening. Knowing this helps direct treatment toward decreasing pain and inflammation. Conversely, patients with more than 20 mm but less than functional opening may require passive, dynamic or static stretching techniques and exercises.

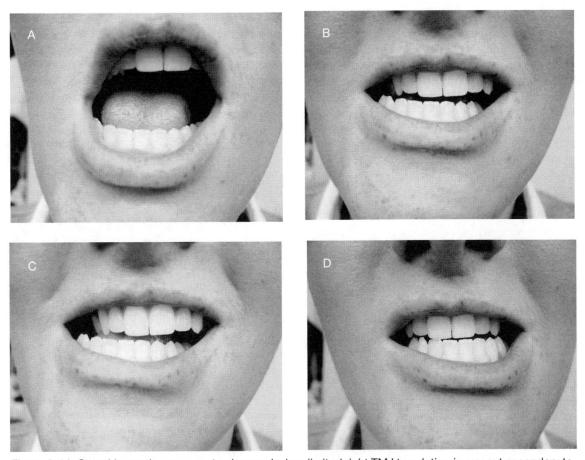

Figure 8-14: Osteokinematic movements observed when limited right TMJ translation is present secondary to fibrous adhesions or Stage II disc displacement: A) Limited opening with right deflection; B) Limited protrusion with right deflection; C) Normal right lateral excursion; D) Limited left lateral excursion.

Section Two—Evaluation and Classification of TMD

The evaluation is intended to identify the *source* of the patient's pain (in other words, which anatomic structure is producing the pain). The evaluation is not intended to identify the etiology.[66] Green states, "...what we have at the individual TMD patient level is nearly always an idiopathic situation—we simply cannot know enough, or cannot measure enough, or cannot precisely determine why each patient has TMD. Even in the absence of a perfect understanding of etiology, we still can provide good conservative care, and we should avoid aggressive and irreversible treatments, especially when they are based on flawed concepts of etiology."[66]

The physical therapy evaluation consists of a history and physical examination. The history and physical examination will uncover most TMD disorders.[29] Adjunctive tests such as imaging studies usually are not needed.[65] Adjunctive tests become necessary if the evaluation findings are questionable or vague, if a fracture or disease is suspected, or if invasive treatment options are being considered.[29]

Following the evaluation, the clinician should be able to determine whether or not TMD is present and should be able to classify it. It is unwise to assume that every patient with TMD will fit neatly into a specific subclassification with a predictable outcome to treatment. Management of TMD can include a myriad of treatments, including anti-inflammatory, analgesic, and antidepressant medications; occlusal appliances, occlusal equilibration and reconstruction; biobehavioral treatments such as biofeedback, hypnosis, cognitive-behavioral therapy and education; arthrocentesis, arthroscopy and arthrotomy surgery; and physical therapy.[50] No evidence-based rationale for selecting among TMD treatments has emerged. Rather, experts agree that treatments for TMD should be reversible and noninvasive.[119,129,132]

History

The history helps the clinician determine whether the TMJ(s) and/or muscles of mastication are the source of the patient's head, face and jaw symptoms. Greene states, "Now you can call me old-fashioned, but I happen to believe that people who are supposed to have jaw problems ought to have pain and dysfunction clearly associated with mandibular function."[65] Though colloquial, Dr. Green's statement appropriately warns clinicians to avoid overdiagnosing TMD.

The main symptoms of TMD are:[39,50,63,109,119,128,129,132]

1. Pain or discomfort in the TMJ and masticatory muscles that is influenced by jaw movement
2. Joint noises during jaw movement
3. Limitation or difficulty in jaw movement

Additional information to obtain during the history includes:

- Whether the onset of symptoms was related to a specific event or was insidious
- Intensity, frequency and duration of symptoms
- Change in symptom behavior over time
- Functional limitations
- Past and/or current treatment results
- Pertinent medical history (medication, surgeries, allergies, etc...)
- Patient's understanding of the condition and what the symptoms mean
- Patient's expectations and goals of treatment

Physical Examination

The physical examination is performed to reproduce or change the patient's symptoms through active movements and provocative tests, and to establish a baseline from which to assess a treatment's effectiveness. To achieve these two objectives, the examination must have an accept-

able level of reliability. *Reliability* is the consistency of a measurement or observation.[145] The clinician's training and experience affects the reliability of measurements and observations.

To identify tissue involvement, tests should be valid. *Validity* means that a test measures what it is supposed to measure.[145] Clinicians need to be responsible with respect to the objectivity of examination methods used, and their appropriate interpretation. Tests or measurements that do not have a high degree of reliability or validity are not necessarily useless. However, acknowledgement of their poor or unknown reliability and validity will keep the clinician honest. Clinicians should avoid using the results of such tests to exaggerate findings to the patient, other health professionals and insurance companies.

The following tests have above average reliability and validity: [39,49,63,65,93]

- Measurement of active jaw movements
- Pain response to muscle palpation
- Pain response to joint palpation
- Assessment of joint sounds

The following tests can be used, but are not as reliable or valid as those listed above. Of the following tests, only compression and force biting are discussed in this text.[39]

- Intraoral evaluation of joint play
- Passive end-feel assessment
- Static resistance tests
- Compression tests
- Force biting tests

Adjunctive Tests

Imaging Studies

The most common TMJ imaging studies are plain radiography, tomography, panoramic radiography, computed tomography (CT), arthrography, and magnetic resonance imaging (MRI). Bone can be visualized with all the techniques, but visualizing soft tissue structures such as the disc requires arthrography or MRI.[49,138] MRI and arthrography tend to overdiagnose TMD disc displacements.[180]

Plain films or conventional radiographs are readily produced in most dental or medical offices. Projections include transcranial, transpharyngeal and transorbital.[138] Each provides limited information of the bony anatomy and no information on soft tissue conditions of the TMJ.[68]

Tomograms are views of a preselected plane of joint anatomy, from .5 to 10 mm thickness. An advantage over plain films is that clear images of the selected joint anatomy can be seen, and abnormalities not seen on plain films can be detected.[11,68]

Panoramic radiography is a modified tomogram that provides an image of the maxilla, mandible and condyle. The mandibular fossa and articular eminence are not well visualized. Common in dental offices, panoramic radiography provides a convenient, relatively low-radiation method of screening the TMJs for bony and dental abnormalities.[11,68]

Computed tomography produces images of both hard and soft tissues, but since TMJ soft tissue resolution is generally poor, CT is mainly used for bony analysis.[11,68]

Arthrography is an invasive procedure that involves the injection of radiopaque contrast medium usually into the lower joint space.[173] Arthrography can be combined with any imaging technique. It is frequently used with lateral transcranial or lateral tomographic views to indirectly evaluate the disc's integrity and position. Contrast medium that flows from the injected lower joint space to the uninjected upper joint space indicates a perforation, usually in the posterior attachment. Arthrography combined with fluoroscopy is useful for dynamic analysis of the disc-condyle complex.[173] Though once considered the gold standard, the arthrographic procedure may distort the joint so that an actual disc displacement looks normal.

Magnetic resonance imaging (MRI) is inferior to CT for bone studies but superior for evaluating TMJ soft tissues, including disc position. MRI is generally accepted as the current gold standard for evaluating TMJ disc position. The disadvantage of MRI is that it is not dynamic.[20] However, echo planar imaging (EPI) is a recent ultrafast MRI technique that can scan a single frame in less than a second.[23] Though EPI is dynamic, the patient must be able to perform slow mandibular movements and some technological issues can lead to unpredictable results.[23]

Electronic Devices

Electronic devices used to evaluate the TMJ include surface electromyography, neuromuscular stimulation, jaw tracking, and sonography. However, results from electronic devices have low specificity, resulting in false positive diagnoses. Evidence does not support the routine use of electronic devices to diagnose TMD or to monitor the patient's response to treatment.[65,185,186]

Surface electromyography is thought to distinguish between normal and abnormal masticatory muscle activity during rest and function. However, it does not discriminate patients from non-patients and should not be used to justify treatment.

Table 8-1: The American Academy of Orofacial Pain's classification system for TMD with ICD-9 CM codes.

Articular Disorders

Congenital or Developmental Disorders

    Aplasia (754.0)

    Hypoplasia (526.89)

    Hyperplasia (526.89)

    Neoplasia [benign] (213.1)

    Neoplasia [malignant] (170.1)

Disc Derangement Disorders (524.63)

    Disc Displacement With Reduction

    Disc Displacement Without Reduction

    Acute Disc Displacement Without Reduction

    Chronic Disc Displacement Without Reduction

TMJ Dislocation [Open] (830.1)

Inflammatory Disorders

    Synovitis and Capsulitis (727.09)

    Polyarthritides (714.9)

Osteoarthritis (Non-Inflammatory Disorders) (715.18)

    Osteoarthritis Primary

    Osteoarthritis Secondary

Ankylosis (524.61)

    Fibrous Ankylosis

    Bony Ankylosis

Fracture (802.21)

Masticatory Muscle Disorders

Myofascial Pain (729.1)

Myositis (728.81)

Myospasm (728.85)

Local Myalgia Unclassified

Myofibrotic Contracture (728.9)

Neoplasia (171.0)

Neuromuscular stimulation is applied to the masseter muscle and may relax the muscles. Proponents of neuromuscular stimulation use it along with jaw tracking analysis.

Jaw tracking devices (mandibular kinesiographs) are used to evaluate jaw mobility or position. A magnet is attached to the anterior mandibular teeth and the patient performs various mandibular movements. The jaw tracking device is said to assess mandibular range of motion, speed and regularity of movement, chewing movements, and other parameters.

Sonography devices are used to enhance the TMJ sounds and monitor the timing of the sounds during mandibular movement. The intent is to record joint sounds from one TMJ. However, the microphone or transducer also records arterial blood flow, ambient room noise, and skin/hair noise.

Physical Therapy Classification of TMD

TMD is a term that was adopted at *The President's Conference on the Diagnosis and Management of Temporomandibular Disorders* in 1982.[9] The American Academy of Orofacial Pain (AAOP), formerly the American Academy of Craniomandibular Disorders, formed a committee of experts to develop a classification system for TMDs.

The AAOP classification system was influenced by and follows closely the *International Headache Society's Classification and Diagnostic Criteria for Headache Disorders, Cranial Neuralgias and Facial Pain.*[67] The International Headache Society lists *Disorders of the Temporomandibular Joint* as one of eight subcategories of the 11 major classifications of pain titled, *Headache or facial pain associated with disorders of the cranium, eyes, ears, nose, sinuses, teeth, mouth or other facial or cranial structures.*[67] The 1982 TMD classi-

fication system was expanded by AAOP's 1993 TMD guidelines, which were updated in 1996[132] and 2004[144] (Table 8-1).

Temporomandibular disorders are classified as TMD arthrogenous disorders (TMD-A), TMD myogeneous disorders (TMD-M), or both.[132] The arthrogenous and myogeneous groupings are subclassified into additional categories. In addition to the AAOP guidelines on TMD, there are eight other published TMD guidelines.[49] However, none of them accurately and comprehensively address physical therapy management issues. Identifying the TMD diagnoses that can be helped by physical therapy will facilitate the appropriate utilization of physical therapists by the dental and medical professions.

The physical therapy TMD classification I propose is similar to the AAOP classification, but specifically identifies TMD conditions that a physical therapist treats (Table 8-2). Modification of this classification system will surely occur over time as research enables better understanding of the physical therapist's role in head and neck pain management.

Table 8-2: Physical Therapy Classification for TMD with ICD-9 CM codes.

Arthrogenous
Inflammation (727.09)
Hypermobility (830.1)
Hypomobility
Disc Displacement without Reduction (524.63)
Fibrous Adhesions (524.61)
Myogenous
Masticatory Muscle Pain (728.5)

Section Three—
Evaluation and Treatment of Myogeneous Involvement (TMD-M)

Muscles of mastication are a primary source of pain related to TMD. Single muscles or groups of muscles may be involved. According to the AAOP guidelines, muscle pain falls under the broad category of masticatory muscle disorders.

The AAOP guidelines list six subclassifications for TMD masticatory muscle disorders (Table 8-1). Establishing reliable and valid criteria to honestly identify each of the muscle conditions listed is difficult.[51,158] Simply understanding the physiology and neurophysiology of muscle pain and its clinical presentation is a challenge.[166]

An increase in muscle activity is postulated to lead to increased muscle tone or spasm and subsequent muscle pain.[89,172] However, there is no experimental proof that increased tone leads to pain.[93,158] Patients with masticatory muscle pain do not always have masticatory muscle hyperactivity as identified by an increase in EMG activity.[22,158,163] Likewise, patients who brux regularly (clench, tap and/or grind the teeth while either asleep or awake) do not always have masticatory muscle pain.[22,40,93,163] Masticatory muscle pain does not always cause a limitation in mandibular dynamics. One study found no differences in mandibular mobility between people who were functionally healthy and those with muscle pain.[167] Clinically, patients with 40 mm of opening may complain of restricted opening, while some patients with less than 40 mm do not have any complaints.

These examples are included to show that there is not necessarily a correlation between mandibular dynamics and masticulatory muscle involvement. However, pain in masticatory muscles is clearly a common finding with TMD.[158,164] The physical therapy diagnosis for pain originating from the muscles of mastication is *masticatory muscle pain (MMP)*. In addition to being a primary problem, MMP may play a role as a predisposing, precipitating and perpetuating factor for TMD arthrogeneous conditions.[127,153]

History

The patient complains of facial or jaw pain and may or may not be aware of bruxism.[29] Patients should be asked if they make contact with their teeth since some patients may not know what bruxism means. The patient may wake at night or in the morning with pain, soreness or tension in the TMJ or jaw muscles.

Physical Examination

Palpation of the muscles of mastication is the primary method of identifying MMP. Palpation is performed to reproduce or increase the patient's symptoms. Depending upon severity or frequency of symptoms, a symptomatic response may not occur at the time of the examination, but the clinician may be able to identify increased tone or tension in the muscles being palpated.

Muscles that elevate the mandible are often the symptomatic muscles and will be the primary muscles to palpate. Of the three muscles that elevate the mandible, the temporalis and masseter muscles can be palpated directly, thereby providing a high level of reliability and validity. Both the temporalis and masseter are palpated extraorally (Fig 8-15).[49] Other sites can be palpated, but with less reliability and validity (Table 8-3).

Table 8-3: Palpation technique for muscles related to the TMJ.[49]

Temporalis	Palpate anterior, middle and posterior fibers located in the temporal fossa
Masseter	Palpate from the zygomatic process to the angle of the mandible
Posterior Digastric	Palpate extraorally, posterior to the angle of the mandible
Anterior Digastric	Palpate extraorally, inferior to the body of the mandible
Medial Pterygoid	Palpate intraorally, along the medial rim of the mandible
Lateral Pterygoid	Palpate intraorally, placing the finger posterior to the third maxillary molar, and palpating in a superior, posterior and medial direction
Temporalis Tendon	With the mouth wide open, palpate intraorally following the ramus of the mandible in a posterior direction until the tip of the coronoid is felt

Treatment for Masticatory Muscle Pain

The challenge is to control the habits that perpetuate MMP. Jaw habits include gum chewing, object, nail, lip or cheek biting, protrusive jaw positioning and diurnal or nocturnal bruxism.[121] Diurnal oral habits can be controlled once the patient is made aware of them. Bruxism, especially noc-

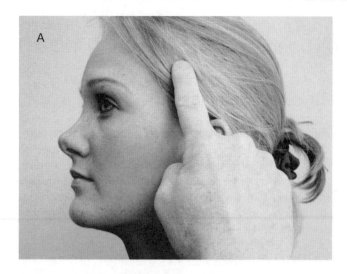

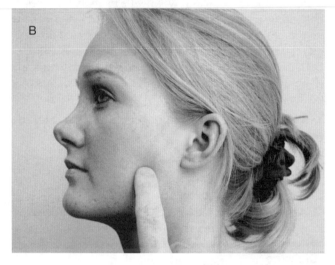

Figure 8-15: Palpation of A) the anterior fibers of the temporalis; and B) the masseter muscle.

turnal bruxism, is one of the more difficult oral habits to manage. Bruxism is more prevalent in TMD patients than in the general population.[89] The etiology of bruxism is multifactorial.[93] The relationship between bruxism and TMD is still unclear.[93,97,166]

Oral Modification and Awareness Training

Clinicians should not assume patients will know that certain oral activities are harmful. Patients should be encouraged to stop biting fingernails, pencils and lips, leaning on their chins, chewing ice and gum, and biting on a smoker's pipe.

Tongue Up—Teeth Apart—Breathe. Teaching the patient the "tongue up, teeth apart and breathe (TTB)" awareness exercise will provide a means of controlling diurnal bruxism that may occur in response to stressful events.

- *Tongue up*—The tongue is composed of various intrinsic and extrinsic muscles. The genioglossus is the main muscle responsible for maintaining the tongue against the palate.[96] The muscles that elevate the mandible (temporalis, masseter, medial pterygoid) have the least amount of activity when the tongue is against the palpate (jaw-tongue reflex).

  The rest position of the tongue, also referred to as the postural position of the tongue, is described in the following way: The anterosuperior tip of the tongue lies just behind the upper central incisors but does not press against them. The rest of the tongue, at least the first half, touches the palate. The patient must be told to not "push" or "poke" the tongue against the palate. It helps to visualize the tongue as floating in this position (Fig 8-16).

  Tongue up may be difficult to achieve in patients who have upper airway disturbances such as colds, allergies, or nasal septum deviations.

- *Teeth Apart*—Teeth apart should naturally follow once the patient's tongue is in the correct rest position.

- *Breathe*—Patients should be taught to breathe through the nose, using the diaphragm. Breathing through the nose makes better use of the diaphragm, the principle driver of respiration. Diaphragmatic breathing promotes general relaxation of the body. Mouth breathing decreases diaphragmatic breathing, increases use of accessory muscles (the scalenes and sternocleidomastoid), and should generally be avoided.

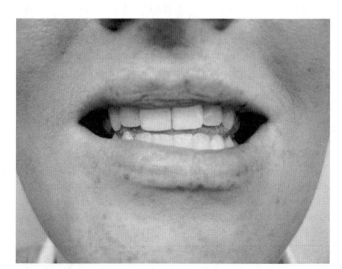

Figure 8-16: The resting position of the tongue for awareness training to control diurnal bruxism.

Tongue Up and Wiggle. Some patients with MMP may not brux during their waking hours. Instead, they brace their mandible with the teeth apart. Patients who are suspected of "bracing" their mandible with their teeth apart should be taught the *tongue up and wiggle* exercise. With the tongue in its rest position, the patient is instructed to oscillate or wiggle the jaw from side to side. The amplitude of side to side movement is kept low—the patient should exert minimal effort. The exercise should be repeated frequently throughout the day. The more the patient wiggles, the less likely he will be bracing. If joint noises occur, the amplitude of the wiggle should be reduced.

Modalities

Modalities are used to decrease pain and to improve healing.[129] Modalities frequently used to treat MMP include:

- Hot or cold packs
- Ultrasound
- Iontophoresis
- Electric Stimulation

Electrical stimulation over the bilateral masseter muscles works particularly well for decreasing muscle pain and increasing mouth opening. The current can be constant but tends to be better tolerated if intermittent (e.g., 12 seconds on and 12 seconds off). The intensity should be high enough to get a contraction of the masseter muscles yet comfortable for the patient. The patient can alternate between actively and passively opening the mouth three or four times when the current is on. The patient should rest with the tongue up when the current is off (Fig 8-17). Active and passive mouth opening during electrical stimulation (stretching with contraction) often achieves decreased pain and increased mouth opening.

Massage to the Muscles of Mastication

Extra-oral or intra-oral massage to tight and painful muscles may provide short or long-term relief of MMP. Detailing specific techniques is beyond the scope of this text.

Therapeutic Exercises

Therapeutic exercises are done to relax or strengthen the muscles of mastication. Relaxing the masticatory muscles is clinically more important than strengthening them.

Muscles that elevate the mandible often need relaxation exercises. Relaxing the elevator muscles can involve contracting the muscles directly (contract-relax) or contracting the antagonist muscle (depressor muscles of the

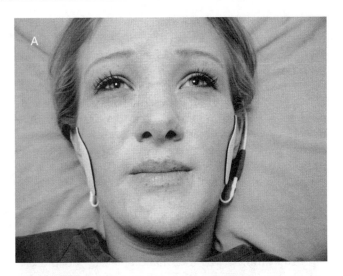
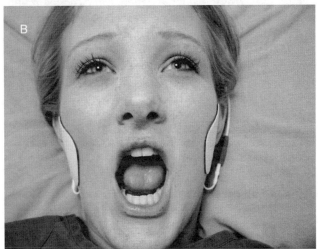
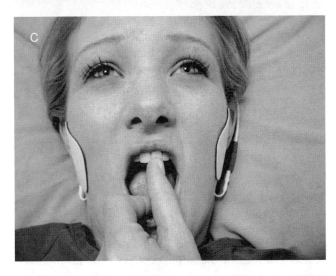

Figure 8-17: Electric stimulation on surge mode for MMP and/or limited opening due to MMP or Stage II disc displacement. A) Current off; B) Patient opens mouth 3-4 times with current on; C) Patient passively stretches mouth 3-4 times with current on.

mandible). A strong contraction is not recommended. Contract-relax technique provides the patient with feedback. The goal is to have the patient identify more with the relaxation portion of the exercise.

Strengthening the muscles of mastication is rarely needed. Furthermore, it is difficult to identify a truly weak masticatory muscle because pain or reflex inhibition may cause a pseudo-weakness, and the masticatory muscles are difficult to isolate. Jaw muscle weakness tends to be the exception rather than the rule. After immobilization following facial trauma, orthognathic surgery or surgery to repair fractures, a return to normal diet is usually adequate to restore strength.

In the rare case where the mandibular elevator muscles need to be strengthened, the patient can close the mouth against resistance by placing the index finger over the lower central incisors and contracting the elevator muscles. A 5-10 second contraction, repeated 10 times, 3-5 sessions per day is usually satisfactory to normalize strength.

Oral Appliance

An oral appliance is a very common treatment for TMD offered by dentists.[31,159] Oral appliances are removable devices usually fabricated in hard acrylic plastic resin, but occasionally made with a soft resilient material. The oral appliance fits on either the upper or lower arch of teeth. There is a wide variety of opinions about the mechanism of effectiveness and the optimum design of the appliance. Five major theories covering an oral appliance's mechanism of action have been described.[31,32]

A detailed discussion of each theory is beyond the scope of this text; they are listed here to illustrate the diversity of opinion about the use of oral appliances:

1. Occlusal disengagement theory
2. Restored vertical dimension theory
3. Maxillomandibular realignment theory
4. TMJ repositioning theory
5. Cognitive awareness theory

Clinicians treating TMD will hear various names for oral appliances, such as stabilization splint, flat plane appliance, Tanner mandibular appliance, Gelb splint, centric related splint, occlusal splint, night guard, and bite guard.[31,159] Some appliances are given names based upon special features of the appliances such as the modified hawley or anterior bite splint,[181] Nociceptive Trigeminal Inhibition (NTI),[16] repositioning splint,[31] pivot appliance,[95] hydrostatic appliance,[91] mandibular orthopaedic repositioning appliance (MORA),[60] and myo-monitor appliance.[80] Physical therapists need not be concerned about the name of the oral appliance, but should be aware of its design, purpose and goals from the dentist's point of view. At a minimum, oral appliances must be comfortable, aesthetic, retentive, functional, and, most importantly, reversible and non-invasive to the occlusion, muscles of mastication and cervical spine.[31,159] A stabilization splint has these features and has the most evidence of effectiveness in the literature.[159] Clinicians treating TMD should become familiar with oral appliance design and theory, and should refer to the reference list for more resources.[104,159]

Why oral appliances work is still unknown.[132,159] All oral appliances have the potential for a positive effect via increased cognitive awareness and/or positive patient expectations.[31,132,159] Though oral appliances are sometimes effective in controlling MMP, symptoms sometimes worsen or do not respond with their use.[130] In such situations, the dentist should investigate whether the patient has cervical involvement that can contribute to MMP and intolerance to the appliance.

Cervical Spine Considerations

The cervical spine is often overlooked in the management of head and jaw pains. The vast majority of patients experiencing neck pain can be classified as having nonspecific neck pain, also termed mechanical neck pain.[87,144] In the rest of this chapter, the term *neck pain* will be used when referring to patients with cervical spine involvement.

Neck pain can originate from various tissues associated with the cervical spine, and has an influence on TMD management for the following reasons:

Neck pain can mimic TMD pain. Pain originating in the cervical spine can be perceived in the head, face, and jaw areas via an area in the brain termed the *trigeminocervical nucleus.*[15] Bogduk describes the trigeminocervical nucleus as the area in the brain where the trigeminal and cervical afferents converge. He states that the trigeminocervical nucleus is the nociceptive nucleus for the entire head and upper neck. Nociceptive information from cervical spine tissues can be transmitted to the trigeminocervical nucleus, giving the patient the perception of symptoms in the head, face and jaw areas.[15,82]

Neck pain often coexists with TMD. The coexistence of neck symptoms with TMD is more prevalent than one might expect and must be recognized if patients with head and neck pain are to be treated successfully.[1,18,25,27,37,38,43,76,84,94,135,178]

Clinical research supports the following statements:

- Neck pain is associated with TMD 70% of the time.[135]
- Bruxism is more common in patients with pain in both the masticatory and cervical spine musculature.[76]
- Patients with TMD complain about neck pain more frequently than patients without TMD.[40]
- Patients with neck pain report more signs and symptoms of TMD than healthy controls.[40]
- Neck pain is more prevalent with myogenous than arthrogenous TMD.[94,43]

Neck pain can cause MMP. It is clear that neck symptoms and TMD coexist. This suggests that treatment will be required for both the neck and the masticatory muscles. The cause of MMP is multifactorial and is not well understood. It is possible that neck pain may be a cause of MMP. Therefore, effective treatment for MMP may, in fact, focus on treatment of the neck. Investigating a cause and effect relationship is one of the most difficult challenges in clinical research, and no one can say for certain the exact relationship between neck problems and MMP. However, two theories are proposed that shed light on how neck problems may precipitate, perpetuate, or predispose one to MMP.

The first theory is that cervical spine neurophysiological influences cause masticatory muscle pain via the tonic neck reflex and/or by the agonist/antagonist relationship of the anterior cervical muscles (including the muscles of mastication) to the posterior cervical muscles.[148]

The second theory postulates that MMP actually occurs in response to neck pain. For example, patients may respond to neck pain by bruxing, which may lead to MMP. A detailed explanation of these theories is beyond the scope of this text, but clinicians are encouraged to seek more information and certainly consider the cervical spine when patients present with head and jaw pain.

Neck Pain and Oral Appliances

Neck pain and an oral appliance both have an influence on the resting position of the mandible and the subsequent trajectory of jaw closure. If the neck and oral appliance affect the resting position of the mandible in different ways, an increase in MMP and a decrease in tolerance to the oral appliance may result.

The rest position of the mandible is defined by Atwood as "the habitual postural position of the mandible when the patient is at ease in an upright position."[7] Mohl states, "we must logically conclude that, if rest position is altered by a change in head position, the habitual path of closure of the mandible must also be altered by such a change."[116] Studies of normal subjects have demonstrated that the resting position of the mandible and the trajectory of mandibular closure into occlusion is affected by the relationship of the head to the cervical spine and gravity.[19,52,62,98,105]

Head and neck mobility and position affect the tension and tone of connective tissues and muscles that traverse from the cervical spine and cranium to the mandible (Fig 8-18). Neck pain with associated altered mobility and positioning of the head and neck is believed to influence mandibular position and the trajectory of jaw closure into centric occlusion or into the oral appliance.

All oral appliances influence the rest position of the mandible. Therefore all oral appliances have an influence on the trajectory of mandibular closure into the oral appliance.[90] Depending on the design of the oral appliance, some can have a significant effect on jaw dynamics. The thickness of an oral appliance may influence head and neck posture. The head may extend on the cervical spine to compensate to the increase in vertical dimension of a thick appliance.[35,143] An oral appliance should be kept as thin as the possible unless an increase in vertical dimension can be justified.

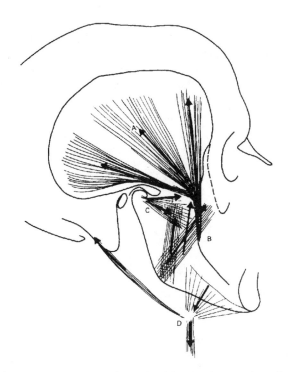

Figure 8-18: The connective tissues and muscles that traverse from the cervical spine and cranium to the mandible. Connective tissue tension and muscle tone can be affected by neck pain, thereby influencing mandibular rest position and the trajectory of jaw closure.

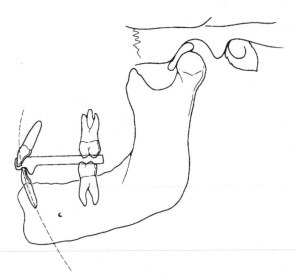

Figure 8-19: An ARA may be used by some dentists to treat a disk displacement with reduction. It positions the mandible forward and down to prevent the disc from displacing anteriorly on mandibular closing.

An example of an oral appliance that influences jaw and neck equilibrium is the anterior repositioning appliance (ARA). An ARA may be used by some dentists to treat disc displacements. The ARA is thicker than other oral appliances, and repositions the mandible in a forward and down position, significantly changing the rest position of the mandible and the trajectory of jaw closure (Fig 8-19).

The patient with neck pain who is wearing an ARA may not respond to its use or may have an increase in neck pain. This results because both the ARA and the cervical spine are competing over influencing mandibular rest position and the trajectory of jaw closure. Other oral appliance designs have more or less similar influences on mandibular rest position, the trajectory of jaw closure, and head and neck position.

In summary, the cervical spine should be considered when the patient's MMP does not improve or worsens with the use of an oral appliance. If the patient perceives that the "bite" is off, but the dentist cannot identify any occlusal factors to account for the perception, the cervical spine should be suspected as influencing the trajectory of jaw closure. If the patient is treated initially with an ARA and does not achieve a favorable response, referral to a physical therapist for evaluation of the cervical spine is appropriate, rather than more prolonged treatment with an ARA or referral to an oral surgeon.

Not all patients with neck pain respond poorly to an oral appliance. Variables to consider are the structural design of the appliance, the technique used by the dentist to balance/adjust the appliance, the degree of acute or chronic neck pain, and the adaptive response of the individual.[144] Reliable criteria do not exist to identify those patients who may adversely respond to an oral appliance secondary to cervical spine influences. Therefore, treatment of neck pain should be done before or at the time of delivery of an oral appliance. The stabilization splint, with proper features, currently represents the best design for oral appliance treatment of TMD with or without neck pain.

Screening for NNP by the Dentist

Dentists should screen for neck problems during the history. Symptoms suggesting neck involvement are grouped by most commonly to least commonly seen (Table 8-4). Although the list in Table 8-4 was compiled from a reference on whiplash injury, it is also useful for neck pain that did not result from a whiplash injury. Patients who have any of the symptoms listed should consult with a physical therapist for a comprehensive evaluation of the cervical spine.

Table 8-4: Symptoms associated with non-specific neck pain (NNP).[160]

GROUP ONE – Most Common
Neck and/or shoulder pain
Reduced and/or painful neck movements
Headaches
Numbness, tingling or pain in arm or hand
Dizziness or unsteadiness
Nausea or vomiting
GROUP TWO
Difficulty swallowing
Ringing in the ears
Memory problems
Problems concentrating
Vision problems
Reduced and/or painful jaw movement
GROUP THREE – Least Common
Numbness, tingling, or pain in leg or foot
Lower back pain

Section Four—
Evaluation and Treatment of Arthrogeneous Involvement (TMD-A)

TMJ Inflammation

TMJ inflammation can involve the capsule, TMJ ligament, lateral and medial collateral ligaments, anterior and posterior bands of the disc and posterior attachment. Tests are not sensitive enough to differentiate between these tissues. Even if such tests were available, the results of the tests would not affect treatment planning.

History — TMJ Inflammation

Symptoms are located in the preauricular area with or without referral into the temporal and mandibular areas. Pain is typically reproduced with chewing, talking and/or yawning. Mandibular dynamics may or may not be affected. Patients with significant joint effusion may be unable to bring their back teeth together on the ipsilateral side.

Physical Examination — TMJ Inflammation

The physical examination includes the provocation tests of palpation and TMJ loading. Whether or not the patient's symptoms are affected depends on the degree of inflammation. With the exception of limited mandibular dynamics and rarely seen joint swelling, provocative tests require the patient's verbal response. The clinician should carefully correlate all elements of the evaluation to properly interpret the patient's verbal response, and avoid over or under-diagnosing TMJ inflammation.

TMJ Palpation

Palpation over the lateral pole. Facing the patient, the clinician uses the index or middle fingers to palpate over and then slightly posterior to the lateral pole with the patient's back teeth together (Fig 8-20). Palpation continues as the patient opens the mouth. A positive test is an increase or reproduction of the symptoms on the ipsilateral side. Targeted tissues are the lateral collateral ligament, capsule, and TMJ ligament.

Palpation via the external auditory meatus. Facing the patient, the clinician inserts his little finger (pad of the finger facing towards the condyle) in the patient's external auditory meatus (EAM) and asks the patient to open the mouth (Fig 8-21). The clinician applies slight pressure forward with his finger as the patient then closes the mouth, bringing the back teeth together. A positive test is an increase or reproduction of the symptoms on the side being palpated. The target tissue is the posterior attachment of the disc.

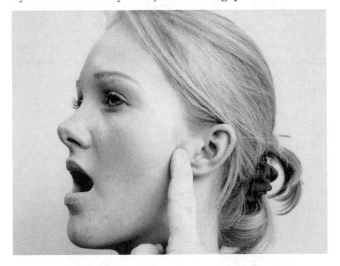

Figure 8-20: Palpation over the lateral pole to provoke the lateral collateral ligament, capsule and TMJ ligament. It is performed with the patient's back teeth together and then with the mouth opened.

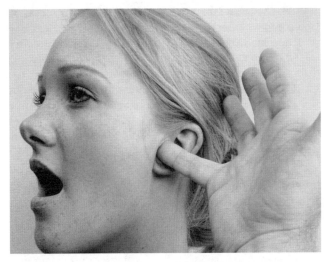

Figure 8-21: Palpation via the external auditory meatus to provoke the posterior attachment of the disc. The clinician inserts his finger with the mouth opened, then asks the patient to close the mouth, bringing the back teeth together.

The clinician should not be concerned about joint noises during this test. If excessive pressure is applied by the finger, the disc position may be influenced enough to produce a joint noise, but it is not significant.

TMJ Loading

Dynamic Loading. Biting with the molars against resistance causes joint loading (compression) on the contralateral side with less compression and possible distraction on the ipsilateral side.[70,73,78,140] Dynamic loading is accomplished by asking the patient to bite hard on a cotton roll placed between the molars on one side. A rolled up 4x4 gauze cut in half can also be used (Fig 8-22). A positive test is an increase or reproduction of the symptoms on the contralateral side.

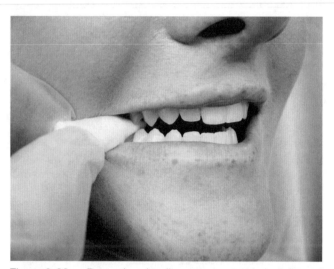

Figure 8-22: Dynamic loading to provoke inflamed intracapsular tissues. The patient bites on a cotton roll placed between the molars to load the contralateral side.

Dynamic loading requires contraction of the elevator muscles of the mandible. Patients can have a false positive response to TMJ loading if MMP is present. Patients can also have both TMJ inflammation and MMP. Asking the patient to point to the location of the pain during dynamic loading can help differentiate. Patients with joint pain will point to the temporomandibular joint; patients with MMP will point to the temporalis, masseter, or both.

Passive Loading. Passive loading of the TMJ involves applying a posterosuperior force to the mandible. The clinician grasps the patient's chin with the index finger and thumb. With the patient's back teeth slightly apart, the clinician applies pressure on the chin in a posterosuperior direction and then in a posterosuperior and slightly lateral direction to the left and right. The opposite hand gives appropriate counterforce on the back of the patient's head

(Fig 8-23). This test is not selective for either the right or left TMJ. A positive test is a reproduction or increase of the patient's TMJ symptoms. A false negative response is possible for patients who are unable to relax the jaw.

Treatment for TMJ Inflammation

The treatment goal is to decrease inflammation in and around the TMJ. Modalities frequently used to treat TMJ inflammation include:

- Hot or cold packs
- Ultrasound
- Iontophoresis
- Electric Stimulation

TMJ inflammation should respond within a relatively short period of time to modality treatment. Patients have

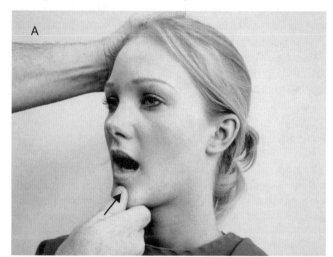

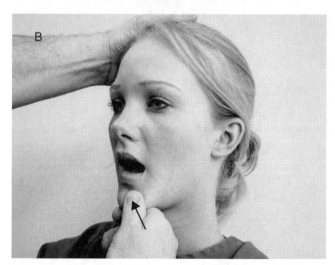

Figure 8-23: Passive loading to provoke tissues posterior and posterolateral to the head of the condyle. A) Posterosuperior loading; B) Posterosuperior and lateral loading—repeat to right and left.

varying responses to modalities, and a variety of modalities can be tried.[129,179] If inflammation persists, MMP or a disc displacement may be present.

TMJ Hypermobility

Hypermobility occurs when the condyle translates excessively beyond the articular eminence onto the articular tubercle.[44] Hypermobility has been thought to cause osteoarthritis and disc displacement. However, studies have not confirmed this relationship.[44,45,46] TMJ hypermobility does not impair function and is often a benign condition.

History—TMJ Hypermobility

The patient may state, "My jaw feels like it goes out of place." The patient may also point to the condyle with mouth opening, demonstrating the excessive movement. The appearance of excessive condyle movement may be magnified in patients with narrow faces. Clinicians must avoid placing undue emphasis on the appearance or sensation of excessive condyle movement, because these perceptions do not always correlate with actual pathology.[161]

The patient may report joint noises. Joint noises do not always occur with hypermobility. The noise typically occurs either at the end of opening (caused by the condyle moving abruptly past the articular crest onto the articular tubercle) or at the beginning of closing (caused by the condyle moving abruptly past the articular crest onto the

articular eminence). The patient may incorrectly believe that the clicking or popping is related to a disc displacement.

The patient may relate short-term episodes of jaw "catching" with mouth closure. This symptom may point to an intermittent dislocation of the condyle. A predisposing factor for dislocation appears to be an articular eminence with a short, steep slope.[10,133]

In the event a patient presents with a dislocated condyle, the diagnosis is straightforward. The patient is unable to close the mouth from a fully opened position. With a unilateral dislocation, the jaw deflects contralaterally (Fig 8-24). The physical therapist rarely sees these patients, because they typically seek emergency treatment. Once the condyle has been reduced, the patient may be referred to physical therapy for treatment of inflammation and control of mandibular opening.

Physical Examination—TMJ Hypermobility

Facing the patient, the clinician uses the index or middle fingers to palpate over the lateral pole as the patient opens and closes the mouth.

The clinician may be able to detect excessive translation of the condyle or feel a "jutter" at the end of mouth opening and beginning of mouth closing (Fig 8-25). The "jutter" is the condyle moving across the articular crest onto the articular tubercle. No consistent deviation or deflection is observed.

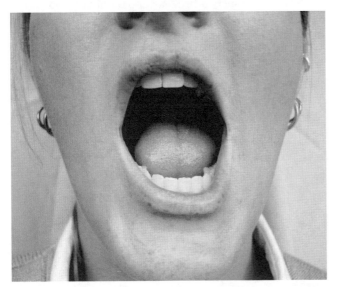

Figure 8-24: Dislocated right condyle. The jaw is deflected to the left and the patient is unable to close the mouth from a fully opened position.

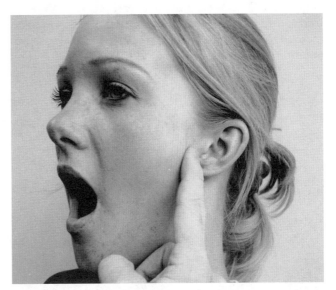

Figure 8-25: Condylar hypermobility is identified by palpating excessive translation of the condyle and/or a "jutter" that occurs at the end of mouth opening and the beginning of mouth closing.

Diagnosing hypermobility via palpation is not reliable or valid. However, since the condition and its treatment are benign, false positives and negatives can be tolerated. The alternative is to request an x-ray, which is not justified.

Treatment for TMJ Hypermobility

Treatment of TMJ hypermobility is important when:

- The patient makes it an issue. Some patients are anxious about the possibility that their jaw will displace or believe that their popping is related to a disc displacement.
- The patient has TMJ inflammation. If hypermobility is not controlled, the joint can be aggravated every time the patient opens wide while eating or yawning.
- The patient has a history of his jaw catching intermittently when closing from an open mouth position that is confirmed on examination.

Treatment focuses on patient education to reassure the patient that there is no severe pathology. Patients should be taught to eat smaller portions of food (avoid large sandwiches) and to place the tongue against the roof of the mouth when yawning to avoid excessive opening (Fig 8-26). Patients should inform their dentists that they have hypermobility so the amount and duration of opening during dental treatment can be minimized.

Treatment for hypermobility very rarely involves surgery. Surgical approaches could include eminectomy, condylotomy, sectioning of the lateral pterygoid muscle, intracapsular injection of sclerosing solutions, and increasing the height of the articular eminence to block anterior movement of the condyle.[56]

Hypomobility, Including Disc Displacements

Hypomobility can be a result of TMD-A or TMD-M involvement. Examples of arthrogeneous hypomobility include disc displacement without reduction (Stage II) and articular adhesions discussed later in this chapter.

There is a high prevalence (34%) of disc displacements in asymptomatic children and young adults.[142] Why some disc displacements are painful and others are not, or why some non-painful disc displacements progress to painful disc displacements is not understood.

Disc displacement or internal derangement has been defined as, "a disturbance in the normal anatomic relationship between the disc and condyle that interferes with smooth movement of the joint and causes momentary catching, clicking, popping or locking."[88] The disc is considered to be displaced when the patient has the back teeth together and the posterior band of the disc is anterior or anteromedial to the head of the condyle (Fig 8-27).[10]

A disc displacement is believed to be caused by laxity of the medial or more likely the thin lateral collateral ligament.[10,133,137,156] Ligamentous laxity allows excessive movement between the disc and condyle, with subsequent loss of the self-seating relationship.[183]

Collateral ligament laxity can result from trauma. It can also result from microtrauma in the form of continuous or repetitive loading from daily functional and parafunctional activities such as bruxism and other oral habits. The health of the disc and articulating surfaces is dependent upon the frequency, duration, magnitude, direction and location of the microtrauma and variations in bony and

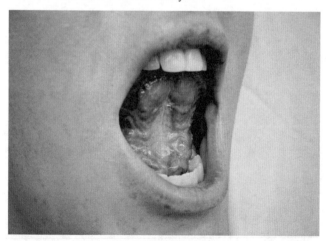

Figure 8-26: The tongue up position to control translation of the condyle during yawning.

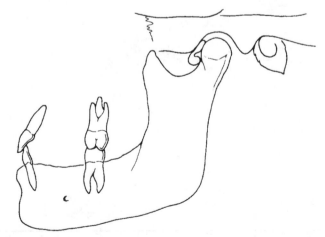

Figure 8-27: Disc displacement. With the back teeth together, the posterior band of the disc is displaced anterior to the condyle.

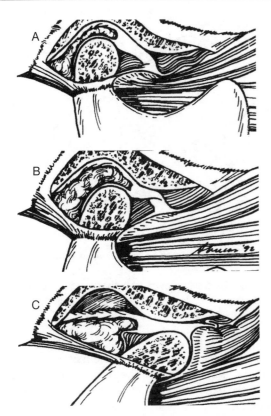

Figure 8-28: Disc displacement with reduction—Stage I. A) With the back teeth together, the disc is displaced anterior to the condyle; B) With opening, translation of the condyle tenses the superior lamina; C) Tension in the superior lamina "snaps" the disc posterior, causing the classic opening "click" (adapted from Okeson).[133]

muscular anatomy.[118] Understanding the etiological events and anatomical changes that contribute to a disc displacement enables the clinician to formulate realistic goals for treatment.

Several classifications of disc displacements have been recorded in the literature.[115,187] I prefer Moffett's classification, which is also used by the AAOP.[115] This classification does not require imaging studies and relies only on the history and physical examination. Moffett's three stages of a disc displacement are:

Stage I—Disc Displacement with Reduction

Stage II—Disc Displacement without Reduction

Stage III—Disc Displacement with Osteoarthritis

A study of the natural history of disc displacements suggests that patients start with a Stage I and progress to a Stage II and III.[42,150] However, many variations from this progression are possible and are not understood.[77] In all stages of disc displacement, the disc is displaced when the patient's back teeth are together.

The history and physical examination help the clinician determine the stage. Except in unusual circumstances (e.g., conservative care has failed and surgery is being considered), MRI, arthrography or other sophisticated assessments are unnecessary to diagnose disc displacement.[169]

Disc Displacement with Reduction—Stage I

When the patient's back teeth are together, the disc is already displaced. As the patient opens the mouth, the condyle rotates on the posterior attachment. Approximately 10 mm into opening, the condyle begins to translate but is initially limited because the disc displacement blocks translation. As translation continues, the condyle pushes against the posterior band of the disc. Additional tension develops in an already stretched superior lamina, which causes the superior lamina to "snap" the disc posterior, causing an opening "click" (Fig 8-28).

A *click* is a distinct sound, of brief and very limited duration, with a clear beginning and end.[49] The disc reduction can occur at various points of mandibular opening, depending upon the amount of tension in the superior lamina.

On closing, the disc displaces anterior to the condyle and is identified by a closing "click". The closing click is softer than the opening click, and occurs at the end of closing. The disc displaces anterior because of laxity in the collateral ligaments, loss of the self-seating relationship of the disc to condyle and by activity of the upper head of the lateral pterygoid muscle. A Stage I is therefore identified by the classic *reciprocal click* (Fig 8-29).[57]

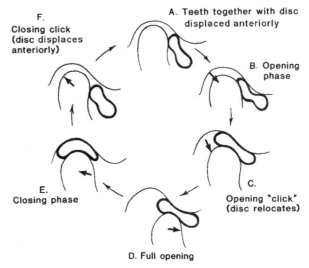

Figure 8-29: Disc displacement with reduction—Stage I is identified by the classic reciprocal click.

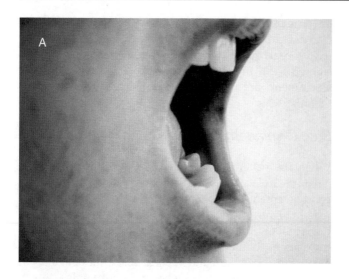

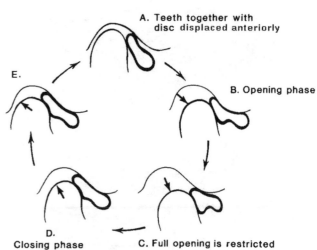

Figure 8-31: Disc displacement without reduction—Stage II. The disc remains displaced through mandibular opening and closing and there is no reciprocal click.

TMJ joint noise is defined as a noise that is heard by the patient and is *always felt* by the clinician. Noises that are heard by the patient but not felt by the clinician may not be significant.

Second, the clinician attempts the elimination of the reciprocal click with the mandible protruded. Starting with the patient's back teeth together, the clinician palpates the patient's lateral poles. The patient is asked to open wide enough to get the opening click and then close forward, bringing the central incisors to an end to end position. Then, the patient is asked to open several times while maintaining this protruded position of the mandible (Fig 8-30). More often than not, the reciprocal click is eliminated because the condyle is not allowed to go back to its original position where the disc displaced anterior to the condyle.[49]

Disc Displacement without Reduction—Stage II

With a Stage II, the disc remains anterior to the condyle throughout the entire phase of opening and closing (Fig 8-31).[169] The disc obstructs condylar translation. The disc is unable to reduce because excessive elongation of the superior lamina has occurred and/or increased activity of the elevator muscles compress the joint space, preventing disc reduction (Fig 8-32).[169]

History—Disc Displacement Stage II

The patient often reports previous joint noises (Stage I), with or without previous episodes of intermittent "locking". There are no current joint noises, but the patient is unable to open the mouth wide and has difficulty performing movements such as chewing and yawning.

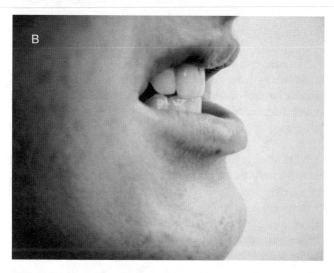

Figure 8-30: Elimination of the reciprocal click from a protruded position of the mandible. Starting with the back teeth in contact, the patient first opens wide enough to cause the opening click (A), then closes with the central incisors at an end to end position (B). From this position, the patient open and closes several times to confirm that the reciprocal click is gone.

History—Disc Displacement Stage I

The patient reports hearing an opening and a closing click during mandibular movements. If noises are not heard by the patient, then a Stage I is not present.

Physical Examination—Disc Displacement Stage I

The physical examination consists of two parts: First, the clinician identifies the reciprocal click by palpating over the lateral poles during mandibular opening and closing. The clinician may not actually hear the noises, but should feel a palpable irregularity. Therefore, in the rest of this text, a

Physical Examination—Disc Displacement Stage II

No joint noises are present. Mandibular dynamics are limited (Fig 8-14).

Chronic Disc Displacement without Reduction—Stage III

Stage III involves the perforation of the posterior attachment, resulting in bone-on-bone contact with associated degenerative changes. The posterior disc may eventually become detached from the postglenoid spine.[48] As the disc becomes more deformed and the posterior attachment degenerates, mandibular dynamics are near normal.[54]

History—Disc Displacement Stage III

The patient may report a history of a Stage I and/or Stage II disc displacement. The patient complains of multiple joint noises (crepitus) with mandibular opening and closing. Crepitus often identifies a Stage III even with no prior history of a Stage I or II. Crepitus is distinguished from the short "click". It is a continuous sound over a longer range of jaw movement.[49] Crepitus is the sound of

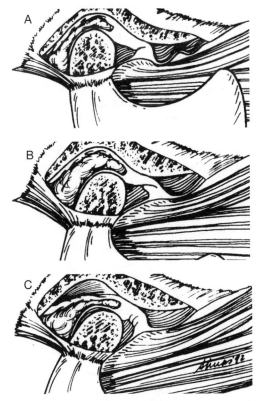

Figure 8-32: Disc displacement without reduction—Stage II. A) With the back teeth together, the disc is displaced anterior to the condyle; B) With opening, translation of the condyle is blocked by the displaced disc; C) The disc acts as a mechanical obstruction causing limited mouth opening (adapted from Okeson).[133]

bone grinding against bone, and is highly indicative of Stage III disc displacement. Osteoarthrosis (OA) and degenerative joint disease (DJD) can also accompany disc displacement.[24] These conditions are likely to be related to each other. Stage III disc displacement, OA and DJD will show radiographic evidence of structural bony change.[75,182] OA and DJD are treated using the same methods as treatment for Stage III disc displacement.

Physical Examination—Disc Displacement Stage III

Mandibular dynamics are normal or near normal. With palpation over the lateral pole during opening and closing, palpable irregularities of crepitus are identified.

Comments on Joint Noises

Three types of joint noises have been discussed:
- A reciprocal click that may occur with hypermobility
- A reciprocal click that occurs with a Stage I disc displacement
- Crepitus that is present with a Stage III disc displacement

Yet another type of joint noise can occur with *deviation in form* (DIF) (ICD 719.68).[132,162] A DIF involves irregular surfaces on the articulating surfaces of the condyle or temporal bone that form obstacles for rotation of the disc against the condyle or translation of the disc against the articular eminence.[132,162] DIF joint noises occur at the exact same condylar position during mandibular opening, closing or both. Palpation reveals a repetitive, non-variable palpable irregularity that cannot be explained by hypermobility or Stage I disc displacement. Noises that are a result of DIF require no treatment other than patient education.

Treatment for Disc Displacements—All Stages

Treatments for disc displacements have historically involved either the use of oral appliances or invasive procedures such as arthrocentesis, arthroscopy or arthrotomy.[8,72,134,191] However, depending on the treatment goal, physical therapy for disc displacements may result in equally good outcomes.

Oral Appliance

Anterior repositioning appliances (ARAs) are used by some dentists to treat Stage I disk displacements (Fig 8-19). As the name implies, an ARA repositions the mandible forward. Repositioning the mandible forward keeps the disc from displacing. The recapture of the disc is confirmed by the elimination of the reciprocal click. The objective of an ARA is to maintain the proper relationship between condyle and disc until sufficient healing of injured tissues (lateral collateral ligament and posterior attachments) has occurred. Often this means the ARA must be worn 24 hours a day for three to six months.

Disadvantages of treatment with ARA include a change in the original bite and jaw position (Fig 8-33), which sometimes requires additional treatment with orthodontics, prosthodontics, equilibration or orthognathic surgery.

Furthermore, treatment with an ARA or other appliance does not result in a permanent corrected position of the disc to condyle, except in a very a small percentage of patients.[99,122,188,165] Proper patient selection with thorough patient education is essential before treating Stage I disc displacement with an ARA. When patients are informed of what may have to occur with their occlusion following treatment with an ARA, they may elect other treatment options such as physical therapy.

For Stage II disc displacements, dentists may use a stabilization appliance and/or intraoral techniques, with the goal of achieving the reciprocal click, indicative of a Stage I disc displacement with functional opening. Then, the dentist may elect to treat the Stage I as previously described or leave it alone if the patient is asymptomatic. For a Stage III disc displacement, the dentist may use a stabilization splint to minimize adverse loading secondary to bruxism.

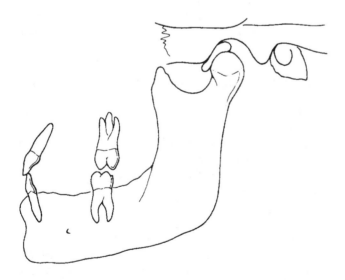

Figure 8-33: Following ARA treatment of a Stage I disc displacement, the patient's mandible is repositioned anteriorly. To bring the molars into contact, a combination of orthodontics, prosthodontics, equilibration and/or orthognathic surgery is often required.

Surgery

Arthrocentesis is lavage and manipulation. This procedure can be done for a Stage II to restore mandibular function or for any stage of disc displacement that involves inflammation.

The joint is anesthetized and the patient is under conscious sedation. In its simplest form, a 1.2 mm needle is used for outflow and is positioned in the anterosuperior joint space.[72] The irrigation is performed with a syringe and a 0.6 mm needle placed in the posterosuperior joint space. One hundred milliliters of isotonic saline solution are slowly injected. The patient is asked to move the jaw during the lavage, with the goal of increasing mouth opening.[72] Though mandibular movement improves, disc displacement to the condyle often remains unchanged.[72] Improvement in mandibular function may have occurred due to elongation of the posterior attachment with further anterior displacement and deformation of the disc.

Arthroscopy is the placement of an arthroscope with camera into the superior joint space. Lavage and lysis of adhesions are performed, and corticosteroid or sodium hyaluronate is injected. This procedure can be done for all stages of disc displacements but is most frequently used for Stage II.[72]

Improvement of mandibular opening and decrease in pain frequently occurs following arthroscopy for a Stage II. However, the improvement is not necessarily a result of restoring the normal disc/condyle relationship.[28,72,124,131,136] Instead, improvement in mandibular function may be due to elongation of the posterior attachment with further anterior displacement and deformation of the disc.

Arthrotomy—Patients who do not respond to conservative care or who have not responded to arthrocentesis and arthroscopy may be appropriate for arthrotomy.

Some authors feel that arthrotomy should be performed only when arthroscopy or arthrocentesis has been tried and has failed, but this point is debated.[6] Arthrotomy can be done for any of the disc displacement conditions. Arthrotomy is also the treatment of choice for ankylosis.

There are many methods of arthrotomy, and none have been shown to have a distinct advantage. Surgical method choices are influenced by the evolving philosophy of the surgeon and long-term results reported in the literature.[8] The results of arthrotomy may be similar to those of arthrocentesis and arthroscopic surgery—disc displacement may still be present despite improved mandibular dynamics and symptoms.[123,147] Physical therapy post-surgery for disc displacements focuses on maintaining the opening achieved from the procedure (see *Physical Therapy Treatment for Fibrous Adhesions* on page 204) and should address any concurrent inflammation or MMP.

Physical Therapy Treatment for Disc Displacements—General Comments

Disc displacements have not been convincingly demonstrated to be entirely pathological.[26,64] Imaging studies have documented the presence of disc displacements in both patient and non-patient populations who have no pain or functional limitations.[55,83] So common are asymptomatic disc displacements that they may be considered a normal anatomic variability.[83,175,184] The long term success of maintaining a "normal" disc to condyle position with oral appliances or surgery is mixed.[6,123]

Given the less than satisfactory long term results with appliance therapy and surgery, it seems unlikely that physical therapy treatment (exercise and manual therapy) can restore disc position. Nonetheless, physical therapists play an important role in the treatment of disc displacements. Physical therapy can facilitate the normal progression of disc displacements. Since the articular tissues of the human TMJ often adapt or remodel in response to disc displacement, the success of physical therapy is not dependent upon the positioning of the disc or the absence of joint noises. Appropriate goals for physical therapy treatment of disc displacements are freedom from pain and improved function. Patients must clearly understand these goals prior to treatment so their expectations are accurate.

Physical Therapy Treatment for a Stage I and a Stage III Disc Displacement

To review, Stage I and Stage III disc displacements present with functional mandibular dynamics and the joint itself may not be painful. Why, then, would a patient with good mandibular function and no TMJ pain seek help? Patients may present with head and neck pain that is originating from other tissues and not from the disc displacement. The patient may mistakenly believe that the clicking or crepitus is the source of the pain. In such cases, the patient's attention should be directed toward the treatment of pain originating from TMJ inflammation, MMP and/or the cervical spine.

TMJ joint pain that accompanies disc displacement is often due to joint inflammation. In fact, the physical therapist should assume that inflammation and disc displacement simply co-exist. Treating the inflammation frequently resolves the pain, even though the Stage I or III disc displacement persists. Sometimes, TMJ inflammation cannot be easily controlled because it is being aggravated

by the disc displacement.[47,126] These are the cases that should be referred to a dentist or oral surgeon.

Physical therapy treatment for Stage I and III should focus on patient education about the meaning of joint noises.[47] Patients should be made aware of other treatment options such as oral appliances and surgery and more importantly, have realistic expectations about the outcome of such treatments (i.e., the unlikelihood that "normal" disc position will be achieved long-term). The physical therapist and dentist who are co-treating a patient must be in philosophical agreement and have good communication to avoid sending the patient mixed messages. Joint noises associated with Stage I are often louder and more disconcerting to patients than joint noises associated with Stage III. Patients with a Stage I may experience occasional catching during opening or closing of the mouth. Therefore, one treatment option for a Stage I is to prevent the disc from relocating on opening by stretching out the already stretched posterior attachment. The electrical stimulation stretching technique described below for Stage II disc displacement can be used. The goal is to allow the condyle to translate with the disc permanently displaced on opening and closing. Essentially, the disc behaves as a Stage III but without crepitus. Crepitus may occur in later years.

Physical Therapy Treatment for a Stage II Disc Displacement

Unlike Stages I and III, patients with Stage II disc displacements with or without pain have functional limitations. Physical therapy objectives for a Stage II are to restore pain free functional mandibular dynamics regardless of the disc position. It is often necessary to treat concurrent TMJ inflammation, MMP and neck pain. Several treatment options are helpful:

Electric stimulation. The electric stimulation is applied over the masseter muscles. The current is intermittent (12 seconds on and 12 seconds off). The intensity should be high enough to get a contraction of the masseter muscle as long as the patient can tolerate the current. The contracting masseter loads the condyle on the posterior attachment. The posterior attachment (which is already stretched) can be further stretched by having the patient actively open or passively stretch the mouth three to four times while the current is on (Fig 8-17). Patients with joint pain seem to tolerate the active and passive stretching better during electric stimulation. The result is often an increase in mandibular opening.

Manual Intraoral Techniques. Intraoral mobilization techniques are used to successfully restore functional mandibular dynamics (Fig 8-34).[58,79,113,154,177] Distraction

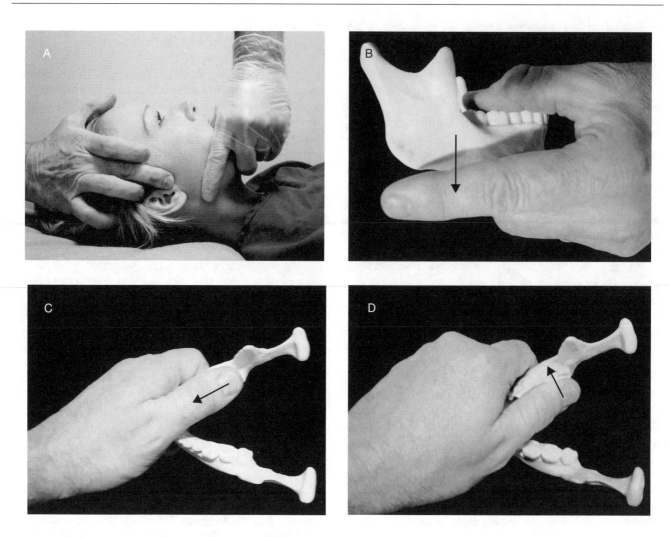

Figure 8-34: Intraoral mobilization techniques for TMJ hypomobility. A) Hand placement with the right hand stabilizing and palpating the condyle, and the left hand mobilizing; B) Distraction technique; C) Translation technique; D) Lateral glide technique.

and translation are the techniques typically used. The lateral glide mobilization also can be used but is usually more effective in the treatment of fibrous adhesions.

Home Exercise Program.   Home exercises can be very effective alone or with the other treatments described, and consist of both dynamic and static stretches.

Some recommended home exercises (Fig 8-35):

A. Finger Spread Stretch—The patient uses the thumb and finger to apply a stretch as shown. Five to ten repetitions are performed 6-8 times/day.

B. Repetitive Protrusion—The patient holds seven tongue depressors horizontally between the upper and lower central incisors. Seven tongue depressors are approximately 10 mm, which is where translation

usually begins. This position improves the patient's tolerance to repetitive protrusion. The patient performs 20-30 repetitions, 2-3 times/day.

C. Touch and Bite—Some patients lose proprioceptive awareness of mandibular lateral excursion and protrusion. The touch and bite exercise helps restore awareness and range of motion. To gain lateral excursion, the patient places a fingertip on the contralateral maxillary canine tooth. The patient is then asked to attempt to bite the index finger. The patient has to move the jaw laterally to accomplish this movement. The finger provides proprioceptive feedback of the direction the jaw is to move. To gain protrusion, the patient touches the maxillary incisors with the index finger and is instructed to attempt to bite the index

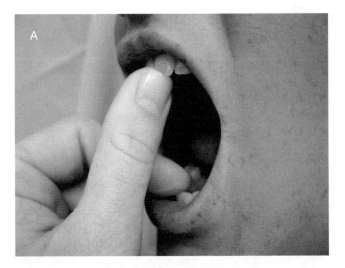
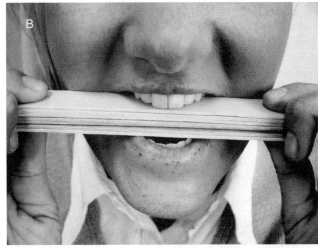
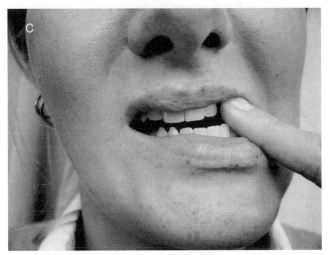
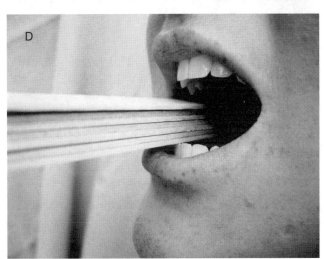

Figure 8-35: Home exercises for TMJ hypomobility. A) Passive finger spread stretch; B) Repetitive protrusion with 7-10 tongue depressors to keep the mouth opened to 10 mm; C) Touch and bite exercise to improve proprioceptive awareness for lateral excursion; D) Static stretch with tongue depressors.

finger. Five to ten repetitions are performed 6-8-times/day.

D. Static Stretch—Stacked tongue depressors are inserted between the patient's ipsilateral molars. The clinician should choose enough tongue depressors to take up the joint slack and provide a slight stretch. A static stretch should be held up to 5 minutes, 2-3 times/day.

It should be noted that increased opening achieved from physical therapy techniques may be due to elongation of the posterior attachment, which causes further anterior displacement and advanced deformation of the disc. When the disc is displaced and the condyle functions on the posterior attachment, the posterior attachment is capable of remolding and fibrosing. In effect, a pseudo-disc develops.[14] Remolding of the posterior attachment is not always successful, or may be inadequate or temporary. If physical therapy, a trial of a stabilization appliance and medication have all failed to restore function and eliminate pain, a surgical consultation is in order.

Fibrous Adhesions

Fibrous adhesions involve tightness of the TMJ capsule and/or TMJ ligament. Fibrous adhesions result from trauma or from a period of joint immobility. Immobility has been well documented to cause physiological changes in the joint capsule,[4,146] with adhesions occurring after as little as two weeks of immobility.[3]

Immobility can be caused by patient apprehension of pain, a Stage II disc displacement, intermaxillary fixation post-orthognathic surgery, trauma or arthrotomy involving a surgical incision into the joint capsule. Limited joint mobility can lead to additional problems. Adhesions can develop in the superior joint space producing decreased movement between the disc and temporal bone.[132] Limited joint mobility can contribute to an accumulation of waste products on the surfaces of the cartilage, leading to cartilage cell dystrophy and potential arthritis.[61] Finally, limited joint mobility can affect mechanoreceptor activity.

Polyarthritic disease is an uncommon cause of fibrous adhesions.[132] Polyarthritides are caused by generalized systemic polyarthritic conditions such as rheumatoid arthritis, juvenile rheumatoid arthritis, spondyloarthropathies, crystal-induced diseases and Reiter's syndrome. Each of the polyarthritides is best diagnosed via serologic tests and managed by a rheumatologist. Physical therapy management may include addressing pain and functional limitations.

Other uncommon causes of adhesions are fibrous ankylosis or bony ankylosis of the TMJ. Fibrous ankylosis is the result of significant trauma or surgery causing hemarthrosis and eventual fibrous adhesions.[10] Bony ankylosis or ossification is even less common than fibrous ankylosis. Ossification is more likely to occur when an infection has been present.[10] Bony ankylosis is often bilateral due to the etiology of infection.

History — Fibrous Adhesions

The history is often the key to identifying fibrous adhesions of the capsule. The clinician should pay particular attention to situations that can cause immobility, which include chronic pain, Stage II disc displacement, intermaxillary fixation, trauma and arthrotomy. An open incision into the joint capsule is a leading cause of fibrous adhesions.

Physical Examination — Fibrous Adhesions

Altered mandibular dynamics are seen with fibrous adhesions, and are the same as for a Stage II disc displacement (Fig 8-14). The key to differential diagnosis is the history.

Physical Therapy Treatment for Fibrous Adhesions

Treatment for fibrous adhesions is essentially the same as treatment for a Stage II disc displacement. The most important difference is how aggressive the treatments are applied and how soon translation is engaged. For example, the physical therapist should be fairly conservative in the early days post-arthrotomy that involved repairing or replacing the disc with autogeneous tissue or alloplastic material.

The physical therapist should tailor the exercises, modalities and manual procedures to a level that is acceptable for healing tissues. If there are any questions as to the arthrotomy procedure done, the physical therapist should consult with the oral surgeon to find out if there are any special precautions required. Exercises, modalities and manual procedures can be applied more aggressively post-arthrotomy for discectomy, bony ankylosis, intermaxillary fixation and total joint prosthesis.

REFERENCES

1. A De Wijer, de Leeuw JR, Michel H. Steenks, et al: Temporomandibular and Cervical Spine Disorders: Self-Reported Signs and Symptoms. Spine 21:1638-1646, 1996.
2. Abdel-Fattah RA: An Introduction to Occlusal Biomechanics in Temporomandibular Disorders. Cranio 15(4):349-350, 1997.
3. Akeson WH, Amiel D, and Woo S: Immobility Effects of Synovial Joints: The Pathomechanics of Joint Contracture. Biorheology 17:95-110, 1980.
4. Akeson WH, Amiel D, LaViolette D, et al: The Connective Tissue Response to Immobility: An Accelerated Aging Response. Exp Gerontol 3:289-301, 1968.
5. Alkofide EA, Clark E, El-Bermani W, et al: The Incidence and Nature of Fibrous Continuity Between the Sphenomandibular Ligament and the Anterior Malleolar Ligament of the Middle Ear. J Orofac Pain 11(1):7-14, 1995.
6. Assael LA: Arthrotomy for Internal Derangements. In: Temporomandibular Disorders, Diagnosis and Treatment. AS Kaplan, LA Assael eds. WB Saunders, Philadelphia 1991.
7. Atwood DA: A Review of the Fundamentals on Rest Position and Vertical Dimension. Int Dent J 9:6-19, 1959.
8. Bays RA. Surgery for Internal Derangement. In: Oral and Maxillofacial Surgery. Temporomandibular Disorders Vol 4, pp 275-300. RJ Fonseca ed.; RA Bays and PD Quinn vol eds. WB Saunders Company, Philadelphia 2000.
9. Bell WE: Classification of TM Disorders. In: The President's Conference on the Examination, Diagnosis and Management of Temporomandibular Disorders, pp 24-29. DM Laskin, W Greenfield, E Gale, et al eds. American Dental Association, Chicago 1982.
10. Bell WE: Temporomandibular Disorders; Classification, Diagnosis and Management, 3rd ed. Year Book Medical Publishers, Inc, Chicago 1990.
11. Benoit PW and Razook SJ: TMJ Imaging. In: Clinics in Physical Therapy; Temporomandibular Disorders, 2nd ed, pp 115-124. SL Kraus, ed. Churchill Livingstone, New York

1994.

12. Bertilsson O and Strom D: A Literature Survey of a Hundred Years of Anatomic and Functional Lateral Pterygoid Muscle Research. J Orofac Pain 9(1):17-23, 1995.

13. Blaustein DI and Heffez LB: Arthroscopic Atlas of the Temporomandibular Joint. Lea and Febiger, Philadelphia 1990.

14. Blaustein DI, and Scapino RP: Remolding of the Temporomandibular Joint Disc and Posterior Attachment in Disc Displacement Specimens in Relation to Glycosaminoglycan Content. Plast Reconstr Surg 79:756-764, 1986.

15. Bogduk N: Cervical Causes of Headache and Dizziness. In: Modern Manual Therapy, pp 289-302. G Grieve, ed. Churchill Livingstone, Edinburgh 1986.

16. Boyd JP, Shankland W, Brown C, et al: Taming the Muscular Forces That Threaten Everyday Dentistry. Postgraduate Dentistry, Nov 2000.

17. Boyd RL, Gibbs CH, Mahan PE, et al: Temporomandibular Joint Forces Measured at the Condyle of Macaca Arctoides. Am J Orthod Dentofac Orthop 97:472-479, 1990.

18. Braun BL, DiGiovanna A, Schiffman E, et al: A Cross-Sectional Study of Temporomandibular Joint Dysfunction in Post-Cervical Trauma Patients. J Orofac Pain 6(1):24-31, 1992.

19. Brenman HS, and Amsterdam, M: Postural Effects on Occlusion. Dental Progress 4:43–47, 1963.

20. Brooks SL, Brand JW and Gibbs SJ, et al: Imaging of the Temporomandibular Joint: A Position Paper of the American Academy of Oral and Maxillofacial Radiology. Oral Surg Oral Med Oral Pathol Oral Radiol Endod 83:609-618, 1997.

21. Burch JG: Activity of the Accessory Ligaments of the Temporomandibular Joint. J Prosthet Dent 24:621-628, 1970.

22. Carlson, CR, Okeson JP, Falace DA et al: Comparison of Psychologic and Physiologic Functioning Between Patients With Masticatory Muscle Pain and Matched Controls. J Orofac Pain 7(1):15-22, 1993.

23. Chen Y-S, Gaallo LM and Meier D, et al: Dynamic Magnetic Resonance Imaging Technique For the Study of the Temporomandibular Joint. J Orofac Pain 14(1):65-73, 2000.

24. Cholitgul W, et al. Clinical and Radiological Findings in Temporomandibular Joints With Disc Perforations. Int J Oral Maxillofac Surg 19:220-225, 1990.

25. Ciancaglini R, Testa M and Radaelli G: Association of Neck Pain With Symptoms of Temporomandibular Dysfunction in the General Adult Population. Scand J Rehab Med 31: 17-22, 1999.

26. Clark GT, and Mulligan RA. A Review of the Prevalance of Temporomandibular Dysfunction. J Gerodontaol 3:231, 1986.

27. Clark GT, Green EM, Doman MR, et al: Craniocervical Dysfunction Levels in a Patient Sample From a Temporomandibular Joint Clinic. J Am Dent Assoc 115: 251-256, 1987.

28. Clark GT, Moody DG, and Saunders B: Arthroscopic Treatment of Temporomandibular Joint Locking Resulting From Disc Derangement: Two-year Results. J Oral Maxillofac Surg 49:157-164, 1991.

29. Clark GT, Seligman DA, Solberg WK, et al: Guidelines for the Examination and Diagnosis of Temporomandibular

Disorders. J Orofac Pain 3(1):7-14, 1989.

30. Clark GT, Seligman DA, Solberg WK, et al: Guidelines for the Treatment of Temporomandibular Disorders. J Orofac Pain 4(2):80-88, 1990.

31. Clark GT: A Critical Evaluation of Orthopedic Interocclusal Appliance Therapy: Design, Theory, and Overall Effectiveness. J Am Dent Assoc 108:359-368, 1984.

32. Clark GTL Occlusal Therapy: Occlusal Appliances. In: The President's Conference on the Examination, Diagnosis and Management of Temporomandibular Disorders, pp 137-146. DM Laskin, W Greenfield, E Gale, et al eds. American Dental Association, Chicago 1982.

33. Clark RF and Wyke BD: Contributions of Temporomandibular Articular Mechanoreceptors to the Control of Mandibular Posture: An Experimental Study. J Dent 2:121-129, 1974.

34. Copray JC, Dibbets JM and Kantomaa T: The Role of Condylar Cartilage in the Development of the Temporomandibular Joint. Angle Orthod 58: 369, 1988.

35. Daly P: Postural Response of the Head to Bite Opening in Adult Male. Am J Orthod 82:157-160, 1982.

36. Dawson P: Evaluation, Diagnosis, and Treatment of Occlusal Problems, 2nd ed. Mosby, St Louis 1989.

37. Kronn S: The Incidence of TMJ Dysfunction in Patients Who Have Suffered a Cervical Whiplash Injury Following a Traffic Accident. J Orofac Pain 7(2):209-213, 1993.

38. De Laat, Meuleman H, Stevens A, et al: Correlation Between Cervical Spine and Temporomandibular Disorders. Clinical Oral Invest 2:54-57, 1998.

39. de Wijer A, Lobbezoo-Scholte AM, Steenks MH, et al: Reliability of Clinical Findings in Temporomandibular Disorders. J Orofac Pain 9(2):181-190, 1995.

40. De Wijer A: Temporomandibular and Cervical Spine Disorders. (Thesis) Utrecht University (Dissertation). Utrecht, The Netherlands, Elinkwijk BV 1995.

41. DeBont LGB, Boering G, Liem RSB, et al: Osteoarthritis and Internal Derangement of the Temporomandibular Joint: A Light Microscopic Study. J Oral Maxillofac Surg 44:634-643, 1986.

42. deBont LGM, Dijkeraaf LC, and Stegenga B: Epidemiology and Natural Progression of Articular Temporomandibular Disorders. Oral Surg Oral Med Oral Pathol Oral Radiol Endod 83: 72-76, 1997.

43. DeLeeuw JRJ, Steenks MH, Ros WJG, et al: Psychosocial Aspects and Symptom Characteristics of Craniomandibular Dysfunction. The Assessment of Clinical and Community Findings. J Oral Rehabil 21:127-143, 1994.

44. Dijkstra PU, de Bont LGM, Leeuw R, et al. Temporomandibular Joint Osteoarthrosis and Temporomandibular Joint Hypermobility. J Craniomandibular Pract 11(4):268-275, 1993.

45. Dijkstra PU, de Bont LGM, Stegenga B, et al: Temporomandibular Joint Osteoarthrosis and Generalized Joint Hypermobility. J Craniomandibular Pract 10(3):221-227, 1992.

46. Dijkstra PU, de Bont LGM, van der Weele LT, et al: The Relationship Between Temporomandibular Joint Mobility and Peripheral Joint Mobility Reconsidered. J Craniomandibular Pract 12:149-154, 1994.

47. Dodson TB: Epidemiology of Temporomandibular Disorders. In: Oral and Maxillofacial Surgery.

Temporomandibular Disorders Vol 4, pp 93-107. RJ Fonseca ed.; RA Bays and PD Quinn vol eds. WB Saunders Company, Philadelphia 2000.

48. Dolwick MF: Diagnosis and Etiology of Internal Derangements of the Temporomandibular Joint. In: The President's Conference on the Examination, Diagnosis and Management of Temporomandibular Disorders, pp 112-117. DM Laskin, W Greenfield, E Gale, et al eds. American Dental Association, Chicago 1982.

49. Dworkin S and LeResche L, eds: Research Diagnostic Criteria for Temporomandibular Disorders: Review, Criteria, Examination and Specifications, Critique. J Orofac Pain 6(4):301-355, 1992.

50. Dworkin SF, Huggins KH, Wilson L, et al: A Randomized Clinical Trial Using Research Diagnostic Criteria for Temporomandibular Disorders—Axis II to Target Clinic Cases for a Tailored Self-Care TMD Treatment Program. J Orofac Pain 16(1):48-63, 2002.

51. Dworkin SF, LeResche L, DeRouen T, and Korff M: Assessing Clinical Signs of Temporomandibular Disorders: Reliability of Clinical Examiners. J Prosthet Dent 63: 574-580, 1990.

52. Eberle WR: A Study of Centric Relation as Recorded in a Supine Position. J Am Dent Assoc 42:15, 1951.

53. Eggleton TM and Langton DP: Clinical Anatomy of the TMJ Complex. In: Clinics in Physical Therapy; Temporomandibular Disorders, 2nd ed, pp 1-40. SL Kraus, ed. Churchill Livingstone, New York 1994.

54. Eriksson L and Westesson PL: Clinical and Radiological Study of Patients With Anterior Disc Displacement of the Temporomandibular Joint. Swed Dent J 7:55, 1983.

55. Eriksson L and Westesson PL: Clinical and Radiological Study of Patients With Anterior Disc Displacement of the Temporomandibular Joint. Swed Dent J 7:55-64, 1983.

56. Esposito C, Clear M, and Veal S: Arthroscopic Surgical Treatment of Temporomandibular Joint Hypermobility With Recurrent Anterior Dislocation: An Alternative to Open Surgery. J Craniomandib Pract 9(3):286-292, 1991.

57. Farrar WB and McCarty WL: Inferior Joint Space Arthrography and Characteristics of the Condylar Path in Internal Derangements of the TMJ. J Prosthet Dent 41:548-555, 1979.

58. Friedman MH: Closed Lock. A Survey of 400 Cases. Oral Surg Oral Med Oral Pathol 75:422-427, 1993.

59. Fukushima S: Function of Temporomandibular Joint During Habitual Opening and Closing Movements. J Jpn Prosthodont Soc 15: 267-290, 1971.

60. Gelb H and Tarte J: A Two-year Clinical Evaluation of 200 Cases of Chronic Headache: The Craniocervical-Mandibular Syndrome. J Am Dent Assoc 91:1230-1236, 1975.

61. Glineburg RW, Laskin DM, and Blaustein DI. The Effects of Immobilization on the Primate Temporomandibular Joint: A Histologic and Histochemical Study. J Oral Maxillofacial Surgery 40:3-8, 1982.

62. Goldstein DF, Kraus SL, Williams WB, et al: Influence of Cervical Posture on Mandibular Movement. J Prosthet Dent 52:421–426, 1984.

63. Goulet JP and Clark GT: Clinical TMJ Examination Methods. CDA Journal 18(3):25-33, 1990.

64. Greene CS, Turner C, and Laskin DM: Long-term Outcome of TMJ Clicking in 100 MPD Patients. J Dent Res 61:218,

1982.

65. Greene CS: Can Technology Enhance TM Disorder Diagnosis? CDA Journal 18(3):21-24, 1990.

66. Greene CS: The Etiology of Temporomandibular Disorders: Implications for Treatment. J Orofac Pain 15(2): 93-105, 2001.

67. Headache Classification Committee of the International Headache Society. Classification and Diagnostic Criteria for Headache Disorders, Cranial Neuralgias and Facial Pain. Cephalalgia: An International Journal of Headache 8(Suppl 7):9-93, 1988.

68. Helms CA and Kaplan P: Diagnostic Imaging of the Temporomandibular Joint: Recommendations for Use of the Various Techniques. AM J Roentgenol 154:319-326, 1990.

69. Hesse JR and Hansson T: Factors Influencing Joint Mobility in General and in Particular Respect of the Craniomandibular Articulation: A Literature Review.J Orofac Pain 2(1): 19-28, 1988.

70. Hesse JR, Naejie M: Biomechanics of the TMJ. In: Clinics in Physical Therapy; Temporomandibular Disorders, 2nd ed, pp 41-69. SL Kraus ed. Churchill Livingstone, New York 1944.

71. Hochstedler JL, Allen BA and Follmar MA: Temporomandibular Joint Range of Motion: A Ratio of Interincisal Opening to Excursive Movement in a Healthy Population. J Craniomandibular Pract 14(4):296-300, 1996.

72. Holmlund AB: Arthroscopy.In: Oral and Maxillofacial Surgery. Temporomandibular Disorders Vol 4, pp 255-274. RJ Fonseca ed.; RA Bays and PD Quinn vol eds. WB Saunders Company, Philadelphia 2000.

73. Hylander WL: An Experimental Analysis of Temporomandibular Joint Reaction Force in Macaques. Am J Phys Anthropol 51:433-456, 1979.

74. Ide Y and Nakazawa K: Anatomical Atlas of the Temporomandibular Joint. Quintessence Publishing Co, Tokyo 1991.

75. Irby WB and Zetz MR: Osteoarthritis and Rheumatoid Arthritis Affecting the Temporomandibular Joint. In: The President's Conference on the Examination, Diagnosis and Management of Temporomandibular Disorders, pp 106-111. DM Laskin, W Greenfield, E Gale, et al eds. American Dental Association, Chicago 1982.

76. Isaccsson G, Linde C and Isberg A: Subjective Symptoms in Patients With Temporomandibular Joint Disc Displacement Versus Patients With Myogenic Craniomandibular Disorders. J Prosthet Dent 61:70-77, 1989.

77. Isberg A, Stenstrom B and Isacsson G: Frequency of Joint Bilateral Joint Disc Displacement in Patients With Unilateral Symptoms: A 5-year Follow-Up Of the Asymptomatic Joint. Dentomaxillofac Radiol 20:73-76, 1991.

78. Ito T, Gibbs CH, Marguelles-Bonnet R, et al: Loading on the Temporomandibular Joint With Five Occlusal Conditions. J Prosthet Dent 56(4):478-484, 1986.

79. Jagger RG: Mandibular Manipulation of Anterior Disc Displacement Without Reduction. J Oral Rehab 18:497-500, 1991.

80. Jankelson B: The Myo-Monitor: Its Use and Abuse. Quint Int 2:47, 1978.

81. Jee W: The Skeletal Tissues. In: Histology, Cell and Tissue Biology. L Weiss ed. Elsevier Biomedical Publishers, New York 1988.

82. Kerr FW: Mechanism, Diagnosis and Management of Some

Cranial and Facial Pain Syndromes. Surg Clin N Am 43:951-961, 1963.

83. Kircos LT, Ortendahl DA, Mark AS, et al: Magnetic Resonance Imaging of the TMJ Disc in Asymptomatic Volunteers. J Oral Maxillofac Surg 45:852-854, 1987.

84. Kirveskari P, Alanen P, Karskela V, et al: Association of Functional State of Stomatognathic System With Mobility of Cervical Spine and Neck Muscle Tenderness. Acta Odont Scand 46:281-286, 1988.

85. Klineberg I: Influences of Temporomandibular Articular Mechanoreceptors on Functional Jaw Movements. J Oral Rehabil 7:307-317, 1980.

86. Klineberg IJ, Greenfield BE and Wyke BD: Contributions to the Reflex Control of Mastication From Mechanoreceptors in the Temporomandibular Joint Capsule. Dent Pract 21:73-83, 1970.

87. Kraus SL: Physical Therapy Management of Temporomandibular Disorders. In: Oral and Maxillofacial Surgery. Temporomandibular Disorders Vol 4, pp 161-193. RJ Fonseca ed.; RA Bays and PD Quinn vol eds. WB Saunders Company, Philadelphia 2000.

88. Laskin DM: Etiology and Pathogenesis of Internal Derangements of the Temporomandibular Joint. In: Oral and Maxillofacial Surgery Clinics of North America: Current Controversies in Surgery for Internal Derangements of the Temporomandibular Joint. pp 217-222. DM Laskin, ed. WB Saunders, Philadelphia 1994.

89. Laskin DM: Etiology of the Pain-Dysfunction Syndrome. J Am Dent Assoc 79:147-153, 1969.

90. Lawrence ES, and Razook SJ: Nonsurgical Management of Mandibular Disorders. In: Clinics in Physical Therapy, Temporomandibular Disorders, 2nd Ed, p 161. SL Kraus, ed. Churchill Livingstone, New York 1994.

91. Lerman M: The Hydrostatic Appliance: A New Approach to Treatment of the TMJ Pain Dysfunction Syndrome. J Am Dent Assoc 89:1343-1350, 1974.

92. Lipp MJ: Temporomandibular Symptoms and Occlusion: A Review of the Literature and the Concept. NY State J Dent 56(9):58-64, 1990.

93. Lobbezoo F and Lavigne GJ: Do Bruxism and Temporomandibular Disorders Have a Cause-Effect Relationship? J Orofac Pain 11(1):15-23, 1997.

94. Lobbezoo-Scholte AM, Leeuw De JRJ, Steenks MH, et al: Diagnostic Subgroups of Craniomandibular Disorders. Part 1: Self-Report Data and Clinical Findings. J Orofac Pain 9(1):24-36, 1995.

95. Lous J: Treatment of TMJ Syndrome by Pivots. J Prosth Dent 40:(2)179-182, 1978.

96. Lowe AA: Tongue Movements—Brainstem Mechanics and Clinical Postulates. Brain Behavior 25:128-137, 1984.

97. Lund JP: Pain and the Control of Muscles. Adv Pain Res Therapy 21:103-115, 1995.

98. Lund P, Nishiyama T and Moller E: Postural Activity in the Muscles of Mastication With the Subject Upright, Inclined, and Supine. Scand J of Dent Res 78:417-424, 1970.

99. Lundh H, Westesson PL, Kopp S, et al: Anterior Repositioning Splint in the Treatment of Temporomandibular Joints With Reciprocal Clicking: Comparison With a Flat Occlusal Splint and an Untreated Control Group. Oral Surg Oral Med Oral Pathol 60:131-136, 1985.

100. MacConaill MA: Studies in the Mechanics Of Synovial Joints. Ir J Med Sc 6:223, 1946.

101. MacConaill MA: The Movements of Bones and Joints. JBJS [Br] 35:290, 1953.

102. Mahan PA, Wilkinson TM, Gibbs CH, et al: Superior and Inferior Bellies of the Lateral Pterygoid Muscle EMG Activity at Basic Jaw Positions. J Prosthet Dent 50:710-718, 1983.

103. Mahan PE: The Temporomandibular Joint in Function and Pathofunction. In: Temporomandibular Joint Problems. WK Solberg and GT Clark eds. Quintessence Publishing Co, Lombard, IL 1980.

104. Major PW and Nebbe B: Use and Effectiveness of Splint Appliance Therapy: Review of Literature. J Craniomandib Pract 15(2):159-166, 1997.

105. Mclean LW, Brenman HS, Friedman MGF: Effects of Changing Body Position on Dental Occlusion. J Dent Res 52:1041–1045, 1973.

106. McNamara JA Jr, Seligman DA and Okeson JP: The Relationship of Occlusal Factors and Orthodontic Treatment To Temporomandibular Disorders. In: Temporomandibular Disorders and Related Pain Conditions, pp 399-427. BJ Sessle, PS Bryant, and RA Dionne eds. IASP Press, Seattle 1995.

107. McNamara JA, Jr: The Independent Functions of the Two Heads of the Lateral Pterygoid Muscle. Am J Anat 138:197-206, 1973.

108. McNamara JA, Seligman DA and Okeson JP: Occlusion, Orthodontic Treatment, and Temporomandibular Disorders: A Review. J Orofac Pain 9(1):73-115, 1995.

109. McNeill C, Danzig WM, Farrar WB, et al. Craniomandibular (TMJ) Disorders—The State of Art. Position Paper of the American Academy of Craniomandibular Disorders. J Prosthet Dent 44: 434-437, 1980.

110. Mennell J: Joint Pain. Little Brown and Company, Boston 1964.

111. Milam SB: Pathophysiology of Articular Disk Displacement of the Temporomandibular Joint. In: Oral and Maxillofacial Surgery. Temporomandibular Disorders Vol 4, pp 46-72. RJ Fonseca ed.; RA Bays and PD Quinn vol eds. WB Saunders Company, Philadelphia 2000.

112. Mills D, Fiandaca D, and Scapino R: Morphologic, Microscopic, and Immunohistochemical Investigations Into the Function of the Primate TMJ Disc. J Orofac Pain 8(2):136-154, 1994.

113. Minagi S, Nozaki S, Sato T, et al: Manipulation Techniques for Treatment of Anterior Disk Displacement Without Reduction. J Prosthet Dent 65:686-691, 1991.

114. Minarelli A, Del Santo M, and Liberti E: The Structure of the Human Temporomandibular Joint Disc: A Scanning Electron Microscopy Study. J Orofac Pain 11(2):95-100, 1997.

115. Moffett BC. Definitions of Temporomandibular Joint Derangements. In: Diagnosis of Internal Derangements of the Temporomandibular Joint, Vol 1. Double-Contrast Arthrography and Clinical Considerations. BC Moffett and PL Westesson eds. Proceedings of a Continuing Dental Education Symposium, Seattle 1984.

116. Mohl N: Head Posture and Its Role in Occlusion. NY State Dent J 42:17-23, 1976.

117. Mohl ND and Dixon DC: Current Status of Diagnostic Procedures for Temporomandibular Disorders. J Am Dent

Assoc, 125:56-64, 1994.

118. Mohl ND: Functional Anatomy of the Temporomandibular Joint. In: The President's Conference on the Examination, Diagnosis and Management of Temporomandibular Disorders, pp 3-12. DM Laskin, W Greenfield, E Gale, et al, eds. American Dental Association, Chicago 1982.

119. Mohl ND: The Anecdotal Tradition and the Need for Evidence-Based Care for Temporomandibular Disorders. J Orofac Pain 13(4)227-231, 1999.

120. Mohl ND: The Temporomandibular Joint. In: Textbook of Occlusion. ND Mohl, GA Zarb, GE Carlsson, et al eds. Pp 81-96, Quintessence Publishing Company, Chicago 1988.

121. Molina OF, Santos JD, Mazzetto M, et al: Oral Jaw Behavior in TMD and Bruxism: A Comparison Study by Severity of Bruxism. J Craniomandib Pract 19(2):114-122, 2001.

122. Moloney F and Howard JA: Internal Derangements of the Temporomandibular Joint III. Anterior Repositioning Splint Therapy. Aust Dent J 31:30-39, 1986.

123. Montgomery MT, Gordon SM, Van Sickels JE, et al: Changes in Signs and Symptoms Following Temporomandibular Joint Disc Repositioning Surgery. J Oral Maxillofac Surg 50:320-328, 1992.

124. Montgomery MT, Van Sickels JE, Harms SE. Success of Temporomandibular Joint Arthroscopy in Disk Displacement With and Without Reduction. Oral Surg Oral Med Oral Pathol 71:651-659, 1991.

125. Morani V, Previgliano V and Schierano G: Innervation of the Human Temporomandibular Joint Capsule and Disc as Revealed by Immunohistochemistry for Neurospecific Markers. J Orofac Pain 8(1):36-41, 1994.

126. Murakami KI, Segami N, Fujimura K, et al: Correlation Between Pain and Synovitis in Patients With Internal Derangement of the Temporomandibular Joint. J Oral Maxillofac Surg 49:1159-1161, 1991.

127. Naeije M, and Hansson TL: Electromyographic Screening of Myogenous and Arthrogenous TMJ Dysfunction Patients. J Oral Rehabil 13:433-441, 1986.

128. Nassif NJ and Talic YF: Classic Symptoms in Temporomandibular Disorder Patients: A Comparative Study. J Craniomandibular Pract 19(1):33-41, 2001.

129. National Institutes of Health Technology Assessment Conference On Management of Temporomandibular Disorders. pp 15-120. Judith Albino, Chairperson. Bethesda, Maryland, April 29 - May 1, 1996.

130. Nicolakis P, Nicolakis M, Piehslinger E, et al: Relationship Between Craniomandibular Disorders and Poor Posture. J Craniomandibular Pract 18(2):106-112, 2000.

131. Nitzan DW, Dolwick MF and Heft MW: Arthroscopic Lavage and Lysis of the Temporomandibular Joint: A Change In Perspective. J Oral Maxillofac Surg 48:798-801, 1990.

132. Okeson JP ed. Orofacial Pain: Guidelines for Assessment, Diagnosis, and Management. Quintessence Publishing Co, Chicago 1996.

133. Okeson JP: The Management of Temporomandibular Disorders and Occlusion. 3rd ed. Mosby, St. Louis 1993.

134. Orenstein ES: Anterior Repositioning Appliances When Used for Anterior Disk Displacement With Reduction — A Critical Review. J Craniomandibular Pract 11(2):141-145, 1993.

135. Padamsee M, Mehtan N, Forgione A, et al: Incidence of

Cervical Disorders in a TMD Population (IADR; Abstract No. 680). J Dent Res 73 1994.

136. Perrott DH, Alborzi A, Kaban LB, et al: A Prospective Evaluation of the Effectiveness of Temporomandibular Joint Arthroscopy. J Oral Maxillofac Surg 48:1029-1032, 1990.

137. Pertes R and Attanasio R: Internal Derangements. In: Temporomandibular Disorders, Diagnosis and Treatment, pp 142-164. AS Kaplan and LA Assael eds. WB Saunders Company, Philadelphia 1991.

138. Pharoah M: The Prescription of Diagnostic Images for Temporomandibular Joint Disorders. J Orofac Pain 13(4): 251-254, 1999.

139. Pinto OF: A New Structure and Function of the Mandibular Joint. J Prosthet Dent 12:95-103, 1962.

140. Pruim GJ, de Jongh HJ and Ten Bosch JJ: Forces Acting on the Mandible During Bilateral Static Bite at Different Bite Force Levels. J Biomech 13:755, 1980.

141. Rees LA: The Structure and Function of the Mandibular Joint. Br Dent J 96:125, 1954.

142. Ribeiro RF, Tallents RH, Katzberg RW, et al: The Prevalence of Disc Displacement in Symptomatic and Asymptomatic Volunteers Aged 6-25 Years. J Orofac Pain 11(1):37-47, 1997.

143. Root GR, Kraus SL, Razook SJ, et al: Effect of an Intraoral Appliance on Head and Neck Posture. J Prosthet Dent 58:90-95, 1987.

144. Rosenbaum RS, ed. Orofacial Pain Guidelines for Assessment, Diagnosis, and Management, 4th ed. Quintessence Publishing. Chicago 2004.

145. Rothstein JM: Measurement and Clinical Practice: Theory and Application. In: Measurements in Physical Therapy, pp 1-46. J Rothstein ed. Churchill Livingstone, New York 1985.

146. Salter RB, Hamilton WH, Wedge JH, et al: Clinical Applications of Basic Research on Continuous Passive Motion for Disorders and Injuries of Synovial Joints, a Preliminary Report of a Feasibility Study. J Orthop Res 3:325-342, 1983.

147. Sanders B and Buonocristiani R. Temporomandibular Joint Arthrotomy, Management of Failed Cases. Oral and Maxillofac Surgery Clinics of North America 1:443, 1989.

148. Santander H, Miralles R, Perex J, et al: Effects of Head and Neck Inclination on Bilateral Sternocleidomastoid EMG Activity in Healthy Subjects and in Patients With Myogenic Cranio-Cervical- Mandibular Dysfunction. J Craniomandibular Pract 18(3):181-191, 2000.

149. Sato H, Strom D and Carlsson G: Controversies on Anatomy and Function of the Ligaments Associated with the Temporomandibular Joint: A Literature Survey. J Orofac Pain 9(4):308-316, 1995.

150. Sato S, Goto S, Kawamura H, et al: The Natural Course of Nonreducing Disc Displacements of the TMJ: Relationship of Clinical Findings at Initial Visit to Outcome After 12 Months Without Treatment. J Orofac Pain 11(4):315-320, 1997.

151. Scapino R: The Posterior Attachment: Its Structure, Function and Appearance in TMJ Imaging Studies. Part 1: J Orofac Pain 5(2):83-94, 1991.

152. Scapino R: The Posterior Attachment: Its Structure, Function and Appearance in TMJ Imaging Studies. Part 2: J Orofac Pain 5(3):155-166, 1991.

153. Schiffman EL, Fricton JR, Haley DP, et al: The Prevalence and Treatment Needs of Subjects With Temporomandibular

Disorders. J Am Dent Assoc 120:295-303, 1999.

154. Segami N, Murakami KI, and Iizuka T: Arthrographic Evaluation of Disk Position Following Mandibular Manipulation Technique for Internal Derangement With Closed Lock of the Temporomandibular Joint. J Orofac Pain 4(2):99-108, 1990.

155. Seligman DA and Pullinger AG: The Role of Intercuspal Occlusal Relationships in Temporomandibular Disorders: A Review. J Orofac Pain 5(2):96-106, 1991.

156. Sharawy M: Developmental and Clinical Anatomy and Physiology of the Temporomandibular Joint. In: Oral and Maxillofacial Surgery. Temporomandibular Disorders Vol 4, pp 1-19. RJ Fonseca ed.; RA Bays and PD Quinn vol eds. WB Saunders Company, Philadelphia 2000.

157. Sheppard SM: Asymptomatic Morphologic Variations in the Mandibular Condyle-Ramus Region. J Prosthet Dent 46:539-544, 1982.

158. Simons DG, and Mense S: Understanding and Measurement of Muscle Tone as Related to Clinical Muscle Pain. Pain 75:1-17, 1998.

159. Sollecito T: Role of Splint Therapy in Treatment of Temporomandibular Disorders. In: Oral and Maxillofacial Surgery. Temporomandibular Disorders Vol 4, pp 145-160. RJ Fonseca ed.; RA Bays and PD Quinn vol eds. WB Saunders Company, Philadelphia 2000.

160. Spitzer WO, Skovron ML, Salmi LR, et al. Scientific Monograph of the Quebec Task Force on Whiplash-Associated Disorders: Redefining "Whiplash" and its Management. Spine 20(8 Suppl) p1S-73S, 1995.

161. Spruijt RJ and Hoogstraten J: Symptom Reporting in Temporomandibular Joint Clicking: Some Theoretical Considerations. J Orofac Pain 6(3):213-218, 1992.

162. Spruijt RJ and Hoogstraten J: The Research on Temporomandibular Joint Clicking: A Methodological Review. J Orofac Pain 5(1) 45-50, 1991.

163. Stohler CS, Zhang X and Lund JP: The Effect of Experimental Jaw Muscle Pain on Postural Muscle Activity. Pain 66:215-221, 1996.

164. Stohler CS: Muscle-Related Temporomandibular Disorders. J Orofac Pain 13(4):273-284, 1999.

165. Summer JD, Westesson PL: Mandibular Repositioning Can Be Effective in Treatment of Reducing TMJ Disk Displacement. A Long Term Clinical and MR Imaging Follow-up. J Craniomandibular Pract 15(2):107-120, 1997.

166. Svensson P and Graven-Nielson T: Craniofacial Muscle Pain: Review of Mechanisms and Clinical Manifestations. J Orofac Pain 15(2):117-145, 2001.

167. Szentpetery A: Clinical Uility of Mandibular Movement Ranges. J Orofac Pain 7(2):163-168, 1993.

168. Tallents RH, Stein SI and Moss ME: The Role of Occlusion in Temporomandibular Disorders. In: Oral and Maxillofacial Surgery. Temporomandibular Disorders Vol 4, pp 194-297. RJ Fonseca ed.; RA Bays and PD Quinn vol eds. WB Saunders Company, Philadelphia 2000.

169. Tennenbaum HC, Freeman BV, Psutka DJ, et al: Temporomandibular Disorders: Disc Displacements. J Orofac Pain 13(4):285-289, 1999.

170. Thilander B: Innervation of the Temporomandibular Disc in Man. Acta Odontol Scand 22:151, 1964.

171. Thilander B: Innervation of the Temporomandibular Joint Capsule in Man. No 7, Transactions of the Royal Schools of Dentistry. Stockholm-Umea, 1961.

172. Travell J, Rinzler S and Herman M: Pain and Disability of the Shoulder and Arm.Treatment by Intramuscular Infiltration With Procaine Hydrochloride. JAMA 120:417-422, 1942.

173. Trumpy I, Erickson J and Lyberg T: Internal Derangement of the Temporomandibular Joint: Correlation of Arthrographic Imaging With Surgical Findings. Int J Oral Maxillofac Surg 26:327-330, 1997.

174. Turell J, and Ruiz G: Normal and Abnormal Findings in Temporomandibular Joints in Autopsy Specimens. J Orofacial Pain 1(4):257-275, 1987.

175. Turell J, and Ruiz HG: Normal and Abnormal Findings in Temporomandibular Joints in Autopsy Specimens. J Orofac Pain 1(4):257-275, 1987.

176. Turp JC, Alt KW, Vach WV, et al: Mandibular Condyles and Rami are Asymmetric Structures. J Craniomandibular Pract 16(1):51-56, 1998.

177. Van Dyke AR, and Goldman SM: Manual Reduction of Displaced Disk. J Craniomandibular Pract 8(4):350-352, 1990.

178. Visscher CM, et al: Cervical Spinal Pain in Chronic Craniomandibular Pain Patients. Thesis prepared at the Department of Oral Function, Section CMD of the Academic Center for Dentistry Amsterdam (ACTA), the combined Faculty of Dentistry of the University of Amsterdam and the Vriji Universiteit, the Netherlands, 2000.

179. Watson T: The Role of Electrotherapy in Contemporary Physiotherapy Practice. Manual Therapy 5(3):132-141, 2000.

180. Watt-Smith S, Sadler A, Baddeley H, et al: Comparison of Arthrotomographic and Magnetic Resonance Images of 50 Temporomandibular Joints With Operative Findings. Br J Oral Maxillofac Surg 31:139-143, 1993.

181. Weinberg L: Treatment Prosthesis in TMJ Dysfunction-Pain Syndrome. J Prosth Dent 39(6):654-669, 1978.

182. Westesson PL, and Rohlin M: Internal Derangement Related to Osteoarthritis in Temporomandibular Joint Autopsy Specimens. Oral Surg Oral Med Oral Pathol 57:17-22, 1984.

183. Westesson PL, Bronstein SL and Liedberg J. Internal Derangement of the Temporomandibular Joint: Morphologic Description With Correlation to Joint Function. Oral Surg Oral Med Oral Pathol 59:323, 1985.

184. Westesson PL, Eriksson L, and Kurita K: Reliability of a Negative Clinical Temporomandibular Joint Examination: Prevalence of Disk Displacement in Asymptomatic Temporomandibular Joints. Oral Surg Oral Med Oral Pathol 68:551-554, 1989.

185. Widmer C, Lund J and Feine J: Evaluation of Diagnostic Tests for TMD. CDA Journal 18(3):53-60, 1990.

186. Widmer C: Evaluation of Diagnostic Test for TMD. In: Clinics in Physical Therapy; Temporomandibular Disorders, 2nd ed, pp 99-114, SL Kraus, ed. Churchill Livingstone, New York 1994.

187. Wilkes C: Internal Derangements of the Temporomandibular Joint: Pathological Variations. Arch Otolaryngol Head Neck Surg 115:469-477, 1989.

188. Williamson EH, and Rosenzweig. The Treatment of Temporomandibular Disorders Through Repositioning Splint Therapy: A Follow-up Study. J Craniomandibular Pract 16(4):222-225, 1998.

189. Wong GV, Weinberg S and Symingen JM: Morphology of

the Developing Articular Disc of the Human Temporomandibular Joint. J Oral Maxillofac Surg 43:565-569, 1985.

190. Yale SH, Allison BD and Hauptfuehrer JD: An Epidemiological Assessment of Mandibular Condyle Morphology. Oral Surg, 21:169, 1966.

191. Zamburlini I, and Austin D: Long-term Results of Appliance Therapies in Anterior Disk Displacement With Reduction: A Review of the Literature. J Craniomandibular Pract 9(4):361-367, 1991.

ACKNOWLEDGEMENTS

To my wife, Pattie, for her love, understanding and patient support; to my daughter Emily Jane, who gives me such joy and happiness; and to my parents, Dottie and Kenneth L. Kraus, my inspiration.

9

CERVICOGENIC HEADACHE

David Groom, GDMT PT

Section One—Differential Diagnosis of Headaches

Headache affects a large proportion of the population. Predominantly benign in nature, headache may nonetheless be the presenting complaint of catastrophic illness such as brain tumor, cerebral hemorrhage or meningitis. Chronic headache, although benign, can be severely disabling and can lead to chronic pain syndromes, psychological disorders and social withdrawal.

Knowledge of the pathophysiology of various headache types has advanced significantly in recent years, but there is still much that is unknown or speculative. Management regimens, both pharmacological and non-pharmacological, have advanced considerably, leading to improved outcomes for headache sufferers.

As headache research continues on many frontiers, it is crucial that clinicians managing headache patients have a thorough understanding of the currently available data.

Understanding the anatomy and physiology of head pain and pain modulator mechanisms helps clinicians in differential diagnosis and therapeutic endeavors. The International Headache Society[16] (IHS) lists a multitude of diagnostic categories for headache. Classifications are numerous, ranging from migraines and tension-type headaches to cervicogenic headaches and headaches related to infection and psychiatric disorders.

Despite the number of different headache classifications, it is important to realize that all headaches have something in common—namely, "pain in the head". When reviewing the anatomy and physiology of headache, a degree of commonality becomes apparent.

Anatomy of Headache

The trigeminal (5th) cranial nerve has its nucleus extend caudally through the pons, medulla and spinal cord down to the C2 spinal level and sometimes as far as C4.[3,17,47] Nociceptive afferents from this nerve, accompanied by somatic afferents from the facial (7th), glossopharyngeal (9th) and vagus (10th) cranial nerves descend in the grey matter of the nucleus to intersect with the grey matter of the upper three cervical segments.[21] This area of intersection of grey matter from the 5th, 7th, 9th and 10th cranial nerves and the upper cervical segments is the trigeminocervical nucleus (TCN).[5] It is the anatomical region through which all head pain is directed.

Somatic afferents from the upper three cervical segments overlap trigeminal afferents in the TCN. Consequently, the spinal nucleus of the trigeminal nerve can also receive afferents from the C1-3 spinal nerves. Any of the structures innervated by the 5th, 7th, 9th or 10th cranial nerves or the C1-3 spinal nerves can therefore be a source of head pain. The pain may be felt locally within the distribution of a specific nerve or may be referred due to convergence of afferent inputs from the various nerves providing input to the TCN. The TCN is the anatomical substrate by which pain from a source in the head can be referred to the neck and vice versa. At an elementary level, this explains why migraine sufferers may develop pain and tightness in neck muscles even though the primary source of pain may be intracranial. Consequently, whether the headache is caused by a neck disorder or intracerebral vascular disorders or is related to migraine headache, it will always be associated with activity in the TCN.

The trigeminal nerve has ophthalmic (V1), maxillary (V2), and mandibular (V3) divisions. The ophthalmic division, supplying the anterior two-thirds of the head including the eye and forehead, has the most caudal distribution of the three divisions within the TCN. The ophthalmic division has the greatest overlap with the upper three spinal nerves. The maxillary division, supplying the maxillary area, has a lesser projection into the spinal cord. The mandibular division, supplying the mandibular area, has the weakest projections of all, lessening the likelihood of structures innervated by this component being a source of head pain.[4]

Knowledge of the nervous anatomy helps explain the source of headaches. For example, an impairment of the upper cervical spine may produce pain or headache in the frontal, orbital or retro-orbital regions because the ophthalmic division of the trigeminal nerve innervates these areas. Similarly, facial pain in the maxillary or mandibular regions is less likely to be referred from the cervical spine because the maxillary and mandibular divisions of the trigeminal nerve have weak or non-existent projections into the TCN. In cervicogenic headache (CGH), pain is often felt in the frontal, orbital and retro-orbital areas corresponding to the distribution of the ophthalmic division.

The trigeminal nerve supplies the skin of the face and forehead, orbit, dura mater and major vessels of the venous sinuses of the middle and anterior cranial fossae, nose, mouth, teeth, and temporomandibular joints (TMJs). The 7th, 9th and 10th cranial nerves innervate the ear, pharynx and larynx and the carotid sinuses and bodies.[4]

Extracranially, the upper three cervical nerves supply the skin over the suboccipital and occipital areas, the ligaments and joints of the first three cervical segments, the C2-3 intervertebral disc, and the prevertebral and postvertebral upper cervical muscles, including the longus capitis, upper portion of longus cervicis, the suboccipital muscles, the upper portion of semispinalis capitis, scalenus medius, trapezius and sternocleidomastoid. Intracranially, they innervate the dura of the posterior cranial fossa and the vertebral artery via recurrent branches that re-enter the posterior cranial fossa via the foramen magnum.[4]

Afferent information from all of the structures innervated by the 5th, 7th, 9th and 10th cranial nerves and the C1-3 segments converges at the level of the TCN. After synapse in the TCN, second order neurons project to various thalamic nuclei for further relay. Connections above the thalamic level are still the subject of further research but in general terms may include projection to the sensory cortex of the parietal lobe for perception of somatic pain, the insula cortex for visceral pain, the temporal lobes for memory search and comparison with previous episodes, and the limbic and prefrontal lobe systems for generation of emotional affect.[7] The key point is realizing that all headache types share some common anatomical pathways and it is this commonality that accounts for overlap of symptomatology between types of headaches and makes differentiation into discrete diagnostic entities sometimes difficult.

Pain Mechanisms of Headache

Most clinicians have an understanding of the mechanisms by which tissue damage causes pain. Peripheral nociceptors of the small diameter Aδ and C fibers are activated by chemical irritation related to inflammation, by mechanical tissue damage or by thermal stimulus. These primary neurons synapse with second order neurones, predominantly in the outer laminae of the dorsal column grey matter.[32] Nociceptive input is then relayed via thalamic, brainstem and cerebellar nuclei to various areas of the brain for perception of pain. When the painful stimulus is from nociceptors in the periphery, the pain is called *peripheral nociceptive pain*. Similarly if the pain arises from a stimulus applied to the peripheral nerves or their meningeal coverings it is termed *peripheral neurogenic pain*.[6]

Less well appreciated by clinicians are the pain modulator mechanisms and the mechanisms by which the central nervous system (CNS) can become excessively sensitive to painful stimuli or by which pain may originate from within the CNS itself. The CNS has its own in-built pain modulation systems or *endogenous pain control systems* that can modulate the pain experience either upward or downward.[6,7] At a simplistic level, these pain control systems are influenced by cognitive processing strategies, thoughts, feelings and emotions, and utilize presynaptic inhibition of noci input and chemical systems, including opioids, serotonin and noradrenaline.[6,7]

Many factors, including genetics, attitudes and beliefs about pain, the context of the pain, and environmental factors, influence the endogenous pain control systems. Normal function requires a balance between noci input and the endogenous pain control systems that allow the perception of pain to be directly related to the degree of pathology. If there is an inhibition of normal endogenous pain control systems it can result in excessive pain being experienced for the degree of pathology. This phenomenon called *disinhibition* is important in the understanding of various types of headaches. It is probable that both migraines and tension-type headaches are associated with varying degrees of disinhibition and consequent sensitization of the CNS, whereby the CNS becomes sensitized to various stimuli, both from peripheral noci input and from emotions, thoughts and feelings. This inhibition of the normal descending pain control systems can lead to the pain experience being disproportionate to the degree of pathology. The phenomenon of CNS sensitization, or *central sensitization* in the case of headache, is likely to be at the level of the TCN.

The basis for sensitization of the CNS is probably neuroplasticity at the synaptic junctions between neurons. The release of amino acids and neuropeptides into synaptic clefts may cause an opening up or awakening of previously silent synapses, a lowering of thresholds for activation, or inhibition of a synapse or an increase in receptive field.[6] A degree of CNS sensitization is normal in response to peripheral noci input, but when the afferent noci input lessens as the tissue heals, the central effects should likewise settle.

In chronic pain, the central sensitization does not dampen down and return to normal. This may occur when any of a number of psychosocial risk factors are present or in the presence of persistent and severe afferent noci input. Kendall et al[20] suggest that psychosocial factors that may predispose the patient to the development of chronic pain include: attitudes and beliefs about pain, fear avoidance behavior, emotions such as anxiety or depression, and compensation, diagnosis and treatment, family and work issues.

An understanding of central pain mechanisms and the predisposing factors for the development of central sensitization helps the clinician recognize when acute pain states are more likely to progress to chronic states so that interventions can be modified appropriately. Central pain mechanisms also help explain the pathophysiology of some of the more chronic forms of headache such as chronic tension-type headache or chronic migraine. In addition to the sensory inputs and cognitive and emotional aspects to pain experience, the nervous system also has *output and homeostatic systems*. The endocrine, immune, motor and autonomic systems are all interrelated output and homeostatic mechanisms.[6] Activation of the sympathetic nervous system (SNS) and its effects on the adrenal cortex may result in secretion of cortisol, adrenaline, and noradrenaline.[6] A chronic excess of cortisol may suppress the immune system, slow tissue healing and create mood

swings. The SNS can make already damaged tissues more sensitive, leading to regional pain syndromes or produce other sympathetic responses of altered sweating, color changes, or hot or cold feelings of a body part.[6] Motor system responses to pain may be overt muscle spasm or more subtle changes in muscle tone or patterning of movement. Evidence of some of these endocrine, immune, motor and autonomic responses may assist the clinician in understanding the pain mechanisms involved in a patient's headache and making a more accurate differential diagnosis.

Classification of Headache Types

Optimal management of headache requires accurate differential diagnosis and identification of contributing factors in order for treatment to be specifically tailored for patients and their headaches. Various forms of headache may display similar features and be difficult to distinguish. For many headache types, valid and reliable diagnostic tests do not exist and so differential diagnosis is reliant on patients' descriptions of their symptoms. A specific diagnosis aids in guiding the treatment approach, but in many cases the clinical features do not fit a precise diagnostic category.

The IHS first published a classification system for headaches in 1988[15] with the completely revised second edition published in 2004.[16] The time taken to update this edition and the number of modifications required are evidence of the difficulty in accurately classifying headaches into discrete entities. The second edition describes 14 possible diagnostic categories for headaches (Table 9-1).

It is worth reflecting upon the various diagnostic categories listed and their links with the previous discussion on anatomy of headache and peripheral and central pain mechanisms. All diagnostic categories involve structures innervated by the 5th, 7th, 9th and 10th cranial nerves or the upper three cervical nerves. The stimulus may be chemical, inflammatory or mechanical and the pain may be nociceptive, neuralgic or central.

The Subjective Examination

A thorough subjective examination is the most important aspect in headache diagnosis. To understand a patient's headache experience requires excellent verbal and non-verbal communication. Non-verbal cues such as eye contact or posture give clues about the patient and the problem. Some patients are attentive and listen to questions while others may be fidgety or not answer the questions asked.

Table 9-1: Diagnostic Categories for Headaches

Primary Headaches
  Migraine
  Tension-type headache
  Cluster headache and other trigeminal-
  autonomic cephalgias
  Other primary headaches

Secondary Headaches
  Headache attributed to head and/or neck trauma
  Headache attributed to cranial and/or cervical
  vascular disorders
  Headache attributed to non-vascular intracranial
  disorder
  Headache attributed to a substance or its
  withdrawal
  Headache attributed to infection
  Headache attributed to disturbance of
  homeostasis
  Headache or facial pain attributed to disorder of
  cranium, neck, eyes, ears, nose, sinuses, teeth,
  mouth, or other facial or cranial structures
  Headache attributed to psychiatric disorder
  Cranial neuralgias and central causes of facial
  pain
  Other headache, cranial neuralgia, central or
  primary facial pain

Maitland[28] recommends listening to patients in an open minded and non-judgmental manner, believing them, yet at the same time questioning them. Using the words and tone of voice that they use helps to build rapport.

Asking questions in an open-ended manner avoids being too suggestive of a desired response. This type of questioning allows patients to give information about what is foremost on their minds. Greatest importance should be attached to information given spontaneously rather than that gained from directed questions.

What patients say may not be everything that is on their minds or troubling them. If they start to sense that they are identified with, they are more likely to open up and reveal more of what they really feel or what some of the real contributing factors may be. This can be likened to peeling back the layers of an onion to find out what is really at the core of the experience. This is where personal, family or work issues are raised and contributing factors to chronic pain are identified. In many instances simply being understood is highly therapeutic.

The subjective examination follows the format outlined in Chapter 4, *Evaluation of the Spine*, but with the addition of the following areas specific to headache.

Headache Types

Patients may experience more than one distinct headache type, each with its own temporal pattern, location, quality, associated features, aggravating and easing factors, and onset. When headache types within the same patient are clearly distinct they can be managed accordingly. Often, however, they are difficult to distinguish because of anatomy and physiology universal to all headaches. An attempt to distinguish discrete headache types assists appropriate intervention. In instances where there appears to be more than one headache type existing but it is not clear cut, intervention directed specifically to one of the possible headache types and subsequent analysis of its effect may provide information as to the presence of one or more type. It is necessary to ascertain the features of each unrelated headache.

Frequency

Establishing the number of headaches per hour, day, week, month or year is important in diagnosis. In some headache types there may be several bursts of severe pain within an hour while in others the headache may last for days or be continuous. The period of time that a patient is free of headache (the headache-free interval) can be useful information. The clinician should establish whether there is a pattern of remission and relapse and if there has been any change in the pattern of headache. If there is an increase in the frequency of headaches in a specific time period, trigger factors preceding or during that time can be looked for.

Intensity

Headache intensity can vary from mild to excruciating and adds valuable information to the diagnostic picture. Ascertaining whether the headache inhibits or prohibits normal activities gives an indication as to the intensity. A ten point ranking scale can be used to rate the severity. Intensity will be a reflection of the pain mechanisms in play and the degree of impairment.

Duration

The length of time a headache lasts with and without treatment should be recorded. Headache duration may be variable or have a set length. Constant headache may indicate a persistent stimulus to nociceptors from chemical or mechanical irritants or may suggest central pain mechanisms or structural abnormalities of a nerve resulting in abnormal impulse generating sites. If the pain is of peripheral origin, as in cervicogenic headache, the pain is likely to vary with the degree of chemical or mechanical irritation of the causative tissue.

Location

In which area does the headache occur? Is it retro-orbital, orbital, frontal, temporal, occipital or in the "'whole head"? Is there radiation from the occipital region up and over the vertex toward the eye, down into the neck or is there pain into the arm, upper back, or lower limb? Are the symptoms unilateral or bilateral? Do they vary in location between attacks or are they always the same? Is the pain superficial or deep? Answers to these questions provide information about the likely source of the pain and the pain mechanisms involved.

Quality

The quality of the headache may give clues as to the source of the pain. Burning or stabbing pains or descriptions of a "red hot poker" may suggest a neuralgic cause. Pulsating or throbbing pain possibly indicates a vascular component and a diffuse ache may imply somatic referred pain.

Associated Features

Does the patient experience any other symptoms associated with the headache? In particular, nausea, vomiting, visual disturbances, loss of concentration, photophobia (sensitivity to lights), phonophobia (sensitivity to noise), and osmophobia (sensitivity to smell) should be noted. Are there any basilar symptoms such as dizziness, light-headedness, dysarthria, or ataxia? Are there any autonomic nervous system symptoms of lacrimation or nasal congestion? Are there any premonitory or warning signs like fatigue, hyperactivity, hypoactivity, depression, craving for special foods, repetitive yawning, phonophobia, photophobia, euphoria or increased thirst? These give clues about the physiological mechanisms involved and the possible diagnostic category.

Trigger or Aggravating Factors

Is there anything that brings on or aggravates the headaches? Specific questions include whether headaches are related to stress, either during or after the stressful period, hormonal factors such as menstrual cycle (typically pre or mid cycle in migraine), or dietary factors.

Specific foods or drinks may precipitate migraine in some patients. Environmental factors such as a change of season with an increase in pollens can trigger an allergic response and headache. Afferent stimuli like strong perfumes, bright lights, and loud noise can also trigger migraine. Is the headache aggravated by physical exercise or is it related to mechanical load on the neck as may occur in cervicogenic headache?

Easing Factors

Is there anything that relieves the headache? Direct suboccipital pressure or a change of neck position may relieve some cervicogenic headaches by lessening noci input from the neck. Typically an untreated migraine will require avoiding environmental stimuli by sleeping in a dark room. If peripheral inflammation is the cause, then non-steroidal anti-inflammatory drugs (NSAIDs) may be effective. If central pain mechanisms are involved, medications that increase serotonin levels such as tricyclic antidepressants may play a role in management. Migraines may disappear completely during pregnancy, indicating a hormonal link. Relaxation or removal of personal, family or work stressors may ease or lessen the frequency of headaches.

Onset

Ascertain the history of each unrelated headache. When did it begin? Was there a specific cause such as a different sleeping posture or motor vehicle accident (possible musculoskeletal component) or did it link with a particularly stressful period? Commonly, the onset of tension-type headaches seem to be related to emotional, personal, school, work or family issues.

Find out which treatments have been tried and their effects. These may include various types of medications, physical therapy, chiropractic, relaxation therapy, natural therapies, dietary modifications, acupuncture, hypnosis and the application of heat or cold. The response to treatments may provide hints about the diagnosis.

Red Flags

Headaches may be equally intense whether their source is benign or malignant and so will often require special investigation to rule out serious pathology. Clinicians need to be aware of the more serious causes of headache that can masquerade as musculoskeletal problems and be able to identify where medical intervention is necessary and when certain mechanical therapeutic interventions are contraindicated.

While clinicians can use palpatory skills to identify musculoskeletal impairments, they must be careful to avoid overdiagnosing cervical problems. Rather, they must be prepared to exclude other possible causes of headache or recognize that musculoskeletal impairments in the neck may only be one component of the problem, a secondary effect of another type of headache, or indeed an incidental finding.

Some important signs to keep in mind are:

- Sudden onset of severe headache with vomiting and neck stiffness (sub-arachnoid hemorrhage, meningitis, encephalitis)
- Headache associated with fever, nausea and vomiting not explained by a systemic illness (meningitis, encephalitis)
- First or worst headache of their life (sub-arachnoid hemorrhage)
- Constant unremitting headache or severe night pain (tumors)
- Headaches accompanied by loss of consciousness, slow pulse, progressive vision failure, memory disturbance, personality change or convulsions
- Sudden change in a chronic headache pattern
- Worsening of head pain over several days
- Headaches of subacute onset aggravated by cough, sneezing or Valsalva's maneuver

Headache Diary

A headache diary may assist in headache diagnosis by identifying circumstances or factors that trigger the headaches and more accurately reflecting the pattern and behavior of the headache. The patient records the characteristics of each headache and the factors associated with it to present to the clinician. This written account of each headache can assist in diagnosis and management. It should include activities undertaken, dietary intake, medications taken, physical and environmental factors, stressful situations, mood, sleep patterns and characteristics of the headache itself.

Migraine

The IHS[16] has six diagnostic categories for migraine:

1. Migraine without aura
2. Migraine with aura: Typical aura with migraine headache, typical aura with non-migraine headache, typical aura without headache, familial hemiplegic migraine, sporadic hemiplegic migraine, basilar-type migraine

3. Childhood periodic syndromes that are commonly precursors of migraine: Cyclical vomiting, abdominal migraine, benign paroxysmal vertigo of childhood
4. Retinal migraine
5. Complications of migraine: Chronic migraine, status migrainosus, persistent aura without infarction, migrainous infarction, migraine-triggered seizures
6. Probable migraine: without aura, with aura or chronic

Migraine without aura and migraine with aura are the most frequently occurring migraine types, and will be discussed below.

Pathophysiology of Migraine

The current hypothesis for the pathophysiology of migraine views it as a neurovascular phenomenon, triggered by various factors and occurring in patients who have a genetic predisposition. For a more detailed description consult Lance and Goadsby[24] on which this account is based.

Genetic Predisposition. Migraine sufferers are genetically predisposed to migraines.[24] In other words they are either wired for it or not. Some forms of migraine such as the familial hemiplegic variety have been linked to specific chromosomal defects.[37] Various other chromosomal abnormalities may account for the genetic susceptibility to other types of migraine in some patients.[29] Magnesium deficiency in the brain may be linked to central hyperexcitability and may make the brain more susceptible to triggering of the spreading depression associated with the aura phenomena (see *The Aura of Migraine* on page 217).[25] These areas are the subjects of continuing investigations.

Many of the premonitory symptoms of irritability, fatigue, hypoactivity, depression, craving for special foods, euphoria, increased thirst, and particularly repetitive yawning are likely to be dopaminergic in origin.[24] Current information suggests a dopamine deficiency in migraine and super-sensitivity of dopamine receptors.

In migraine sufferers, the endogenous pain control systems are defective, leading to an unstable TCN complex. This unstable system becomes excessively susceptible to stimulation from the cortex such as in response to stressful situations, psychological processing, emotions, thoughts or feelings.[24] A specific trigger or combination of trigger factors then sets in motion a series of events on an already susceptible system.

Trigger Factors. A combination of endogenous factors (e.g., biological clock) and/or exogenous factors (e.g., flashing lights, loud sounds, perfumes and psychological stress) can provide a neurological trigger. Vascular triggers such as the ingestion of vasodilator agents appear to act on the cranial blood vessels, providing excessive afferent input to an already unstable TCN. The resultant headache is likely due to activation of the nociceptive trigeminovascular system and subsequent cranio vascular afferent input to further excite the unstable TCN.[24]

The Aura of Migraine. Most migraine patients experience migraine without aura. For those that do experience an aura, it is typically followed by headache. Occasionally, the aura is not followed by a headache. To what extent the aura and headache are linked is still somewhat uncertain.

At the onset of aura, cerebral blood flow is reduced, initially in the occipital region, progressively spreading forward as a *spreading oligaemia*.[36] In animal experiments Leão described a progressive shutdown in cortical function known as *spreading depression*.[27] These waves of inhibition (often preceded by excitation) of cortical function progress at 2-3 mm per minute and last for 5-60 minutes. It is likely that cortical spreading depression is responsible for the aura symptoms. Thus aura symptoms arise from the visual cortex and not from the retina. Aura symptoms are described in detail on page 218 .

Brain Stem Nuclei in Migraine. At the pathophysiologic core of migraine is the brain stem, with its descending and ascending projections from the brain stem nuclei.[43] The upstream projection from these brain stem nuclei to the cortex can regulate blood flow and the downstream projections play an important part in blood flow, the nociceptive trigeminovascular system, and in modulation of the endogenous pain control systems. [24]

Blood Flow in Migraine. Vascular changes associated with migraine are likely secondary to brain stem activity and not the primary cause of headache. Recent evidence points to perturbation of neural activity within the serotonergic and noradrenergic systems as an important precursor to migraine. In animal experiments, activity in the locus coeruleus induces *intracerebral vasoconstriction*.[11] Subsequent ischemia of the occipital cortex followed by cortical spreading depression is the likely precursor to the visual aura of migraine with aura. Locus coeruleus activation can also influence the extracranial circulation producing *extracranial vasodilation*, likely mediated by parasympathetic outflow in a branch of the facial nerve.[12] Animal experiments also show that stimulation of the nucleus raphe dorsalis can produce *vasodilation in both intracranial and extracranial circulation*, again mediated by

the parasympathetic outflow in a branch of the facial nerve.[13, 14] Although extracranial circulation (e.g., in the superficial temporal artery) may increase during migraine attack, this alone is rarely the sole cause of the head pain experienced in migraine.

This neurovascular reaction not only produces constriction or dilation of intracranial and extracranial arteries but also activates the nociceptive trigeminovascular system.

Nociceptive Trigeminovascular System. The activation of the trigeminal system, either centrally or peripherally, causes release of vasoactive neuropeptides including substance P, calcitonin gene-related polypeptide and neurokinin A, an outcome that results in a neurogenic or sterile inflammation of the blood vessels.[34] These inflamed blood vessels are a likely source of the pain in migraine. Medications such as serotonin agonists (e.g., sumatriptan) and the ergots (e.g., ergotamine) may act to block the release of these neuropeptides, thereby preventing or inhibiting an attack of migraine.[33] As discussed later, these drugs may also have actions on the central pain pathways and/or the cranial blood flow. These inflamed blood vessels then provide afferent input to the already sensitized TCN, producing the severe pain of migraine headache.

Endogenous Pain Control Systems in Migraine. The downstream projection of the locus coeruleus to the thoracic sympathetic outflow could cause the release of noradrenaline into the systemic circulation, setting in motion the platelet release of 5-hydroxytryptamine (5-HT, serotonin). Following a phase of monoaminergic excitation, subsequent monoamine depletion could free the endogenous pain control pathway[24] and facilitate the perception of pain in the head, occasionally radiating down the body on the same side, implicating the spinothalamic pathway as well as the trigeminal system.

Migraine without Aura

Diagnostic Criteria. The IHS[16] lists the following diagnostic criteria for migraine without aura:

1. At least five attacks fulfilling criteria 2-5 below, less than 15 days/month.
2. Duration
   - 4-72 hours (untreated)
   - May be as short as 1 hour in children
3. At least two of:
   - Location: predominantly unilateral, frontotemporal or temporoparietal although may be

bilateral in 40%. Often bilateral in young children. Occipital headaches in young children are rare and call for diagnostic caution.
- Quality: pulsating
- Intensity: moderate-severe (prohibits activity)
- Aggravated by routine physical activity like walking or climbing stairs

4. During headache at least one of (associated features)
   - Nausea and/or vomiting
   - Photophobia and phonophobia
5. Not attributed to another disorder

An understanding of the pathophysiology of migraine headache, where inflamed blood vessels provide nociceptive input to an already sensitized TCN, helps the clinician appreciate the clinical features of migraine. The pulsating pain and severe intensity of pain are linked to the inflamed vascular structures and can be aggravated by routine movements that mechanically load or vibrate the vessels.

Other Clinical Features. Migraines are approximately three times more common in females than in males, but the precise incidence varies between studies.[24] An episode of migraine can be separated into five phases: premonitory, aura (if present), headache, resolution and recovery. An individual attack can consist of any or all of these phases of the clinical spectrum.

Premonitory symptoms occur in 50-80% of cases, hours to a day or two before a migraine attack.[45] Patients will often be aware that a migraine headache is about to occur. Symptoms may include neck stiffness, fatigue, hyperactivity, hypoactivity, depression, craving for special foods, repetitive yawning, osmophobia, phonophobia, photophobia, euphoria, increased thirst, and similar atypical symptoms.[45] Some of these may be linked to activation of dopaminergic systems. If abortive medications are to be used this is typically the optimal time to do so.

Migraines in some instances may be aggravated or triggered by foods containing nitrates and nitrites (usually in processed meats), food additives such as monosodium glutamate (MSG), tyramine, and sulphites. Canned or processed foods, Asian foods, tenderizers and seasonings such as soy sauce may contain MSG. Dairy products including milk, cream and aged cheeses may contain tyramine and sulphites, and dried fruits (in particular apricots) may contain sulphites. This lists is far from comprehensive. A headache diary may assist in detecting the presence of any specific food triggers for a particular patient.

Emotional stress, either during or after the stressful period has passed, can trigger an attack in some people.

Similarly, hormonal factors probably associated with fluctuating estrogen levels can cause migraine. Typically migraines may occur mid cycle or in the pre-menstrual phase, sometimes disappearing completely during pregnancy.

Environmental stimuli, bright lights, sun glare, excessive loud noise, or strong scents like perfumes can also precipitate an attack. In some instances neck strain appears to set off an episode of migraine with patients noticing that the headache appears to begin with stiffness and pain in the top of the neck. This is probably due to nociceptive input to the TCN in patients already predisposed to migraine.

Migraine with Aura

Migraine with aura is characterized by aura symptoms, which are reversible focal neurological symptoms that develop over 5-20 minutes and last less than 60 minutes.[16] Headache as described above usually follows the aura symptoms. Less commonly, headache may not have migrainous features or may be completely absent.

Diagnostic Criteria. The IHS[16] lists the following diagnostic criteria for migraine with aura:

1. At least two attacks fulfilling criterion 2 below
2. Migraine aura fulfilling specific criteria for subforms of typical aura, hemiplegic aura or basilar aura
3. Not attributed to another disorder

Aura Symptoms. Most migraine sufferers will exclusively have attacks without aura and those who have attacks with aura may also have attacks without. The most common aura symptoms are visual. Visual aura symptoms include fortification spectra, resembling a zigzagged top wall of a fortress, typically bright and shimmering, that slowly drift across the visual field leaving in their wake a band of visual blurring or loss. This area of visual field loss is often surrounded by a bright rim and is called a *scintillating scotoma*. Other patients experience photopsias that are poorly formed brief flashes or sparks of light that usually remain in the same part of the visual field or are scattered across both visual fields.

Most patients (65%) having visual aura symptoms experience a combination of phenomena, but the majority (72%) have only one usual manifestation.[42] Aura symptoms arising from areas of the cortex other than the visual cortex are much less common. Other aura symptoms include sensory disturbances of unilateral pins and needles and/or numbness spreading from the point of origin to one side of the body or face, speech disturbances of aphasia or unclassifiable speech difficulty, and motor disturbances of unilateral motor weakness.

Basilar aura symptoms originate from the brain stem or both occipital lobes, and include dysarthria, vertigo, tinnitus, decreased hearing, double vision, ataxia, or decreased levels of consciousness. Again, they are infrequent in comparison to the frequency of visual aura symptoms.

Differential diagnosis is evident from careful history taking, particularly in respect to duration and onset of aura. Specific aura diagnostic categories in the IHS classification include those with a typical aura comprising visual and/or sensory and/or speech symptoms but no motor weakness. They are categorized as typical aura with migraine headache, typical aura with non-migraine headache and typical aura without headache. Familial hemiplegic migraine includes the aura of motor weakness and requires at least one first or second degree relative to have migraine aura with motor weakness. Sporadic hemiplegic migraine involves motor weakness but no first or second degree relative having the symptoms. Basilar-type migraine involves aura symptoms that clearly originate from the brain stem or from simultaneous affection of both hemispheres and where no motor weakness is present.

Migraine Management

There are two goals when treating migraine: pain relief and prevention of future attacks. Currently no cure exists for migraine, although control can be achieved for most patients. It is reassuring to explain to patients that they were born with a sensitive neurovascular system that over-reacts to internal changes or external stimuli and that their conditions can probably be controlled with non-pharmacologic and/or appropriate pharmacologic treatment.

Non-pharmacological treatment may begin with a general wellness program. This may include lifestyle modifications such as regular exercise, relaxation, good sleeping habits, regular nutritious meals, not overeating, moderate alcohol intake and avoidance of smoking. Specific trigger factors that have been identified need to be addressed. Wearing sunglasses, avoiding bright lights, loud noises, strong perfumes and odors or hormonal intervention may be beneficial. If a cervical spine or TMJ dysfunction is linked to the onset of migraines, then these must be addressed with appropriate therapy. Similarly, if eyestrain is a factor, appropriate referral and management that may include new or different eyeglasses should be sought. Education as to the pathophysiology of migraine assists the patient in understanding the importance of self-responsibility for general well being, managing trigger factors and taking medications as prescribed.

For mild to moderate attacks, pharmacological treatment may include simple analgesics, combination analgesics, or NSAIDs. For moderate to severe attacks, abortive medications like serotonin receptor agonists (e.g., sumatriptan) and the ergots are the agents of choice. Alternatives include corticosteroids and possibly opioid analgesics. Anti-emetics may be prescribed to control vomiting. Preventive medications may include adrenergic or beta-blockers such as propranolol, serotonin antagonists such as pizotifen, tricyclic anti-depressants, calcium channel blockers and anti-convulsant medication. Supplements such as oral magnesium are reported to help in some cases.

Medications used in the management of headache can act in the periphery (e.g., NSAIDs, ergots), can block nociceptive transmission at the dorsal horn (e.g., opioids), decrease neural sensitivity (e.g., membrane stabilizers), or normalize levels of neurotransmitters involved in descending pain inhibition of the dorsal horn/TCN. Descending inhibition of the TCN utilizes mainly noradrenaline and serotonin although dopamine may also have a role in inhibiting nociceptive activity.

Tension-Type Headache

The IHS[16] has four diagnostic categories for tension-type headache related to the frequency of attacks.

1. Infrequent episodic tension-type headache (less than 12 per year): with and without pericranial tenderness

2. Frequent episodic tension-type headache (12-180 per year): with and without pericranial tenderness

3. Chronic tension-type headache (15 days per month or more): with and without pericranial tenderness

4. Probable tension-type headache: infrequent, frequent or chronic

Diagnostic Criteria

The IHS[16] lists the following diagnostic criteria for tension-type headache:

1. Frequency as outlined above

2. Duration (30 minutes—7 days)

3. At least two of:
   - Location: bilateral (typically occipital ± fronto-temporal)
   - Quality: pressing, tightening, non-pulsating

- Intensity: annoying, mild to moderate (inhibits, not prohibits activity)
- Not aggravated by routine physical activity like walking or climbing stairs

4. No nausea; photophobia or phonophobia (but not both) may occur

5. Not attributed to another disorder

Other Clinical Features

Episodic tension-type headaches occur randomly and are often the result of temporary stress, anxiety, fatigue, or anger. Chronic tension-type headaches may be related to depression, physical problems, or psychological issues. Environmental factors, excessive afferent stimuli (loud noise, bright lights), and occlusal problems including TMJ dysfunction causing abnormal activity of masticatory muscles can initiate a headache of this type. Similarly, impaired sight causing overuse of eye and periorbital muscles and cervical spine muscle disorders can precipitate a tension-type headache.

There may be symptoms of anxiety, trouble falling asleep, insomnia, morning nausea, light-headedness and poor concentration. If associated with depression, patients may awaken frequently, awaken too early in the morning, or sleep excessively (hypersomnia). There may be other physical symptoms of depression, including shortness of breath, constipation, nausea, weight loss, ongoing fatigue, decreased sexual drive, palpitations, dizziness, unexpected crying and menstrual changes. Emotional symptoms of depression could include feelings of guilt, hopelessness, unworthiness, fear of mental or physical disease or death, poor concentration, little ambition, no interest in life, indecisiveness or poor memory. Symptoms of chronic muscle contraction such as pericranial, suboccipital, neck and interscapular aching and tightness are also commonly found.

Pathophysiology of Tension-Type Headache

Various authors report a low platelet content of 5-HT in tension-type headache sufferers.[1,44] It is possible that low platelet 5-HT reflects a 5-HT deficiency in brain stem endogenous pain control pathways. Tension-type headache is thus probably a central disinhibitory phenomena associated with neurotransmitter changes in the brain stem.

Underlying psychosocial factors as discussed earlier may be linked to this central sensitization. Muscular overactivity may be a primary phenomenon of this type of headache or more likely a secondary effect of the central sensitization. Excessive use of analgesia may also diminish platelet content of 5-HT, leading to rebound headache and predisposing patients to chronic tension-type headache or chronic daily headache.[24]

Tension-Type Headache Management

Episodic headaches can usually be kept under control by using simple analgesics, relaxation and attention to general well-being. Chronic headaches will typically not be relieved by simple analgesics and the pain may seem constant and unrelenting.

If specific physical impairments are present they should be addressed. Occlusal problems or TMJ dysfunction may require dental work, alteration of bite mechanics with appropriate splinting, or techniques discussed in Chapter 8, *Temporomandibular Disorders*. Impaired vision may require corrective lenses to lessen eyestrain. Cervical spine impairments should be addressed as discussed in the section on cervicogenic headaches. Lifestyle risk factors such as poor posture, faulty living and working habits, ergonomic issues and lack of general fitness may need to be considered.

Psychosocial risk factors including lowered mood, stress, anxiety, depression, and personal, work and family issues, may need to be addressed and patients can sometimes benefit from psychologic or psychiatric intervention. Typically, psychosocial issues precipitate tension-type headaches and headaches will probably recur if these issues are not addressed.

Pharmacological treatment may be aimed at either relieving the immediate pain of headache or at preventing future attacks. Abortive treatment medications may include simple analgesics, NSAIDs and muscle relaxants. Overuse of analgesics should be avoided for reasons discussed earlier. Preventive treatment may include medications such as tricyclic anti-depressants, selective serotonin re-uptake inhibitors or other medications used in the management of migraine. The serotonin medications may act centrally to address the 5-HT deficiency in endogenous pain control pathways.

Non-pharmacological interventions include avoiding or minimizing triggers, self-help measures such as biofeedback, meditation or relaxation exercises, acupuncture, spinal mobilization, massage and psychological counseling. Spinal mobilization, massage and acupuncture directed to the upper cervical structures will provide neural input to the sensitized TCN. This may assist in restoring regular neuronal activity.

Cluster Headache and Other Trigeminal-Autonomic Cephalgias

Cluster headaches derive their name from the phenomenon of groups of attacks separated by intervals of complete remission. Recent diagnostic categories, however, list chronic forms without remission. Episodic cluster headaches occur in periods lasting seven days to one year, separated by pain free periods lasting one month or more. Chronic cluster headaches occur for more than one year without remission or with remissions lasting less than one month. The IHS[16] identifies the following subcategories within this diagnosis:

1. Cluster headache: Episodic and chronic cluster headache
2. Paroxysmal hemicrania: Episodic and chronic paroxysmal hemicrania
3. Short-lasting unilateral neuralgiform headache with conjunctival injection and tearing (SUNCT)
4. Probable trigeminal autonomic cephalgia: cluster headache, paroxysmal hemicrania, SUNCT

Presented here are some features of cluster headache. For more detail on the other trigeminal-autonomic cephalgias consult the IHS classification and Lance and Goadsby.[24]

Diagnostic Criteria for Cluster Headache

The IHS[16] lists the following diagnostic criteria for cluster headache:

1. At least five attacks fulfilling criteria 2-4
2. Severe unilateral orbital, supraorbital, and/or temporal pain lasting 15 to 180 minutes if untreated
3. Headache is accompanied by at least one of the following signs that have to be present on the side of the pain:
    *   Conjunctival injection and/or lacrimation
    *   Nasal congestion and/or rhinorrhea
    *   Eyelid edema
    *   Forehead and facial sweating
    *   Miosis and/or ptosis
    *   Restlessness or agitation
4. Frequency of attacks: from one every other day to eight per day
5. Not attributed to another disorder

Other Clinical Features

The incidence of cluster headache is significantly less than the incidence of migraine, but reports vary as to the precise incidence. They are approximately five times more common in males than females.[14]

Nocturnal attacks that disrupt sleep are common. There may be a link with alcohol or long-term smoking and they may be more prevalent during changes in the seasons. There is no familial link and psychological stress does not appear to be related.

Pathophysiology of Cluster Headache

The region of the ipsilateral hypothalamic grey matter is likely to be the primary driving or permissive area for cluster headache. Some patients become aware that an attack is about to start due to twinges of pain in the susceptible areas. Others detect a watering eye and stuffy nostril for half an hour or so before the pain begins. The pain and the autonomic phenomena are separate variables, although one usually follows the other. They are compatible with paroxysmal discharge of central trigeminal, parasympathetic and sympathetic pathways.[24]

Dilation of parts of the internal and external circulations are likely to be secondary to activity in vascular projections from the brain stem, and intensify pain by increasing input to the brain stem through trigeminal and upper cervical afferent fibers into the TCN. The fact that episodic pain may continue after surgical lesions of the trigeminal nerve indicates the primary defect is a central disturbance.[24]

Management of Cluster Headache

Medications that are also used for migraines can be used to try to abort an acute attack or for prophylaxis. Medications can be directed at the dilated arteries or at central mechanisms.[24] Optimal treatment involves the use of medications to prevent further attacks within a bout. Alcohol should be avoided during a bout.

Cervicogenic Headache

A cervicogenic headache (CGH) can be defined as "referred pain perceived in any part of the head caused by a primary nociceptive source in the musculoskeletal tissues innervated by cervical nerves".[51] Cervicogenic headaches are listed by the IHS under a subsection of "headache or facial pain attributed to disorder of cranium, neck, eyes, ears, nose, sinuses, teeth, mouth or other facial or cranial structures".

Diagnostic Criteria

The IHS[16] lists the following diagnostic criteria for CGH:

1. Pain, referred from a source in the neck and perceived in one or more regions of the head and/or face, fulfilling criteria 3 and 4

2. Clinical, laboratory and/or imaging evidence of a disorder or lesion within the cervical spine or soft tissues of the neck, known to be, or generally accepted as a valid cause of headache

3. Evidence that the pain can be attributed to the neck disorder or lesion, based on at least one of the following:

   • Demonstration of clinical signs that implicate a source of pain in the neck

   • Abolition of headache following diagnostic blockade of a cervical structure or its nerve supply using placebo or other adequate controls

4. Headache resolves within three months after successful treatment of the causative disorder or lesion

Detection of clinical signs of cervical musculoskeletal physical impairment, such as articular instability or hypomobility or muscular deficit in the presence of headache, does not prove that cervical structures are the cause of the headache. The cervical physical impairment in the presence of headache may be:

Causative. True cervicogenic headache, wherein the headache is caused by the cervical spine. Sometimes, but not always, a cervical spine investigative procedure reproduces the headache.

Coexisting. Cervicogenic headache may coexist with another headache type.

Incidental. Cervical disorder may have no link to any headache.

Contributory. Cervical disorder may contribute to the headaches. In this scenario treatment directed to the cervical musculoskeletal physical impairment will provide measurable improvement in the headaches but will not completely cure the headache, as it is only a partial cause of the headache.

Trigger. Cervical disorder may be a trigger for headache of another type such as migraine.

In clinical practice, diagnostic blockade is unlikely to be readily available. Reassessment after cervical spine treatment is the best approximation available in most clinical environments. If reassessment after treatment shows relief or lessening of the headache, a cervicogenic component is likely. Reassessment may include noting headache

intensity, frequency, severity, and duration, or may involve the use of functional disability questionnaires or other outcome measures. The Neck Disability Index[48] (NDI) or Northwick Park Neck Pain Questionnaire[26] can be used as appropriate in the clinic.

Other Clinical Features

Unlike migraines, cervicogenic headaches usually occur on a continual basis either daily or several times per week and have a variable duration. They are unlikely to prohibit activity, while an untreated migraine will typically prohibit activity.

Most cervicogenic headaches are reported to be frontal, occipital, temporal and retro-orbital, correlating with the distribution of the C1-3 nerves and the distal projection of the ophthalmic division of the trigeminal nerve. The headache may originate in the neck and spread into the occipital region or extend up and over the head. This is in contrast to a migraine, which is more likely to originate in the head and then spread to the neck.

Cervicogenic headaches are typically unilateral but may be bilateral if the cervical disorder is bilateral. In contrast to migraines they do not alternate from one side to the other. The pain of cervicogenic headache is usually described as a dull ache consistent with musculoskeletal or somatic referred pain. The area of headache alone however is insufficient to implicate a specific cervical segment.

Dizziness, light headedness, nausea, tinnitus or vague visual disturbances such as ipsilateral blurring or difficulty focusing may exist but are not necessarily associated with cervicogenic headache. Cervicogenic headache may be associated with neck postures or movements or neck pain and stiffness, but this is not always the case. Long sitting or driving may aggravate a headache of neuromeningeal origin. Relieving factors are often difficult to identify. Some patients gain relief by lying down, changing posture or applying direct pressure to the suboccipital area, while others find analgesics and anti-inflammatory drugs to be beneficial.

It is important to look for predisposing lifestyle or extrinsic factors such as poor posture, poor ergonomics, faulty living and working habits, loss of physical conditioning or lack of variety of movement. Poor sleeping posture with an unsupportive pillow can trigger cervicogenic headaches on waking. Prolonged sitting in a forward head posture or incorrect workplace design puts excessive load on the cervical spine, possibly triggering cervicogenic headache. Repetitive and loaded neck movement as well as sustained postures can overload the musculoskeletal tissues. Sports requiring neck movements may lead to headaches. An example would be a sport like freestyle swimming. Poor head turning technique can place excessive load on the upper cervical structures.

Genetic, biomechanical and intrinsic factors can also predispose one to cervicogenic headaches. Intrinsic factors refer to potential causes that are internal characteristics of the patient, rather than external factors such as working or living conditions.

Examples of intrinsic factors include rheumatoid arthritis of the upper cervical spine and other medical conditions that may lead to upper cervical inflammation or ligamentous laxity. Mid or lower cervical spine hypomobility, possibly caused by osteoarthritis, congenital or surgical fusion may place excessive load on the upper cervical spine and predispose one to cervicogenic headaches.

Other intrinsic risk factors may be prior cervical spine trauma or altered spinal biomechanics, possibly related to leg length discrepancy or a disorder of the thoracic or lumbar spine.

Pathophysiology of Cervicogenic Headache

Any musculoskeletal structures innervated by the C1-3 spinal nerves can be a source of cervicogenic headache. Irritation of musculoskeletal structures can produce head pain locally within the afferent distribution of the C1-3 nerves or may lead to referred head pain into the trigeminal nerve distribution due to convergence in the TCN.

The pain mechanisms of cervicogenic headache are predominantly peripheral, whereas migraine and tension-type headaches are related to central sensitization.

Sensations of dizziness, light-headedness and some visual disturbances may be caused by altered proprioceptive impulses arising from impairment of upper cervical joints and muscles.

The neurologic basis for nausea, tinnitus, and other sometimes bizarre symptoms that rarely occur with cervicogenic headache is probably the extensive interconnection with the 7th, 9th and 10th cranial nerves and the superior cervical ganglion via the trigeminocervical nucleus.

Section Two—Physical Examination for Cervicogenic Headache

Cervicogenic headaches are caused by physical impairments in the joints, muscles or neuromeningeal tissues innervated by the C1-3 nerves. The physical examination assesses for movement abnormalities. Reproducing part or all of the symptoms helps to implicate a specific structure. Should the physical examination not reveal movement abnormalities in the cervical spine then the headache is less likely to be cervicogenic in origin.

If and when a specific diagnosis of the tissues responsible for the headache can be established, it guides selection of appropriate treatment and helps to improve accuracy of prognosis. Unfortunately, diagnostic tests for detecting specific abnormalities are not available in the typical clinical setting. If a specific diagnosis is not possible, therapeutic intervention is applied to an identified physical impairment with subsequent reassessment to ascertain its benefit.

The physical examination should also help identify lifestyle and extrinsic risk factors, genetic, biomechanical,

and intrinsic risk factors, and evidence of central or peripheral pain mechanisms. Physical examination for cervicogenic headache may require a general examination of the entire musculoskeletal system but more specific attention is directed to the upper cervical spine and its related structures because of their anatomical significance in causation of cervicogenic headaches.

In the following discussion, many of the examination techniques are also appropriate as treatment techniques. Where appropriate, general guidelines for adapting testing procedures for treatment are given.

Observation

Posture in standing can be analyzed for abnormal alignment in the feet, legs, hips, pelvis or spine. With the patient seated, the clinician observes from the front, side and behind for muscular deficits and postural abnormalities such as protracted or winging scapulae, rounded shoulders, an elevated shoulder girdle, increased cervicothoracic kyphosis, and forward head posture. A forward head posture is of particular significance as it places the upper cervical spine in extension, compressing articular structures and placing muscles under excessive loads, possibly leading to muscle imbalance.

The postural examination provides information about extrinsic and intrinsic risk factors. Correcting poor posture, improving core stability, addressing a thoracic or lumbar disorder, or correcting a leg length discrepancy or foot malalignment may remove excessive load on the upper cervical structures and cure a cervicogenic headache if it is a primary causative factor. Chapter 4, *Evaluation of the Spine*, provides a more detailed account of postural assessment.

Mobility Testing

Mobility testing is done routinely to detect possible movement impairments of the upper cervical spine. In evaluating mobility, the clinician is looking for pain response including possible reproduction of headache, total range of movement and specific areas of instability, hypomobility or hypermobility. Deficits identified can be used for reassessment after application of a specific therapeutic intervention. Absence of movement deficits on mobility testing or inability to reproduce the headache do not rule out the cervical spine as a source of headache. In fact, articular hypomobility or a loss of holding capacity of the cervical spine stabilizing muscles may still be present, even with full mobility. It is not uncommon to have pain-free active mobility of the cervical spine and be unable to reproduce the headache with manual examination but to still ameliorate or abolish the headache with mobilization or muscle strengthening techniques applied to the upper cervical spine.

The standard cervical spine active mobility tests detailed in Chapter 4, *Evaluation of the Spine*, can be modified to localize and place greater stress on the upper cervical segments. Mobility testing more specific to the upper cervical spine is detailed here. *The vertebral artery test described in Chapter 4 should be performed prior to all cervical spine tests described in this section.*

Upper Cervical Flexion — Nodding

The patient is instructed to nod the head as if saying "yes", and the movement is observed. To apply overpressure, the clinician stands in front of the patient, placing his left elbow on the front of his body with the left palm facing upward. The patient's chin is placed in the web space between the left thumb and index finger as shown (Fig 9-1). The fingers of the clinician's right hand reach over the patient's head to

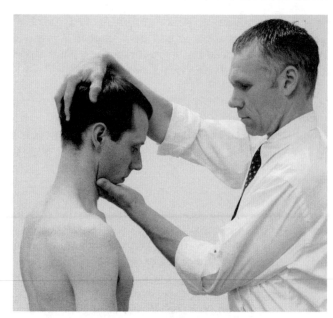

Figure 9-1: Upper cervical flexion — nodding.

grasp beneath the occiput. The clinician then guides the patient's head into a nodding motion, being careful to localize the movement to the upper cervical spine. Both hands work together to over-press this movement.

Upper Cervical Flexion — Retraction

The clinician stands on the patient's left side, placing his right hand on the back of the patient's head and resting his right forearm along the upper thoracic spine. The left hand is positioned so that the web space between the thumb and index finger rests on the front of either the patient's mandible or maxilla.

In this position the clinician's left forearm should be perpendicular to the desired line of motion. The clinician instructs the patient to tuck the chin in, and assists by guiding the movement. Overpressure as necessary can be performed with the left hand, guiding the neck into a retracted position (Fig 9-2). Overpressure can be applied through the maxilla to avoid pressure through the TMJ.

Upper Cervical Extension

The clinician stands to the patient's left side so that his body is in contact with the patient's left shoulder to prevent slouching. The fingers of the clinician's right hand are placed over the top of the patient's head so that they rest just above the eyebrows. The web space of the clinician's left hand comes to rest beneath the mandible. The patient is instructed to poke the chin forward while the clinician guides the movement into upper cervical extension. This is best performed with the clinician using his left hand to pull

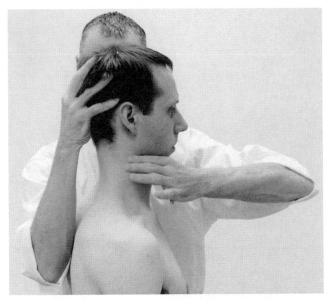

Figure 9-2: Upper cervical flexion—retraction.

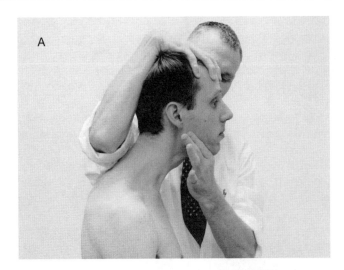

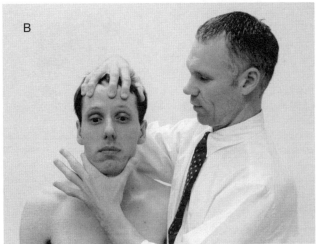

Figure 9-3: Upper cervical extension. A) Lateral view; B) Anterior view.

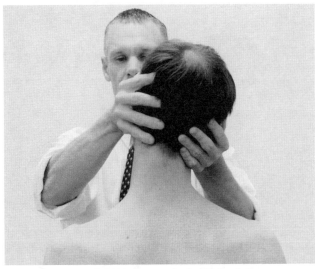

Figure 9-4: Upper cervical side flexion.

up and forward and right hand to pull down and back, adding some degree of compression to the upper cervical joints (Fig 9-3). Care needs to be taken with this motion, as the compression force loads the upper cervical spine.

Upper Cervical Side Flexion

The clinician stands in front of the patient, positioning the ulna side border of both hands on the lateral aspect of the patient's cervical spine at the desired level. The hands rest comfortably on both sides of the cervical spine. The clinician assists the patient into a side flexion position using the ulna side border of one hand as a pivot point while the other hand lifts the cervical spine in an up and over direction, being careful to produce side flexion at and above the desired level only (Fig 9-4). Overpressure can be localized to upper, mid or lower cervical segments depending on the position of the clinician's hands.

Rotation Differentiation of Upper and Lower Cervical Spine

The clinician stands to the left side of the patient with his right forearm behind the patient's left shoulder girdle to fix the trunk. The clinician's right hand rests on the left side of the patient's head and the left hand rests on the right side of the head above the mandible to avoid pressure on the TMJ. The clinician grasps the head so that the patient is still able to hear any instructions (Fig 9-5).

Once overpressure has been applied to the rotation component, an attempt can be made to differentiate symptoms arising from the upper or lower cervical segments. If

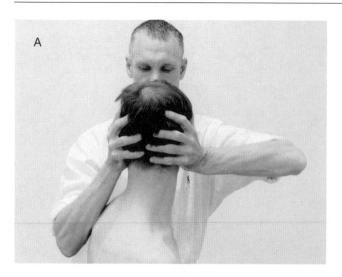

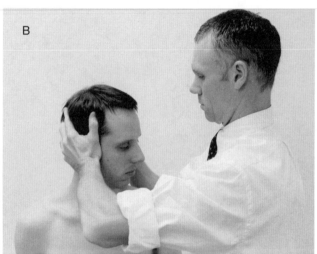

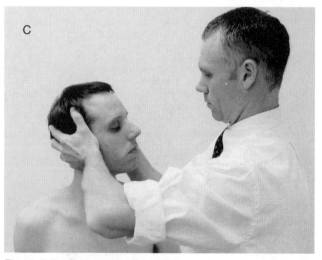

Figure 9-5: Rotation differentiation of upper and lower cervical spine. A) Standard overpressure; B) Addition of upper cervical flexion; C) Addition of upper cervical extension.

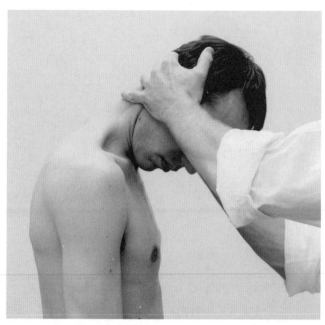

Figure 9-6: Rotation in full cervical flexion.

this rotation movement has reproduced symptoms and it is unclear whether they are arising from the upper or lower segments, the principle is to maintain the lower cervical segments in the identical position while moving the upper cervical segments. This is performed by the clinician applying a very slight upper cervical flexion and/or extension to the patient's head while maintaining the lower cervical segments in the identical position. Any change in symptoms is more likely to implicate the upper cervical segments.

Rotation in Full Cervical Flexion

This test may produce a different response than testing of rotation in the neutral position and may localize rotation more to the C1-2 segment. The clinician stands in front of the patient and asks him to bring the chin fully down to the chest. The clinician then places both hands over the sides of the patient's head. The patient is asked to keep the chin right down to the chest as the clinician assists with active rotation in full cervical flexion (Fig 9-6).

Rotation in Cervical Retraction

Rotation with the cervical spine held in a retracted position may more specifically test segments at C2-3 and below. The clinician stands in front of the patient and instructs him to tuck the chin. The position can be maintained by the clinician's thumbs (Fig 9-7). The clinician asks the patient to slowly rotate the head to one side while maintaining the full retraction position. Resting the thumbs on the anterior aspect of the patient's mandible maintains the cervical spine retraction.

Upper Cervical Quadrant

The upper cervical quadrant is a combined movement of upper cervical extension, ipsilateral rotation, and contralateral or ipsilateral side flexion. By design it is a highly provocative test and should only be attempted when other test movements are full range and the clinician is not concerned about aggravating the presenting condition (Fig 9-8).

For the left quadrant, the clinician stands to the patient's left side so that the right side of his body can prevent the patient from slouching. The fingers of the right hand are placed over the top of the patient's head resting just above the eyebrows. The web space of the clinician's left hand rests beneath the mandible. The patient pokes the chin forward while the clinician guides the movement into upper cervical extension. Overpressure is applied and maintained to the upper cervical extension component.

The second component to add is ipsilateral rotation. This is produced by the clinician simultaneously radially deviating both left and right wrists approximately 5-10° until resistance is felt in the upper cervical segments. While maintaining this position, the third component of ipsilateral upper cervical side bending is added. The clinician produces this by very slightly moving his right hand toward himself and the left hand away until a compression is felt through the upper cervical segments on the left side.

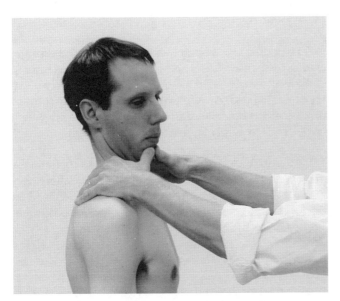

Figure 9-7: Rotation in cervical retraction.

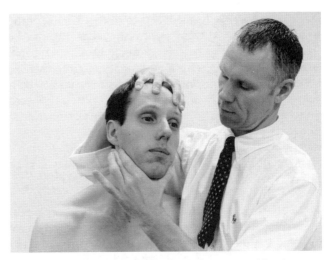

Figure 9-8: Left upper cervical quadrant—combined upper cervical extension, ipsilateral rotation, and ipsilateral side flexion.

Alternatively, contralateral upper cervical side bending can be added as the third component.

Articular System Examination

Articular disorders causing cervicogenic headache may be due to mechanical or inflammatory processes. Manual examination techniques are one method employed in the clinic to detect articular dysfunction that may be a cause of cervicogenic headache. Mechanical disorders of the articular system that can cause cervicogenic headache may be associated with articular movement restriction (hypomobility) or the loss of normal articular restraint mechanisms (instability).

Articular hypomobility can be due to movement restriction of joint capsule and ligaments, abnormal muscle activity or protective muscle spasm. It may also be associated with inflammatory and arthritic conditions. Spinal instability occurs when a vertebral segment displaces further than normal before resistance is encountered and/or displaces beyond its normal range and muscular activity or tension does not control the abnormal movement.[39] This may occur as a result of trauma to articular restraint mechanisms, disease processes, excessive mechanical loads, and inflammatory or arthritic processes.

Upper Cervical Instability Tests

In the upper two cervical segments, capsuloligamentous structures provide a primary restraint mechanism and are aided by the muscular system. Important ligaments in the upper cervical spine are the transverse and alar ligaments and the tectorial membrane.

The transverse ligament acts to restrict flexion of the head and anterior displacement of the atlas.[10] It may be injured by a blow to or a fall onto the back of the head. Examples include falls from gymnastics or motor vehicle accidents. The alar ligaments limit axial rotation to both sides but particularly to the contralateral side.[38] They also limit lateral flexion. They are under greatest tension in rotation and flexion, but can also limit extension.[9] The tectorial membrane is the continuation of the posterior longitudinal ligament. It limits flexion and rotation[35] and may also be important in stabilizing the head vertically.[40]

Upper cervical instability may be caused by inflammation, congenital abnormalities, or excessive mechanical loads and trauma.[2,46] Rheumatoid arthritis, pharyngeal or other infection may lead to inflammation and subsequent laxity of the upper cervical ligaments. Congenital causes may include congenital fusion of two segments placing excessive strain above or below, or syndromes such as Downs syndrome where the transverse ligament may be lax.[2] Clinically it is important to remember that there is a wide spectrum of instability ranging from frank fracture/dislocations to minor instability caused by ligamentous or muscular deficits. Minor instabilities may present with complaints of headache, neck pain or feelings of neck weakness. On palpation examination, the unstable segment may have restricted movement due to muscle guarding. Recognizing upper cervical instability is important because it may change the management approach. Instability may require medical or surgical intervention, may contraindicate manual therapy, or cause the need for special care with manual techniques. The difficulty lies in detecting the instability and then deciding whether it is related to the presenting complaint. At the present time there is little evidence that clinical tests detect the minor instabilities that may present to clinicians.

Findings in the subjective examination that may alert the clinician to the possibility of upper cervical instability include a history of trauma, history of infection or inflammatory disorder like rheumatoid arthritis, clunking or clicking of the upper cervical spine or cord signs associated with neck movement. Care should be taken in performing any of the following clinical tests as they carry certain risks and may be contraindicated.

Sharp-Purser Test . Upper cervical flexion will tend to create an anterior displacement force for the occiput and atlas on the axis. Loss of ligamentous restraints such as insufficiency of the transverse or alar ligaments may create an anterior instability of the atlantoaxial segment. If the transverse ligament of the dens lacks structural integrity the dens may compress the upper cervical spinal cord during cervical spine flexion, eliciting spinal cord signs and

symptoms. More serious pathology such as a fractured dens may also produce a similar clinical presentation.

To perform the test the patient is seated with the neck relaxed in a semi flexed position. The clinician cradles the patient's head with one hand while the other hand stabilizes the tip of the spinous process of the axis with an index finger/thumb pincer grip. The head (taking the atlas with it) is passively moved posteriorly by the clinician, thereby relocating the atlas from its potentially subluxed position on the dens. Any giving way or clicking (dens against anterior arch) or easing of spinal cord symptoms is considered a positive test for atlantoaxial instability.[2,41] This test can be performed from the same position by stabilizing the head and applying a posteroanterior pressure on the spinous process of the axis.

Directing a force to increase the stress on these structures can also assess transverse ligament and dens integrity. In the sitting position, the patient actively flexes the cervical spine as outlined above. The head is then stabilized and a posteroanterior pressure is applied on the posterior arch of the atlas. Any aggravation of symptoms is considered a positive test. Care is needed, as this maneuver will tend to increase any existing subluxation created by the cervical flexion. If the Sharp-Purser test is positive it is suggested not to perform this latter test.

Alar Ligament Test. Upper cervical side flexion should cause an immediate rotation of the axis to the same side due to alar ligament tension. This can be palpated as a deviation of the spinous process of the axis contralateral to the direction of side flexion. Put simply, as soon as the head is taken into left side flexion, the spinous process of the axis should move to the right.

To perform the test the patient is seated. The clinician cradles the patient's head and palpates the spinous process of the axis with the other hand. The clinician laterally flexes the patient's head. Any delay in movement of the spinous process to the opposite side is indicative of alar ligament laxity. The test is then repeated to the other side.

Alternatively the clinician can stabilize the spinous process and lamina of the axis with a thumb-index finger grip. Passive lateral flexion is then applied to the head on the neck in three positions of neutral, flexion, and extension. Movement should be absent or minimal.

Posteroanterior Pressures

Posteroanterior directed pressures are commonly used in manual examination of the upper cervical segments. They may detect hypomobility, provoke localized pain, or reproduce the headache. An unstable spinal segment is usually protected by muscle guarding or spasm that restricts the mobility of that segment. This may mimic hypomobility even though the underlying problem is actually instability.

The detection of movement abnormalities or reproduction of the headache increase the likelihood that cervical structures either cause or contribute to the headache. Mobility findings and symptom and tissue responses are compared to adjacent segments and to what would be expected for that person. At the same time the clinician is questioning for pain reproduction either at the site of palpation or referred to the head or other areas. The contact pressure with the skin may be very broad or very precise depending on the desired effect. Unnecessarily sharp contact pressure may be painful and mask symptom reproduction, so it is important to check that pain reported is not due to sharpness of the contact pressure.

Central P/A Pressure C2.   Posteroanterior pressure over the C2 spinous process may elicit pain or reproduce a headache but will produce only a small amount of movement due to impaction of the dens against the anterior arch of the atlas. The technique is performed with the patient in prone, the cervical spine in slight flexion, and the clinician standing at the head of the plinth. The clinician places his thumbs together over the C2 spinous process or rests one thumb on top of the other over the C2 spinous process (Fig 9-9).

The clinician should begin by establishing if there is any pain at rest. He then gently leans into the movement, applying downward pressure over the C2-3 joint while looking for onset of symptoms. The clinician's thumbs and arms should remain fixed and the transfer of body weight should produce the movement, continuing until the end of range unless limited by spasm, pain or pathology. Does the segment feel restricted or hypomobile? Is it limited by muscle spasm? Is there any pain provocation? The findings assist the clinician in making a clinical diagnosis. This technique can also be performed as a gentle or firm mobilization.

Unilateral Pressure O-C1.   The clinician stands at the head of the plinth with the patient positioned in prone as far up the plinth as possible. With both thumbnails together, the clinician rests the tips of the thumbs over the posterior aspect of the occiput at the level of the O-C1 facet joint. Next the thumbs are slid slightly inferiorly so they can still maintain contact with the occiput. The clinician then leans forward, aligning the forearms and thumbs so that the force will be directed toward the patient's eye on the same side (Fig 9-10).

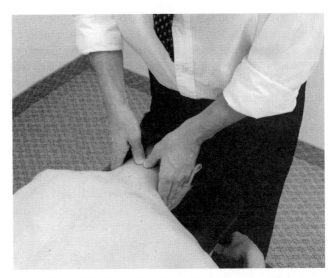

Figure 9-9: Central posteroanterior pressure C2.

To examine unilateral mobility at O-C1, the clinician gently applies pressure over the O-C1 joint by leaning into the movement while looking for onset of symptoms. The clinician's thumbs and arms should remain fixed with the transfer of body weight producing the movement. Pressure continues until the end of range unless limited by spasm, pain or pathology. Does the segment feel restricted? Is the mobility the same as the opposite side? Is there muscle spasm or pain provocation?

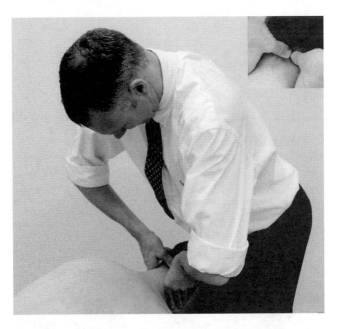

Figure 9-10: Unilateral pressure O-C1. The clinician bends forward to achieve the proper angle. The thumb and forearms are directed toward the patient's eye. Inset shows thumb placement.

Applying unilateral pressure to O-C1 may be easier from the side because less forward bending is required. The clinician stands at the side of the plinth with the patient in prone and close to the clinician. Ideally, the clinician will have one foot positioned in front of the other so the movement can be produced by transference of body weight. The clinician aligns both thumbs so that the thumbnails rest together and the thumbs and forearms are angled toward the patient's eye on the same side (Fig 9-11). The pads of the thumbs are applied just beneath the occiput to either the O-C1 facet joint or different points along the posterior arch of the atlas. The graded pressure is performed using the clinician's body and trunk rather than thumb or forearm musculature. This procedure is described as a test of articular motion but it applies force through several layers of muscle as well. Any abnormalities encountered may be related to muscle spasm, tightness or trigger points rather than definitively identifying an articular disorder. This technique can also be performed as a gentle or firm mobilization.

Unilateral Pressure C1-C2. The clinician stands to the side of the plinth with the patient in prone and close to him. The spinous process of C2 is located as a bony landmark. From the C2 spinous process, the clinician moves his thumbs toward himself to identify the articular pillar over the C2-3 facet joint. To identify the C1-2 joint, the clinician moves his

thumbs further laterally toward himself and then angles the pressure superiorly to access the C1-2 joint, which lies anterior to the rest of the cervical articular pillar. It is often easier to have one thumb as the contact point with the skin and the other thumb reinforcing the movement. At this point the thumbs will be just inferior to the transverse process of the C1 segment (Fig 9-12).

Graded manual pressure is applied using the clinician's body weight rather than movement of the thumbs. The technique is usually applied with a superior and medial inclination, but many different angles should be tried in an effort to reproduce the headache or find the most restricted area. As the vertebral artery crosses this area extreme care should be taken not to provoke any symptoms that may be related to the vertebral artery. This technique can also be performed as a gentle or firm mobilization.

Unilateral P/A Pressure C2-3. Unilateral posteroanterior pressure over the C2-3 facet joint is one of the most valuable manual examination and treatment techniques available to manage cervicogenic headaches. The clinician stands to the side of the plinth with the patient in prone and close to him. The spinous process of C2 is located as a bony landmark. From the C2 spinous process, the clinician moves his thumbs toward himself to identify the articular pillar over the C2-3 joint (about ¾" lateral from the C2 spinous process). It is more readily palpated if the paravertebral muscles are moved medially. The inferior articular process of the C2 segment may be identifiable as a small ridge. The clinician's fingers rest on the opposite side of the neck (Fig 9-13). The thumbs should be perpendicular to the desired

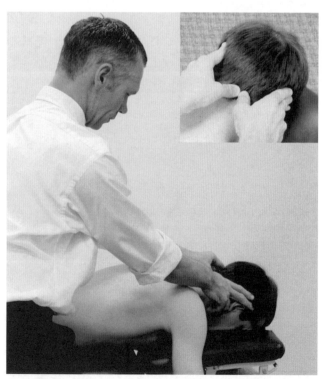

Figure 9-11: Unilateral pressure O-C1, alternate position from the side. The thumb and forearms are directed toward the patient's eye. Inset shows thumb placement.

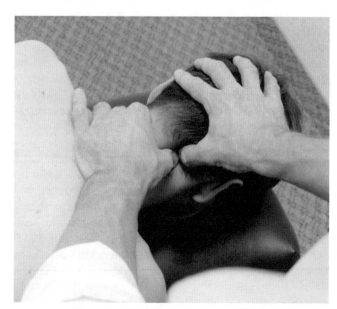

Figure 9-12: Unilateral pressure C1-2.

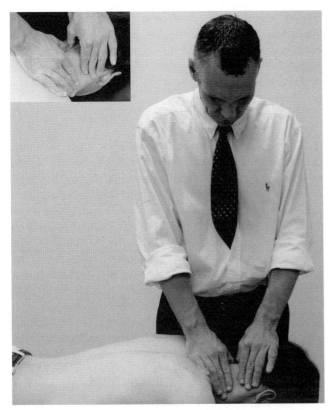

Figure 9-13: Unilateral pressure C2-3. Inset shows thumb placement.

line of movement. Often it is easier to have one thumb as the contact point with the skin and the other thumb reinforcing the movement.

The clinician should begin by establishing if there is any pain at rest. He then gently leans into the movement, applying downward pressure over the C2-3 joint while looking for onset of symptoms. The clinician's thumbs and arms should remain fixed with the transfer of body weight producing the movement. Pressure may be angled in a superior or inferior direction to increase the detail of the examination. Adding a superior inclination to the glide will simulate the movement that occurs with flexion and rotation or lateral flexion in the opposite direction from the side of palpation. Adding an inferior inclination may simulate the movement of extension or rotation or side flexion toward that side. Pressure over the articular pillars can also be angled medially or laterally to further increase the detail of the examination.

Pressure should continue until the end of range, unless limited by spasm, pain or pathology. Does the segment feel restricted? Is the feel at end range one of muscle spasm or is it springy? Mobility findings, symptom and tissue

responses are compared to adjacent segments and to what would be expected as normal for that person.

As well as being a valuable assessment procedure, unilateral P/A pressures over the C2-3 facet joint are often used to treat cervicogenic headaches. Typically they are employed when restricted mobility is present. When there is a predominance of muscle spasm, they should be performed gently and at the beginning of range until there is a noticeable decrease in muscle guarding (sometimes after just a few minutes of mobilization). When there is a significant articular restriction, the technique may need to be very firm, provoking considerable localized discomfort.

P/A Pressure C2 in Rotation.   Posteroanterior pressure applied over the C2 articular pillar will likely influence both the C1-2 and C2-3 joints. In an attempt to differentiate symptoms originating from the C1-2 joint from those arising from the C2-3 joint, a posteroanterior pressure over the C2 articular pillar is tested in both neutral and in approximately 30° of ipsilateral rotation.

The patient is positioned in prone with his forehead in the palms of his hands. Posteroanterior pressure is then applied over the C2 segment in a neutral position as described earlier. This pressure should be to about half the full range of posteroanterior motion. The clinician then stops the pressure and asks the patient to turn his head approximately 30° toward the clinician by putting his eye approximately in the palms of his hands. The clinician then performs the same pressure to the same depth, questioning the patient about any change in symptomatic response and assessing for any change in articular movement (Fig 9-14).

With the cervical spine in 30° of rotation, the articular mechanics change. Since the first 30° of rotation will involve predominantly movement at the C1-2 joint, it is likely that increasing the rotation will have changed the position of the C1-2 joint more than that of the C2-3 joint. Therefore, it can be assumed that any change in symptoms is due to the change in position of the C1-2 joint. This test provides one means to possibly differentiate symptoms arising from the C1-2 and C2-3 segments. Whether the test is able to reliably differentiate symptoms is debatable. Nonetheless, a posteroanterior pressure over C2 in rotation may reproduce symptoms of headache that were not reproducible in the neutral position. This technique can be valuable in both examination and mobilization.

Transverse Pressure C1

Although the predominant movements occurring at the O-C1 segment are flexion and extension, and the predom-

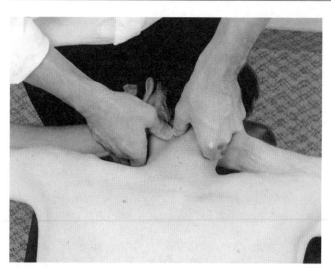

Figure 9-14: Posteroanterior pressure of C2 in rotation.

inant movement at the C1-2 segment is rotation, all these movements are accompanied by small degrees of rotation, side bending and translations. A transverse pressure applied to the transverse process of the C1 segment can assess for minor degrees of transverse glide at C1 segment and for any symptom reproduction.

The patient is positioned in side lying with a towel roll under the head to position the cervical spine in neutral. The clinician stands at the head of the plinth and positions the pad of one thumb over the tip of the C1 transverse process (Fig 9-15). This location is midway between the angle of the jaw and the mastoid process, and is often deep to the sternocleidomastoid muscle. If the contact point is extremely tender, the clinician can move the thumbs slightly posteriorly.

Graded manual pressure is applied using the clinician's body weight rather than movement of the thumbs or forearms. This examination technique may sometimes reproduce headaches and can also be used as an articular mobilization technique.

Distraction Maneuvers

Upper Cervical Distraction in Supine. This technique is primarily used to treat spasm or overactivity of the upper cervical musculature, or when symptoms are thought to arise from inflammation of the upper cervical segments. Upper cervical joint inflammation can occur when an instability underlies the muscle spasm.

Upper cervical distraction is a gentle technique and can be used in conjunction with other soft tissue techniques described later in this chapter. The patient is positioned in supine with the clinician seated at the head of the plinth. The clinician places the fingertips of both hands firmly under the patient's occiput (Fig 9-16). A distraction force is then applied using the fingertips up against the base of the occiput. The position is held for approximately ten seconds before resting and reapplying. The number of repetitions of the distraction technique will vary depending on the clinical indications but in total may last for several minutes.

Upper Cervical Distraction in Prone. This technique is valuable to treat cervicogenic headaches when symptoms arise from overactivity of posterior cervical muscles or inflammatory conditions of the joints. Although it looks difficult for the clinician it is usually quite comfortable for both clinician and patient.

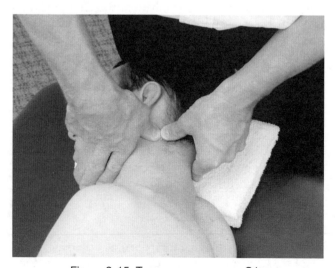

Figure 9-15: Transverse pressure, C1.

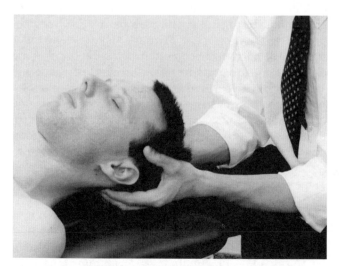

Figure 9-16: Upper cervical distraction in supine.

The patient is positioned in prone with the clinician at the head of the plinth. The clinician leans forward over the patient's body, positioning the ulna side border of each hand under the patient's occiput. The clinician's forearms should be oriented in an upward direction to optimize the mechanics of the movement (Fig 9-17). This technique requires good clinician shoulder mobility. The clinician applies the distraction technique through the forearms and hands. This technique will often apply a stretch to the posterior cervical musculature as well. Being able to perform a distraction mobilization in prone can mean less change of patient position during treatment.

The same technique can be applied from the side, when the clinician has difficulty performing the technique from the head of a plinth. The patient lies in prone with the clinician to the side of the plinth. The clinician should position one leg in front of the other and place the thenar eminences of both hands under the patient's occiput with the fingers resting comfortably over the back of the patient's head (Fig 9-18). The clinician performs the mobilization or stretching technique by transferring his body weight gently from the back foot to the front foot.

Distraction in Sitting.   Distraction is performed in sitting when muscle guarding or inflammatory joint changes are thought to be the predominant cause of headache. The patient sits on either the plinth or on a stool. The clinician stands behind with the thenar eminences of both hands under the posterolateral aspect of the patient's occiput (Fig 9-19). The clinician orients his forearms in the direction of the desired line of motion. The clinician lifts the patient's head to perform the technique. This technique may be useful either as a quick test to ascertain the value of distraction treatment or as a mobilizing technique when a patient is unable to lie down.

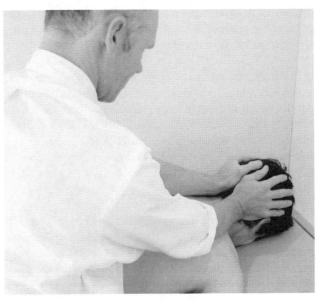

Figure 9-18: Upper cervical distraction in prone, alternate technique from the side.

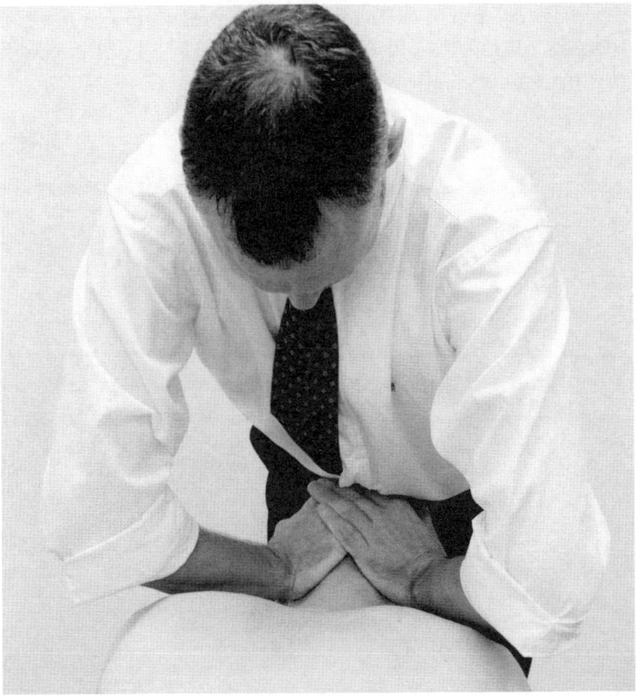

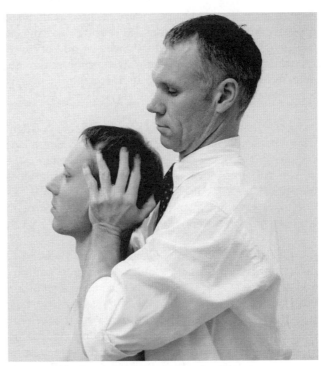

Figure 9-17: Upper cervical distraction in prone.

Figure 9-19: Distraction in sitting.

Muscular System Examination

Muscular system impairments can be a direct cause of cervicogenic headache or may predispose the patient to the development of cervicogenic headache. Impairments of the muscular system may also occur with tension-type headaches or coexist with other headache types, including migraine. Muscular system impairment may involve imbalance between muscles or muscle groups, faulty muscular contraction patterns, or tenderness or trigger points in the muscles themselves.

Muscles innervated by the C1-3 nerves can be a direct source of cervicogenic headache. These include the longus capitis, upper portion of longus cervicis, suboccipital muscles, upper portion of semispinalis capitis, scalenus medius, trapezius and sternocleidomastoid. Muscle dysfunction further down the kinetic chain may predispose the patient to cervicogenic headaches by increasing the load on the upper cervical joints or muscles.

Muscle dysfunction may be caused by a range of extrinsic or lifestyle factors such as poor posture, poor ergonomics or faulty living and working habits. There are many genetic, biomechanical, and intrinsic factors that may predispose to muscular system impairments in cervicogenic headache. These include trauma to the cervical spine and its muscles or to areas further down the kinetic chain. Inflammatory joint disorders such as rheumatoid arthritis may predispose to muscular dysfunction. Altered biomechanics away from the upper cervical spine can place excessive load on cervical muscles causing cervicogenic headache. Hypomobility of the thoracic or mid or lower cervical spine or shoulder girdle dysfunction may place excessive requirements on the muscles thereby increasing the mechanical load on the upper cervical structures.

Other headache types including migraine and tension-type headache may lead to altered function of the muscles of the upper cervical spine. In this instance the person suffering tension-type headaches or migraines may develop secondary tightness of the cervical muscles due to the anatomical and physiologic linkage through the trigeminocervical nucleus.

Evaluation of the muscular system is intended to detect muscular imbalance, faulty contraction patterns, and tender or trigger points. Typical patterns seen in cervicogenic headache are of tightness or overactivity of the upper cervical posterior muscles, often associated with overactivity of the levator scapulae and upper trapezius. There may be poor holding capacity of scapular stabilizing muscles such as the mid and lower trapezius and the serratus anterior. Coupled with poor holding capacity of the scapular stabilizing muscles may be poor functioning of the cervical spine stabilizing muscles

The assessment for muscular dysfunction in cervicogenic headaches includes evaluation for extrinsic risk factors regarding posture, ergonomics and living and working habits. Specific postural evaluation includes analysis of skeletal positioning and muscular definition. When possible, muscular palpation is used to assess for trigger or tender points in muscles. Specific tests can be used to evaluate muscle length and the holding capacity of specific stabilizing muscles.

Posterior Upper Cervical Muscles

Palpation. This technique examines for tightness, tenderness or spasm of the posterior upper cervical muscles and can also be a valuable treatment technique for these deficits. Specifically, it examines the occipital insertion of the upper trapezius and semispinalis capitis muscles, and the deep suboccipital muscles, the rectus capitis posterior major and minor, and the superior and inferior obliques.

The patient lies in prone with the clinician positioned at the side of the plinth. The clinician positions his thumbs side by side on the muscles at the base of the occiput with the fingers pointing away (Fig 9-20). Using both thumbs to sink deeply into the soft tissues, the clinician applies a medially directed force to assess for areas of tightness, tenderness, or spasm. Sustaining the pressure for several seconds allows the clinician to get a good feel of the posterior upper cervical muscles and their responses.

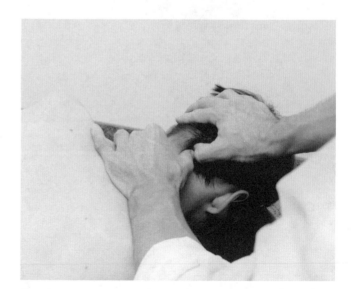

Figure 9-20: Palpation of the posterior upper cervical muscles.

This technique can also be applied as a gentle or strong treatment, depending on the desired effect. When muscle spasm is the predominant finding the technique should be performed slowly and gently with sustained holds until a decrease in spasm is detected. When tightness is the main finding it is often of a long-standing nature and the technique is performed strongly, often in conjunction with stronger stretching techniques and strong articular mobilization procedures.

Cross-Fiber Stretching Technique. This technique can be used in assessment but is mainly used in treatment to address tightness, tenderness or spasm of the posterior upper cervical muscles.

The patient lies in supine with the clinician positioned at the head of the plinth. The clinician places the fingers of both hands just distal to the patient's occiput with the index and middle finger in contact with the skin (Fig 9-21). Using one hand at a time or both hands together, the clinician sinks the fingers deeply through the superficial soft tissues in an attempt to get to the depth of the suboccipital muscles. The most comfortable motion is usually of sinking in deeply and then maintaining the pressure while moving the fingers laterally to apply a cross-fiber stretch to the deep suboccipital muscles. If this is done alternately using left and right hands, a gentle reciprocal rotation motion of the cervical spine can be produced that is both relaxing and therapeutic. This technique will often relieve symptoms of upper cervical pain or headache caused by overactivity of the posterior upper cervical muscles. Symptom relief typically coincides with a palpable decrease in muscle tension beneath the clinician's fingers.

Contract-Relax Technique. Contract-relax techniques are mainly used for hypersensitivity, overactivity or spasm of the posterior upper cervical muscles. The overactivity may

be protecting inflamed or injured articular structures or may be a response to an underlying instability.

The clinician sits or stands at the head of the plinth and places his fingers beneath the patient's occiput in firm contact with the muscles of the suboccipital region. The hands cradle the patient's head. The patient is asked to look up toward the clinician without raising the eyebrows. The clinician should detect a contraction of the muscles beneath his fingertips. After a five to ten second hold the patient returns his eyes to the neutral position, which should cause the posterior upper cervical muscles to relax. This technique may be repeated a number of times until relaxation of the suboccipital muscles is obtained.

If there is no muscle contraction palpated when the patient raises his eyes, or to get a progressively stronger contraction, the patient is asked to lift the eyebrows up at the same time as raising the eyes (Fig 9-22). The clinician should now detect a contraction of the muscles. After maintaining the position for five to ten seconds, the patient is again instructed to relax while the clinician palpates for muscle relaxation. If necessary a more forceful contraction

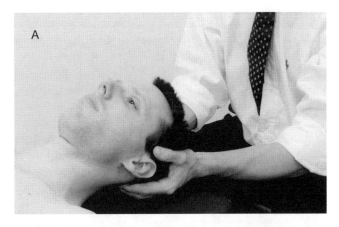

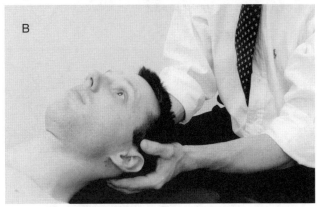

Figure 9-22: Posterior upper cervical muscle contract-relax technique. A) Starting position; B) Contracting by raising the eyebrows.

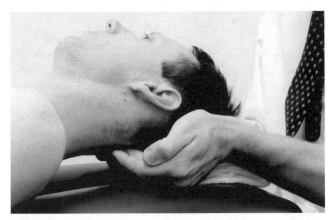

Figure 9-21: Cross-fiber stretching technique for posterior upper cervical muscles.

can be obtained. To do this the patient is instructed to gently tilt the head backward into the resistance of the clinician's hands, without actually moving the head. This is again followed by a hold period and then a relaxation of the contraction. The goal is to get relief of headache caused by overactivity of the upper cervical muscles. The less contraction required to achieve subsequent relaxation and headache relief, the better.

Strong Longitudinal Stretch. This technique can be used to assess for or treat tightness or overactivity of the posterior upper cervical muscles. These muscular impairments occur commonly as a result of long-term poor posture, chronic articular hypomobility, or as a component of other headache types including tension-type headaches and migraine. It can achieve a strong stretch and is not recommended for acute conditions.

The clinician stands at the head of the plinth placing the left hand beneath the patient's occiput and the right hand over the patient's forehead. Ideally the clinician extends the right arm for optimal body positioning (Fig 9-23). Using both hands in a coordinated fashion, the clinician creates a nodding motion of the upper cervical spine. The bottom hand pulls up and backward while the top hand provides a reciprocal down and forward motion. Patients with tightness of the posterior upper cervical region will feel a firm stretch. The stretch should be maintained for about ten seconds and can be repeated several times. It is often used in conjunction with other firm soft tissue and articular techniques.

Oblique Stretch. The oblique stretch technique can be used in assessment or treatment of tightness or overactivity of the posterior upper cervical muscles. Unlike the longitudinal stretch, it stretches one side only. Like the

longitudinal stretch, it can achieve a strong stretch and is not recommended for acute conditions.

The patient lies in supine with the clinician at the head of the plinth. To stretch the left upper cervical region the clinician places the base of his left index finger under the patient's head between the occiput and the left side of the arch of the atlas. The patient's head rests on his left hand, which is resting on the plinth. The patient's head is then positioned into approximately 30° left rotation. The clinician places the heel of his right hand over the patient's right zygoma with the fingers directed toward the floor. The patient's head should then be resting comfortably between his hands.

Using both hands, the clinician radially deviates his wrists to impart upper cervical flexion. Keeping the elbows relatively straight, the clinician applies upper cervical right side bending in the left rotated position by pushing down with the heel of the right hand while pulling up with the left hand until tension is felt in the left cervical region (Fig 9-24). Patients with tightness of the posterior upper cervical region will feel a firm stretch.

Cervical Stabilizing Muscles

The deep cervical muscles are thought to be important for providing stability and postural control to the cervical spine.[8,22,23,30,31,49,50] In contrast to the more superficial muscles that act phasically, the deep muscles are required to act continuously or tonically for prolonged periods of time.

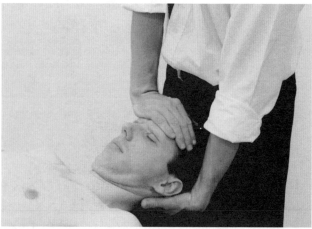

Figure 9-23: Strong longitudinal stretch for the posterior upper cervical muscles.

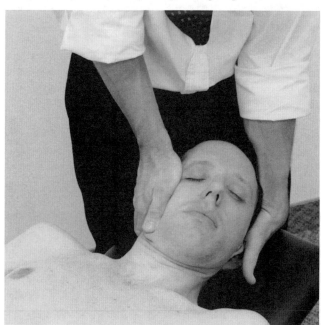

Figure 9-24: Oblique stretch for the posterior upper cervical muscles.

These deep muscles include the deep cervical flexors, the longus colli and longus capitis, and the deep cervical extensors, including the posterior suboccipital extensors, semispinalis capitis, and semispinalis cervicis. Because of painful inhibition, prolonged poor posture and other extrinsic factors, some cervicogenic headache sufferers cannot continuously hold a tonic contraction in the deep cervical muscles.

Deep Flexors—Testing and Retraining. Activation and holding capacity of the deep cervical flexors is difficult to detect and measure due to the deep location of these muscles in the cervical spine. The craniocervical flexion test (CCFT) is an indirect method that seeks to establish their holding capacity.[18,19] With the patient lying in supine with the cervical spine in a neutral position, the motion of upper cervical flexion or nodding can be performed. In theory the superficial and/or deep muscles may perform this movement. If, however, the superficial muscles (sternocleidomastoid, platysma and hyoids) are palpated and found to be inactive it can be reasoned that the muscles performing this movement are in fact the deep cervical flexors.

When this nodding motion is performed with the patient in supine, there will be a decrease in the cervical spine lordosis, as evidenced by a reduced space between the plinth and the back of the patient's neck. The degree of loss of lordosis will be related to many factors including the patient's age and natural flexibility.

The CCFT uses a pressure sensor placed beneath the mid/upper cervical spine to measure the degree to which the space between the back of the patient's neck and the plinth is reduced. This gives both clinician and patient feedback regarding the ability to obtain and maintain a specific position of upper cervical flexion. It can be used both in testing and in retraining of the deep cervical flexors.

The patient lies supine with the head and cervical spine in a neutral position. A folded towel may be placed beneath the patient's head to obtain a neutral position if necessary. The patient is instructed regarding the purpose of the test and the different functions of both the superficial and deep cervical flexors. Emphasis is placed on the fact that the movement of upper cervical flexion or nodding should be gentle and controlled and should feel easy.

To ensure the correct motion is understood, the clinician may use his hands on the patient's head to demonstrate the movement (Fig 9-25). The motion can be likened to nodding as if saying "yes". If the patient has trouble reproducing the movement, a larger range of flexion/extension can be demonstrated. Sometimes an instruction to slide the head down along the surface of the towel can help the patient visualize the proper movement.

The patient is instructed to place the tip of the tongue on the roof of the mouth and keep the jaw relaxed. This prevents the patient from fixing the jaw and substituting with the hyoid muscles. The pressure sensor or pressure biofeedback unit (PBU) is prepared by folding the unit into three and clipping it together. The PBU is then inflated to a baseline pressure of 20 mmHg and squeezed several times to distribute the air in the bag evenly. If the pressure drops after distributing the air in the bag it should be readjusted to the baseline pressure. The folded PBU is then placed beneath the mid/upper cervical spine while the clinician checks the dial to see it still reads 20 mmHg.

Initially it is best for the patient to practice the motion without viewing the PBU gauge and just to focus on the gentle, controlled nodding motion. The superficial anterior neck muscles can be palpated to ensure they are relaxed and the hyoid bone can be passively moved side to side to ensure the hyoid muscles are inactive. The patient is instructed to gently nod the head down without activating the superficial muscles and then maintain this position. The pressure at which the patient can maintain the position without any loss of pressure for ten seconds is the level at which the holding capacity will be tested. Ideally the patient should be able to obtain a pressure increase to at least 26 mmHg, but 28 to 30 mmHg is even better.

For testing the holding capacity, the patient is told to perform ten repetitions of ten second holds at the predetermined pressure (Fig 9-26). If the patient has poor holding capacity, he will tend to substitute by using the superficial muscles or the pressure will fluctuate in a jerky fashion. A common trick movement to be alert for is substitution of the correct movement with a chin tuck or axial extension of

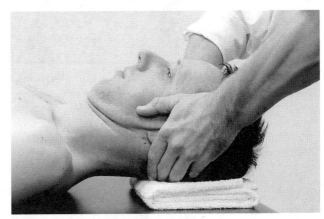

Figure 9-25: Teaching the patient how to correctly perform upper cervical movements to train the deep cervical flexors.

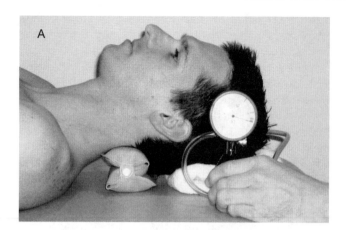

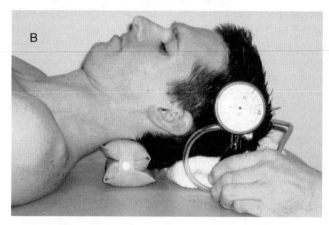

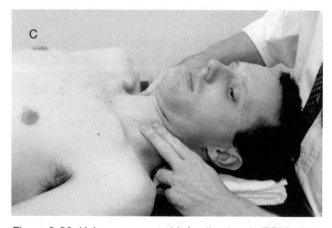

Figure 9-26: Using a pressure biofeedback unit (PBU) while strengthening the deep cervical flexors. A) Starting position; B) Contracting the deep cervical flexors; C) Palpating the muscles during training to ensure no substitution is occurring. (Stabilizer™ Pressure Biofeedback unit from Chattanooga Group, Chattanooga, TN.)

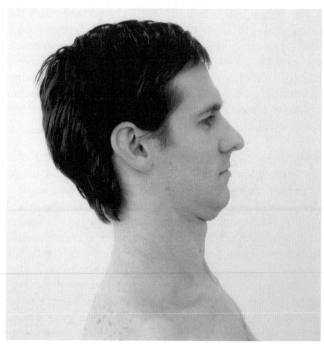

Figure 9-27: Axial extension to retrain the deep cervical stabilizing muscles.

undertakes to perform the exercises in a structured manner at least twice per day. Whenever possible, the goal should be to perform ten sets of ten repetitions at the stated pressure. It may be necessary, however, to begin with fewer repetitions or a shorter hold period. Patients should be taught to monitor the position of the superficial cervical muscles themselves and should also practice with the PBU at home when feasible. An advanced technique involves moving from one pressure level to another. For example, the patient may hold at 26 mmHg and then increase to 28 mmHg, hold for five seconds, and then gradually drop to 26, 24, then 22 mmHg.

The retraining of the deep cervical flexors can be progressed by using the motions of protraction and retraction or cervical flexion and extension in the sitting position. The activity of cervical spine retraction or axial extension involves coordination of both cervical spine flexors and extensors. The patient should be seated with good lumbar spine lordosis and appropriate activation of the deep abdominals and scapula muscles. Performance of a chin tuck or axial extension motion followed by a moderate degree of protraction completes the exercise (Fig 9-27). A suggested dosage is ten sets of ten repetitions.

The movement of full range cervical spine flexion and extension places significant load on the cervical spine articular structures. It is a higher-level activity and is usually only performed once a good level of control has been achieved. In a good sitting posture, the patient is instructed

the neck. It is important to get the correct movement of upper cervical flexion or nodding.

As with any rehabilitation program, it is essential that the patient understands the purpose of the activity and

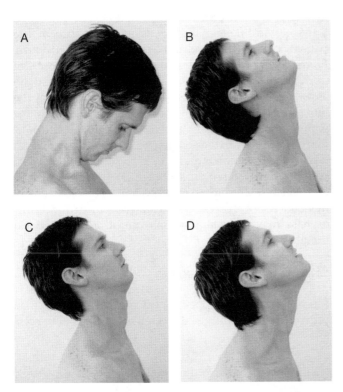

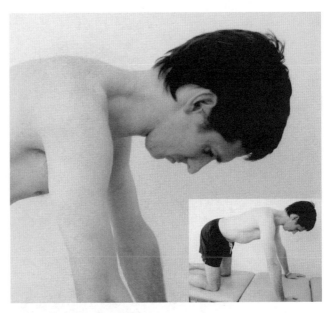

Figure 9-29: Quadruped position to retrain the holding function of the cervical extensors.

Figure 9-28: Controlled cervical flexion/extension. A) Flexed position; B) Extended position; C) Return from extended position showing correct activation of the cervical flexors with segmental rolling; D) Return from extended position showing incorrect activation of cervical flexors, including overactivity of the sternocleidomastoid muscles.

to roll the head down into a fully flexed position from the neutral position. From this fully flexed position, the patient then slowly unwinds the cervical spine to obtain a fully extended position, trying to extend one segment at a time. This should be performed without pain and only when not limited by pathology. The most difficult part of the exercise is returning to the neutral position from the fully extended position.

The goal is to initially flex the upper cervical spine and roll the head down on the neck to return to the neutral position. If patients have inadequate control of the deep cervical flexors, they will tend to initiate the movement from the cervicothoracic junction with overactivity of the sterno-cleidomastoid and superficial muscles (Fig 9-28).

Deep Extensors—Testing and Retraining. Many activities in the work and home environments call for sustained neck postures in a semi-flexed position. This position requires prolonged activation of the cervical stabilizing muscles, including the deep cervical extensors. Loss of holding capacity of the deep cervical extensors may occur as a result of painful inhibition, poor posture or excessive amounts of

time spent with the head and neck in a semi-flexed position.

The four-point kneel or quadruped position can be used for both testing and retraining of the cervical extensor muscles. The patient is positioned in quadruped with the knees beneath the hips, the hands beneath the shoulders and the trunk in a neutral position. The initial task is simply to maintain the cervical spine in a neutral position for a ten second hold (Fig 9-29). This activity is repeated ten times.

Once this is accomplished, slightly greater demands can be placed on the cervical extensors by requiring cervical spine protraction followed by retraction (Fig 9-30). It is important to maintain perfect technique with this exercise, which works the cervical extensors both concentrically and eccentrically. This exercise progression can be used both for testing and retraining. A suggested dosage is ten repetitions with a five to ten second hold.

The addition of cervical spine rotation makes the exercise even more difficult. In the same quadruped position, the patient first obtains a neutral cervical spine position. Maintaining this position, he rotates the head slowly to the left and right, while maintaining a neutral flexion/extension position (Fig 9-31). Rotation to each side should take approximately five seconds to perform and a suggested dosage is ten repetitions to each side. A loss of holding capacity of the deep cervical extensors is evidenced by the patient losing the neutral flexion/extension position and dropping into protraction of the cervical spine.

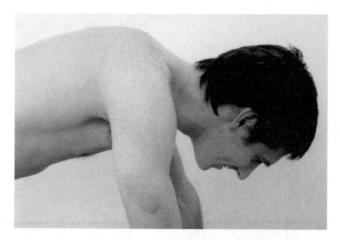

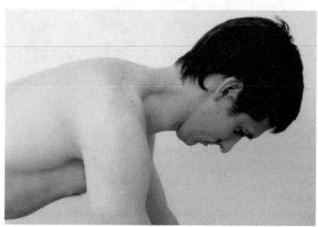

Figure 9-30: Cervical protraction/retraction in quadruped to retrain the holding function of the cervical extensors.

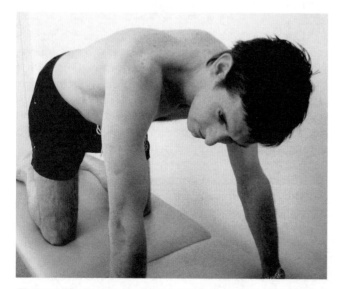

Figure 9-31: Cervical rotation in quadruped to retrain the deep cervical extensors. A loss of holding capacity causes inability to maintain neutral flexion/extension. Protraction of the cervical spine will occur.

An even more difficult and complex exercise involves active cervical flexion and extension in quadruped. The patient begins in the quadruped position described above. From the cervical spine neutral position, an upper cervical flexion motion is performed. If necessary, the clinician can assist with his hands to give the patient an idea of the motion. From the upper cervical flexion position the patient slowly "unfolds" the neck to look up into the position of maximum extension (Fig 9-32). This motion should take five to ten seconds and should be performed only in a pain free range of motion. A dosage of ten repetitions with each cycle taking approximately ten seconds is recommended. A loss of precise segmental movement during this exercise may indicate a lack of control of deep cervical extensor muscles.

Shoulder Girdle Muscles

Muscles such as the upper trapezius and levator scapulae provide a direct linkage between the scapula and the cer-

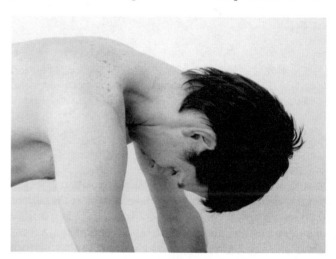

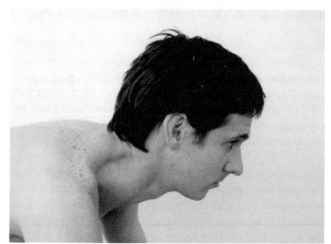

Figure 9-32: Cervical flexion/extension in quadruped—an advanced exercise that must be performed precisely.

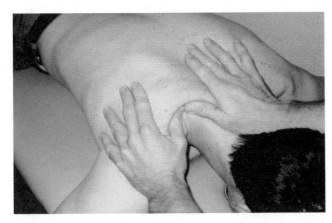

Figure 9-33: Palpating for tightness or trigger points in the upper trapezius.

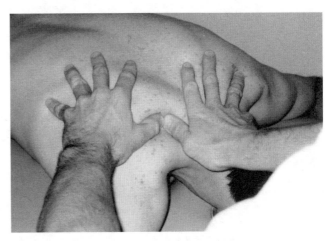

Figure 9-34: Palpating for tightness or trigger points at the scapula attachment of the levator scapulae.

vical spine. Inadequate function of any of the shoulder girdle muscles may place abnormal loads on the cervical spine. Muscular dysfunction may be due to trigger or tender points in the muscles, faulty contraction patterns, or imbalance. Impairment of the shoulder girdle muscles may contribute to cervicogenic headache. Clinical findings for some cervicogenic headache sufferers are trigger or tender points in the levator scapulae and upper trapezius muscles. Other observations include a poor ability to control the position of the scapula, alerting the clinician to poor contraction patterns with possibly inadequate stabilizing function of specific muscles. Scapula winging or protraction is a common finding; this may be associated with poor holding capacity of the serratus anterior and mid and lower trapezius muscles.

Upper Trapezius. The patient lies in prone with the clinician positioned at the head of the plinth slightly to one side. The clinician uses the thumbs or fingers to palpate directly onto the upper trapezius, feeling for areas of tightness or tenderness (Fig 9-33). Stretching and palpatory techniques can be applied to treat tight or tender areas.

Levator Scapulae. The patient lies in prone with the clinician positioned at the head of the plinth slightly to one side. Remembering that the levator scapulae lies deep to the fascia and upper trapezius muscle, the clinician palpates along the line of the levator scapulae for tightness or tenderness. Palpation at the scapular insertion of the levator scapulae will often reveal areas of tenderness and tightness (Fig 9-34). This may be related to overactivity of the levator scapulae in an effort to stabilize the cervical spine during a forward head posture. Techniques to unload the levator scapulae as well as stretching and palpatory techniques can be used.

Middle and Lower Trapezius. Initial exercises should aim to isolate and facilitate the stabilizing muscles. Exercises to

facilitate the middle and lower trapezius can begin in sitting or prone. In a sitting position, the patient is taught to simultaneously retract and depress the scapulae. This can be done unilaterally or bilaterally as appropriate.

Techniques to aid with facilitation include taping, demonstration by the clinician, and positioning of the clinician's thumbs beneath the inferior angle of the scapulae to provide a guide. Another useful facilitation technique is to palpate the coracoid process and instruct the patient to gently retract and depress the scapula by just moving the coracoid process away from the palpating fingers (Fig 9-35). The clinician should monitor for excessive scapula retraction or medial rotation, indicating overactivity of the rhomboids.

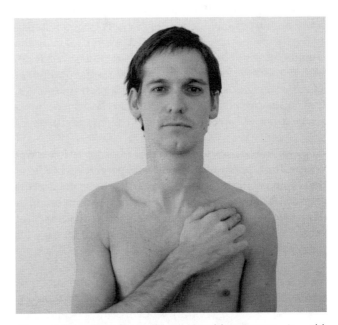

Figure 9-35: Palpating the coracoid process to aid performance of scapular retraction/depression.

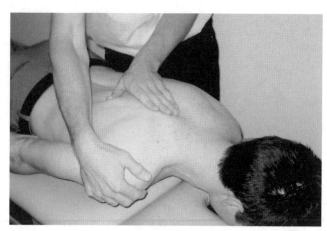

Figure 9-36: Clinician assisting to achieve correct scapula position for activation of mid and lower trapezius.

In prone, the patient is asked to gently pull the shoulder blades back and down. It may be helpful for the clinician to position the scapula appropriately to begin with and ask the patient to hold the position (Fig 9-36). Initially this is performed with the patient's arms at his side at about 30% of the maximum contraction capacity.

A guideline for initial treatment is to aim for ten steady contractions for ten seconds each. The clinician should palpate the relative activity of the upper and lower trapezius muscles with the aim being to minimize or avoid contraction of the upper trapezius. Techniques to facilitate the correct contraction such as visual imagery, use of manual cues, and clinician feedback can be helpful.

Once the patient is able to adequately stabilize the scapulae, bilateral shoulder extension with scapula stabilization in prone can be attempted. While maintaining scapula retraction/depression, the patient is asked to lift both arms a few inches off the plinth into the position of shoulder extension. Shoulder horizontal extension in varying degrees of abduction can then be added. Functional positions can be added as the patient progresses.

Tape can be used to facilitate the middle and lower trapezius. The tape is applied from the superolateral border of the scapula, across the medial border or inferior angle of the scapula. This tape is applied with the scapula in a depressed and retracted position (Fig 9-37). Reassessment is used to evaluate the optimal positioning of the tape for the specific patient.

Serratus Anterior and Scapula Stabilizers. Serratus anterior facilitation may begin in sitting or supine. The first step is to gain an isolated contraction of the muscle and then retrain its holding capacity. Functional tasks are added as the patient improves. Serratus anterior activation is diffi-

cult to perform in isolation and can sometimes be facilitated if the patient palpates the serratus anterior on the rib cage. The motion is of scapula protraction with a small degree of lateral rotation. Once activation is achieved, a program of ten repetitions with ten second holds can be set.

The addition of weight bearing often helps facilitation of the serratus anterior. Initially, the patient can be taught to take some weight through an extended arm resting on a table, while palpating the muscle activity against the rib cage (Fig 9-38).

To further increase weight bearing, the patient is asked to position both hands against a wall with his feet away from the wall. A small push up maneuver against the wall should be performed with the clinician observing the patient's ability to control the scapula position (Fig 9-39). These exercises can be used in both assessment and in rehabilitation where the aim is to control winging of the scapula.

The scapula stabilizers can also be retrained in the four point kneel or quadruped position. The patient assumes the quadruped position with good control of the lumbar spine, scapula and cervical spine posture. Weight shifting, cervical spine or limb movements are added, while the patient maintains core stability (Fig 9-40).

A modified push up from the knees is another good activity for assessment and treatment of scapula stability. During this movement, right and left scapula position and control is compared (Fig 9-41). Slow eccentric contraction

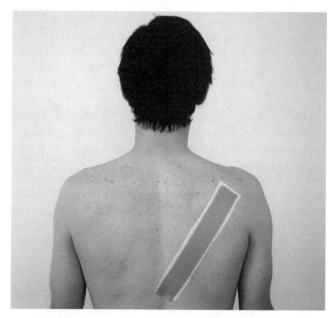

Figure 9-37: Taping to facilitate activation of the mid and lower trapezius.

will often reveal muscular fatigue and lack of control. Exercises can be progressed from easier positions to more difficult ones.

In patients with chronic neck problems and associated headaches, the existence of muscle system impairments is very likely. These patients will often require a considerable length of time to correct faulty patterns of movement. Motor skill learning principles such as practice, rest periods, beginning gently, not exercising when fatigued, clinician feedback, and the use of tape are valuable.

Diagnosis and Treatment of Cervicogenic Headache Summarized

In managing musculoskeletal disorders, identification of a specific pathological entity using valid and reliable diagnostic tests assists implementation of an optimal management regimen. It also assists in determining an accurate prognosis. Wherever possible, a specific diagnosis should be sought.

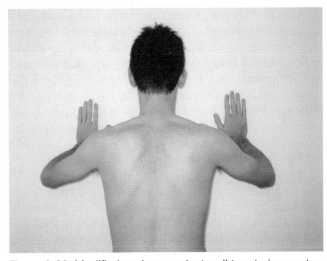

Figure 9-39: Modified push up against wall to retrain serratus anterior and scapular stabilizers.

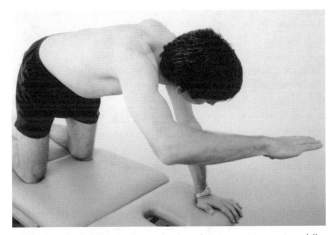

Figure 9-40: Addition of cervical and arm movements while maintaining core stability.

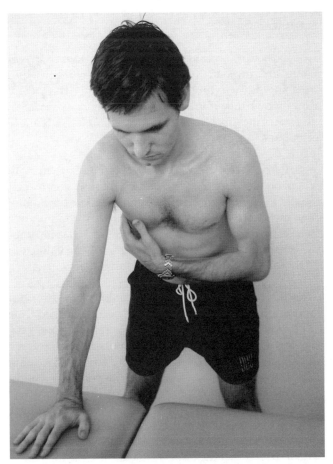

Figure 9-38: Activation of serratus anterior with mild weight bearing and palpation on the rib cage.

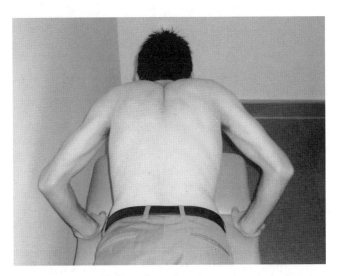

Figure 9-41: Modified push up from knees to retrain serratus anterior and scapular stabilizers.

For patients presenting with headache, the subjective examination assists in identifying whether the headache fits the profile of cervicogenic headache. Often a headache will have some components that are compatible with a cervicogenic cause, but the picture isn't perfectly clear. Other symptoms less commonly associated with cervicogenic headache may also be present. The physical examination of articular and muscular systems seeks to identify specific physical impairments that may be related to or consistent with cervicogenic headache.

Even if a headache can be categorized as a cervicogenic headache on the basis of IHS classification, subjective criteria, and evidence of specific physical impairments, this does not necessarily identify the specific structures at fault. The IHS's diagnostic criteria for cervicogenic headache states that it should be possible to abolish the headache with diagnostic blockade of the causative tissues or their nerve supplies. In typical clinical practice, however, it is not practical to use these procedures.

Nonetheless, patients presenting with headache still require management. The clinician should not shy away from treating identifiable problems that may contribute to cervicogenic headache, just because a definitive diagnosis cannot be made. On the other hand, test/retest procedures should be used to make sure any treatment is having its intended effect. Otherwise, the assumption that the headache is cervicogenic in origin must be challenged.

Specific guidelines for clinical decision-making are found below. These guidelines help identify contributing factors and appropriately manage cervicogenic causes of headache. Keep in mind that migraines, cluster headaches, and tension-type headaches can involve a cervical component. The guidelines below can be used for physical therapy management of any headache that involves the cervical spine, even if the primary cause is not cervicogenic.

Be Alert for Red Flags

The clinician should always watch for conditions not appropriate for mechanical therapy, and should identify when certain physical interventions are contraindicated or where medical intervention is necessary. Precautionary signs and symptoms have been discussed in this chapter and in *Chapter 3, Medical Screening*.

Make a Diagnosis When Possible

Ascertain from the subjective examination if the headache fits the profile of cervicogenic headache. If it does, establish from the physical examination if mechanical impairments are present that are consistent with cervicogenic headache. If a specific diagnosis can be made, commence treatment accordingly. If a specific diagnosis is not possible, mechanical intervention is based on the physical impairments detected. It is often necessary to administer three or four sessions of treatment to determine whether a cervical impairment is contributing to or causing the headache.

It is important to remember that a cervical impairment in the presence of headache may be causative, coexisting, incidental, contributory, or a trigger.

Treat Musculoskeletal Impairments

Articular System. With instability, articular techniques will usually be gentle, directed to relief of muscle spasm. If hypomobility is present, techniques usually include firm or strong articular mobilization procedures.

Muscular System. If the patient has posterior upper cervical muscle spasm, tenderness or overactivity, gentle palpation, cross-fiber stretching or contract-relax techniques work well.

If posterior upper cervical muscle tightness or trigger points are present, strong palpation techniques and stretching of these muscles are appropriate. The patient using his own fingers to apply soft tissue massage or digital pressure to the suboccipital region can complement clinical techniques.

If the deep cervical muscles lack holding capacity, activation of the deep cervical flexors should commence, initially in supine with emphasis on the tonic function of these muscles. The PBU can be used to test and improve exercise performance. Exercises are progressed to incorporate activation of the cervical extensors and are tailored to fit the patient's specific functional requirements.

When the scapular muscles lack holding capacity, activation of the specific muscles should be emphasized. This will typically include the mid/lower trapezius and possibly the serratus anterior, with the emphasis on their tonic function. Exercises can be progressed as required to more difficult tasks and to suit the patient's functional demands.

Sometimes, scapular muscle overactivity, trigger points or tightness will be detected. The levator scapulae or upper trapezius muscles are typically involved, and may benefit from stretching or palpation techniques.

Address Lifestyle and Extrinsic Risk Factors

Posture. Because sleeping posture can aggravate cervicogenic problems, proper sleeping postures and the appropriate use of pillows should be reviewed. Postural awareness exercises and re-education of postural muscle groups, including scapula stabilizers and deep abdominals, may be helpful.

Ergonomics. Occupational positions and workplace design should be reviewed. Patients should be instructed to take breaks from sustained postures and perform home exercises that reverse stressful positions at work or otherwise help promote an overall balanced posture.

Variety of Movement. A variety of activities requiring different patterns of movement and activation of different muscle groups can be beneficial for people whose work and daily living activities are highly repetitive. Many patients benefit from participation in new sports or activities such as yoga.

Address Genetic, Biomechanical, and Intrinsic Risk Factors

Altered mechanics of lumbar, thoracic or cervical segments or the thoracic cage and related musculature may need to be treated. Other biomechanical factors such as poor foot mechanics or leg length discrepancies also may need to be addressed. Although some genetic and intrinsic risk factors cannot be changed, the simple recognition that these factors contribute may help both clinician and patient understand the cause of the headaches and why they may be resistant or slow to respond to treatment.

Address Psychosocial Risk Factors

Psychosocial factors that may predispose the patient to chronic pain include attitudes and beliefs about pain, fear avoidance behaviors, anxiety or depression, and compensation, family and work issues. If these factors are present and interfering with successful treatment, referral to other practitioners may be advised. The physical therapist may play a role in wellness education, encouraging relaxation, good sleep habits, a balanced diet and appropriate physical exercise.

Address Pain Mechanisms

The primary pain mechanism of cervicogenic headache is due to irritation of the tissues innervated by the peripheral nervous system, but inflammatory and central components to cervicogenic or other headache types may need to be addressed with appropriate medications and therapies.

Special Considerations for Rheumatoid Arthritis and Upper Cervical Instability

Rheumatoid arthritis and upper cervical instability are two specific diagnostic entities that require special mention, since some of the more aggressive treatment techniques used to treat cervicogenic headache may be contraindicated.

Rheumatoid arthritis can be easily detected medically, and most patients are aware of their diagnosis prior to being seen in the physical therapy clinic. Upper cervical instability, on the other hand, is not reliably detected from diagnostic or clinical testing. Clinicians should be alert to a history of a blow or fall on the back of the head coupled with a headache that is aggravated by cervical spine flexion. This combination of symptoms may be indicative of laxity or damage to the transverse ligament or tectorial membrane, with possible excessive anterior mobility of the occiput and atlas on the axis. Other physical findings likely with upper cervical spine instability are protective guarding of the posterior upper cervical muscles, onset of headache with upper cervical flexion, and articular mobility limited by pain and muscle guarding.

If the clinical features are consistent with those described above, a working diagnosis of upper cervical instability can be made. Initial treatment may include immobilization in a collar. Very gentle techniques directed toward protecting the posterior upper cervical muscles and relieving muscle guarding may be indicated. Gentle soft tissue palpatory or cross-fiber stretches or the contract-relax technique described earlier can be used. Patients should be instructed to avoid cervical spine flexion in daily activities. Deep cervical flexor retraining is usually contraindicated and even the gentlest attempts to perform it tend to create severe aggravation of the symptoms.

Once the acute symptoms have settled, gentle stabilizing exercises in a neutral position can be attempted, but these can also provoke symptoms. The inability to sustain cervical spine flexion may necessitate the avoidance of occupations requiring prolonged computer work or head down positions.

Headache in a patient with rheumatoid arthritis presenting with the same symptoms is assumed to be related to upper cervical spine instability, since rheumatoid arthritis leads to laxity of these same ligaments. Thus, management is the same. This principle also applies to any other systemic or genetic disorder that may cause ligamentous laxity, such as Down's syndrome or pharyngeal infection.

Physical Therapy Management of Headache Patients Summarized

Cervicogenic Headache

In cases where the sole cause of the headache is abnormal function of the muscles or joints of the cervical spine, treatment directed toward these impairments forms the mainstay of management. The clinician can use specific interventions in an attempt to correct articular and muscular mechanical impairments. These physical impairments are said to be *causative* of the headache. If there is an inflammatory component to the cervical spine pathology this may be addressed concurrently with appropriate medications.

Although the IHS suggests that treatment must result in complete abolition of the headache within three months, this does not always occur clinically. Pathologies may indeed be ongoing or there may be underlying instability or articular hypomobility caused by degenerative changes. Similarly there may be structural changes further down the kinetic chain that continue to place excessive load on the upper cervical segments. These conditions may prolong the resolution of cervicogenic headache. Nonetheless, where there is a true cervicogenic headache, physical therapy is the main focus of treatment for the mechanical component of these headaches.

Other Headache Types

Because of the complex anatomy and physiology involved in head pain, separation of headaches into specific diagnostic categories as suggested by the IHS is not always possible. The clinical picture may be complicated, with many factors contributing to the presenting headache. Many headache types that do not fit the specific IHS criteria for cervicogenic headache respond well to manual therapy directed to the upper cervical spine.

When the headache's primary cause is due to central disinhibitory phenomena, dietary or hormonal factors or allergies, physical therapy may be less beneficial. When there are cervical spine abnormalities detected on physical examination but appropriate treatment directed to these does not cause any change in the presenting headache, these physical signs are said to be *incidental* to the headache.

When the presenting headache is a mixed pattern or primarily fits a tension-type or migraine headache pattern, some features suggestive of a cervicogenic component such as tightness in the upper part of the neck may also be present. A trial of three or four physical therapy treatments is indicated to ascertain whether impairments of the upper cervical articular or muscular structures are contributing to the presenting headaches. In many instances, treatment directed to the cervical spine has a beneficial effect on parameters such as the frequency, intensity or possibly duration of the headaches. When treatment of the cervical spine has a clearly beneficial effect on what is predominantly a migraine, mixed or tension-type headache, the cervical spine impairment is deemed to be *contributory* to the overall headache presentation.

Sometimes after an episode of migraine, a patient will present with neck stiffness and residual head pain that is different from his normal migraine pain. Physical therapy directed to the neck will often help to completely resolve the headache. In this case, the migraine resolves, leaving a headache that is purely cervicogenic in origin. This is an example of two discrete headache entities *coexisting*.

It is not uncommon for patients to present with a long history of migraines where over time, they notice neck stiffness with a corresponding marked increase in migraine headache frequency. Physical therapy directed to the musculoskeletal impairments will often reduce the frequency of migraines to their previous level. In this situation we would say that the cervical spine was a *trigger* for another type of headache. The goal of physical therapy is to remove the trigger.

Part of the Team

The more clinicians understand the pathophysiology of all headache types, the various factors that can trigger them, and the pharmacological and non-pharmacological interventions available, the more they will be able to help improve the quality of life of their patients.

Physical therapists who can accurately differentially diagnose headaches and assess and treat articular and muscular impairments with specific intervention strategies form a valuable part of the team. Physical therapists are primary practitioners for treating the mechanical components of cervicogenic headache, but they should realize that appropriate mechanical intervention to cervical spine structures could also play a valuable role in treating other types of headache, such as migraine and tension-type headache. Chronic headache sufferers experience severe lifestyle restrictions. With appropriate management of all the various components by experts in each specific discipline, chronic headache sufferers can usually continue a full and relatively normal lifestyle. Being able to assist with overall management strategies and being the clinician of choice for managing the musculoskeletal component of headache can be a most rewarding experience.

REFERENCES

1. Anthony M, Lance JW: Plasma Serotonin in Patients with Chronic Tension Type Headaches. J Neurol Neurosurg Psychiatry 52:182-184, 1989.
2. Aspinall W: Clinical Testing for the Craniovertebral Hypermobility Syndrome. J Orthop Sports Phys Ther 12(2):47-53, 1990.
3. Bogduk N: Anatomy and Physiology of Headache. Biomed Pharmacother 49(10):435-445, 1995.
4. Bogduk N: Anatomy of Headache. In: Proceedings of Headache and Face Pain Symposium, M Dalton, ed. pp 1-16. Manipulative Therapists Association of Australia, Brisbane 1989.
5. Bogduk N: Cervical Causes of Headache and Dizziness, Chapter 22. In: Modern Manual Therapy of the Vertebral Column, 2nd ed. JD Boyling and N Palastanga, eds. pp 317-331. Churchill Livingstone, Edinburgh 1994.
6. Butler DS: The Sensitive Nervous System. Noigroup Publications, Adelaide 2000.
7. Charman RA: Pain and Nociception: Mechanisms and Modulation in Sensory Context, Chapter 18. In: Modern Manual Therapy of the Vertebral Column, 2nd ed. JD Boyling and N Palastanga, eds. pp 253-270. Churchill Livingstone, Edinburgh 1994.
8. Conley MS, Meyer RA, Bloomberg JJ, et al: Noninvasive Analysis of Human Neck Muscle Function. Spine 20:2505-2512, 1995.
9. Dvorak J, Panjabi MM: Functional Anatomy of the Alar Ligaments. Spine 12(2):183-189, 1987.
10. Dvorak J, Schneider E, Saldinger P, et al: Biomechanics of the Craniovertebral Region: The Alar and Transverse Ligaments. J Orthop Res 6(3):452-461, 1988.
11. Goadsby PJ, Lambert GA, Lance JW: Differential Effects on the Internal and External Carotid Circulation of the Monkey Evoked by Locus Coeruleus Stimulation. Brain Res 249:247-254, 1982.
12. Goadsby PJ, Lambert GA, Lance JW: Effects of Locus Coeruleus Stimulation on Carotid Vascular Resistance in the Cat. Brain Res 278:175-183, 1983.
13. Goadsby PJ, Piper RD, Lambert GA, et al: The Effect of Activation of the Nucleus Raphe Dorsalis (DRN) on Carotid Blood Flow. I. The Monkey. Am J Physiol 348:R257-R262, 1985.
14. Goadsby PJ, Piper RD, Lambert GA, et al: The Effect of Activation of the Nucleus Raphe Dorsalis (DRN) on Carotid Blood Flow. II. The Cat. Am J Physiol 348:R263-R269, 1985.
15. Headache Classification Committee of the International Headache Society: Classification and Diagnostic Criteria for Headache Disorders, Cranial Neuralgias and Facial Pain. Cephalalgia 8 (Suppl 7), 1988.
16. Headache Classification Subcommittee of the International Headache Society (IHS): The International Classification of Headache Disorders, 2nd ed. Cephalalgia 24 (Suppl 1), 2004.
17. Humphrey T: The Spinal Tract of the Trigeminal Nerve in Human Embryos Between 71/2 and 81/2 Weeks of Menstrual Age and its Relation to Early Fetal Behavior. J Comp Neurol 97:143-209, 1952.
18. Jull G: Headaches of Cervical Origin. In: Clinics in Physical Therapy: Physical Therapy of the Cervical and Thoracic Spine. 2nd ed. Grant R, ed. pp 261-285. Churchill Livingstone, New York 1994.
19. Jull G: Management of Cervical Headache. Manual Therapy 2(4):182-190, 1997.
20. Kendall NAS, Linton SJ, Main CJ: Guide to Assessing Psychosocial Yellow Flags in Acute Low Back Pain: Risk Factors for Long Term Disability and Work Loss: Accident Rehabilitation and Compensation Insurance Corporation of New Zealand and the National Health Committee, Wellington 1997.
21. Kerr FWL: Structural relation of the Trigeminal Spinal Tract to Upper Cervical Roots and The Solitary Nucleus in the Cat. Experimental Neurology 4:134-148, 1961.
22. Keshner E, Campbell D, Katz R, et al: Neck Muscle Activation Patterns in Humans during Isometric Head Stabilization. Exp Brain Res 75:335-344, 1989.
23. Keshner E, Peterson B: Mechanisms Controlling Human Stabilisation. 1. Head-Neck Dynamics during Random Rotations in the Horizontal Plane. J Neurophysiol 73:2293-2301, 1995.
24. Lance JW, Goadsby PJ: Mechanism and Management of Headache. 6th ed. Butterworth Heinemann, Oxford 1998.
25. Lauritzen M: Pathophysiology of Migraine Aura. The Spreading Depression Theory. Brain 117:199-210, 1994.
26. Leak AM, Cooper J, Dyer S, et al: The Northwick Park Neck Pain Questionnaire, Devised to Measure Neck Pain and Disability. Br J Rheumatol 33:469-474, 1994.
27. Leão AAP: Spreading Depression of Activity in Cerebral Cortex. J Neurophysiol 7:359-390, 1944.
28. Maitland GD, Hengeveld E, Banks K, et al: Maitland's Vertebral Manipulation. 6th ed. Butterworth Heinemann, Oxford 2000.
29. May A, Ophaff RA Terwindt, GM, et al: Familial Hemiplegic Migraine Locus on Chromosome 19p13 is Involved in Common Forms of Migraine With and Without Aura. Human Genet 96:604-608, 1995.
30. Mayoux-Benhamou MA, Revel M, Vallee C, et al: Longus Colli has a Postural Function on Cervical Curvature. Surg Radiol Anat 16:367-371, 1994.
31. Mayoux-Benhamou MA, Revel M, Vallee C: Selective Electromyography of Dorsal Neck Muscle in Humans. Exp Brain Res 113(2):353-360, 1997.
32. Meyer DER, Snow PJ: Distribution of Activity in the Spinal Terminals of Single Hair Follicle Afferent Fibers to Somatopically Identified Regions of the Cat Spinal Cord. J Neurophysiol 56:1022-1038, 1986.
33. Moskowitz MA: Neurogenic Versus Vascular Mechanisms of Sumatriptan and Ergot Alkaloids in Migraine. Trends Pharmacol Sci 13:307-311, 1992.
34. Moskowitz MA: The Neurobiology of Vascular Head Pain. Ann Neurol 16:157-168, 1984.
35. Oda T, Panjabi MM, Crisco JJ, et al: Role of Tectorial Membrane in the Stability of the Upper Cervical Spine. Clin Biomech 7(4):201-207, 1992.
36. Olesen J, Larsen B, Lauritzen M: Focal Hyperemia Followed by Spreading Oligemia and Impaired Activation of rCBF in Classic Migraine. Ann Neurol 9(4):344-352, 1981.
37. Ophoff RA, Terwindt, GM, Vergouwe, MN, et al: Familial Hemiplegic Migraine and Episodic Ataxia Type-2 are Caused by Mutations in the Ca^{2+} Channel Gene CACNLA4.

Cell 87:543-552, 1996.

38. Panjabi MM, Dvorak J Crisco J, et al: Effects of Alar Ligament Transection on Upper Cervical Spine Rotation. J Orthop Res 9(4):584-593, 1991.

39. Panjabi MM: The Stabilizing System of the Spine, Part II. Neutral Zone and Instability Hypothesis. J Spinal Disord 5(4):390-397, 1992.

40. Penning L: Functional Pathology of the Cervical Spine. Excerpta Medica Foundation 1968.

41. Pettman E: Stress Tests of the Craniovertebral Joints. In: Modern Manual Therapy of the Vertebral Column, 2nd ed. JD Boyling and N Palastanga, eds. pp 529-537. Churchill Livingstone, Edinburgh 1994.

42. Queiroz LP, Rapoport AM, Weeks RE, et al: Characteristics of Migraine Visual Aura. Headache 37(3):137-141, 1997.

43. Raskin NH: On the Origin of Head Pain. Headache 28:254-257, 1988.

44. Rolfe LH, Wiele G, Brune GG: 5-Hydroxytryptamine in Platelets of Patients with Muscle Contraction Headache. Headache 21:10-11, 1981.

45. Silberstein SD, Lipton RB: Overview of Diagnosis and Treatment of Migraine. Neurology 44(Suppl 7):S6-S16, 1994.

46. Swinkels R, Beeton K, Alltree J: Pathogenesis of Upper Cervical Instability. Manual Therapy 1(3):127-132, 1996.

47. Torvik A: Afferent Connections of the Sensory Trigeminal Nuclei, the Nucleus of the Solitary Tract and Adjacent Structures. J Comp Neurol 106:51-141, 1956.

48. Vernon H, Moir SA: The Neck Disability Index: A Study of Reliability and Validity. J Manipulative Physiol Ther 14:409-415, 1991.

49. Vitti M, Fujiwara M, Basmajain J, et al: The Integrated Roles of Longus Coli and Sternocleidomastoid Muscles: An Integrated Electromyographic Study. Anat Rec 177:471-484, 1973.

50. Winters JM, Peles JD: Neck Muscle Activity and 3-D Head Kinematics During Quasi-Static and Dynamic Tracking Movements. In: Multiple Muscle Systems: Biomechanics and Movement Organisation, JM Winters and SL-Y Woo, eds. pp 461-480. Springer-Verlag, New York 1990.

51. World Cervicogenic Headache Society. http://www.cervicogenic.com/definit1.htm July 15, 2003.

10

JOINT MOBILIZATION

H. Duane Saunders, MS PT and Robin Saunders Ryan, MS PT

Joint mobilization and manipulation techniques are passive movements applied to joints in a specific manner to normalize joint motion. Physical therapists often use the term *manual therapy* to encompass the wide variety of techniques used. Manual therapy is an art that has been practiced since prehistoric times. It was first documented by Hippocrates (460 BC - 375 BC). He taught his students to apply a vertical manipulative thrust on a gibbus (prominent vertebra) and to give exercises afterward. Galen describes manipulation of the spine for misalignment in a patient following trauma to the neck.[35]

For many centuries in England, bonesetters practiced manipulation as a family tradition. People consulted them to have their painful joints manipulated. Bonesetters still exist today in many European countries. In 1876, Sir James Paget (1814-1899), the renowned British surgeon, published his famous lecture, *Cases That Bonesetters Cure*, in the British Medical Journal. Paget delineated the types of cases that were responsive to manipulative therapy. He exhorted his readers to "Learn them...imitate what is good and avoid what is bad in the practice of bonesetters." Paget's words fell on deaf ears. Orthodox medicine of the day found the rationale behind bonesetting untenable, an attitude probably justified in part even though patients who had visited bonesetters attested to their skill.[35]

Two joint mobilization/manipulation schools of thought are osteopathy and chiropractic. Superficially, these two schools bear certain resemblances to each other with regard to the mechanistic approach to illness but beyond that, their scopes and philosophies are quite different.[35]

The history of osteopathy is intimately connected with Andrew Taylor Still (1828-1917). He studied medicine at the College of Physicians and Surgeons in Kansas City, Missouri. Still lost three of his sons in an epidemic of spinal meningitis, even though they had the best medical treatment available. Still became disillusioned with orthodox medicine as it was practiced during his day. A deeply religious man, the idea of osteopathy came to Still like a "revelation." He concluded that the human body possessed self-healing properties, that efficient functioning was dependent on unimpaired structure, and that proper nerve and blood supply to the tissues was necessary for health maintenance. These concepts were contained in his "Rule of the Artery" which he proclaimed in 1874 and which became the basic concept of osteopathy. He founded the American School of Osteopathy in 1892 in Kirksville, Missouri.[35] Today, osteopathic physicians (DO's) may be found in virtually every field of medicine and surgery as their backgrounds have expanded to encompass both osteopathic and allopathic knowledge.

Chiropractic began in Davenport, Iowa with Daniel David Palmer, a grocer. Palmer, having read some of Still's work, reported in 1895 that he cured the deafness of a janitor after he adjusted the latter's misaligned vertebra. Palmer's belief was that the spinal column was the controller of the human machinery and that all diseases could be traced to it. He formulated "The Law of the Spinal Nerve" as the basis for chiropractic. Palmer founded the first chiropractic school in Davenport in 1897. His adolescent son was its first graduate. Today there are 16 colleges that are accredited by the Council on Chiropractic Education, a specialty accreditation program recognized by the US Department of Education.

The basis of chiropractic philosophy is the theory of subluxation. Chiropractors claim that subluxation in the spinal column interferes with nerve function and that this is the significant factor in disease causation. Manipulation of the appropriate area of the spine restores the natural alignment of the spine, which relieves the symptoms. Statements regarding the adjustment of the spine for disorders such as diabetes, various intestinal disorders, heart trouble and cancer are quite common in chiropractic literature.[35]

There is still no consensus as to the rationale behind spinal manipulation, but there exists a wealth of theories. Each school of thought has advanced its own rationale and has evolved manipulative techniques consistent with it.

The number of allopathic physicians (MD's) who have recognized and used manipulative principles is growing, and several physicians have made remarkable contributions to its conceptualization. James Mennell published a book in 1952 entitled *The Science and Art of Joint Manipulation*. He pointed to the facet joints, postural strain and adhesions as causative factors in back pain. Later, his son John enunciated the concepts of joint play and joint dysfunction.[35]

More than any other physician, James Cyriax has demonstrated the usefulness of manipulation to the medical profession. His book, *Textbook of Orthopædic Medicine*, first published in 1954, is a valuable resource.[11] Because of his ardent belief in the disc as a source of back pain problems, most of Cyriax's manipulative techniques are designed to reduce disc herniation. It is thought that his rotatory maneuvers apply a torsional stress on the spine that exerts a centripetal force that reduces the bulging disc material if the longitudinal ligaments are intact.[35]

The driving force behind a Scandinavian school of thought is Freddie Kaltenborn, who is a physiotherapist, a chiropractor and an osteopath. His philosophy is a synthesis of what he considers to be the best in chiropractic, osteopathy and physical medicine. He uses some of Cyriax's methods to evaluate the patient and mainly employs specific osteopathic and sometimes chiropractic techniques for treatment.[35] His refinement and development of treatment techniques is a vast contribution to understanding manual therapy.

In 1964 Australian physical clinician Geoffrey Maitland published his book, *Vertebral Manipulation*, now in its 5th edition.[30] He distinguished between mobilization and manipulation and put heavy emphasis on mobilization. His techniques are fairly similar to the "articulatory" techniques used by osteopaths, and involve oscillatory movements performed within the patient's available range of movement. Because his techniques are gentler and easy to learn, they have appealed to physical therapists and have gained much recognition, especially in the United Kingdom and Australia. By using the word mobilization instead of manipulation, Maitland has successfully eliminated the emotional aspects surrounding the subject, which has led to its better acceptance among members of the medical profession.

Theory

One must have a basic appreciation of joint mechanics to effectively employ manual therapy techniques. The reader should review Chapter 2, *Spinal Biomechanics* for a complete discussion of spinal biomechanics and a review of Fryette's Laws of Spinal Motion.

Joint play motions, first described by Mennell,[31] are involuntary, interarticular motions present in all synovial joints. Joint play is necessary for painless, unrestricted, voluntary motion. Examples of joint play motion include distraction and P/A glide of the cervical spine facet joints during active cervical flexion. Joint play can be thought of as normal joint laxity or slack. Manual therapy techniques employing joint play motions include long axis distraction, tilts, glides and rotations.

Component motions are generally thought of as extra-articular movements that normally accompany active motions and are necessary for full range of movement. Examples of component motions include spreading of the mortise of the ankle in dorsiflexion or the sliding of the radius along the ulna during elbow extension.[36]

Articular position of the joint as described by MacConaill and Basmajian[29] must be considered when performing joint mobilization. The close-packed position is at the extreme of one of the most habitual movements of the joint. It is the position in which the concave surface (smaller area) is in complete congruence with the convex surface (larger area). The capsule and ligaments are maximally taut and the two bones of the articular unit cannot be separated by traction across the joint surface. Joint mobilization should not be performed in the maximal close-packed position. If joint motion is to be avoided, the close-packed position can be useful during treatment. For example, the spinal segments above and below a segment to be mobilized can be "locked" into a close-packed position to isolate the mobilizing force to the desired level between.

Any position that is not close-packed is considered loose-packed. The articular surfaces are not totally congruent and some parts of the capsule are lax. The maximum loose-packed position is often described as the resting position of the joint, and is the best position for early mobilization. Subsequent treatments may be performed in positions nearer the close-packed position, but they are never performed in the maximum close-packed position.

Generally speaking, rotation will cause a close-packed position. Likewise, extremes of all motions will tend to place the joint into more of a close-packed position, whereas mid-range of a joint movement will be closer to the loose-packed position. Full extension is the maximum close-packed position of the spine.[30]

The joint capsule is a richly innervated structure that is made up of two layers, the synovial lining on the inside and an external layer of dense, irregular collagen connective tissue. This outer layer of collagen fiber is somewhat thickened and immobile in joints that have a *capsular* pattern of hypomobility. This may be caused by increased collagen fiber that is laid down in response to injury or inflammation, or a binding together of the individual collagen fibers. These collagen fibers cannot be stretched like the yellow elastic fibers; rather, they must be mobilized in a subtler manner and allowed to rearrange and loosen over a period of time. Therefore, certain manual therapy techniques work better than others for stretching collagen fibers.

Soft tissue massage, contract-relax techniques, passive stretching and active and passive range of motion exercises all increase the mobility of soft tissue in general. However, with the exception of certain contract-relax techniques, their effectiveness in mobilizing the joints is limited to stretching the contractile (muscle-tendon) tissue. Specific and general joint mobilization techniques are more effective in restoring mobility of the joints because they act specifically on the inert structures (capsule, ligament, cartilage and intervertebral disc). They offer an additional advantage because they can be applied with the joint in a comfortable mid-range position rather than at the painful limit of range of motion.[37]

Indications

The Agency for Health Care Policy and Research (AHCPR) has generated an increased interest in joint mobilization by supporting its use.[7] The AHCPR reviewed the literature and concluded that the use of manipulation was justified in persons with acute low back pain without evidence of neurologic injury during the first four weeks of treatment. Use of mobilization in persons with chronic low back disorders was not definitively recommended because of the lack of research that had shown its effectiveness. However, mobilization and manipulation techniques are widely used for both acute and chronic spinal pain.

The main goal of joint mobilization techniques is restoration of normal motion, in joints that are hypomobile,

impinged or subluxed. However, joint motion is thought to have a pain inhibiting effect, so joint mobilization techniques can be useful for painful joints that are moving normally. Joint mobilization may also increase circulation to a joint or disc, thus promoting the healing process.

Joint mobilization is particularly valuable in subacute stages of soft tissue injuries. As soft tissue injuries and inflammations heal, stiffness is inherent. Left alone, the joints may become hypomobile. The untreated hypomobile joint will soon begin to show signs of joint degeneration. Obviously, a muscle cannot be fully rehabilitated if the underlying joints are not free to move, and conversely, a muscle cannot move a joint that is not free to move. To avoid this pathological chain of events, mobilization techniques and exercise must be used. The earlier they are started in the treatment regime, the more benefit obtained, provided they are not aggravating to any soft tissue pathology present.

Joint mobilization has become a widely known and accepted treatment modality. However, it is not a panacea. There are clear reasons to use joint mobilization techniques, but soft tissue mobilization and proper exercise and functional rehabilitation techniques should be employed as necessary for optimum restoration of function.

Contraindications

Joint mobilization techniques should not be used on any joint where movement is contraindicated. Specifically, joint manipulation using a high velocity, low amplitude thrust is contraindicated in cauda equina syndrome, myelopathy, congenital or acquired bleeding disorders, aneurism, hypermobility syndromes such as Downs or Ehlers-Danlos, primary joint disease such as rheumatoid or infectious arthritis, aseptic necrosis, malignancy, osteoporosis and metabolic bone disease.[5] There is controversy over the use of high velocity manipulation with diagnoses of spondylolisthesis or acute herniated disc. We prefer to use other types of therapy to treat these conditions.

Adverse effects of high velocity manipulation reported in the literature include local discomfort, headache, and, much less commonly, nausea and dizziness.[38] The rare incidence of vertebrobasilar artery (VBA) dissections resulting from cervical spine manipulations has been reported.[26] One study compared cervical manipulation to mobilization and found that mobilization was as effective as manipulation in reducing neck pain and disability.[26] Since mobilization has fewer contraindications and less risk of adverse side effects, it makes sense to use mobilization techniques when possible.

Effects

The effects of manual therapy are both neurophysiologic and mechanical. The work of Wyke and others[18,24,37] in the area of joint mechanoreceptors explains why mobilization techniques can be effective in relieving pain, causing reflex inhibition of muscles and promoting relaxation. Both manipulation and mobilization have been shown to cause a regional inhibitory effect on alpha-motoneuron excitability.[12,14] One study used transcranial magnetic stimulation techniques to show a transient but significant central motor facilitation caused by lumbar spine manipulation.[13]

Since joint mobilization is performed to increase movement, one would expect increased movement as a result. An immediate increase in cervical active range of motion has been measured after cervical spine manipulation.[41] Increased C2-C7 segmental mobility has also been documented by pre and post manipulation radiographic examination.[42] However, one study showed that sacroiliac joint manipulation did not alter the position of the sacroiliac joint, even though positional testing performed pre and post-manipulation had changed.[40]

When mobilization techniques are employed into the range of restriction, they are moving into the area of plastic deformation of the soft tissue (collagen). Simply stated, if a tissue is stretched only in its elastic range, no permanent structural change will occur. When the tissue is stretched into the plastic range and beyond, permanent structural changes can occur.

It is important to realize that the effects of joint mobilization will vary between clinicians and patients. One study looked at the forces applied during manual therapy.[10] Ten physical clinicians applied central P/A mobilization techniques to 80 patients with low back pain. The forces were measured, and attempts were made to characterize the type and force of the mobilizations. There was high variability in the forces used for each grade of mobilization. The force used related not only to patient characteristics, but also to physical therapist characteristics. Interestingly, current pain intensity and nature of symptoms did not affect the forces used.

The clinical efficacy of manipulative techniques remains controversial. Several review articles have been written, with differing conclusions.[4,15,16,27,39] Interestingly, a 1995 review of the review articles indicated that the majority of reviews were positive toward spinal manipulation. Furthermore, reviews with a higher methodological quality tended to have more positive reviews. Still, the authors bemoaned the general poor quality of all the reviews and the clinical trials published.[2]

In a 2003 meta-analysis, authors compared the effectiveness of spinal manipulation to individual therapies and sham therapy. They concluded that there is no evidence that spinal manipulation is more effective than other therapies advocated for acute and low back pain, including analgesics, exercises, physical therapy and back schools. Spinal manipulation was more effective than sham therapy and therapies shown in previous studies to be ineffective. Thus, they recommend that future studies on spinal manipulation focus on its relative cost-effectiveness compared to other therapies. The authors indicated that the reason for the difference in their conclusions compared to previous reviews was that they included more recent studies, and they more precisely compared spinal manipulation with specific therapies rather than pooling the results of studies in a less-specific manner.

Despite the continued debate about the effectiveness of manipulation, specific clinical effects of various manual techniques have been reported. It is worthwhile to consider some of the individual study results. One randomized trial with a small sample size showed cervical manipulation had no effect on episodic tension-type headache.[8] An earlier trial with one of the same authors had shown a dramatic effect on cervicogenic headache.[34] The authors stressed the importance of accurate assessment of the headache's cause before using manipulative techniques. A trial comparing the results of cervical spine manipulation to amitriptyline for treating migraines showed comparable results, suggesting manipulation can be helpful in treating migraines.[33]

One study showed that low back pain patients receiving osteopathic manipulative techniques required significantly less medication than patients receiving standard medical care. Otherwise, outcomes were similar.[1] Another study showed that high velocity, short amplitude manipulation provided better short term results in patients with chronic back pain than acupuncture or medication.[20]

Comparisons of manual therapy to exercise results show mixed opinions. One study of patients with chronic low back pain claimed better short and long-term effects of manual therapy compared to exercise.[6] Studies on mechanical and chronic neck pain show the best short and long term effects result from a combination of manipulation and exercise.[9,17,23] One study compared joint manipulation, myofascial therapy and back school results in treating subacute low back pain. No significant differences were seen.[25] Since all of these studies had different subjects, methods, and interventions, no global conclusions can be drawn. We believe the literature as a whole has shown adequate justification to use manual therapy for certain spinal problems, despite individual study limitations and the conflicting recommendations of published reviews and meta-analyses. Clinicians must use sound judgment and compare the advantages of using manual therapy techniques to other techniques at their disposal when developing a treatment plan.

Techniques

Joint mobilizations are also called graded passive movements or joint articulations. The most commonly used grading system is one proposed by Maitland, which has five grades of movement:[30]

- Grade 1 – slow, small-amplitude movements performed at the beginning of the range
- Grade 2 – slow, larger-amplitude movements performed through the range, but not reaching the end of range.
- Grade 3 – slow, large amplitude movements performed to the limit of the range.
- Grade 4 – slow, small-amplitude movements performed at the limit of the range and into the resistance.
- Grade 5 – fast, small-amplitude, high-velocity movement performed beyond the pathological limitation of range.

Grades 1 through 4 are commonly considered mobilization techniques and generally use oscillatory movements. Grades 1 and 2 are used primarily to maintain joint mobility, promote tissue healing and relieve pain in the acute and subacute stages of healing. Grades 3 and 4 are used to increase joint mobility in more advanced stages of hypomobility or with joint impingement. Grade 5 articulations are the quick thrusting maneuvers usually referred to as manipulations, and are especially helpful when their purpose is to mobilize a subluxed or impinged joint.

Although many techniques use oscillatory movements at end range, *stretch* articulations are also helpful. The slack in the joint is slowly taken up, and a gentle but firm stretch at end range is held for several seconds. Another technique variation involves *progressive* articulations, where progressively increasing grades of movement are used in a gentle, step-wise fashion (Fig 10-1).

Another form of manual therapy is manual traction. Manual traction techniques can be used with passive range of motion to impart general mobilization to the spine. They are particularly effective in the cervical spine.

Muscular contract-relax techniques can also be effective in mobilizing joints. The joint is carefully positioned into the direction of restriction, and the patient exerts a muscular effort, causing the joint to move. These principles are also called osteopathic *muscle energy techniques (METs)*. METs can be very general or specific to one joint, depending upon the degree of localization achieved by joint positioning. At the end of this chapter, we introduce the principles of METs and provide two examples. A more advanced discussion is beyond the scope of this text; a thorough exploration can be found in textbooks specifically addressing the osteopathic evaluation scheme and METs.[21,28,32]

Principles to Remember

Because of pain, mobilization cannot always be performed in the most restricting direction. In such a case, it is performed in directions other than, or possibly opposite to, the direction of restriction. Restoration of mobility in one direction will usually increase mobility in other directions as well. For example, a rotational mobilization is likely to increase range of motion in all other planes of motion. Often, the first mobilization treatment consists of gentle tractions applied to the joint structures with five to ten second holds. The purpose is to relieve the pain. Gradually, the mobilization may be increased to meet other goals, such as improved mobility.

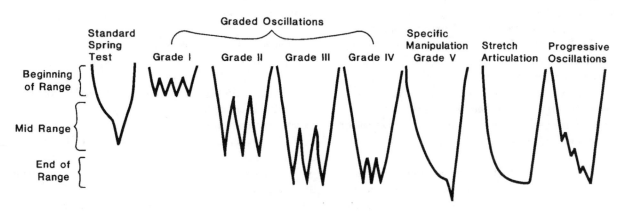

Figure 10-1: Grades of mobilization.

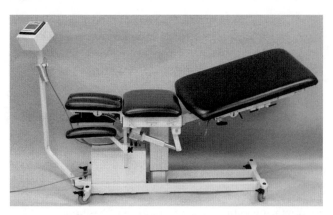

Figure 10-2: A three-dimensional (3D) mobilization table (The Saunders Group, Inc.) The lower half of the table can be positioned in flexion/extension, rotation and side bending to enhance mobilization techniques.

The rules of mobilization are as follows:[31]

1. The patient and clinician must be relaxed.
2. The procedure should be relatively pain free.
3. When possible, the clinician should stabilize one bone and move or mobilize the other.
4. The first treatment should be gentle to observe the patient's reaction.
5. The clinician should always compare and observe the vertebral levels above or below to gain knowledge of individual patient differences.
6. When possible, the clinician should examine one joint and one movement at a time.
7. Lever arms of force should be kept as short as possible.
8. Consider contraindications and precautions when deciding to use joint mobilization techniques.

A three-dimensional (3D) mobilization table can enhance the effectiveness and convenience of many of the techniques we describe (Fig 10-2). A 3D table has many potential uses, including positional stretching, mobilization and traction, and many clinicians consider them indispensable in the treatment of spinal patients. The use of a 3D table and a basic understanding of spinal biomechanics allows for endless options in joint mobilization. The 3D table allows the clinician to work on passive range of motion in all planes in an unweighted position. It can be used to position a patient to make accessory mobilization more specific to a physiologic motion. Finally, it can be used very effectively in combination with traction to find the position of most relief or maximize the centralization of lumbar herniated nucleus pulposus (HNP) symptoms.

Mobilization, like any other evaluation or treatment skill, cannot be learned or developed entirely by the reading of a textbook. There is no substitute for clinical practice and experience. It is reasonable to assume that the

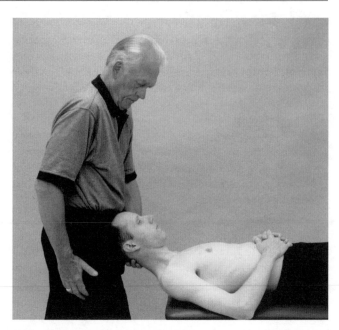

Figure 10-3: The patient's head rests against the clinician's anterior hip for cervical mobilization techniques.

beginner will feel some insecurity and uncertainty when attempting these techniques for the first time. With perseverance, these techniques can be perfected. It is often beneficial to bring a spinal model into the treatment room to help both with patient education and to remind the clinician where his or her hand placement should be. Patients will appreciate the explanation and will not be aware the clinician is using the model as a guide!

Cervical Spine

Before attempting to mobilize the cervical spine, the clinician should perform the vertebral artery test to ensure that cervical movements will not compromise the circulation of the vertebral artery. Most clinicians are taught to perform the vertebral artery test during the initial examination, but we retest prior to each manual therapy session. A detailed description of the vertebral artery test is found in Chapter 4, *Evaluation of the Spine*.

Thirteen basic cervical mobilizations are presented. The first five techniques are similar to the segmental mobility tests described in Chapter 4, *Evaluation of the Spine*: forward bending/gliding, backward bending, rotation, side bending and side gliding. For each of these techniques, the patient is positioned supine with the head extending over the end of the treatment table, resting on the clinician's hip (Fig 10-3). The clinician's hands cradle the patient's head and neck with the index fingers supporting the articular pillars superior to the segment to be mobilized (Fig 10-4). Graded passive movements and stretch articulations are most effective with these techniques.

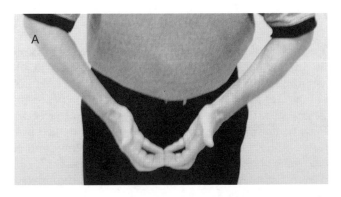

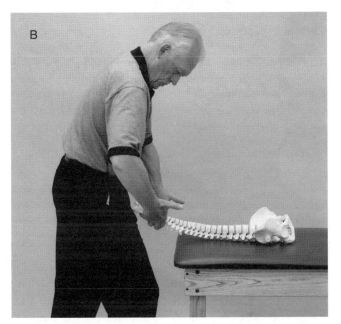

Figure 10-4: Position of the clinician's hands for cervical mobilization. A) Front; B) Side.

Cervical Forward Bending/Gliding

Lifting the head and neck straight upward with both hands causes a forward bending/gliding mobilization. The patient's cervical spine should be flexed to about 30. To start, the clinician's knees should be somewhat flexed. The clinician then alternately extends and flexes the knees slightly to keep the patient's head in correct position as the mobilization force is applied (Fig 10-5). The mobilizing force is directed through the index fingers, but maximal hand contact is maintained with the neck and head so they are carried along with the movement. Using the proximal interphalangeal joints (PIPs), the principle contact is made with the index fingers against the articular pillars of the neck. One should be careful not to use the fingertips with these techniques to avoid discomfort.

Cervical Backward Bending

For cervical backward bending, the patient's neck is held in a neutral, mid-range position. The backward bending mobilization is similar to forward bending except that the head and the portion of the neck superior to the point of contact of the index fingers is not carried along with the movement. Rather, as the mobilizing force is applied upward by the index fingers, the head and the portion of the neck superior to the force are allowed to fall into backward bending. Thus, backward bending of the cervical joints superior to the contact occurs. This effect is most pronounced at the segment immediately superior to the contact point (Fig 10-6). The cervical backward bending technique is also very effective in the first two or three segments of the thoracic spine.

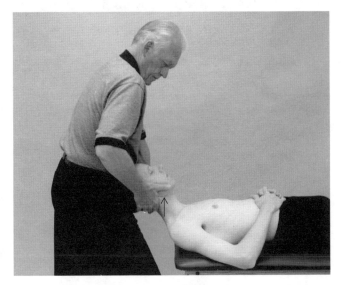

Figure 10-5: Cervical forward bending mobilization.

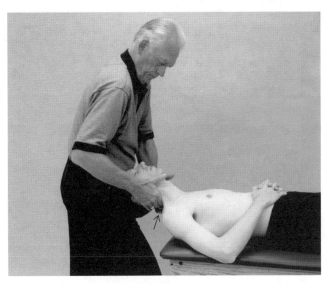

Figure 10-6: Cervical backward bending mobilization.

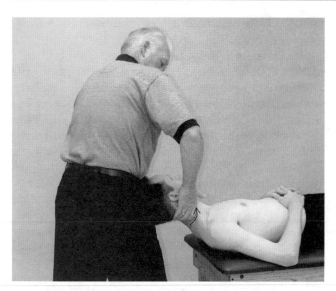

Figure 10-7: Cervical rotational mobilization.

Cervical Rotation

The cervical rotation mobilization is similar to the forward bending technique, but it is done unilaterally with the head and neck held in a neutral, mid-range position. To perform left rotation, the PIP contact of the right hand lifts upward onto the right articular pillar while the left hand supports the head and neck. As the upward mobilizing force is initiated against the right articular pillar, the clinician will immediately sense that left rotation is occurring. The clinician continues the movement, following the arc of rotation that naturally occurs. The head and neck are carried along with the movement (Fig 10-7).

Cervical Side Bending

The cervical side bending mobilization uses the same positioning as the cervical techniques previously described. The neck is held in a neutral, mid-range position. The radio-palmar surface of the index finger near the metacarpophalangeal joint (MCP) is placed against the lateral aspect of the articular pillar. The mobilization force is applied in a medial and slightly inferior direction, causing the segment below the point of contact to side bend to the same side as the mobilizing force. The opposite hand supports the head and neck (Fig 10-8).

Cervical Side Gliding

The cervical side gliding mobilization also uses the same basic position previously described. The mobilizing force is applied in a medial direction through the index finger as it contacts the lateral aspect of the articular pillar. Movement occurs at the segment below the contact. The point of contact on the index finger is on the palmar surface of the MCP joint. The main difference between this technique and that of cervical side bending is that in the side gliding technique, the patient's head is carried to the side with the movement. This is accomplished by a shift of the clinician's hips in the direction of the movement (Fig 10-9). In the side bending technique, the head and neck actually tilt as side bending occurs around the fulcrum created by the clinician's index finger.

Most clinicians agree that cervical side gliding is an easy technique to learn and it is one that is usually comfortable for the patient. Side gliding is a technique with which an inexperienced clinician can gain confidence. It is also a good technique to use if the patient is apprehensive or uncomfortable with the idea of having the head and neck

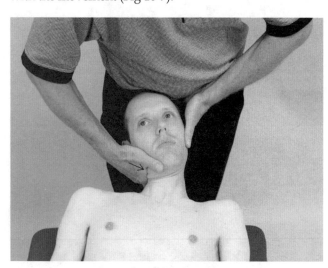

Figure 10-8: Cervical side bending mobilization.

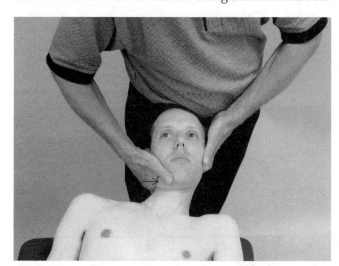

Figure 10-9: Cervical side gliding mobilization.

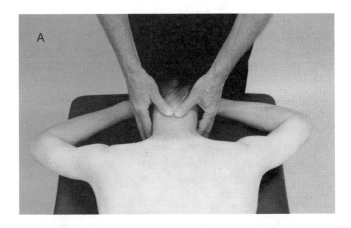

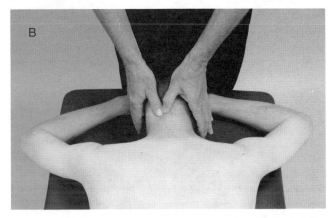

Figure 10-10: Cervical P/A mobilizations. A) Central P/A; B) Unilateral P/A.

moved passively by the clinician. This technique can be used to demonstrate to the patient that some movement can occur without discomfort.

Cervical P/A Accessory Mobilization

Unlike the five cervical techniques described above, P/A accessory mobilizations do not use physiologic motion (flexion, extension, rotation or side bending). P/A accessory mobilizations are palpatory techniques and were also used to assess segmental mobility in Chapter 4, *Evaluation of the Spine*. One advantage to P/A accessory mobilizations is that they are segment specific and allow the therapist to detect changes in the joint feel during performance of the technique. P/A accessory mobilizations are performed with the patient lying prone with the spine in neutral. Either central or unilateral techniques can be employed (Fig 10-10). A central technique is performed by placing the thumbs together and applying an anterior force on the spinous process of a vertebra. Unilateral P/A techniques are performed by using the same thumb contact, but applying the pressure lateral to the midline on the articular

pillar. The thumb contact on the spinous process should be as broad as possible to avoid sharp contact pressure.

Upper Cervical Rotation (C1-2)

Rotation is the major motion of C1-2. Approximately 40-45° of cervical rotation to either side occurs at this joint. When a rotational restriction of C1-2 is found, contract-relax or METs are the easiest methods of treatment.

According to Fryette's Laws of Spinal Motion, full flexion of the cervical spine decreases its ability to rotate. Therefore, fully flexing the cervical spine can be used to isolate a rotational technique to C1-2. The patient lies supine. Holding full cervical flexion, the clinician rotates the patient's head toward the restriction, taking up slack. The clinician's thumbs are holding firmly along the patient's maxilla on both sides. The patient is then asked to rotate in the opposite direction (Fig 10-11).

The force needed varies from patient to patient. If the patient contracts too hard, it helps to ask the patient to look only with the eyes—this gently activates the suboccipital musculature. The clinician should hold against the patient's resistance for a count of five. The patient relaxes and the head is turned further into the motion restriction. After two or three repetitions, the clinician should recheck active range of motion to determine the effect of treatment. Improved range of motion is often dramatic.

Manual Cervical Traction

Manual traction can be done with a straight midline pull, or can be used in combination with passive range of motion in any plane. A towel or strap can be used to assist the cli-

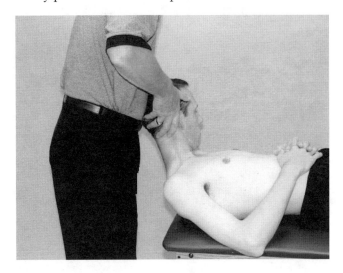

Figure 10-11: Upper cervical rotational mobilization. The cervical spine is fully flexed before upper cervical rotation is performed.

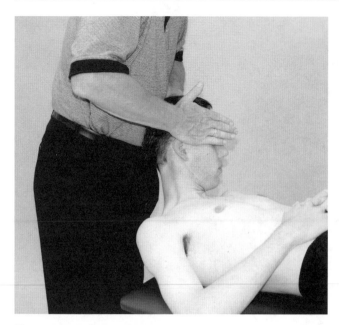

Figure 10-12: Cervical contract-relax technique. The patient shown lacks cervical left rotation and flexion. The clinician positions the patient toward the motion barriers, then asks the patient to turn the head toward the right.

nician. Inhibitive manual traction is a mobilization technique that applies mild traction to the cervical muscles and spine and incorporates a muscle relaxation technique via direct pressure on the suboccipital muscle/tendon origins. It is also called *upper cervical distraction* or *occipital release*. Specific manual traction techniques are described and illustrated in Chapter 12, *Spinal Traction*.

Cervical Contract-Relax Techniques

In the cervical spine, contract-relax or METs are quite effective forms of mobilization. The cervical spine can be specifically positioned in a combination of the three planes of motion (flexion/extension, rotation and side bending) to "lock" a specific segment prior to the patient exerting a muscular effort.

Contract-relax techniques can also be more general, with the clinician positioning the patient's cervical spine toward the restriction, without incorporating all three planes of motion to affect a specific segment. When the patient exerts muscular effort, the effect is at multiple levels. Either single plane motions or a combination of motions can be effective.

For example, if the patient lacks left rotation and flexion, the patient's cervical spine can be positioned into the "barrier" (into left rotation and then flexion as much as possible without recreating the symptoms). The patient then performs a gentle to moderate muscular contraction into right rotation (Fig 10-12). When the patient relaxes, the clinician repositions the cervical spine into more left rotation and flexion as tolerated, and repeats the contraction two or three times.

Cervical Self-Mobilization Techniques

Cervical self-mobilization is done by having the patient grasp and stabilize the cervical spine as shown (Fig 10-13). The points of stabilization are the vertebrae below the segment to be mobilized. For example, if level C2-3 is to be mobilized, the patient stabilizes the C3 vertebra and does not allow movement to occur from that point inferiorly. Then, the patient performs active forward and backward bending, rotation or side bending. The greatest mobilizing force is concentrated at the level just superior to the stabilization. The patient may vary the level of mobilization by moving the stabilization superiorly or inferiorly.

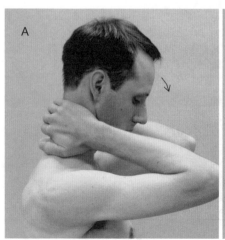
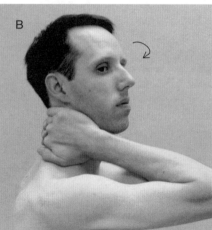
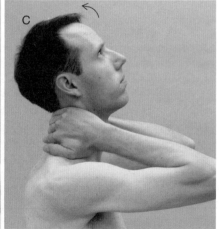

Figure 10-13: Cervical self-mobilization. A) Upper cervical flexion to stretch the suboccipital muscles; B) Upper cervical rotation; C) Mid-cervical extension.

Upper Thoracic Spine and 1st Rib

Four upper thoracic mobilizations are presented. One is an extension technique, two are rotational techniques and one is a side bending technique. The techniques discussed for the 1st rib are similar to the 1st rib segmental mobility tests discussed in Chapter 4, *Evaluation of the Spine*.

Upper Thoracic Extension–Prone

A backward bending mobilization force can be given via direct pressure on a spinous process in prone (Fig 10-14). The patient should be positioned prone in thoracic extension with pillows, a bolster or a 3D table. The clinician's uses a pisiform contact to press anterosuperiorly on a spinous process. The mobilization occurs at the segment inferior to the spinous process contact. Graded passive movements, stretch articulations and thrusts can be used with this technique.

Upper Thoracic Extension–Sitting

Upper thoracic extension also can be performed in sitting. The clinician can either stabilize the segment below the desired level and mobilize the head and neck back over it or can stabilize the head and mobilize the desired segment anteriorly.

The clinician forms a "V" with the thumb and forefinger, which is flexed at the PIP and DIP joints. The points of contact are the thumb and PIP of the forefinger on the transverse processes below the level to be mobilized. The spinous process is located in the notch of the "V". The patient sits at the edge of a chair and the clinician cradles the head with the chest and forearm. The clinician hugs the patient's head to the chest. The patient's nose should be in the bend of the elbow and the clinician's volar forearm cradles the opposite side of the head. The clinician's little finger cups the patient's occiput. The patient's head should be held gently, not squeezed. To move the head, the clinician shifts weight, rather than pushing with the arm. The arm simply holds the patient's head to the chest.

In one technique, the left hand stabilizes with enough force anteriorly to not allow any motion of the trunk posteriorly. The clinician transfers weight from the right to left foot to move the head and neck back over the stabilizing hand (Fig 10-15). In an alternate technique, the head is held steady with the contact hand pushing in an anterior direction so that the trunk moves under the head and neck. Work on postural awareness can be added to this technique. The patient is asked to actively achieve a lumbar lordosis while the head is held stationary. Thus, the patient gets an idea of the effect of improved sitting posture and helps the clinician so that less anterior force is required with the contact

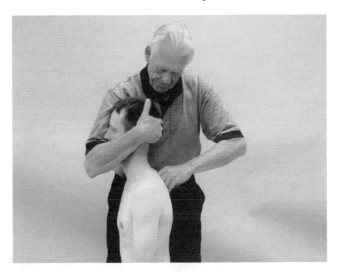

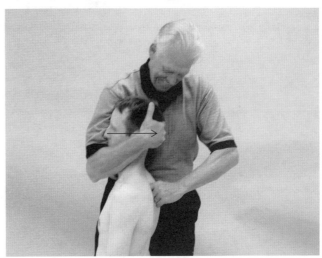

Figure 10-15: Upper thoracic extension technique. A) Starting position; B) The clinician pushes the head and neck posteriorly by transferring his weight from the right to left foot while stabilizing firmly with the left hand.

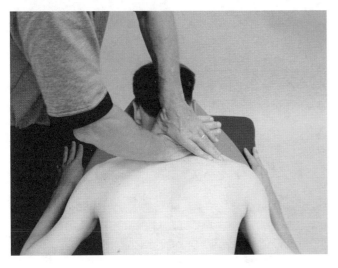

Figure 10-14: Upper thoracic extension in prone.

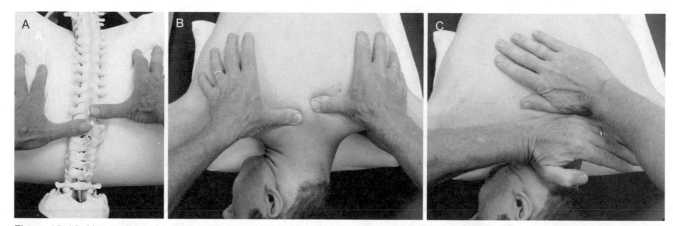

Figure 10-16: Upper thoracic right rotation technique. A and B) The inferior thumb stabilizes as the superior thumb directs a lateral force against the spinous processes; C) A contact using the pisiform and thumb MCP joint is often more comfortable for the patient and clinician.

hand. The clinician can add slight distraction to either technique by standing up slightly or extending the knees.

Upper Thoracic Rotation–Prone

For this technique, the patient lies prone with pillows under the chest. A 3D mobilization table can be positioned to flex the thoracic spine instead of using pillows. Lateral pressure in opposite directions is applied to the spinous processes at two adjacent levels. The inferior segment, or base, is the segment stabilized, and the mobilizing force is applied to the spinous process of the superior segment. The superior spinous process is moved in the opposite direction of the rotational movement desired (move the superior spinous process right to cause left rotation) (Fig 10-16). Graded passive movements and stretch articulations can be used with this technique. Thumb contacts are effective

when mild or moderate specific mobilization is desired. However, thumb contacts are sometimes uncomfortable if strong pressure is exerted. Therefore, pisiform (mobilizing) and thumb MCP joint (stabilizing) contacts are more effective if vigorous mobilization is desired. For maximum effect the patient's head should be turned in the same direction as the desired mobilization.

Upper Thoracic Rotation–Sitting

A second upper thoracic rotation technique is done with the patient sitting with the clinician's hands positioned as shown (Fig 10-17). With neck rotation, the spinous processes move in the direction opposite the movement. For example, with left rotation, each thoracic spinous process moves to the right on its base. If a specific segment is manually blocked from moving, the rotational movement is

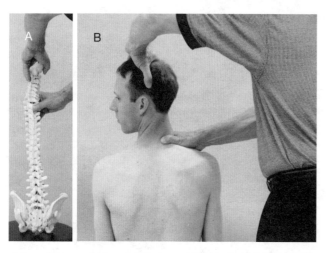

Figure 10-17: Upper thoracic left rotation technique. A) The thumb stabilizes laterally against the inferior spinous process; B) The patient's head is rotated to the left to take up slack, then the mobilization force is directed through the thumb.

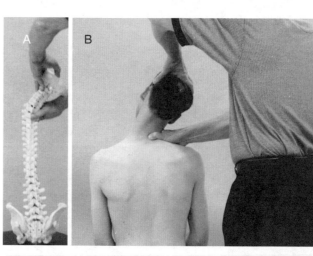

Figure 10-18: Upper thoracic right side bending technique. A) The thumb stabilizes laterally against the inferior spinous process; B) The patient's head is side bent right to take up slack, then the mobilization force is directed through the thumb.

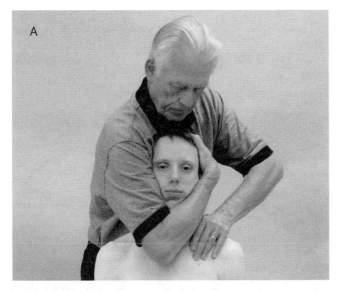
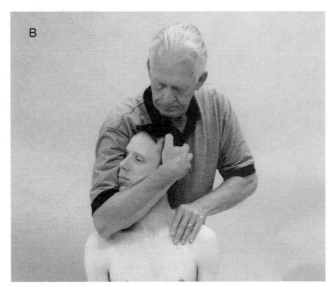
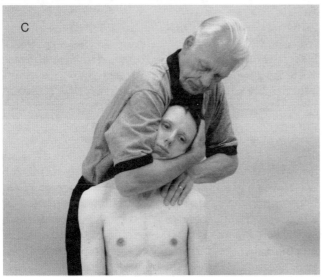
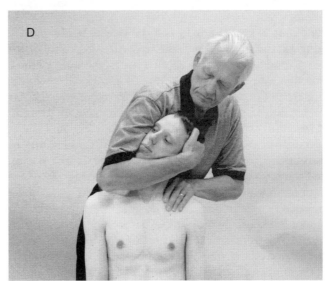

Figure 10-19: Upper thoracic rotation and side bending techniques using an alternate stabilization method. A) The clinician's thumb still stabilizes, but by cradling the patient's head, the clinician has greater control over cervical movements; B) Rotation; C) Side bending; D) Side bending and rotation combined.

prevented from occurring below that point and a greater rotational force can be directed to the segment above the point of stabilization. The thumb stabilizes firmly against the lateral aspect of the spinous process, as the opposite hand rotates the patient's head and neck to the opposite side to take up slack. The mobilizing force is then directed through the thumb. Graded passive movements and stretch articulations can be used with this technique.

Upper Thoracic Side Bending–Sitting

The side bending mobilization technique for the upper thoracic spine is similar to the rotational technique discussed above. With the patient seated, the clinician side bends the head and neck while blocking movement of the spinous process with the thumb at the selected level (Fig 10-18). Normally the spinous processes move in the same direction as the physiological movement. The thumb prevents this movement from the point of stabilization inferiorly and directs an increased side bending force to the segment above the point of stabilization. This technique should be done in three distinct steps as follows: 1) Stabilize with the thumb; 2) Take up slack by passively side bending the head and neck; and 3) Mobilize with the thumb. Graded passive movements and stretch articulations can be used with this technique.

The two previous techniques can be modified by cradling the patient's head in the clinician's arm and against the chest (Fig 10-19). This method allows more head control

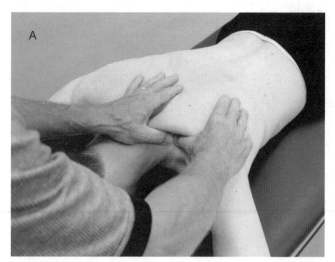
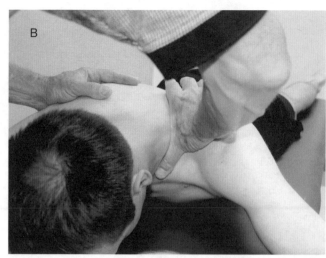

Figure 10-20: Caudal glide of the 1st rib in prone. A) The thumb is placed anterior to the upper trapezius muscle belly and a caudally directed pressure is applied. The first firm resistance felt is the 1st rib; B) Alternate technique using the web space of the hand.

and enables greater force to be applied. Side bending in one direction with rotation in the opposite direction may be combined to increase the effectiveness of these techniques.

Caudal Glide of the 1st Rib–Prone

We perform caudal glide of the 1st rib with the patient lying prone, but the techniques can also be done in sitting or supine. In prone, the clinician palpates the 1st rib by placing a thumb underneath (anterior to) the muscle belly of the upper trapezius right next to the cervical spine. A caudally directed pressure is applied (Fig 10-20). The first firm resistance felt caudally will be the 1st rib. The clinician then applies pressure onto the 1st rib. Either a prolonged stretch or graded passive movements are effective. The mobilization can be fine-tuned by changing the placement of the thumb slightly and applying the mobilization force in a slightly more anterior-caudal or posterior-caudal direction as desired.

A more general technique involves the clinician placing the web space of the hand over the upper trapezius with the thumb anterior and the fingers posterior. A caudal force can then be applied (Fig 10-20).

With either of the above techniques, the patient's neck can be positioned in side bending toward the side of mobilization to put the anterior and middle scalenes on slack, or away from the side of mobilization to put the scalenes on stretch. The clinician can also ask the patient to inhale deeply, as the clinician resists the pump handle motion of the 1st rib during inhalation. As the patient exhales, the clinician can follow the rib inferiorly to take up the slack. Either a prolonged stretch or oscillation can be performed or the deep breath can be repeated as desired.

Mid and Lower Thoracic Spine

Six techniques appropriate for the mid and lower thoracic spine are described: forward bending, rotation, backward bending, traction/backward bending, and P/A accessory mobilization.

Thoracic Forward Bending–Prone

To achieve forward bending, the patient's thoracic spine is flexed over a pillow or bolster, or a 3D table is used. When anterior pressure is directed to the transverse processes of a thoracic vertebra, it causes that vertebra to forward bend on the vertebra inferior to it. The clinician's fingertips contact the transverse processes of the desired segment. The hypothenar eminence of the opposite hand is placed over the fingertips, and anterior pressure is exerted (Fig 10-21).

A crossed-hand method using the pisiform bones as contacts is an alternative many clinicians prefer (Fig 10-22). The transverse processes are located approximately one level higher than the spinous processes of their corresponding segments. The transverse processes can only be palpated indirectly so their approximate position must be determined in relation to the spinous processes. Thus, the transverse processes of a vertebra can be found at one level higher and approximately one-inch lateral to the midline. Graded passive movements, stretch articulations and thrusts may be used with these techniques.

Thoracic Rotation–Prone

The forward bending techniques just described are modified to produce rotation by placing the fingertip contacts on the transverse processes at *adjacent* levels. The

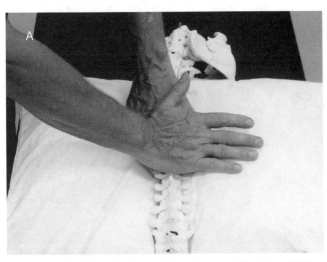

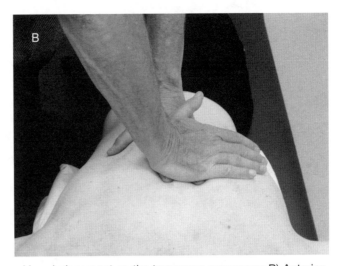

Figure 10-21: Thoracic forward bending mobilization. A) Finger and hand placement on the transverse processes; B) Anterior pressure directed by the opposite hand.

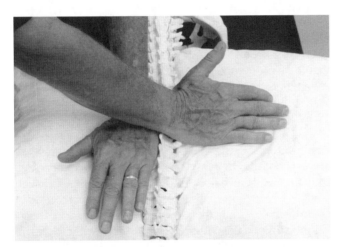

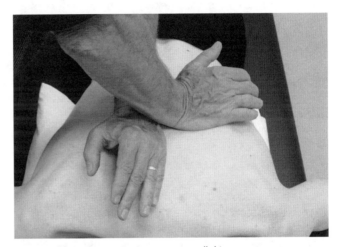

Figure 10-22: Thoracic forward bending mobilization using pisiform contacts. Note the contacts are on parallel transverse processes.

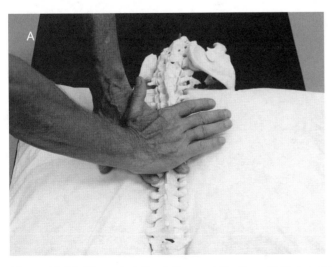

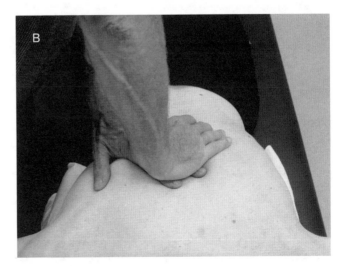

Figure 10-23: Thoracic left rotation mobilization. A) Finger placement on adjacent transverse processes; B) Anterior pressure directed by the opposite hand.

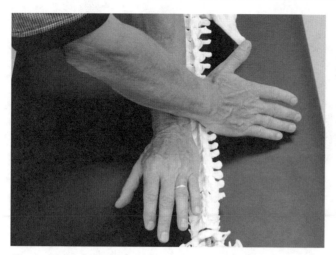 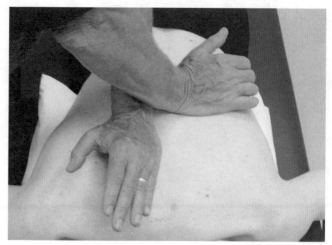

Figure 10-24: Left thoracic rotation mobilization using pisiform contacts. Note the contacts are on adjacent transverse processes.

rotation produced is in the direction of the inferior contact (Fig 10-23). If a more forceful technique is required, the crossed-hand pisiform contact method can be used (Fig 10-24).

Thoracic Rotation–Supine

In this thrust technique, the clinician makes a fist and places it so that the thenar eminence contacts the transverse process on one side and the flat surfaces of the middle phalanges (knuckles) contacts the transverse at the opposite adjacent level. The spinous processes lie in the hollow created between the fingers and the thenar eminence (Fig 10-25). This contact is maintained as the clinician applies a mobilizing thrust through the patient's arms and chest as he rolls the patient over the fulcrum produced by the fisted hand. Rotation is in the direction of the thenar eminence.

Thoracic Backward Bending

A backward bending mobilization force can be given via direct pressure on a spinous process (Fig 10-26). The patient should be positioned in prone thoracic extension with pillows, a bolster or a 3D table. The clinician's hand is rolled in slightly toward the palm so that the contact point is on the hypothenar eminence rather than on the bony pisiform so that patient and clinician comfort is maximized. The mobilization occurs at the segment inferior to the spinous process contact. Therefore, it is important to avoid contact with the segment below the pisiform contact so that it remains free to move. The clinician can ensure correct technique by making sure that the thumb of the contact hand is pointing toward the patient's head. That way, the segment below is free to move. Graded passive movements, stretch articulations and thrusts can be used with this technique.

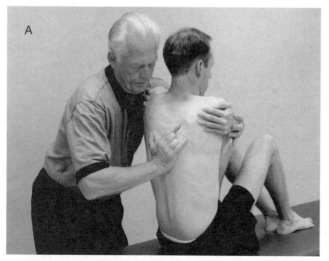 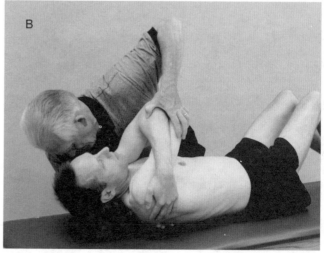

Figure 10-25: Thoracic left rotation mobilization. A) Hand placement on transverse processes; B) As the patient lies down over the fulcrum, the clinician directs a posterior thrust.

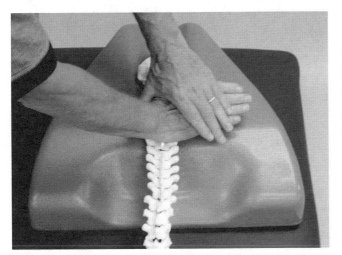
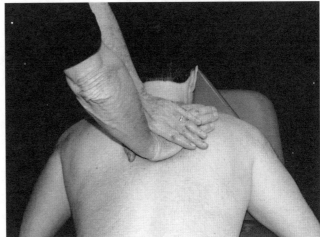

Figure 10-26: Thoracic backward bending mobilization.

Thoracic Backward Bending/Traction

With this technique, a rolled bath towel or pillow stabilizes the level above the segment to be mobilized. Depending upon the level being mobilized and the height of the clinician and patient, it may be necessary for the clinician to stand on a stool or platform to obtain the correct position. The patient crosses the arms with hands on opposite shoulders. The clinician reaches around the patient with both arms and grasps the patient's elbows and lifts upward and slightly backward (Fig 10-27). The amount of backward bending can be varied. The technique is effective when done as a slow stretch and may involve a thrust at the end of the stretch. The thrust is done by the clinician raising on tiptoes, and then suddenly dropping onto the heels. The patient's weight is totally or partially supported by the clinician. This technique can also be done with the patient sitting on a stool. Mennell describes an alternate technique that involves the clinician standing back to back with the patient to effect the mobilization at the lumbar level. In this instance, the clinician's hip acts as a fulcrum as the patient is lifted into extension with traction.[31]

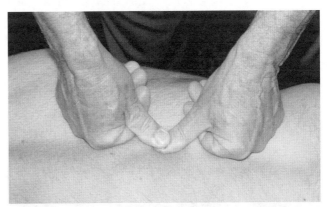
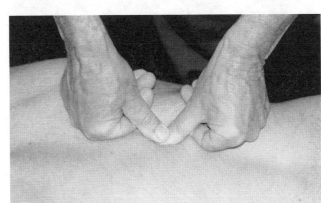

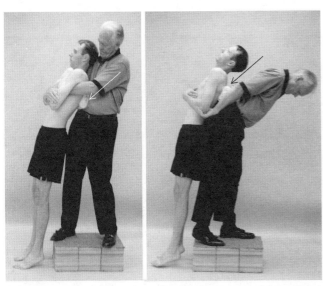

Figure 10-27: Thoracic and lumbar traction/backward bending technique. Arrow points to a 4" rolled towel placed horizontally across the patient's back to act as a fulcrum.

Figure 10-28: Thoracic P/A mobilization. A) Central P/A; B) Unilateral P/A.

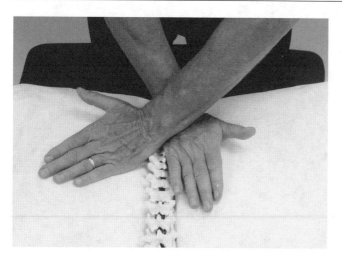
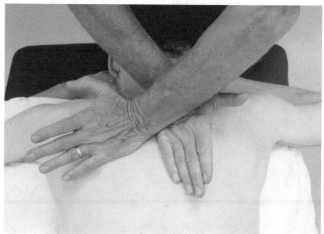

Figure 10-29: Rib P/A glide.

Thoracic P/A Accessory Mobilization

Thoracic central P/A's are performed in the same manner as the thoracic extension mobilization, but the patient is positioned in neutral rather than extension. Unilateral P/A's in the thoracic spine are done using the thumbs over the transverse processes (Fig 10-28). It should be noted that in the thoracic spine the transverse process is approximately a finger width lateral to the spinous process. To obtain a pure P/A glide of an intervertebral joint with the patient lying prone, it is often necessary to angle the pressure cephalically, caudally, medially or laterally to take into consideration the curves of the spine.[22]

Ribs

P/A Glides

P/A accessory mobilization of the ribs is done with the patient lying prone over pillows under the chest. The transverse processes are stabilized with the hypothenar eminence placed parallel to the spine on the opposite side of the rib to be mobilized. The clinician's forearms are crossed and the mobilization force is directed anteriorly and laterally through the hypothenar eminence that contacts the posteromedial aspect of the rib (Fig 10-29). Graded passive movements, stretch articulations or thrusts may be used with this technique.

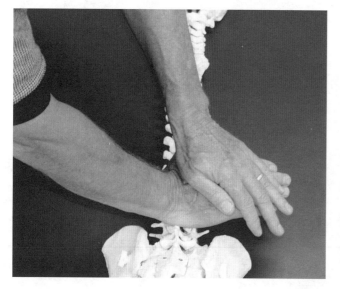
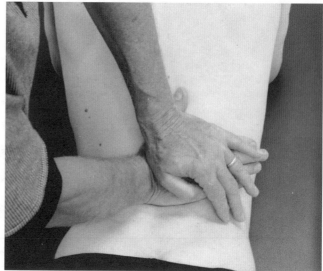

Figure 10-30: Lumbar backward bending mobilization.

Working with the patient's breathing can also augment the mobilization. The clinician can resist rib movement during inhalation or can follow the rib anteriorly and perform an oscillation, a thrust or a prolonged stretch at end range during exhalation.

Lumbar Spine

Eight basic techniques for the lumbar spine are presented: four rotational techniques, one extension technique, one side bending technique, one side bending/rotation technique, and P/A accessory mobilizations. The thoracic backward bending techniques shown in Figures 10-26 and 10-27 are also effective mobilization techniques for the lumbar spine.

Lumbar Backward Bending–Prone

A 3D mobilization table, pillows or the "elbow prop" position can be used to pre-position the patient into varying degrees of extension, depending upon the amount of force desired. The clinician uses a pisiform contact as shown (Fig 10-30). The mobilization occurs at the segment inferior to

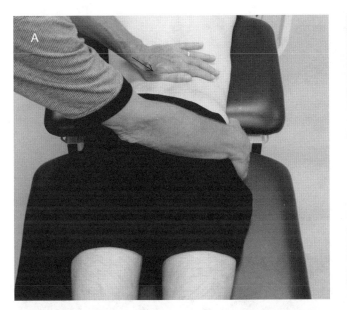
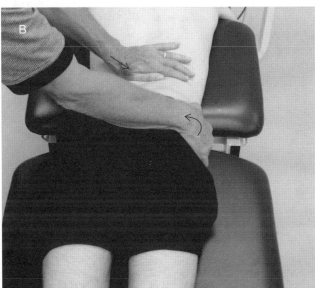
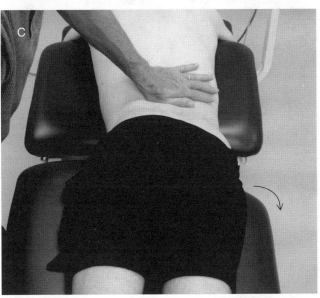
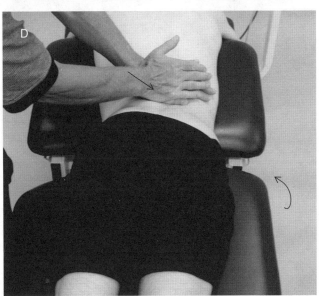

Figure 10-31: Lumbar left rotation mobilization. A) The left hand stabilizes against the spinous process; B) The right hand takes up slack by pulling the ilium posteriorly, then the mobilizing force is applied with the left hand; C) Alternate technique: The table is pre-positioned in right rotation; D) The clinician moves the table to take up the slack, while holding firmly with the left hand, then the mobilizing force is applied with both hands. A stabilization belt over the hips makes the latter technique more effective.

the spinous process being contacted. Therefore, it is important to avoid contact with the segment below the pisiform contact so that it remains free to move. The clinician can ensure correct technique by making sure that the thumb of the contact hand is pointing toward the patient's head. Graded passive movements, stretch articulations and thrusts can be used with this technique.

Lumbar Rotation-Prone

The prone lumbar rotation mobilization technique can be used to effectively isolate the lower segments. This technique is imporant because a high percentage of back pain complaints are at L4-5 and L5-S1. Clinically, one often sees patients who have functional extension mobility (i.e., they can perform a press up or standing backward bending exercises), but upon closer examination have stiffness from L4 to S1 (see Chapter 4, *Evaluation of the Spine*). Mobilizing rotation assists with general mobility of the stiff segments and is very beneficial for these patients.

The lateral aspect of the MCP joint of the thumb is used to stabilize the lateral aspect of the selected spinous process. The thenar eminence and heel of the hand also stabilize along the lateral aspect of the spinous processes superior to the MCP stabilization. The clinician's other hand grasps the anterior rim of the ilium of the side opposite the stabilization and lifts upward and medially to take up the slack. The mobilizing force is then given with the hand that is stabilizing against the lateral aspect of the spinous processes (Fig 10-31A and B).

This technique is specific to the L5-S1 segment if the L5 vertebra is being mobilized. Although this technique becomes less specific as the mobilization force moves superiorly, the greatest mobilizing force is always directed to the segment just inferior to the contact point of the MCP joint of the thumb. For example, if the third lumbar spinous process is contacted, the mobilization force is directed to the three segments between L3 and S1 with the L3-4 segment receiving the greatest force. Graded passive movements and stretch artic-

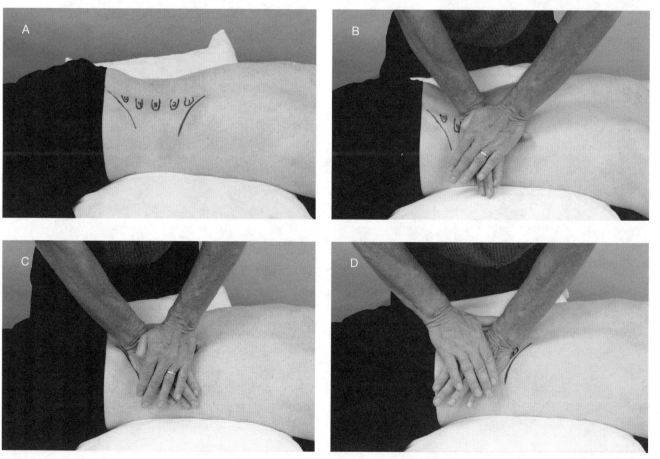

Figure 10-32: Lumbar left rotation mobilization. A pisiform contact is used to direct force anteriorly onto the transverse process. A) Approximate locations of the transverse processes; B) Contact on the L4 transverse process; C) Contact on the L3 transverse process; D) Contact on the L2 transverse process.

ulations are effective with this technique. Thrusting is usually not used. This technique can also be effective in the lower and mid-thoracic spine. It is most effective when done in three steps: l) Stabilize against spinous processes; 2) Take up slack by rotating the pelvis: and 3) Mobilize with the hand that is stabilizing against the spinous processes.

A 3D table enhances the effectiveness of this technique. For maximum effect, the clinician should use the table to rotate the spine in the opposite direction before stabilizing. This way the clinician is in better control and has greater range in which to take up slack (Fig 10-31C and D). This technique can be combined with the side bending technique shown in Figure 10-35. If the patient is in neutral flexion/extension, the rotation and side bending are usually in opposite directions. If the patient is positioned in flexion or extension, the rotation and side bending are usually in the same direction.

Lumbar Rotation-Prone

The mobilizing force is directed through the transverse process with a pisiform/hypothenar eminence contact. The transverse process of L1 is smaller and partially shielded by the 12th rib and the iliac crest usually shields the L5 transverse process. Therefore, hand placements for L2, 3 and 4 are shown, since only these transverse processes are prominent enough to be contacted by the hypothenar eminence (Fig 10-32). Since the transverse processes can only be palpated indirectly through soft tissue, this technique is semi-specific.

Each transverse process is contacted by placing the hypothenar eminence perpendicular to the spine. The L4 transverse process is slightly medial and superior to the posterior rim of the iliac crest. The L2 transverse process is found slightly inferior to the 12th rib. The L3 transverse process is midway between the L2 and L4 contacts. The pisiform contact should always be as close to the spinous process as possible, and the mobilizing force should be directed posteroanteriorly. This causes the vertebra to rotate on its base.

Note that when the L4 transverse process is the contact, the L4-5 segment receives most of the mobilization force. If the contact is on the left side, the direction of the mobilization is right rotation. Graded passive movements and stretch articulations are effective with this technique and it is especially useful when gentle, semi-specific mobilization is indicated for general lumbar hypomobility.

Lumbar Rotation–Supine

This rotational technique is another semi-specific technique that can be effective in the mid and lower thoracic

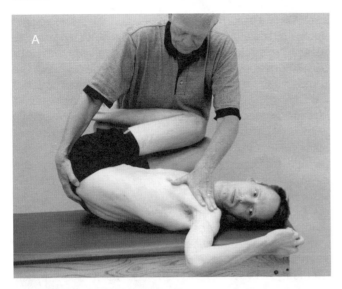
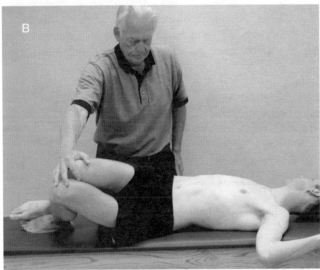
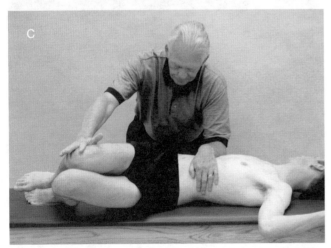

Figure 10-33: Rotation techniques. A) Left mid and lower thoracic mobilization; B) Right lumbar mobilization; C) Right lumbar mobilization with added stabilization across the lower ribs.

spine and in the lumbar spine. It can also be used as an effective self-mobilization or home treatment technique. The patient lies supine with the knees and hips flexed as the pelvis is rotated (Fig 10-33). The degree of knee and hip flexion determines the general level of spinal mobilization. If the knees and hips are flexed completely to the chest, the mobilization is directed into the mid-thoracic spine. As the amount of flexion is decreased, the level of the mobilization moves lower into the thoracic and the lumbar spine. If the patient's lower rib cage is stabilized, the mobilization becomes specific to the lumbar spine. Graded passive movements and stretch articulations are most effective with this technique. Gentle to moderate hold-relax and contract-relax techniques are also useful.

Lumbar Rotation–Supine "Lumbar Roll"

This rotational technique is the classic "lumbar roll" mobilization. Graded passive movements, stretch articulations or thrusts can be used. It is a specific technique because one segment can be isolated with ligamentous locking and facet apposition. The patient is positioned on the side opposite the desired direction of mobilization. The clinician faces the patient and palpates between the desired spinous processes with the cephalad hand. With the caudal hand, the clinician gains a secure hold on the patient's lower leg. The patient's spine is passively flexed by flexing the patient's hip and knee using the clinician's own hip as a balance point for the patient's knee. The clinician is actually shifting his pelvis to move the patient's lower body. With the palpating hand, the clinician feels for flexion to occur at the desired segment. When the clinician feels the inferior spinous process begin to move, he or she stops and lowers the leg to the table, "locking" the spine in flexion at that point. The clinician then rotates the trunk to cause rotation at the specific segment. This is done by pulling the patient's inferior arm forward and/or pressing the superior shoulder backward (Fig 10-34). Rotation is stopped when movement is palpated at the superior spinous process of the desired segment. In effect, this "locking" of the lower segments in flexion and upper segments in rotation causes the mobilizing force to be focused at the one desired level

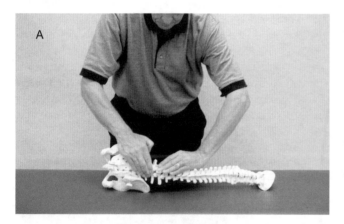

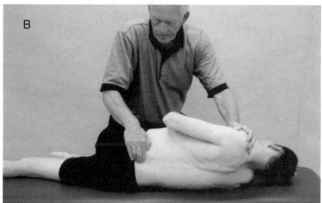

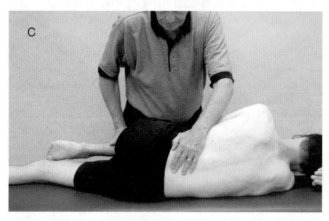

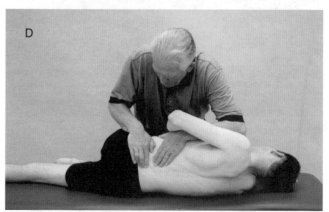

Figure 10-34: Lumbar left rotation technique - the "lumbar roll". A) Position of palpating hands; B) Flexion of the lumbar spine by flexing the patient's hip until the clinician feels the inferior segment move; C) Rotation of the patient's spine until the clinician feels the superior segment move; D) Force is imparted by rotating the lower segments toward and the upper segments away from the clinician.

The actual mobilization is accomplished by rotating the pelvis and lower segments toward the clinician and the shoulder and upper segments away from the clinician. Some of the mobilizing force is directed through the clinician's forearms to the patient's pelvis and shoulder, but it is important to concentrate as much force in the fingers as possible when doing this mobilization, to keep the lever arm as short as possible. The fingers are moved to the lat-eral aspects of the spinous processes to produce the rotational force. The fingers in contact with the inferior spinous process are on its lateral aspect closest to the table. The fingers in contact with the superior spinous process are on its lateral aspect above it. The clinician pulls the pelvis and inferior spinous process toward him, and pushes the superior spinous process and shoulder away. The thumb may be used instead of the fingers for the superior contact.

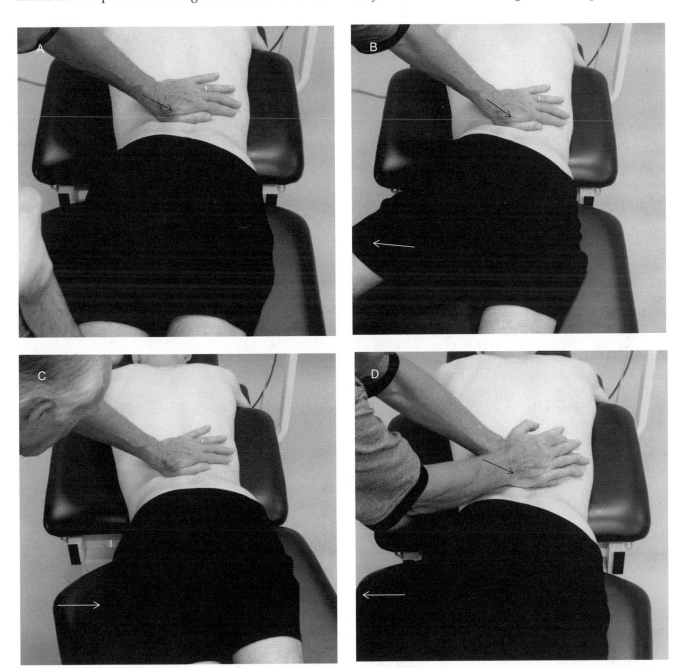

Figure 10-35: Lumbar left side bending technique. A) The left hand stabilizes; B) The hip is abducted to take up slack before mobilization, then the mobilizing force is applied with the left hand; C) Alternate technique pre-positioning the table in right side bending; D) The clinician moves the table back to the left to take up slack before mobilizing. The latter technique works best with a stabilization belt across the patient's hips.

Lumbar Side Bending-Prone

As the hip abducts, the lumbar spine side bends. If a stabilizing force is placed against the lateral aspect of the spinous process, side bending is prevented from that point superiorly. The lateral aspect of the MCP joint of the thumb is used to stabilize the lateral aspect of the selected spinous process. The thenar eminence and heel of the hand also stabilize along the lateral aspect of the spinous processes superior to the MCP stabilization. The technique is done in three steps: 1) The lateral aspect of the MCP joint, the thenar eminence and the heel of the hand are used to *stabilize* along the lateral aspect of the spinous processes; 2) The hip is abducted to *take up slack*; and 3) The clinician applies force against the spinous processes to *mobilize* (Fig 10-35 A and B). This technique concentrates the greatest side bending force at the segment just inferior to the point of contact of the MCP joint. If the patient is large or if vigorous mobilization is necessary, it may be necessary to use one clinician to stabilize and mobilize and an assistant to maintain abduction of the patient's leg. If both legs are carried along in the desired direction, more force can be imparted. This is accomplished easily with the use of a 3D mobilization table.

For maximum effect using a 3D table, the clinician should use the table to side bend the spine in the opposite direction before stabilizing (Fig 10-35 C and D). This way the clinician is in better control and has greater range in which to take up slack. This technique can be combined with the rotation technique shown in Figure 10-31. If the patient is in neutral flexion/extension, the rotation and side bending are usually in opposite directions. If the patient is positioned in flexion or extension, the rotation and side bending are usually in the same direction.

Lumbar Side Bending/Rotation—Side Lying Positional Stretch or Unilateral Traction

The side lying positional stretch involves side bending and may also incorporate rotation (Fig 10-36). The patient is positioned in side lying over a six to eight inch roll. The roll is positioned between the crest of the ilium and rib cage to achieve the maximum amount of side bending at a specific area. As the spine bends over the roll, the facet joints are separated and the muscles and ligaments are stretched on the superior side. If the pelvis is allowed to roll forward and the shoulder backward, a rotational component is added and even more separation and stretching is achieved. Even more stretch can be obtained if the patient's top leg is allowed to hang over the edge of the treatment table.

Because this technique opens the neural foramen on the superior side, it is a type of unilateral traction to the

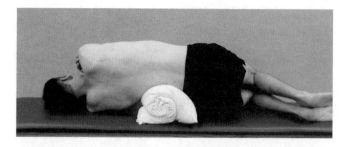

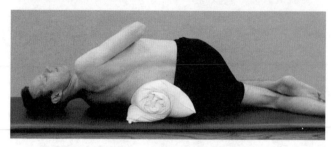

Figure 10-36: Positional stretch. A) Left side bending; B) Left side bending and right rotation.

superior joints. Therefore, it can be used for nerve root impingement problems and for joint hypomobility and muscular tightness. When used for nerve root impingement, one must distinguish between an impingement arising from a disc protrusion with a lateral shift and an impingement caused by narrowing, thickening, osteophyte formation (lateral spinal stenosis) or a disc fragment in the intervertebral foramen. In the latter instance, the patient should be placed with the side of the impingement up. In the former instance, the treatment goal is to correct the lateral shift. This would be accomplished by placing the patient on the side of pathology. This technique to correct a lateral shift should be done only if centralization of the patient's symptoms occurs (see discussion of HNP in Chapter 5, *Treatment by Diagnosis*). Positional stretches are usually done up to a maximum of ten minutes. They are also effective self-treatment techniques.

Lumbar P/A Accessory Mobilization

The central P/A accessory mobilization differs from the prone backward bending technique because the spine is positioned in neutral. The advantage of the technique is that it can be used to relieve pain and improve joint play in relatively acute cases.

Lumbar P/A techniques are the same as the thoracic techniques in Figure 10-28, except that in the lumbar spine the transverse process is at least a finger width lateral to the spinous process. The transverse process may not actually be felt, since lumbodorsal fascia and erector spinæ muscles cover it. The inability to feel the transverse processes directly

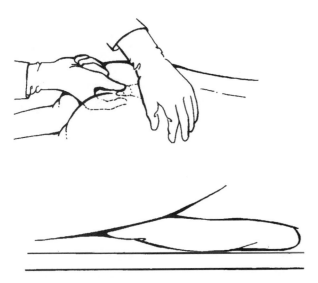

Figure 10-37: Coccyx mobilization.

does not make this a poor technique. The clinician will be able to visualize and feel differences in P/A mobility through the soft tissue. To get a pure P/A glide of an intervertebral joint with the patient lying prone, it is often necessary to angle the pressure cephalically, caudally, medially or laterally to take into consideration the curves of the spine.[22]

Coccyx

If the coccyx is positioned in abnormal extension, mobilization can be an effective form or treatment (Fig 10-37). An internal mobilization is performed with the patient prone over one or two pillows under the pelvis. The index finger is inserted internally into the rectum and the thumb is placed externally to grasp the coccyx. P/A glides and traction can both be effective. An external mobilization is performed with the pisiform or thumbs pressing anteriorly on the coccyx.

Muscle Energy Techniques— An Osteopathic Treatment Approach

Muscle Energy Techniques for joint mobilization are popular among clinicians who have advanced mobilization skills. METs for the sacroiliac joint were introduced in Chapter 7, *Pelvic Girdle Dysfunction*. METs have been promoted primarily by osteopathic physicians, most notably Drs. Fred Mitchell Sr. and Jr and Phillip Greenman.[21,32] These techniques can be quite complicated without first-hand instruction. Therefore, our purpose in this section is to introduce the reader to the concepts of osteopathic METs to stimulate further reading and continuing education.

The mobilization techniques discussed up to this point are primarily passive in nature. Although specific positioning is required, the clinician is the operator and the patient is passive and relaxed.

METs, on the other hand, are active in nature. METs may be likened to PNF contract-relax techniques except that METs for joint mobilization tend to be gentle, isometric contractions rather than maximal isometric contractions, which can tighten and compress joints. The safe and effective use of METs depends upon a thorough understanding of the osteopathic evaluation schemes described by Mitchell, Moran and Pruzzo, by Phillip Greenman and by others.[21, 28, 32] The basic concepts for the employment of METs are summarized as follows:

After a positional diagnosis has been made based on the assessment of motion restrictions, the patient is placed in a position that engages the motion barrier in all three planes. The patient is then asked to actively perform a series of submaximal isometric contractions in a specific direction against a distinct counterforce applied by the clinician so as to facilitate motion. These techniques are particularly safe and gentle, especially in the upper cervical spine where risk of vertebral artery compromise is present with thrust and rotatory techniques.

Manual therapy techniques for the spine are usually taught to the beginner via assessment through the spinous processes because they are easily palpated. Problems sometimes arise using this method when one is trying to determine whether a joint dysfunction is on the left or right side.

For example, palpating the T5 spinous process to be offset to the left of T6 determines only that the vertebral body may be rotated to the right. By palpating between the spinous processes, one might detect that two adjacent spinous processes are closer together than the spinous processes of two other adjacent segments. Does this mean that the superior element is backward bent or that the inferior element is forward bent?

To clarify this problem, osteopaths indirectly palpate the transverse processes through fascial planes to determine the exact position of the facets as well as their ability to move in all three planes of motion. Thus, the lesion can be precisely defined and a treatment maneuver prescribed that exactly corresponds to the dysfunction. The basic principles governing the use of METs are outlined as follows:

Motion Barriers—Normal joints all have physiological barriers to motion at opposite ends of their ranges of motion. These barriers are produced by the protective resiliency and elasticity of the soft tissues. Any other factor impeding the free motion of the joint between these range limits is considered to be pathological. In the normal spine, both in backward and forward bending, the facets at each segment should glide symmetrically in superior and inferior directions (open and close). This means that in flexion, the facets on each side should fully open and in extension the facets should fully close (Table 10-1).

Positioning—Motion takes place in all three planes simultaneously. Positioning of patients for both active and passive techniques should account for motion in all planes. Fryette's Third Law of Spinal Motion applies here in that if motion is introduced into a segment in any plane, motion in the other planes is reduced. This means, for example, that if a spinal segment is positioned in extension, the available range for side bending and rotation is reduced. If the segment is positioned in both extension and side bending, the available range for rotation is even further reduced.[32]

Diagnosis and Treatment—Assessment and treatment of a spinal segment by MET is based on the positional diagnosis as determined by its motion restriction. The motion restriction is what the segment is observed not to be able to do in response to spinal movement. The dysfunctional position is usually opposite that of the motion restriction. Lesioned segments are thus named by their dysfunctional position—either flexed or extended, rotated and side bent to the right or to the left. Designations of such lesions for communication and documentation purposes may be signified, for example, as FRS_R or ERS_L (see *A Diagnostic Example* below for further explanation).

A Diagnostic Example

It is possible for two very different lesions to appear identical (Fig 10-38). However, from a treatment aspect, they can be very dissimilar. In Figure 10-38A, the left facet will not close. Positionally, the lesion is described as flexed, right side bent, and right rotated (FRS_R). Its motion restriction will be into extension, left side bending and left rotation. In Figure 10-38B, the right facet will not open. Positionally, this lesion is described as extended, right side bent and right rotated (ERS_R). Its motion restriction will be into flexion, left side bending and left rotation.

Table 10-1: Normal Facet Function.

Direction of Motion	Facet Function
Forward Bending	Facets Open
Backward Bending	Facets Close
Side Bending Right	Right Facet Closes Left Facet Opens
Side Bending Left	Right Facet Opens Left Facet Closes

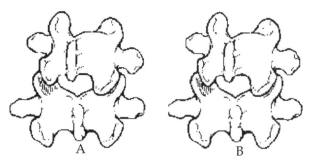

Figure 10-38: A) Lumbar facet lesion in which the left facet will not close; B) Lumbar facet lesion in which the right facet will not open. The two lesions appear identical but are approached very differently in treatment.

Since positionally, the two lesions appear identical, the clinician must palpate the transverse processes with the spine moving through the arc of forward and backward bending to make a proper diagnosis. In the case of an FRS_R, the right transverse process will become more prominent in *backward* bending but the transverse processes will be more equal in forward bending. In the case of an ERS_R, the right transverse process will become more prominent in *forward* bending but the transverse processes will be more equal in backward bending.

The clinician should develop a deductive thought process while making the assessment of segmental position and motion by asking the questions, "Where do I find the segment? What is the segment doing? What is the segment not doing?" in response to forward and backward bending movements.

Using the illustration in Figure 10-38 as an example, the clinician might approach the problem in this manner:

1. In prone (neutral), the spinous process is found to be to the left and the right transverse process is more prominent. From this, the presumption of a segment rotated to the right exists.

2. The patient then assumes a backward bent position (prone on elbows or Sphinx position). If the right transverse process is noted to become more prominent in this position, a presumptive diagnosis of an FRS_R restriction is made. This is deduced on the theory that the right facet is free to move and is being carried along as motion is introduced through the segment but the left facet is unable to extend (close) in response to the same movement. If, however, the transverse process becomes more symmetrical with backward bending, the presumptive diagnosis of an ERS_R lesion is made.

3. The diagnosis is confirmed by the patient assuming a forward bent position (prayer position). If the right transverse process becomes more symmetrical, the presumption is that the lesion is an FRS_R as the theory would indicate that the right facet is opening. There is no presumption that the left facet has moved in the direction of closure.

    Once the motion restriction has been identified, the correct technique can be applied to the motion barrier to facilitate segmental movement. To illustrate this, two MET techniques are presented so that the reader may appreciate the differences.

Treating a Lumbar FRS$_R$

Review: The left facet will not close. It is diagnosed by the posterior prominence of the right transverse process when the spine is in a hyperextended position. It is described as flexed, right rotated and right side bent (FRS_R).

1. The patient is side lying on a table on the side of the more posterior transverse process. The clinician stands at the side of the table facing the patient. The patient is close to the edge of the table.

2. A pillow supports the patient's head and the lower leg is straight with the upper leg flexed at the hip and knee.

3. The clinician's left hand palpates the interspinous space of the involved segment while the right hand extends the patient's lower leg at the hip joint until the extension movement is localized to the lesioned segment (Fig 10-39A).

4. The clinician repositions his hands, placing the right hand in a position to palpate movement of the spine while the left hand introduces rotation down to the segment by pulling the patient's lower arm as shown. Alternately, the clinician can press the upper shoulder backward. The patient is instructed to inhale then exhale. The rotation is produced during exhalation, localizing movement to the segment. The patient is then instructed to grip the edge of the table behind her (Fig 10-39B).

5. The clinician stabilizes the knee against his hip to create a pivot point and may cradle the leg, supporting the ankle at the elbow (Fig 10-39C). Alternately, the clinician can grasp the ankle if the leg is adequately supported with contact at the clinician's hip.

6. The clinician lifts up on the patient's leg (pivoting at the hip) to achieve side bending to the proper level.

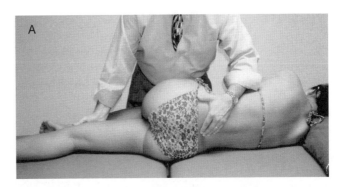

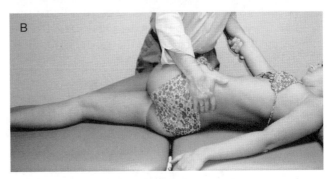

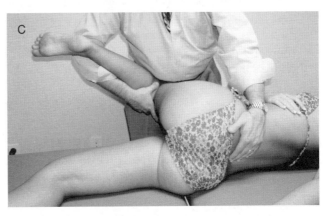

Figure 10-39: Lumbar muscle energy technique for segment that is flexed, right rotated and right side bent (FRS_R). A) Localization of extension; B) Localization of left rotation (the patient grasps the table to stabilize); C) Final localization of side bending, rotation and extension.

7. The patient is instructed to push the ankle down toward the floor against the fixed position and counterforce applied by the clinician. After a 5-10 second contraction, the patient is told to relax and the clinician takes up any slack created by the contraction.

8. The clinician relocalizes motion to the segment.

9. Steps 7 and 8 are repeated three to four times. Segmental motion is then retested and treatment is repeated if necessary.

Treating a Lumbar ERS$_R$

Review: The right facet will not open. It is diagnosed by the posterior prominence of the right transverse process when the spine is in a hyperflexed position. It is described as extended, right rotated and right side bent (ERS$_R$).

1. The patient lies in side lying. The prominent transverse process is on the top side (in this case, the patient is in left side lying).

2. The clinician stands at the side of the table facing the patient. The clinician's right hand palpates the interspinous space below the vertebra to be treated, while the left hand flexes the hips so that flexion is localized to the involved segment (Fig 10-40A).

3. While supporting the knees against the body, the clinician lowers the patient's feet until side bending to the left is localized to the segment (Fig 10-40B).

4. The patient is then asked to reach toward the floor until rotation to the left is localized to the segment (at times, this step can be omitted since rotation may be localized simultaneously with side bending).

5. The clinician instructs the patient to lift her feet up toward the ceiling against the fixed position and counterforce applied by the clinician. After a 5-10 second contraction, the patient is told to relax and the clinician takes up any slack created by the contraction. The force required is approximately five pounds.

6. The clinician relocalizes motion to the segment.

7. Steps 5 and 6 are repeated three to four times. Segmental motion is then retested and treatment is repeated if necessary.

While a beginner may initially have difficulty performing the two lumbar muscle energy techniques described, the purpose of these brief examples has been to show the nearly opposite approaches that are employed for two different types of dysfunctions.

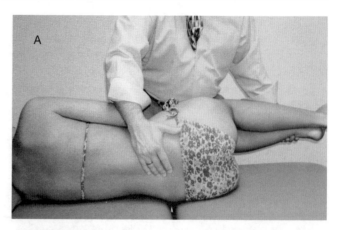

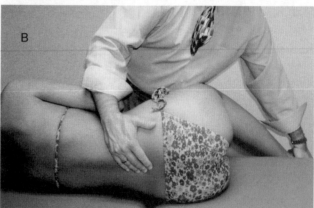

Figure 10-40: Lumbar muscle energy technique for segment that is extended, right rotated and right side bent (ERS$_R$). A) Localization of flexion; B) Localization of side bending.

The clinician unfamiliar with the MET approach may apply the same mobilization treatment to two very different joint dysfunctions just because they may appear similar. That is not necessarily bad. In many cases, a simple rotational mobilization or stretch successfully normalizes movement at a spinal segment. However, there are cases where graded passive movements, stretch articulations or thrusts are not effective. In such cases, the MET evaluation and treatment scheme may be more effective when gentle specificity is needed.

REFERENCES

1. Andersson G, Lucente T, Davis A, et al: A Comparison of Osteopathic Spinal Manipulation with Standard Care for Patients with Low Back Pain. New England J Med 341(19):1426-1431, 1999.

2. Assendelft W, Koes B, Knipschild P, et al: The Relationship Between Methodological Quality and Conclusions in Reviews of Spinal Manipulation. JAMA 274(24):1942-1948, 1995.

3. Assendelft W, Morton SC, Yu EI, et al: Spinal Manipulative Therapy for Low Back Pain. A Meta-Analysis of Effectiveness Relative to Other Therapies. Ann Intern Med 138:871-881, 2003.

4. Astin J and Ernst E: The Effectiveness of Spinal Manipulation for the Treatment of Headache Disorders: A Systematic Review of Randomized Clinical Trials. Cephalalgia 22:617-623, 2002.

5. Atchison J: Manipulation for the Treatment of Occupational Low Back Pain. Occup Med 13(1):185-197, 1998.

6. Aure O, Nilsen J and Vasseljen O: Manual Therapy and Exercise Therapy in Patients with Chronic Low Back Pain. Spine 28(6):526-532, 2003.

7. Bigos S, Bowyer O, Braen G, et al. *Acute Low Back Problems in*

Adults. AHCPR publication 95-0642. Rockville, Md: Agency for Health Care Policy and Research, Public Health Service, US Dept of Health and Human Services; 1994.

8. Bove G and Nilsson N: Spinal Manipulation in the Treatment of Episodic Tension-Type Headache, a Randomized Controlled Trial. JAMA 280(18):1576-1579, 1998.

9. Bronfort G, Evans R, Nelson B, et al: A Randomized Clinical Trial of Exercise and Spinal Manipulation for Patients with Chronic Neck Pain. Spine 26(7):788-799, 2001.

10. Chiradejnant A, Latimer J, and Maher C: Forces Applied During Manual Therapy to Patients With Low Back Pain. J Manipulative Physiol Ther 25(6):362-369, 2002.

11. Cyriax J: Diagnosis of Soft Tissue Lesions. Textbook of Orthopædic Medicine, Vol 1, 8th edition. Bailliere-Tindall, London 1982.

12. Dishman J and Bulbulian R: Spinal Reflex Attenuation Associated with Spinal Manipulation. Spine 25(19):2519-2525, 2000.

13. Dishman J, Ball K, and Burke J: First Prize: Central Motor Excitability Changes After Spinal Manipulation: A Transcranial Magnetic Stimulation Study. J Manipulative Physiol Ther 25(1):1-9, 2002.

14. Dishman J, Cunningham B, and Burke J: Comparison of Tibial Nerve H-Reflex Excitability after Cervical and Lumbar Spine Manipulation. J Manipulative Physiol Ther 25(5):318-325, 2002.

15. Ernst E and Harkness E: Spinal Manipulation: A Systematic Review of Sham-Controlled, Double-Blind Randomized Clinical Trials. J Pain and Symptom Management 22(4):879-889, 2001.

16. Ernst E: Does Spinal Manipulation Have Specific Treatment Effects? Family Practice 17(6):554-556, 2000.

17. Evans R, Bronfort G, Nelson B, et al: Two-Year Follow-up of a Randomized Clinical Trial of Spinal Manipulation and Two Types of Exercise for Patients with Chronic Neck Pain. Spine 27(21):2383-2389, 2002.

18. Freeman M and Wyke B: The Innervation of the Knee Joint: An Anatomical and Histological Study in the Cat. Joul Anat 101:505-532, 1967.

19. Giles L and Muller R: Chronic Spinal Pain Syndromes: A Clinical Pilot Trial Comparing Acupuncture, a Nonsteroidal Anti-inflammatory Drug and Spinal Manipulation. J Manipulative Physiol Ther 22(6):376-381, 1999.

20. Giles L and Muller R: Chronic Spinal Pain Syndromes: A Randomized Clinical Trial Comparing Medication, Acupuncture and Spinal Manipulation. Spine 28(14):1490-1503, 2003.

21. Greenman, P: Principles of Manual Medicine, 3rd ed. Lippincott Williams & Wilkins, Baltimore 2003.

22. Groom D: Cervical Spine and Shoulders. The Saunders Group, Minneapolis MN 2003 Course Manual.

23. Gross AR, Kay TM, Kennedy C, et al: Clinical Practice Guideline on the Use of Manipulation or Mobilization in the Treatment of Adults with Mechanical Neck Disorders. Manual Therapy 7(4):193-205, 2002.

24. Halata Z: The Ultrastructure of the Sensory Nerve Endings in the Articular Capsule of the Knee Joint of the Domestic Cat (Ruffini Corpuscles and Pacinian Corpuscles). Joul Anat 124:717-729, 1977.

25. Hsieh C, Adams A, Tobis J, et al: Effectiveness of Four Conservative Treatments for Subacute Low Back Pain. A Randomized Clinical Trial. Spine 27(11):1142-1148, 2002.

26. Hurwitz E, Moregenstern H, Harber P, et al: A Randomized Trial of Chiropractic Manipulation and Mobilization for Patients with Neck Pain: Clinical Outcomes friom the UCLA Neck-Pain Study. Amer Joul Pub Health 92(10):1634-1641, 2002.

27. Koes B, Assendelft W, van der Heijden G, et al: Spinal Manipulation for Low Back Pain, An Updated Systematic Review of Randomized Clinical Trials. Spine 21(24):2860-2871, 1996.

28. Lee D: Principles and Practice of Muscle Energy and Functional Techniques. In Modern Manual Therapy of the Vertebral Column. G Grieves, ed. Churchill Livingstone, London 1986.

29. MacConaill M and Basmajian J: Muscles and Movements. Williams and Wilkins, Baltimore MD 1969.

30. Maitland G: Vertebral Manipulation, 5th ed. Boston, Butterworths, 1986.

31. Mennell J: Back Pain. Little-Brown, Boston MA 1964.

32. Mitchell F, Moran P and Pruzzo N: An Evaluation and Treatment Manual of Osteopathic Muscle Energy Procedures. Mitchell, Moran and Pruzzo Associates, Valley Park MI 1979.

33. Nelson C, Bronfort G, Evans R, et al: The Efficacy of Spinal Manipulation, Amitriptyline and the Combination of Both Therapies for the Prophylaxis of Migraine Headache. J Manipulative Physiol Ther 21(8):511-519, 1998.

34. Nilsson N, Christensen H, and Hartvigsen J: The Effect of Spinal Manipulation in the Treatment of Cervicogenic Headache. J Manipulative Physiol Ther 20:326-330, 1997.

35. Nwuga V: Manipulation of the Spine. Williams and Wilkins, Baltimore MD 1976.

36. Paris S: The Spine. Atlanta Back Clinic. Atlanta GA 1975. Course Notes.

37. Polacek P: Receptors of the Joints: Their Structure, Variability and Classification. Acta Fac Med Univ Brunensis 23:1-107, 1966.

38. Senstad O, Leboeuf-Yde C, Borchgrevink CF. Frequency and Characteristics of Side Effects of Spinal Manipulative Therapy. Spine 22:435-441, 1997.

39. Shekelle P, Adams A, Chassin M, et al: Spinal Manipulation for Low-Back Pain. Annals of Internal Medicine 117(7):590-598, 1992.

40. Tullberg T, Blomberg S, Branth B, et al: Manipulation Does Not Alter the Position of the Sacroiliac Joint. A Roentgen Steriophotogrammetric Analysis. Spine 23(10):1124-1129, 1998.

41. Wittingham W and Nilsson N: Active Range of Motion in the Cervical Spine Increases after Spinal Manipulation (Toggle Recoil). J Manipulative Physiol Ther 24(9):552-555, 2001.

42. Yeomans S: The Assessment of Cervical Intersegmental Mobility before and after Spinal Manipulative Therapy. J Manipulative Physiol Ther 15(2):106-114, 1992.

SOFT TISSUE MOBILIZATION AND NEUROMUSCULAR TRAINING

Andrew J. Kerk PT, OCS, CFMT, ATC
Gregory S. Johnson, PT, FFCFMT
James R. Beazell, MS PT, OCS, FAAOMPT, ATC

Creating efficiency of human posture and movement is a primary goal in the treatment of neuromusculoskeletal dysfunction. When patients seek treatment for pain that appears mechanical in origin, clinicians are challenged to find and treat the source. This chapter describes soft tissue mobilization (STM) techniques for the connective tissue system blended with proprioceptive neuromuscular facilitation (PNF) techniques to treat the interplay of the mechanical and neuromuscular systems.

Inherent in all treatment systems is a thorough evaluation that includes adequate history, range of motion, strength, and special tests. This chapter includes a specialized evaluation intended to be combined with the more traditional evaluation components outlined in Chapter 4, *Evaluation of the Spine*. The evaluation system presented is intended to assess both structural and functional abnormalities.

Structural dysfunction can be defined as any alteration in the mechanical condition of the musculoskeletal system. For the soft tissue system it is defined as restriction of connective tissue extensibility or elasticity. Structural dysfunction is palpated manually and judged by the clinician to have an inelastic or restricted end feel. The management of structural dysfunctions through STM is described in detail.

In contrast, *functional dysfunction* can be defined as a deficit in neuromuscular control, strength, balance, or coordination. An overview of PNF will provide a means for addressing these functional deficits. Finally, STM and PNF will be combined into one technique termed *functional mobilization*™ (FM).[22,27,43] Functional mobilization is a time-efficient technique for blending treatment of structural and functional dysfunction.

Rationale

Soft tissue restriction is defined as an abnormal end feel to motion assessment. Clinicians can learn to manually palpate alterations in the end feel of joint[37] and soft tissue mobility. The specific histological changes of soft tissue restrictions are unknown. Miller has provided an excellent review of theoretical concepts based on current knowledge and research, but as he states, "The exact nature of the pathologic changes in myofascial tissues has not been elucidated".[36]

Joint capsules can certainly be a source of dysfunction as identified by Mennell, Cyriax, Maitland, and others.[28] A loss of capsular extensibility can be considered one type of soft tissue restriction. The clinician makes a qualitative assessment of this joint restriction by moving the joint through accessory or physiological motion to its end range and identifying its end feel as "abnormal" if it is too firm, inelastic, without recoil, or perhaps limited by pain.[33,45] In the case of extremity joint capsules, one can compare end feel to the opposite extremity. The clinician's assessment of a dysfunctional or abnormal end feel has been validated.[11,21,38,44,46] End feel assessment of joints, neural tissues, muscles, and the related connective tissues should be combined with a comprehensive evaluation. End feel assessment provides valuable information to help measure treatment outcomes and effectiveness.

In addition to joint capsule soft tissue restrictions, the patient may have restrictions of mobility between the basement membrane of the skin and superficial musculature and bony prominences, between two adjacent muscles, in the peritendinous tissue around a tendon or aponeurosis, within a musculotendinous junction, along the margin of a tendon blending into its bony attachment, between a tendon and its surrounding sheath, between a bursa and its surrounding structures, between neurovascular structures and their surrounding tissue matrixes, between adjacent visceral organs, and along visceral organ surfaces in contact with muscles and bone.

The following overview of fascial anatomy and connective tissue histology provides a foundation for the evaluation and treatment principles described. The focus of STM treatment is on the fascia. Fascia can be dense or loose, and provides a support network for musculoskeletal, visceral, and neurovascular structures. The regular connective tissue that makes up tendons and ligaments will also be considered.

It is helpful to recall gross anatomy dissection and the time-intensive labor required to remove and discard the pervasive connective tissue membranes. The removal of the fascia formed from the irregular connective tissue permits the anatomist to visualize and study the muscular, neurovascular, and skeletal structures. It is an interesting analogy to consider soft tissue mobilization as blunt dissection through the skin. The manual contact attempts to separate structures that are meant to move on one another. Again, recall separating the parallel seams of muscles such as the dorsal forearm or hamstrings in cadaver dissection lab. The dissector typically uses a blunt probe or finger, much like we use a finger contact in our soft tissue mobilization methods. The visualization and physical handling of fascia in the anatomy lab is an invaluable tool for understanding the function of the fascial system discussed here. Knowledge of the physiology and structure of fascia also helps the clinician understand the impact that mobilizing and conditioning this system can have on posture and movement.

Anatomical Considerations of Fascia

Figure 11-1 illustrates a lower extremity dissection with the fascia left intact. This unique perspective allows us to visualize many aspects of fascia that may otherwise be overlooked. First, fascia provides a separation of adjacent structures to allow independent movement. In 1938 Gratz described such separation in the abdominal peritoneal fascial planes, calling the interfaces "functional joints".[16] This term is also useful to describe areas within and between musculoskeletal structures that must move in varying directions on one another. In the healthy state,

fascia provides a slippery interface, or "space built for motion",[40] between skin and superficial muscle layers, in the seams between adjacent muscles, and between superficial and deep muscles. This individual muscle mobility can be termed *muscle play*.[24] One of the goals in manual treatment is to restore lost muscle play with specific pressure or contact along these fascial planes or "functional joints" between the tissues. The assessment and treatment of muscle play is described in *Muscle Play* on page 292.

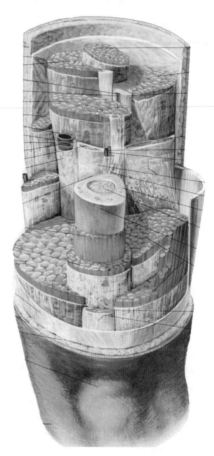

Figure 11-1: Illustrated anatomic dissection that leaves the fascia intact, providing a visualization of the "functional joints" between adjacent structures (From Lopez-Antunez, 1971, with permission from Elsevier).[32]

Fascia connects structures to allow mechanical force absorption, attenuation, and transference. Examples of this fibrous network can be found in the endomysium surrounding individual muscle fibers, the perimysium surrounding groups or bundles of muscle fibers, and the epimysium forming an envelope around an entire muscle. These three components of fascia are part of the myofascial network that is continuous within and between contractile fibers of a muscle. These layers correspond and are continuous with the endotendon, peritendon, and epitendon layers of a tendon, and the subsequent attachment into the periosteum of bone, or perichondrium of cartilage. This myofascial network also blends into the more regular connective tissue of ligamentous joint capsules. The myofascial origins and insertions thereby impart the muscle's contractile tension into movement of joints. Mobilization that alters the tension within the myofascial weave can also affect the neurosensory input from both the muscle spindle units and Golgi tendon organs and could explain the broad changes in postural muscle tone, alignment, and proprioception that are observed clinically after myofascial mobilization.

Fascia also forms tunnels for passage of nerves, arteries, veins, and lymphatic vessels. Mechanically, the neurovascular structures must be able to slide and move separate from the adjacent matrix to prevent their lumen from being collapsed, pinched, or stretched. Butler[9,10] and Elvey[13,14,20,39] have identified these fascial tunnels as potential sources of restricted mobility. Korr[30,31] has shown that an impinged spinal nerve will result in decreased collagen production along the nerve's distribution. The case study at the end of this chapter utilizes mobilization along the sciatic nerve tract and into the distal lower extremity to alleviate persistent tissue restriction and paresthesia after lumbar disc decompression surgery (see *Case Study* on page 296).

In a healthy state, the fascial planes within the body provide a pathway for diffusion of interstitial fluids and materials. If necessary, the fascia can provide a wall to contain bleeding or infection. However, this mechanism for containment can also have an adverse effect on posture and movement if interstitial fluid flow is blocked by dehydration and bogginess in the fascial membranes. Swelling that occurs with injury and inflammation can alter movement patterns—both from the patient's pain avoidance, and from mechanical tension within the fascia itself. As the condition becomes subacute and chronic, the fluid accumulation can become fibrous and eventually restrict mobility. The soft tissue mobility restrictions that result can be addressed with manual mobilization methods and thoughtful exercise and movement training.

Histological Considerations of Fascia

The microscopic study of fascia reveals a network of fibers embedded in a matrix of ground substance. Collagen is the most predominant fiber and is very tough and unyielding. Collagen fibers are woven adjacent to other fibers, each having an interface for movement or a functional joint as described above. This motion between fibers can be limited by development of cross links, which are fibrous bridges of small diameter collagen strands. With immobility there is

a drop in hyaluronic acid proportionate to chondroitin 4 & 6 sulfate resulting in a decrease in water content and greater viscosity of ground substance. This relative dehydration coincides with a decrease in volume of ground substance and a reduction in critical fiber distance. Subsequently, there is greater opportunity for development of cross links. In time, the weave of collagen fibers becomes tighter and more complex, and the range of movement or excursion of tissue decreases.[1,2,3,4,5,7,8,47]

Theoretically, controlled movement imparted to tissue via a clinician's hands and with specific exercise may prevent such cross links from forming simply by moving the matrix of fibers within ground substance, possibly stimulating hydration and assisting in the maintenance of critical fiber distance.

An important cellular element in connective tissue is the fibroblast. Fibroblasts are responsible for producing the other elements present in fascia, namely collagen fibers, elastin fibers, and ground substance. Fibroblasts respond to the mechanical stresses placed on tissue by producing the appropriate elements and arranging them within the fascial network in a manner that allows the tissue to withstand such stress. In healing tissue, it has been noted that immobilization results in fibroblasts that are arranged in multiple directions, causing collagen fibers to be laid down in a more random fashion.

In contrast, healing tissue in which controlled movement takes place has fibroblasts arranged parallel to the direction of movement.[6] The resultant collagen fiber direction is along the lines of stress and in line to withstand the movement. Wolf's Law, which applies to bone, states that trabeculae direction and mineral deposition are arranged in an optimal fashion to best withstand the forces present.

Since bone is a specialized type of connective tissue, this same principle can be expanded to fascia. It is well accepted that tissue responds to mechanical stress with structural transformation.[1,2,3,4,5,6,45,47] Therefore, the concept of applying controlled stresses to the musculoskeletal system as part of a rehabilitation program is well-founded.

Viscoelastic Properties of Soft Tissue

Viscoelasticity is a property exemplified in connective tissue that explains its response to mechanical manipulation, and provides direction for skilled technique application. A stress/strain curve illustrates various levels of stress (pressure of the clinician's finger, or manual contact) and the strain (quantity of tissue excursion or range of motion) that can result (Fig 11-2). Pressure that is too firm or rapid may result in tissue failure or tearing, injury to the

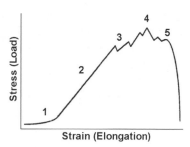

Figure 11-2: Manual stress (load) applied to tissue into areas 1 and 2 (elastic region) will not result in strain (elongation) after release of pressure. Soft tissue mobilization that loads the tissue with enough stress to enter area 3 (plastic deformation) will result in a change in tissue length after pressure is released. Areas 4 and 5 represent tissue failure, which should be avoided.

clinician's phalangeal joint, slipping of the finger off of the targeted tissue, or numbness and subsequent inadequate sensitivity of the clinician's treating finger. The ideal pressure or stress enters the plastic region of the stress/strain curve so that when the pressure is released, the tissue has a greater excursion or more elastic end feel.

Functional Assessment

The testing described in this section is designed to evaluate vertical alignment of the body with advancing compressive loads, and dynamic stabilization responses to gravity, inertia, and manually applied force. Going beyond visual observation of posture allows the clinician to evaluate how the patient's system behaves when balance and stability are challenged. The astute clinician can also move beyond these tests and develop individualized evaluative maneuvers that replicate the physical stresses and loads unique to the particular patient problem, region of dysfunction, and patient's activity demands. Such individualized assessment tools attempt to reveal posture and movement dysfunction more clearly to the patient and clinician, and offer immediate retesting measures to determine treatment effectiveness. These clinical tests also blend into treatment by creating an opportunity for the pain patient to tune into kinesthetic sensations rather than focus excessively on symptoms.

Our functional assessment builds on a foundation of neutral posture alignment. For our purposes, *neutral* refers to a spinal column and extremity joints that are aligned in mid range positions with no buckling or shifting in the presence of a compressive load. This compressive load may be in the form of gravity, a manually applied force, or from inertia during movement. Balance and stability are best established with all body segments stacked vertically

from the lower extremity base of support to the torso, cranium, and upper extremities.

Rolf's analogy of a stack of blocks is a helpful visualization for understanding how alignment affects stability.[40] If the blocks are arranged in a straight vertical relationship to one another, the stack will more easily remain stable and upright within the field of gravity. However, if one of the blocks is displaced slightly, the stack above it and the integrity of the entire column is less stable and at risk of collapse (Fig 11-3).

A person whose posture is aligned vertically with all joints in neutral requires little or no muscular effort to remain standing, and there are no localized segments ready to buckle or collapse. The visual comparison of different bodies in neutral posture, as we have defined it, can vary and still be considered normal and efficient for the given set of circumstances. In general, the clinician should be less concerned with textbook descriptions of perfect posture and more focused on efficiency and optimal physical performance.

The body's blocks, or articulating segments, relate to one another as a kinetic chain. In a state of optimal alignment, forces can be loaded, transferred, dissipated, and stored as kinetic energy in the muscles and elastic tissue components. One can picture ground reaction forces in an extremity being spread from distal to proximal in a closed kinetic chain. These forces are efficiently transferred at each link in the chain of articulations toward the trunk which, if aligned in neutral, can best transfer the kinetic energy back

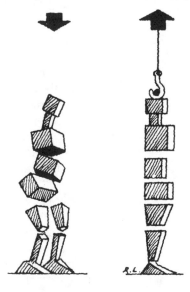

Figure 11-3: Rolf describes the body as a model of blocks or segments that when misaligned are unstable. Balanced vertical alignment creates stability and postural ease.[40]

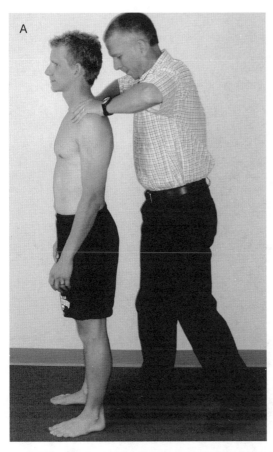 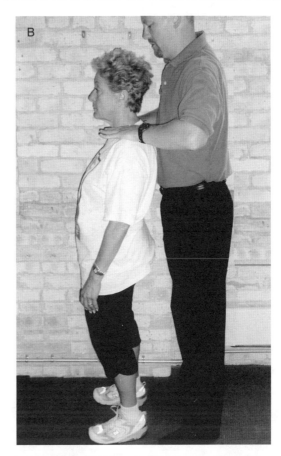

Figure 11-4: Comparing an efficient and inefficient vertical compression test. A) Efficient—Balanced vertical alignment with a solid end feel and efficient force transfer into the base of support. B) Inefficient—Extended spinal posture with thoracic cage posterior to the pelvis and buckling into hyperextension.

down the extremity from proximal to distal for propulsion or open kinetic chain movement. The forces can transfer in either direction along the bony skeleton and along the spiral, winding arrangement of the fascial planes.

Johnson developed the *Vertical Compression*, *Elbow Flexion*, and *Lumbar Protective Mechanism* tests as evaluative tools to determine efficiency in postural alignment, dynamic stabilization abilities, strength, and neuromuscular control.[25,27,41] Additional functional tests described below have been adapted from Gray's work in evaluating the trunk and extremities in closed kinetic chain patterns.[17,18] All of the tests involve movement of forces along the links in the kinetic chain and observation of how efficiently loads are transferred, dissipated, and absorbed.

Vertical Compression

The patient is instructed to stand relaxed with natural posture. The clinician applies a gentle, even, downward force through the upper torso with hand contact in the superior scapula and upper rib cage region.

In optimal well-aligned posture, the clinician will feel a qualitative solid end feel into the feet and will notice the patient's torso remains upright without signs of buckle or collapse. In other words, in an efficient state of alignment the clinician's vertical pressure will be transferred down through the patient's body and passed from the base of support into the feet and ground. In a dysfunctional state with less than optimal alignment, the clinician will feel a giving way in the patient's body, in the form of buckling or movement shift. Dysfunctional movements that may be seen include, but are not limited to, hyperextension of the lumbar spine with anterior tilting of the pelvis, hyperflexion of the thoracic spine, shearing of the pelvis in any direction, or rotational collapse of the torso or pelvis (Fig 11-4).

Repeating the test after treatment intervention determines whether improved vertical posture alignment was achieved. Pain with a postural dysfunction component will often be reproduced during the vertical compression test. If better postural alignment is achieved with treatment, symptoms also may improve. This provides immediate motivation to both the patient and clinician and retrospec-

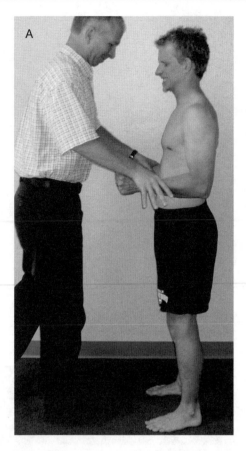 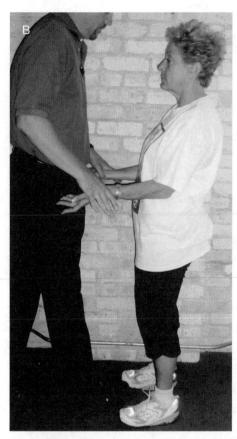

Figure 11-5: The elbow flexion test. A) Efficient—The spine is well-aligned vertically, with shoulder girdles well positioned in posterior depression. B) Inefficient—The thoracic cage moves further into posterior displacement and the shoulders make an inefficient attempt to stabilize with protraction, thereby losing their foundation of support from the rib cage.

tively identifies the postural dysfunction as a probable source of pain.

Elbow Flexion

The elbow flexion test is closely related to the vertical compression test. Instead of pressing down on the upper torso, the clinician applies a downward force through the patient's forearms with the elbows flexed 90°. The elbow flexion test allows assessment of force transfer from the upper extremities through the shoulder girdle into the rib cage and torso. The elbow flexion test also relates to the lumbar protective mechanism described below, since it tests the patient's dynamic stabilization response to manually applied force. If the elbow flexion test is negative, the patient's torso remains solid without buckling and stable contact is maintained between the clavicle and rib cage anteriorly and the scapula and rib cage posteriorly. A positive elbow flexion test is characterized by one or both shoulder girdles moving into elevation with over-contraction of the upper trapezius, shoulder girdle protraction, winging of the medial scapular border, or any movement

that reduces full surface area contact of the clavicles and scapulae on the rib cage. If shoulder girdle instability is seen, concurrent cervicothoracic and lumbopelvic buckling or loss of vertical alignment is often seen (Fig 11-5).

Lumbar Protective Mechanism

The lumbar protective mechanism is a more dynamic test of trunk stability. The patient is instructed to stand relaxed and balanced with one foot in front of the other. The clinician stands within the diagonal that matches the patient's foot position and commands the patient with, "Hold. Don't let me move you." Manual contact is made with the palms of the clinician's hands in the infraclavicular region pushing into a posterior diagonal. Pressure is light in an effort to allow the patient to respond to the force and hold the torso stable over the pelvis. If the patient is able to initiate an opposing contraction and remain stable and vertical, the force may be increased slightly to assess strength. If the patient continues to remain stable without movement out of vertical alignment, the therapist can hold the force for a longer period of time to assess endurance.

A positive test involves the patient losing vertical alignment (Fig 11-6). For a complete test, the same procedure is repeated in both directions in both diagonals. The lumbar protective mechanism test provides a good baseline for repeated testing before and after individual treatment interventions, treatment sessions, or over a number of sessions. Normal responses vary between subjects, but serial testing of the same subject after manual therapy treatment and exercise training should reveal improved stabilization abilities if treatment is effective.

Other Trunk and Extremity Loading Tests

There are other simple, yet informative functional tests that can be done to evaluate the closed kinetic chain in terms of segmental stability and force transfer, dissipation, and storage. Extremity loading tests are a simple expansion of the vertical compression and lumbar protective mechanism tests. For example, during gait the foot pronates in response to ground reaction forces and subsequent loading occurs from distal to proximal. Each segment of the kinetic chain should go through an optimal range of physiological or accessory motion in the process of

loading. Loading, or vertical compression, stores and spreads kinetic energy in the spiral arranged musculature and fascia. The body is then prepared for unloading, or propulsion, which it accomplishes with supinatory movements that occur from proximal to distal from the trunk into the extremities. In this sense, pronation becomes a term synonymous with loading and supination becomes synonymous with unloading.[17,18]

The efficiency of this well-timed mechanism depends on factors such as alignment of segments and joint surfaces, mobility of joint capsules, fascia, and other connective tissue, strength and responsiveness of musculature, and neuromuscular control. As stated previously, the basic tests can serve as a framework for the creative development of patient-specific tests that assess work, sport, or activity demands. In designing functional tests for patients, the clinician must place safety first and avoid over-challenging individuals beyond their abilities. Start with tests and challenges that are easier and progress to more advanced activities as the patient succeeds. Consistency is critical in any testing, so clear documentation of methodology is imperative.

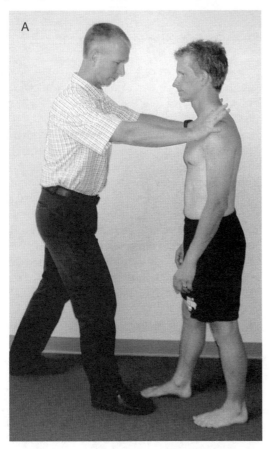 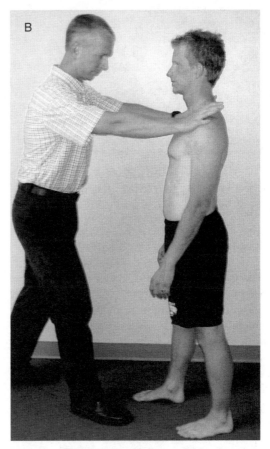

Figure 11-6: Comparing an efficient and inefficient lumbar protective mechanism. A) Efficient—Stabilization of the trunk in a neutral vertical alignment. B) Inefficient—Less activation of the anterior stabilizing musculature, which results in an inefficient shift into hyperextension.

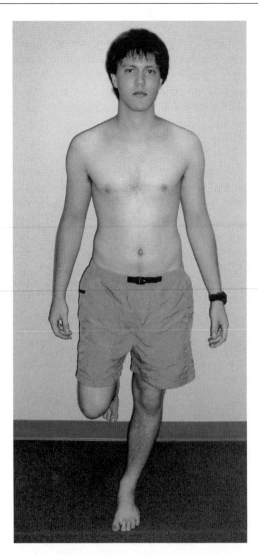

Figure 11-7: Inefficient single leg balance, with excessive pronation or over-loading at the subtalar joint combined with an under-loaded, outwardly rotated proximal tibia and knee.

Single Leg Balance

This test challenges a component of gait and supplements basic gait observation. McPoil and Cornwall[34] noted that the degree of subtalar pronation in balanced single leg stance is essentially equal to the maximal pronation that is reached during gait. While actual walking is more dynamic, we can utilize single leg balance to observe the loading of each link in the kinetic chain.

Ideally, the foot and ankle should be slightly pronated with a mild lowering of the longitudinal arch. The tibia should follow the talus into slight internal rotation, and the knee should slightly flex and tip into valgus. The femur should slightly internally rotate with the patella remaining in the frontal plane. The hip should flex slightly with

internal rotation and varus angulation. The pelvis should remain horizontal in the frontal plane and the trunk should be vertical without excessive rotation or side bending.

With the single leg balance test, the clinician frequently observes a link along the chain that is excessively loaded, rotated, or as Gray and Tiberio describe, overpronated. [17,18] In Johnson's description of vertical compression, he refers to a "buckling of transitional zones leading to a mechanical stress points". [22,23,24] Over time these points can develop a hypermobility (with absorption of too much force) with hypomobility (under-loaded segments) above or below.

A classic example illustrated is overpronation at the subtalar and midtarsal joint with excessive tibial varus (Fig 11-7). The tibia has less internal rotation than expected and in fact appears externally rotated (especially at the proximal portion). Similarly, the knee appears more in varus and extended than one would expect. In this case, the midtarsal is overpronated and the knee is supinated and inadequately loaded. The single leg balance test is an excellent pre and post treatment test to show the presence or absence of symptoms and as a qualitative test to compare sides.

Double and Single Leg Squat

The squat tests serve to increase the load demands of the single leg balance test and challenge more dynamic stability and control. The patient is instructed to place feet hip distance apart and squat downward keeping the feet flat. From the front, the clinician observes whether the patient's knees track toward the second toe and whether ankle dorsiflexion occurs without excessive pronation or supination. From a lateral view, the degree of ankle dorsiflexion, knee flexion, and hip flexion can be noted, as well as the ability to maintain a neutral lumbopelvic alignment. Figure 11-8 illustrates the double leg squat test. The single leg squat test demonstrates the same features, but adds greater resistance and challenges the gluteus medius to maintain a level pelvis and vertical trunk. The right side can be compared to the left to check for asymmetries.

Double and Single Leg Hop

Clinical testing can proceed to double and single leg hop if the patient has succeeded in single leg balance, and double/single leg squat with no symptoms, good alignment, strength, and control. The patient is asked to jump with a submaximal effort straight upward and land softly at the take-off point. The clinician can note alignment of the joints during both the concentric propulsive phase as well as during the eccentric landing phase. The patient can also

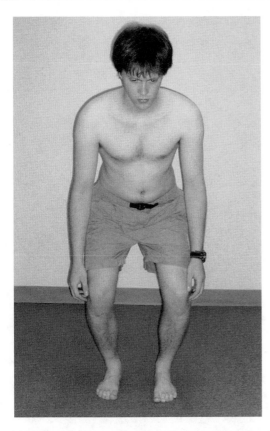

Figure 11-8: Double leg squat with unbalanced kinetic chain loading. Increasing the lower extremity load with a functional squat results in overpronation at the subtalar joints and increased varus angulation at the knees.

note any symptoms that may be present. It can be helpful to videotape this test for repeated observation in slow motion and freeze frame since the movement occurs quickly. The test can be made more advanced by adding a maximal height hop, landing on the same spot, or even hopping a short distance in any direction. The single leg hop is quite advanced, but it can be very revealing, especially when multiple directions are compared. Again, the key is to find the test that reveals the patient's movement dysfunction, and to perform it consistently as a method of retesting to assess treatment effectiveness.

Double and Single Arm Closed Chain Testing

The same procedures used for lower extremities can be applied to upper extremity weight bearing. The classic wall push up position can be performed with double and single arm balance, progressing to a short arc push up. Resistance can be advanced with a counter or waist-height push up (Fig 11-9), hands on a stair step, knee push up on the floor, or a traditional floor push up. As in the lower extremity, a double or single arm hop can be added as a more advanced test activity. Crawling or walking with the hands on a

treadmill is another advanced test. Closed kinetic chain activities of the upper extremity can assess wrist extension range of motion and segmental loading along each link in the chain.

A common observation is lack of shoulder girdle stability in full contact against the rib cage, both with the clavicle anteriorly and scapula posteriorly. Poor proximal stability is a dysfunction that leads to subacromial impingement and rotator cuff breakdown, as well as forearm and hand overuse syndromes such as medial and lateral epicondylitis, wrist and hand tendonitis, and some carpal tunnel syndromes.

Basic Soft Tissue Mobilization

Once a soft tissue restriction is identified, treatment is initiated. Important factors to consider for successful treatment include the proper localization of pressure, the quantity of pressure to use, clinician body mechanics, patient preparation and positioning, and skin preparation.

Localization

Success in the use of soft tissue mobilization begins with a skilled palpation evaluation. The skin should be dry with no lubricant to allow movement of superficial and deeper layers without slipping. Soft tissue restrictions are identified very specifically in terms of direction and depth. First, superficial fascia is evaluated in a specific direction utilizing a broad, flat hand moving the tissue completely through its range of excursion, followed by gentle overpressure to assess end feel. Normal accessory play, or end feel, has a quality of recoil, or elasticity. Abnormal end feel is firm and without recoil, indicating a soft tissue restriction.

Once the direction of restricted end feel is determined with a broad hand, it is localized to a single fingertip. Varying the angle of the finger in relation to the patient's body identifies the specific depth of the restriction. If the angle of the treating finger is parallel to the patient's body, more superficial fascia is assessed. As the angle of the treating finger becomes more perpendicular, deeper layered tissue interfaces are palpated. A common clinician error is to attempt palpation of deeper layers by using more pressure, rather than by increasing the angle of contact. Typically several soft tissue restrictions are identified in an area and treatment is applied to the firmest restrictions first.

Quantity of Pressure

It is imperative to understand how much pressure to use in both evaluation and treatment of soft tissue restrictions. As

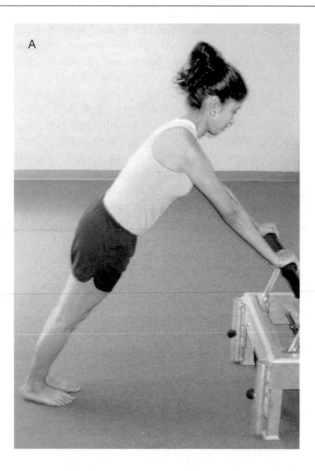 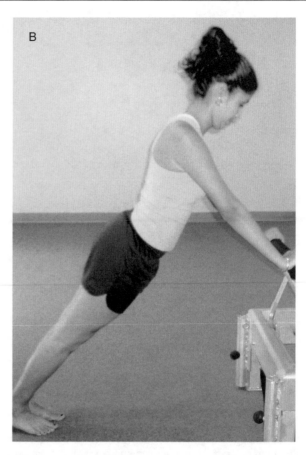

Figure 11-9: Comparing an efficient and inefficient lumbar protective mechanism. A) Efficient—Neutral spinal alignment and stable shoulder girdles in the posterior depressed position. B) Inefficient—Lumbar hyperextension and lack of adequate scapulothoracic contact.

in all methods of treatment, patient tolerance is the primary consideration. It is good practice to repeatedly remind the patient to report excessive tenderness or ask the clinician to decrease pressure at any time. Patient guarding and increased muscle tension is counterproductive. An important mechanical consideration is the viscoelastic quality of connective tissue. The clinician respects viscoelasticity by maintaining a slow speed of contact when gliding into connective tissue. If the finger presses in too quickly, the tissue will respond with a fluid quality of hardness. The result could be tearing and trauma to the tissue, or the finger may slip over the surface of the tissue and be ineffective in assessing the mobility within the matrix. Another disadvantage of using too much pressure is that the clinician's tactile abilities will be inhibited, and he will be less able to evaluate the end feel quality.

Body Mechanics

Alignment of the clinician's body from the lower extremities and trunk through the upper extremity into the finger joints is critical for sensitive palpatory information gathering, success in treatment, and protection of the clinician's body. The same principles of body mechanics apply to the application of PNF and functional mobilization discussed later.[27]

The clinician should maintain a wide base of support with knees unlocked, often with one foot ahead of the other. The feet and pelvis should face the direction of pressure or movement with the spine in neutral alignment. The clinician's scapulae are stable against the rib cage, the elbow is unlocked, and the wrist and fingers are all in a straight-line neutral relationship to transfer force through the clinician's kinetic chain to the tip of the finger without buckling or undue stress at specific joints. Clinicians who do not align their bodies appropriately may eventually develop deviation at the wrist, hyperextension or flexion deformity of the finger joints, and disabling tendonitis and joint instability. The use of proper body mechanics allows the clinician better control of forces so that the techniques are more effective and safer for both the clinician and patient.

Patient Preparation

It is important to communicate certain points to patients prior to the application of soft tissue mobilization. As in all treatment methods, patients should be aware that they can ask the therapist to stop, decrease, or modify manual contact at any time that they become uncomfortable. Certain points of contact may be tender but patients should feel as though they are still able to relax and not feel traumatized. Patients should usually feel either comfortable pressure, or tenderness that is often described as "a good hurt". A guideline often communicated in manual therapy circles is to "use the least amount of force necessary to achieve a desired result". If a patient communicates a desire to have the pressure decreased, or if the therapist notes muscle guarding, pressure is reduced to the patient's comfort level.

Guarding may also prompt the clinician to use a Grade I oscillation technique, or stop treating the restriction and use other methods. Patients should be advised to expect minor soreness at or near areas treated for 12–24 hours after the session. The soreness is usually different from the original complaint and can be described as the sensation of exercising in a different way. Tenderness may be present, but there should be no bruising. Most commonly patients feel more mobile and have more ease with posture and movement.

Hydration of ground substance was discussed above as a possible mechanism by which fascia becomes more mobile. For this reason, patients should also be instructed to increase their water intake and reduce beverages such as alcohol, coffee, or tea that have a diuretic effect.

Patient Positioning

Initial positioning of the patient is based on comfort and the concept of neutral alignment of the skeleton with tissues placed on slack. This allows the clinician to discriminate between tissue restrictions that are mainly structural from those that might be a result of muscles contracting or being placed on stretch. As treatment progresses, soft tissue mobilization may be done with tissues in more lengthened positions, during weight bearing, and during functional movements.

The patient may be placed prone over a pillow extending lengthwise from the upper chest to the anterior superior iliac spines of the pelvis. The pillow will allow the head and neck to drop slightly forward with contact of the forehead on a rolled towel, or table face cradle. The pillow should also allow the pelvis to drop into a slight posterior tilt. In this position, both the cervical and lumbar facet joints are slightly disengaged and unloaded to prevent compression and assist in relaxation. A small pillow under the feet and ankles will help place the hamstrings on slack. Rolled towels under the anterior aspect of each shoulder will also place the medial scapular muscles in a relaxed position and keep the thoracic fascia from appearing artificially taut. The arms can hang over the sides of the table, or be placed at the patient's side.

When evaluating and treating anterior structures of the chest, abdomen, anterior extremities, and craniocervical regions, the patient may be placed supine. One to two pillows may be positioned under the proximal thighs and ischial tuberosities to assure that the lumbar facets are slightly disengaged. The head and neck can be lifted and positioned over a folded towel of appropriate thickness for the cervical facets to be in a neutral position. Rolled towels can also be placed under the posterior shoulders and possibly elbows to position the pectoral fascia on slack.

The side lying position is quite useful as it allows the clinician to palpate and treat the anterior and posterior aspects of the body, and allows manual treatment to efficiently blend into PNF and functional mobilization techniques described below.[27] In subjects with pelvis and shoulders significantly wider than the mid torso, a pillow is placed under the rib cage to prevent the spine from hanging into a side bent position. A doubled pillow under the head is necessary to allow neutral cervical alignment, as well as allowing a trough for the underside shoulder to lie without compressing the shoulder girdle into the rib cage and upper thoracic region. A third pillow between the knees comfortably flexed to 45–90° keeps the hips in neutral so that both anterior and posterior hip fascia are on slack.

Skin Preparation

Most soft tissue mobilization methods are performed with the skin dry. When assessing and treating the mobility of skin and superficial fascia, the skin must move with the clinician's hands and not slip at the interface. The skin of either the patient or the clinician may need to be frequently dried with a towel or small amount of powder to prevent slipping. Dry methods are also used for treatment of deeper layers along bony contours and layered musculature. If the clinician judges that the skin is too dry and is being irritated or scratched, a small amount of lubricant can be applied to the fingers and hand. A good choice is a combination of beeswax and coconut oil. Lanolin based products, oils and other materials are often too greasy and the clinician should be aware that allergic reactions can occur.

Treatment Progression and Specific Techniques

As discussed above, treatment begins with the clinician placing the treating finger at a localized area of restriction. The soft tissue is taken to the end of the available range of excursion. An initial mobilization force, termed *sustained pressure*, is held until a softening or giving way of the firm end feel is noted.[22,24]

If no change in tissue mobility is palpated in a practical length of time (perhaps 5–30 seconds), then the assisting hand may apply *shortening* or *lengthening* to the surrounding soft tissue matrix. This shortening or lengthening is performed within 1–2" of the treating finger and is applied from any direction around the treating finger and is specific to the same depth of the restriction. If the tissue restriction under the treating finger begins to soften, the treating finger can slide or move further through the tissue, often encountering additional aspects of the original restriction that are then treated in the same manner.

Occasionally, the tissue restriction does not ease with sustained pressure and shortening or lengthening with the assisting hand. One alternative is to apply an *unlocking spiral*.[22,24] An unlocking spiral starts with sustained pressure as described above, and adds rotation along the longitudinal axis of the treating finger and arm. While maintaining pressure in the direction of the restricted end feel, the finger is rotated clockwise and counterclockwise a few degrees, noting which rotation feels easier. The treating finger and arm then rotate in this direction of ease and hold, maintaining the sustained pressure in the direction of the restriction while waiting for the tissues to soften.

Other assistive techniques that aid in the release of a soft tissue restriction are associated and direct oscillations. *Associated oscillations* are movements applied by the assisting hand to oscillate the patient's body.[22,24] *Direct oscillations are* imparted directly through the treating finger.[22,24] The direct oscillation can be performed in the same fashion and for the same indications as the joint mobilization techniques discussed in *Chapter 10, Joint Mobilization*. A Grade I direct oscillation is effective for reducing pain and tenderness over a tissue restriction and can be followed by a Grade IV direct oscillation to gain mobility.

Perpendicular strumming is another soft tissue evaluation and mobilization technique that is applied to muscle and will be described in more detail in *Muscle Play* on page 292.[22,24]

Precautions and Contraindications

Following is a list of conditions that may require special consideration. Soft tissue techniques may need to be modified, or may actually be contraindicated. The most obvious contraindication is a healing skin graft or surgical procedure that could be irritated by increased tissue mobility. Soft tissue mobilization should be avoided over or near areas where increased blood circulation is undesirable, such as in the case of malignancy within the tissue. Close communication with all members of the treatment team is essential to ensure that treatment outcomes are not counterproductive to the overall management of the patient's condition.

Conditions that require special consideration include but are not limited to:
- Malignancy
- Inflammatory skin conditions
- Fractures
- Sites of hemorrhage
- Obstructive edema
- Localized infections
- Aneurysm
- Acute rheumatoid arthritis
- Osteomyelitis
- Advanced osteoporosis
- Advanced diabetes
- Fibromyalgia (during flared symptoms stage)
- Increased symptoms
- Utilization of blood-thinning medications

Regions of STM Application

Skin and Superficial Fascia

Evaluation and treatment with soft tissue mobilization is best sequenced from superficial to deep. The clinician should therefore start with the skin and superficial fascia. The skin is often overlooked in favor of the more common methods of deeper palpation and treatment between myofascial layers. Although the latter techniques are important, they will not automatically restore lost motion to the skin overlying the deeper structures. The skin should be addressed because connective tissue is continuous. It starts from the basement membrane of the skin, connects the planes of fascia between muscles, blends into tubular shaped neurovascular tracts, and weaves into joint capsules and periosteum of bone.

The superficial fascia provides a major component of sensory feedback into the proprioceptive system. The skin can be considered a large sensory organ that is intimately invested in the overall fascial system. Rarely does a patient report a sensation of tightness in the skin, but improving skin mobility has a profound effect on postural alignment, range and quality of movement, and related pain syndromes. Given that the meshwork of superficial connective tissue blends and is continuous with the myofascial layers, one can appreciate how superficial tightness can affect mechanical input to the Golgi tendon organs and muscle spindle mechanisms, and negatively influence overall postural tone and proprioception.

Skin palpation assessment is performed to localize a fingertip-sized area that represents the greatest restriction in mobility. The clinician begins with broad, flat, two-hand contact and slides the skin through its full functional excursion followed by gentle overpressure at the end range to assess quality of end feel. This is done in multiple directions (visualize following the numbers of a clock face). The assessment proceeds by defining a single hand-sized area that contains the most restricted end feel in the region. With the direction of restriction now identified, a single finger is used to glide through the hand-sized region to find the specific epicenter of restricted tissue end feel. As the single finger glides through the skin in search of the specific point of restriction, a thicker quality of viscosity or flow of tissue is noted. When the treating finger encounters the specific restriction, bogginess is palpated and the finger is caused to slow in its glide. The clinician will note an easier glide of the finger proximal and distal, as well as medial and lateral to this point. Once the point of soft tissue restriction is localized the clinician can treat it with sustained pressure and unlocking spiral techniques described above. Occasionally, skin and superficial fascia restrictions may present over a broad area and be difficult to localize to a single finger point for treatment. In this case, full hand or other broad contact may be utilized in a sustained pressure method. Typically, this broad contact method can then be followed by better localization of more specific points.

Bony Contours

Establishing full mobility of fascia where it attaches to bony contours is another method of restoring efficient posture and movement, and easing pain that is mechanical in origin. A common area to consider is along the iliac crests. Structures that attach to the crests from superficial to deep are the thoracodorsal fascia, paraspinals, latissimus dorsi, internal and external oblique abdominals, and quadratus lumborum. These layered muscles and their fascial envelopes are in close proximity and have variable fiber directions as they converge into the iliac crests. One can appreciate the importance of elasticity and independent sliding function of these layers. Improving mobility in bony contour areas creates tissue tension changes along the entire span of muscles that originate or insert in these loca-

tions. It is not uncommon to treat soft tissue restrictions along the iliac crest and immediately obtain improved vertical posture alignment, restoration of segmental lumbopelvic motion, or perhaps greater range of motion in the shoulder.

The sacral sulcus is another key bony contour to clear of soft tissue restrictions in patients with back pain. Anatomically, the posterior surface of the sacrum is a key insertion for the multifidus muscle. The multifidus has been identified, along with the transverse abdominus, as a critical factor in lumbopelvic dynamic stability. Development of strength and coordinated contraction of this muscle may be adversely affected if there is fascial soft tissue adherence at this critical anchor point. It is also common to note tissue restrictions in the sacral sulcus in conjunction with sacroiliac dysfunction.

There are many other bony contour locations in the body that can be assessed and treated with soft tissue mobilization. For example, the clinician can influence spinal mobility by clearing restrictions along the spinous processes, laminar grooves, transverse processes, and anterior vertebral bodies (palpated and treated from the anterior abdominal surface). Also, changes in rib cage mobility can be profound after clearing along the contours of each individual rib and intercostal space. In the upper extremity, mobilization should always include the medial and lateral scapular border, spine of the scapula, acromion, coracoid process, elbow epicondyles and carpals and metacarpals. In the lower quarter, restrictions commonly accumulate around bony contours such as the greater trochanter, patella, tibial tubercle, posteromedial tibia, malleoli, calcaneus, and on the plantar fascia attachment to the calcaneus. By considering the muscles that originate or insert on these various bony surfaces, the clinician can influence function in corresponding structures.

In contrast to superficial fascia, where skin is moved tangent to the rest of the body, evaluating and treating along bone edges involves a dimension of depth. The treating finger glides along the bone at a flat angle to assess and treat the more superficial tissue attachments, and moves to deeper layers by increasing the angle of contact as described previously. Depending on the type of bone surface being treated, the clinician can use the tip of an index or middle finger to glide along the bony edge with half of the fingertip on the bone surface, and the other half engaging the connective tissue converging on the attachment. This is typical along an edge such as the iliac crest. If the bony contour is more of a flat surface with overlying soft tissue, such as the sacral sulcus, the tip of the finger glides through the tissue in various directions similar to that of superficial fascia. However, in contrast to superficial fascia, flat bony areas are assessed with varying angles toward perpendicular. Evaluation progresses from superficial to deeper layers. As in superficial fascia assessment, the gliding finger is noting either ease of movement through the tissue or areas where the tissue thickens, slowing down the finger glide. Care is taken to move slowly enough for the viscoelastic quality of tissue to allow the finger to stay engaged in the tissue substance and not just slide over the surface of a potential restriction.

When a soft tissue restriction along a bony contour is encountered, the clinician must first localize more specifically the depth and direction of the restriction. For example in the iliac crest, the finger will engage thickening or bogginess along the rim of the pelvis. Time is taken to assess end feel at this same point in a very slight caudal variation toward the crest, or slightly cephalad away from the crest. The clinician may also vary the angle of contact slightly more perpendicular without moving off the specific point. The depth and direction are thereby fine-tuned three dimensionally to be as specific as possible to the point of maximal tension. With the restriction well localized, the treatment can be initiated with a sustained pressure, waiting for the tissue restriction to soften. Release of the restriction can be further facilitated with a shortening of the surrounding tissue by pressing in a cephalad direction on the ilium with the assisting hand. Conversely, the surrounding tissues may be lengthened by drawing pressure in a caudal direction on the ilium while maintaining contact on the restriction with the treating finger. Other treatment methods such as the unlocking spiral and direct or associated oscillations described earlier may be applied as needed.

Muscle Play

John Mennell referred to the accessory motions in joints as *joint play*.[35] A similar term applied to muscle would be *muscle play*. A muscle must be capable of broadening during a shortening concentric contraction and drawing narrower during a lengthening eccentric contraction. Adjacent muscles also have differing fiber directions with independent sliding functions. The separation or seam between muscles is defined by the fascial coverings or perimysium.

The seams between muscles can be evaluated and mobilized with manual contact that is directed perpendicular to the muscle fibers or along the seam in a parallel orientation. Depth can be varied with a flat angle of pressure directed toward the more superficial aspects of the muscle border, and a more vertically angled contact engaging the deeper layers of muscle separation. As hardness and restricted end feel is encountered, the clinician

makes every effort to localize depth and direction with a single treating finger. Then treatment can proceed to the various techniques outlined above, including sustained pressure, shortening and lengthening with the assisting hand, unlocking spiral, direct oscillations, and associated oscillations.

Another useful technique for evaluating and treating muscle play is called *perpendicular strumming*.[22,24] Perpendicular strumming is performed by aligning the finger tips in a straight row and placing the two hands together to form one tool. The row of finger tips forms a straight edge and slides at a depth and perpendicular direction that engages the border of muscle. The muscle border is deformed like a guitar string being strummed, and then snaps lightly under the fingertips. It is at this brief moment that the clinician has the opportunity to assess the end feel of the muscle being deflected with a perpendicular force. In real time, the strumming is done repeatedly with a steady oscillatory rhythm with systematic movement along the entire border of a muscle. Once a length of muscle has undergone perpendicular strumming, the clinician has gained overall perspective of end feel and can return to more localized single finger-sized areas for more specific localization and treatment. Later, perpendicular strumming can be repeated as a treatment tool for mobilization of broader soft tissue restrictions that may remain.

Common areas of soft tissue dysfunction in the thoracolumbar myofascial tissues are along medial and lateral borders and in seams between the paraspinal muscles, quadratus lumborum, latissimus dorsi, and the smaller segmental units of multifidi, and rotatores. Osteopathic physicians note segmental "tissue texture changes" in these smaller muscles corresponding with segmental facet motion restrictions.[19]

Special attention is drawn to the iliopsoas because of the high incidence of dysfunction found. Anterior spinal structures like the iliopsoas are often overlooked and seem to be key areas of soft tissue dysfunction in many patients with mechanical back pain. Ellis has reported localized restrictions of the psoas at corresponding levels of lumbar facet closing and opening restrictions.[12]

With the patient positioned supine, the hips are supported with pillows to remove tension on the abdominal fascia and relax the hip flexors. Initially the abdominal superficial fascia should be assessed and cleared of any soft tissue restrictions. The clinician can then place the treating finger medial to the ASIS and sink gently into the iliac fossa, while assessing and treating with sustained pressure any restrictions encountered within the iliacus. Unless dense iliacus restrictions are encountered, the tip of the treating finger will follow the contour of the iliac fossa changing direction gradually from a posterior to a medially directed gentle pressure. The lateral border of the psoas will be encountered and should be evaluated for an elastic end feel. Frequently the end feel is inelastic and restricted at this point due to dysfunctional muscle play at the fascial interface between the iliacus and psoas. At this level, the muscles are not yet blended into the single iliopsoas and must have independent mobility on one another.

Another entry point to evaluate and treat the lateral border of the psoas is just lateral to the rectus abdominus at the level of the umbilicus (corresponding with L3) and more caudal at L4 and L5 (Fig 11-10). The fingers sink slowly into the abdominal fascia with a slight medial angulation.

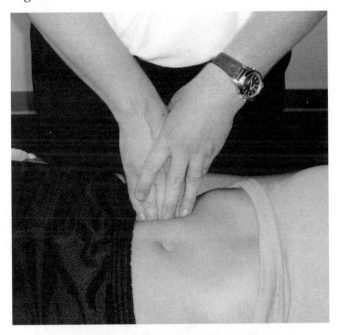

Figure 11-10: Palpation of the psoas.

If arterial pulsation is noted, the aorta or iliac arteries may be under the palpating finger. Carefully redirect the manual contact to avoid occluding these arteries. It is generally safe to feel the arteries pulsating adjacent to the treating finger, but not trapped under the tip. Once the lateral border of the psoas is contacted, the patient is asked to flex the corresponding hip to detect contraction of the psoas. Active contraction of the psoas is helpful in affirming that the psoas is being palpated, and is an excellent mobilization method once a restricted end feel is localized. Once the lateral psoas border and belly are identified, it is relatively simple to move the contact to the medial border of the psoas and gently deflect it laterally to assess the muscle play.

When soft tissue restrictions are encountered and localized, they are treated with the cascade of techniques that includes sustained pressure, shortening or lengthening surrounding tissues (in this case can be done by varying the degree of hip flexion), unlocking spiral, associated or direct oscillations, and possibly strumming as the tenderness and tightness are resolving. In this example sustained pressure may be combined with a light contraction of the psoas with active hip flexion to facilitate a release of the restriction.

Functional Mobilization™

Proprioceptive Neuromuscular Facilitation Foundation

Johnson coined the term *Functional Mobilization*™ (FM) and defined it as "the integrated use of soft tissue and joint mobilization combined with the dynamic principles of proprioceptive neuromuscular facilitation (PNF)". Functional mobilization is a "step-by-step evaluation and treatment approach combining mobilization and stabilization with neuromuscular reeducation".[23,27] This section will present a PNF model of the body, and describe basic principles of PNF evaluation and treatment of the trunk with the shoulder and pelvic girdles. A foundation of STM developed above and the PNF methods that follow set the stage for techniques of functional mobilization that are utilized to blend structural mobilization with neuromuscular training. The result is a time-efficient process for the successful treatment of movement dysfunction that transitions well into an individualized home exercise program.

Rationale for the Diagonal Nature of Human Movement

PNF techniques developed by Knott and Kabat and the related methods of FM later developed by Johnson operate on the basic premise that bodies move in diagonal patterns.[29] Rarely does the human body move in pure cardinal plane patterns, yet clinicians often emphasize such movements during evaluation and treatment. The following discussion is intended to support the use of diagonal, triplanar movement in neuromusculoskeletal rehabilitation.

The muscles and fascia are arranged in a spiral direction around the trunk and extremities. This orientation facilitates angles of pull that are naturally in diagonal directions. Knott and Kabat further observed that movements of the trunk emanate from diagonal patterns at the shoulder and pelvic girdles around three-dimensional patterns of anterior depression, posterior depression, posterior elevation, and anterior elevation.[29]

The right pelvis moves into anterior depression at heel strike, posterior depression at push off, posterior elevation at lift off, and anterior elevation at the end of forward swing. Simultaneously, the left pelvis guides the left lower extremity through a reciprocal gait pattern. At any given freeze frame of the gait cycle, the right and left pelvis will be in the exact opposite quadrants to each other within the diagonal quadrant model.

Expanding this observation to the simultaneous movement of the shoulder girdles reveals similar reciprocal movement patterns with arm swing. Gait that has symmetrical range of movement of both shoulder and pelvic girdles with optimal alignment and timing results in a spine that appears relatively stationary around a neutral position, but is actually mobile, yet balanced, in an incredible state of dynamic stability. Efficient gait is generally not found in patients suffering from back pain. What's more, movement dysfunctions often persist after the pain has subsided, requiring specific treatment to regain a more efficient state.

It is also fascinating to observe diagonal movement patterns in photos from sporting events with athletes running, jumping, reaching, throwing, and catching (Fig 11-11). Athletic movements provide us with classic examples of full body activation into diagonal movement patterns, revealing how the body is able to integrate and coordinate as a whole functional unit. In addition, the image of the trunk acting as a thoroughfare for kinetic energy into and from the extremities underscores the importance of neutral trunk alignment for efficient force transfer described previously.

Inefficiencies in movement that hamper performance and lead to injury are typically a lack of full body integration. For example, a golfer who does not efficiently transfer force from the lower extremities into the hips and trunk tends to overuse the upper extremities, leading to shot inaccuracy and shoulder or back injury. The clinician evaluating such a golfer has the task of identifying if the lack of use of the lower extremities and trunk is from a structural limitation of mobility in the joints and fascia, or from a functional origin such as strength, coordination or balance.

The good golf pro is skilled at teaching the golfer to swing more efficiently within the body's constraints. The treatment outcome (and golf score) might be even more positive if functional mobilization techniques are incorporated to actually change the body's structure and neuromuscular control.

Basic PNF Techniques for the Trunk

This is a brief overview of PNF assessment and treatment techniques specific to the trunk, utilizing the pelvic and shoulder girdles with the patient positioned in side lying. What follows is a procedural framework that allows for many variations. We begin with assessment and treatment of shoulder and pelvic girdles with passive range of motion, followed by training of eccentric and concentric muscle contractions through the diagonal ranges of movement. The side lying position allows for better control of alignment, and compressive loads are minimized for the patient with a painful or irritable condition. The patient

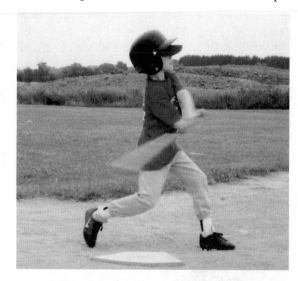

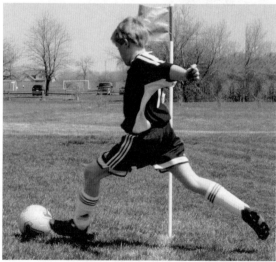

Figure 11-11: Athletic movements show the natural, reciprocal diagonal motions that occur in the shoulder and pelvic girdles.

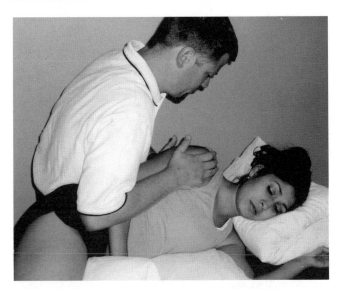

Figure 11-12: Manual contact for PNF techniques for the shoulder girdle.

should be set up in neutral spinal alignment, usually with a pillow under the lateral torso, a doubled pillow under the head, and possibly one pillow between the knees. The hips and knees should be flexed to 90° with the frontal plane of the body perpendicular to the table.

Establishing full passive range of motion is the first goal. Manual contact should firmly encompass the anterior and posterior shoulder (Fig 11-12). The clinician's body should be facing the direction that the shoulder girdle will be pushed or pulled. The following sequence is then followed: Move the shoulder girdle passively to the end range diagonal of anterior elevation and posterior depression, while assessing end feel at these two points. The motion should be along a curved arc that follows the shape of the rib cage and the diagonal should be very narrow near the mid-axillary line.

Repeat the end feel assessment at both ends of the diagonal of posterior elevation and anterior depression. Place the shoulder girdle at the end range of the most restricted diagonal and utilize hold-relax or contract-relax techniques to gain range of motion and establish an elastic end feel.

Once range of motion is restored, the next step is to evaluate and train neuromuscular control of the shoulder girdle through the diagonal range of motion. The patient with efficient neuromuscular control is able to generate coordinated, maintained *isometric* holds as well as smooth *eccentric* and *concentric* contractions through a full range of motion. As a group, these types of muscle contractions are called a *combination of isotonics*.[27,42,43]

The clinician evaluates by placing the shoulder girdle at the newly established end range of motion and assessing the patient's ability to hold it there isometrically. The following sequence is then followed: Train the isometric holding ability as needed in the new range with a sustained hold contraction. Next, have the patient start with the isometric hold at end range and then allow movement through the diagonal arc while resisting with eccentric and concentric control.

Typically the clinician will note points in the range where the eccentric movement is not smooth, giving way with a ratchet type of feeling. These points can be retrained with isometric holds and short arc eccentrics to restore smooth neuromuscular control. The next feat is for the patient to pull against the clinician's resistance through the diagonal arc with a concentric contraction. The clinician should identify any points where the concentric contraction stalls or loses the proper path, and train these points with isometric holds, eccentrics, and short arc and full arc concentrics, in that order.

A similar procedure is applied to the pelvis in side lying by contacting the ischial tuberosity with one hand and anterolateral iliac crest with the other hand (Fig 11-13). The clinician should passively move the pelvis to end range in both directions of both diagonals through a curved arc that follows the head of the opposite femur. The arc of movement at the pelvis is much smaller than at the shoulder girdle. The clinician should be alert for a restricted end feel and treat with hold-relax and contract-relax as needed. Utilizing appropriate manual contacts, the therapist then performs a progression similar to that described for the shoulder girdle to train isometric, eccentric, and concentric contractions.

One of the most remarkable and clinically useful outcomes of this PNF-based method of training is the far-reaching effects beyond the body part under direct contact. Recall from the discussion above that the opposite sides of the body and the upper and lower body participate in these diagonal movements with reciprocal patterns. Therefore, gaining range of motion and improving balance and control in right shoulder girdle posterior depression can facilitate and activate left shoulder girdle anterior elevation, right pelvis anterior elevation and left pelvis posterior depression. This is, of course, the pattern of movement that occurs in efficient gait and other functional movements.

The clinician can amplify this full body effect by combining work on the shoulder girdle and pelvis simultaneously (Fig 11-14). In right side lying, the clinician can provide overpressure of the left shoulder girdle into

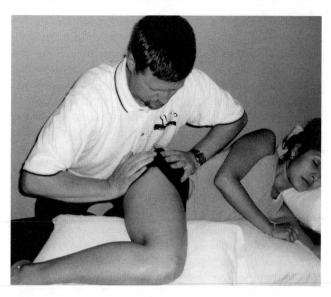

Figure 11-13: Manual contact for passive motion evaluation of the pelvis.

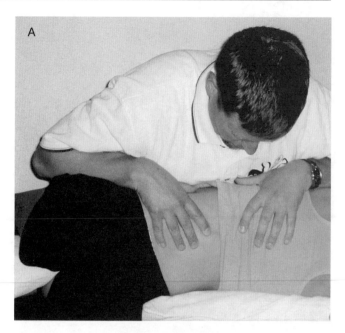

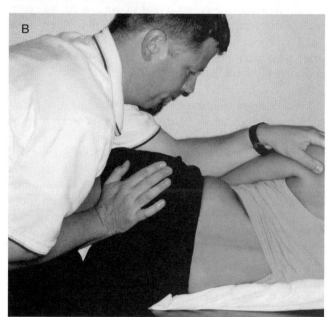

Figure 11-14: A) Side lying elongation method for the left trunk, incorporating left shoulder anterior elevation with left pelvis posterior depression; B) Side lying shortening method for the left trunk, incorporating left shoulder posterior depression with left pelvis anterior elevation. Note the opposite shoulder and pelvic girdles are being moved into the reciprocal quadrants.

anterior elevation while at the same time stretching the left pelvis into posterior depression . The patient can then pull the right shoulder and pelvis toward each other against the clinician's resistance, affording an excellent post-isometric relaxation for stretching the left quadratus lumborum, internal oblique, and latissimus dorsi. The clinician can then reverse contact on the shoulder and pelvic girdles moving into a left torso shortening pattern. This position can then be used for training diagonal left side bending with a *combination of isotonics* involving eccentric and concentric contractions against resistance. This is truly a full body exercise, generating force from the trunk (core) that is often an objective when training patients with spinal dysfunction.

PNF Integrated Into Functional Mobilization™

The technique of functional mobilization[23] combines soft tissue and joint mobilization with traditional PNF patterns of trunk and extremity movement and *functional movement patterns*[22,26] adapted from "Awareness Through Movement" lessons by Moshe Feldenkrais.[15] Dysfunction is identified through passive or active motion palpation. The treating finger maintains contact on the restriction with a specific depth and direction. Mobilization becomes dynamic as the body part is guided through passive, active, or resistive movement. Once the restriction has resolved, neuromuscular reeducation occurs through continued active and resisted movement with *combinations of isotonics* (isometric, eccentric, and concentric) (Fig 11-15). Functional mobilization also leads the clinician to logical and appropriate home exercises that are most relevant to the patient's condition.

Case Study

The patient was a 34–year old male computer consultant with an 18–month history of right lumbar radiculopathy. Symptoms consisted of pain in the right sciatic notch, pos-

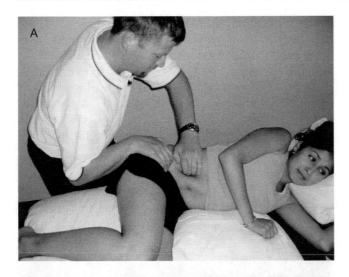

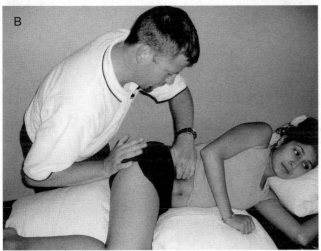

Figure 11-15: A) Functional mobilization along the lateral border of the right psoas with right pelvic passive posterior depression and resisted anterior elevation; B) Functional mobilization along the lateral border of the right psoas with right pelvic passive anterior elevation and resisted posterior depression.

terior thigh, and right inguinal region, as well as aching and burning in the right lateral lower leg. The patient was able to work full time, but symptoms were aggravated with sitting greater than five minutes, walking greater than one block, or if attempting to ride his bicycle with road racing handlebars.

He had been diagnosed by his orthopedist shortly after symptom onset with L4–5 right posterior disc herniation (confirmed by MRI). One year prior to this evaluation he underwent a series of three epidural steroid injections, and had received three months of acupuncture treatments, which reduced his symptom intensity by 50%. The patient verbalized goals of returning to recreational cycling

without symptoms, avoiding lumbar disc surgery, and continuing his occupation, which required prolonged periods of sitting.

Initial Clinical Findings

Observation of posture revealed a slight right side bent torso with concavity noted along the right lateral trunk wall, and a shortened appearance in his right abdomen and lumbar paraspinal region compared to his left. Vertical compression testing caused buckling into lumbar hyperextension and right side bending, and reproduced right lower extremity symptoms slightly. Lumbar protective mechanism testing elicited poor stabilization response and lumbar back bending. He walked with a mild Trendelenburg drop of the left pelvis during right mid stance, and compensated for this with accentuated right trunk side bending. This pattern was more obvious during right single leg balance and hop tests, which also reproduced his right lower extremity symptoms.

Manual muscle testing was normal in the lower extremities and he did not demonstrate sensory deficits. Supine straight leg raise test was positive on the right with sciatic symptoms produced at 30° of hip flexion with the knee extended. Left straight leg raise reproduced right sciatic notch symptoms at 70° of hip flexion. Active range of motion was full and painless into backward bending and right side bending, but forward bending was limited to 50% of normal with finger tips reaching his patellae and symptoms reproduced throughout his right lower extremity. Left side bending appeared stiff below L1, and reproduced his right inguinal pain and tightness. Motion testing using osteopathic principles revealed an FRS left dysfunction at L4–5 (loss of right facet closing at L4–5 with extension) (see discussion in Chapter 10, *Joint Mobilization*).

Moderate soft tissue restrictions were noted at the medial border of the right psoas at L4, the lateral border of the right quadratus lumborum, along the right iliac crest and sacral sulcus, and along the lateral border of the middle and lower right rectus abdominus. The skin and superficial fascia was restricted in mobility in a superior and medial direction from the right posterolateral lumbar and pelvic region into the right lateral hip, thigh, and lateral lower leg. Very dense and tender soft tissue restrictions were encountered with gliding in a superior parallel direction along the central right posterior thigh to the sciatic notch.

Treatment Procedures and Outcomes

The first visit consisted of soft tissue mobilization directed exclusively at the skin and superficial fascia of the right lumbopelvic region, thigh, and lower leg. Immediately after treatment, full left straight leg raising was possible without right lower extremity symptoms and the right straight leg raise increased to 45° before right sciatic symptoms were experienced. Muscle energy technique was applied to L4–5 in left side lying to mobilize right facet closure with extension. The patient was instructed in an active movement exercise in left side lying to facilitate this facet closure with combined right shoulder girdle depression and right pelvic girdle elevation.

At the patient's second and third visits he presented with no further FRS dysfunction at L4–5. Straight leg raise tests demonstrated the same improvements as at the conclusion of his first visit. Sitting still produced symptoms at five minutes, but they were reduced in intensity by 50%. Superficial fascia restrictions were no longer evident, so soft tissue mobilization was directed along the right iliac crest and sacral sulcus, right medial border of the psoas at L4, right lateral border of the quadratus lumborum, and right lateral border of the rectus abdominus. These areas were treated with functional mobilization methods with the patient positioned in left side lying.

Treating finger contact was localized and maintained on multiple soft tissue restrictions while the patient was guided through passive, active, and ultimately resisted patterns of diagonal movement of the right shoulder and pelvic girdles. The functional mobilization techniques led to another home exercise in left side lying over a pillow to stretch and elongate his right torso along a diagonal of right shoulder girdle anterior elevation and right pelvis posterior depression. He noted temporary relief of his right lower leg symptoms after this stretch, and he was told to stretch frequently while sitting or standing by reaching his right shoulder girdle into anterior elevation while actively stretching his right pelvis into posterior depression.

By the patient's sixth visit, his sitting tolerance was improved to nearly 30 minutes. Active left side bending was equal to the right with full segmental recruitment to the sacrum. Active forward bending was now 75% of normal, with his finger tips reaching the mid tibia. The right straight leg raise was 75° without sciatic symptoms. The vertical compression test was painless and solid without buckling. Lumbar protective mechanism testing did not elicit any instability with strong maintenance of neutral spinal alignment.

At this point, the patient was still not able to cycle without symptoms. All joint and soft tissue restrictions were cleared with the exception of the dense restrictions extending along the sciatic nerve tract in the right central posterior thigh extending to the sciatic notch. Access to this area was gained in left side lying as shown in Figure 11-16. Multiple soft tissue restrictions were localized and mobilized along the sciatic nerve tract with methods of sustained pressure, shortening of the surrounding tissue with the assisting hand, as well as lengthening with passive, active, and resistive knee flexion and extension. This position was also used for home stretching of the posterior thigh compartment with a minimal lumbar disc load.

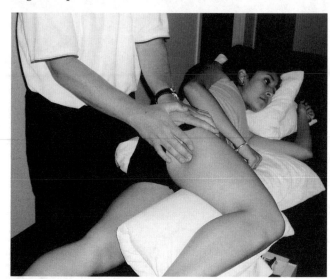

Figure 11-16: Position for assessing and treating sciatic nerve tract tissue mobility.

Functional exercise was initiated with dynamic neutral alignment training. The patient progressed through single leg balance, double and single leg squat, and eventually lunges and single leg hops in multiple directions. A logical progression of his cycling program was developed. He first focused on sustained duration cycling on flat terrain in lower gears, and progressed gradually to hills and higher gears as his symptoms allowed.

Final Treatment Outcome

The patient was seen twice per week for three weeks, once per week for an additional three weeks, then once every 2–3 weeks for a total of 15 visits. At his last visit, he was able to sit for 60–90 minutes without symptoms as long as he performed his right trunk lengthening stretch occasionally. His right straight leg raise was equal to his left at 75° without sciatic symptoms. He demonstrated full active range of motion in all directions without symptoms. No Trendelenburg drop was noted during gait. Right single leg balance, single leg squat, and hop were equal to left. He was able to cycle for 90–120 minutes, 1–3 times per week, with occasional short, intense rides, and complained only of a mild sciatic area "stiffness" that he could relieve with brief rest and stretching.

This case study demonstrates how several different techniques can be combined to effectively and efficiently address a complex problem. Treatment of acute and chronic neuromusculoskeletal disorders is most successful and cost effective if an eclectic approach is used. The ideal approach combines the skilled use of manual therapy techniques with thoughtful, individualized exercise and training. It takes time, patience, and persistence for the clinician to develop these skills, but does not necessarily take excessive clinical time to treat with this model. Advancements in technology and demands for time efficiency have created a need, now more than ever, for clinicians to hone their skills and develop the art and science of therapeutic manual treatment and movement training.

REFERENCES

1. Akeson WH, Amiel D, Mechanic GL, et al: Collagen Cross-Linking Alterations in Joint Contractures: Changes in the Reducible Cross-Links in Periarticular Connective Tissue Collagen After Nine Weeks of Immobilization. Conn Tissue Res 5:15-9, 1977.

2. Akeson WH, Woo SL, Amiel D, et al: Biomechanical and Biochemical Changes in the Periarticular Connective Tissue During Contracture Development in the Immobilized Rabbit Knee. Connect Tissue Res 2:315-23, 1974.

3. Akeson WH, Woo SL, Amiel D, et al: The Connective Tissue Response to Immobility: Biochemical Changes in Periarticular Connective Tissue of the Immobilized Rabbit Knee. Clin Orthop 93:356-62, 1973.

4. Amiel D, Frey C, Woo SL, et al: Value of Hyaluronic Acid in the Prevention of Contracture Formation. Clin Orthop 306-11, 1985.

5. Amiel D, Woo SL, Harwood FL, et al: The Effect of Immobilization on Collagen Turnover in Connective Tissue: A Biochemical-Biomechanical Correlation. Acta Orthop Scand 53:325-32, 1982.

6. Arem JA, Madden JW: Effects of Stress on Healing Wounds. I. Intermittent Noncyclical Tension. J Surg Res 20:93, 1976

7. Buckwalter JA and Grodzinsky AJ: Loading of Healing Bone, Fibrous Tissue, and Muscle: Implications for Orthopaedic Practice. J Am Acad Orthop Surg 7:291-9, 1999.

8. Buckwalter JA, Einhorn TA, Bolander ME, et al: Healing of Musculoskeletal Tissues. In: Fractures in Adults, 4th ed, Rockwood and Green, eds. Lippincott-Raven, Philadelphia 1996.

9. Butler D, Shacklock M, Slater H: Treatment of Altered Nervous System Mechanics. In: Grieve's Modern Manual Therapy: The Vertebral Column, 2nd ed, pp 693-704. J Boyling, N Palastanga, G Jull, et al, eds. Churchill Livingstone, Edinburgh 1994.

10. Butler D: Mobilisation of the Nervous System. 1st ed, Churchill Livingstone, Melbourne 1991.

11. Christensen H, Vach W, Vach K et al: Palpation of the Upper Thoracic Spine: An Observer Reliability Study. JMPT 25:285-92, 2002.

12. Ellis J: Lumbopelvic Integration: Course Notes, 1993.

13. Elvey R: Physical Evaluation of the Peripheral Nervous System in Disorders of Pain and Dysfunction. J Hand Ther 10:122-9, 1997.

14. Elvey R: The Investigation of Arm Pain: Signs of Adverse Responses to the Physical Examination of the Brachial Plexus and Related Neural Tissues. In: Grieve's Modern Manual Therapy: The Vertebral Column, 2nd ed, pp 577-86. J Boyling, N Palastanga, G Jull, et al, eds. Churchill Livingstone, Edinburgh 1994.

15. Feldenkrais M: Awareness Through Movement. Harper & Row, New York 1977.

16. Gratz C: Fascial Adhesions in Pain in the Low Back and Arthritis. JAMA 3:1813, 1938.

17. Gray G, Tiberio D: Golf Reaction: Course Notes, 1999.

18. Gray, G: Chain Reaction Festival: Course Notes, 1996.

19. Greenman, P: Principles of Manual Medicine, 3rd ed. Lippincott Williams & Wilkins, Baltimore 2003.

20. Hall T, and Elvey R: Nerve Trunk Pain: Physical Diagnosis and Treatment. Manual Therapy 4:63-73, 1999.

21. Huijbregts P: Spinal Motion Palpation: A Review of Reliability Studies. J of Manual and Manipulative Therapy 10:24-39, 2002.

22. Johnson GS. Soft Tissue Mobilization. In: Orthopedic Physical Therapy. 2nd ed, RA Donatelli and MJ Wooden, eds. Churchill Livingstone, New York 1994.

23. Johnson G: Functional Mobilization: Course Notes, 2004.

24. Johnson G: Functional Orthopedics I: Course Notes, 1999.

25. Johnson G, Saliba V: Lumbar Protective Mechanism. In: The Conservative Care of Low Back Pain. A White and R Anderson eds. Williams and Wilkins, Baltimore 1991.

26. Johnson GS: Functional Orthopedics II: Course Notes, 2002.

27. Johnson GS, Saliba Johnson V: The Application of the Principles and Procedures of PNF for the Care of Lumbar Spinal Instabilities. J of Manual and Manipulative Therapy 10(2):83-105, 2002.

28. Jull G, Bogduk N, and Marsland A: The Accuracy of Manual Diagnosis for Cervical Zygapophysial Joint Pain Syndromes, Med J Aust 148:233-6, 1988.

29. Kabat, Knott, Voss: Proprioceptive Neuromuscular Facilitation. 2nd ed, Harper & Row, New York 1968.

30. Korr I, Wilkinson P, and Chornock F: Axonal Delivery of Neuroplasmic Components to Muscle Cells. Science 155:342-5, 1967.

31. Korr I: Proprioceptors and Somatic Dysfunction. J Am Osteopath Assoc 74:638-50, 1975.

32. Lopez-Antunez L: Atlas of Human Anatomy, 1st ed, W B Saunders, Philadelphia 1971.

33. Maitland GD: Vertebral Manipulation. 6th ed. Butterworth Heinemann, 2001.

34. McPoil TG, Cornwall MW: Relationship Between Three Static Angles of the Rearfoot and the Pattern of Rearfoot Motion During Walking. J Orthop Sports Phys Ther 23(6):370-375, 1996.

35. Mennell J: Joint Pain. Little, Brown and Company, Boston 1964

36. Miller B: Manual Therapy Treatment of Myofascial Pain and Dysfunction, In: Myofascial Pain and Fibromyalgia, ES Rachlin ed. Mosby, St. Louis 2002.

37. Olsen K, Paris S, Spohr C, et al: Radiographic Assessment and Reliability Study of the Craniovertebral Sidebending Test. J of Manual and Manipulative Therapy 6:87-96, 1998.

38. Powers C, Kulig K, Harrison J, and Bergman G: Segmental Mobility of the Lumbar Spine During a Posterior to Anterior Mobilization: Assessment Using Dynamic MRI. Clin Biomech 18:80-3, 2003.

39. Quintner J: A Study of Upper Limb Pain and Paresthesia Following Neck Injury in Motor Vehicle Accidents: Assessment of the Brachial Plexus Tension Test of Elvey. Br J Rheumatol 28:528-33, 1989.

40. Rolf I: Rolfing: The Integration of Human Structures. Harper and Row, New York 1977.

41. Saliba VL: Back Education and Training: Course Notes, Feb 2003.

42. Saliba VL: Proprioceptive Neuromuscular Facilitation I: Course Notes, Feb 2003.

43. Saliba VL, Johnson GS, Wardlaw C: Proprioceptive Neuromuscular Facilitation. In: Rational Manual Therapies. JV Basmajian and R Nyberg, eds. Williams and Wilkins, Baltimore 1993.

44. Smedmark V, Wallin M, and Arvidsson I: Inter-Examiner Reliability In Assessing Passive Intervertebral Motion of the Cervical Spine. Man Ther 5:97-101, 2000.

45. Threlkeld AJ: The Effects of Manual Therapy on Connective Tissue. Phys Ther 72:893-902, 1992.

46. Wainner RS, Fritz JM, Irrgang JJ, et al: Reliability and Diagnostic Accuracy of the Clinical Examination and Patient Self-Report Measures for Cervical Radiculopathy. Spine 28:52-62, 2003.

47. Woo SL, Matthews JV, Akeson WH, et al: Connective Tissue Response to Immobility: Correlative Study of Biomechanical and Biochemical Measurements of Normal and Immoblized Rabbit Knees. Arthritis Rheum 18:257-64, 1975.

12

SPINAL TRACTION

H. Duane Saunders, MS PT and Robin Saunders Ryan, MS PT

Section One — General Traction Theory

Spinal traction is a valuable treatment technique for certain neck and back disorders. Reference to the use of traction forces to treat back problems can be found in antiquity, including the writings of Hippocrates. The word traction is a derivative of the Latin *tractico*, which means a process of drawing or pulling. To achieve separation between two objects or surfaces, two opposing forces are required — traction and countertraction. Various authors have suggested the word *distraction* as being more descriptive. In the spine, the movement produced at the segment is actually a combination of distraction and gliding. Recently, some traction equipment manufacturers have used the term, *decompression*, meaning, "unweighting due to distraction and positioning."

Whatever the term used, a perusal of the medical literature on traction yields mixed opinion. Inconsistencies in subject characteristics, forces, positions, protocols, and other variables make traction study results difficult to compare. Lumbar traction is currently out of favor in the literature. Review articles and guidelines have been published that conclude traction research is generally poorly done, and there are no randomized, controlled trials that conclusively show its effectiveness.[3,72,80,84]

Certainly, many physicians, therapists and patients recall the poor results of the continuous, or "bed" traction that was common for many years. These poor results caused many physicians and therapists to become uninterested in using spinal traction. Several studies have shown either poor results of treatment or that the positive effects of traction were of limited or marginal significance.[1,8,49,69,86,87,89] However, numerous authors claim that traction is an effective and beneficial method of treatment.[12,15,16,21,24,28,31,32,33,34,35,36,38,39,42,48,54,60,64,65,66,67,68,71,73,74,75,76,77,78,82,92,94]

Perhaps the conflicting results reported are due to the wide variety of traction techniques used, and the variety of criteria used for patient selection.[79] In several articles, the traction method and patient selection criteria are poorly described.

For example, the authors of one randomized clinical trial concluded that traction is of no benefit, but didn't even report the amount of traction force used in the trial.[13]

Another randomized clinical trial concluded that there is no support for the claim that traction is efficacious for low back pain.[1] The study was well designed, but the subjects studied had non-specific low back pain. No effort was made to describe or categorize the symptoms or possible mechanism of pain. It would be interesting to repeat the study using subjects who have a diagnosis for which traction is commonly thought to be helpful (e.g., herniated nucleus pulposus).

Readers are cautioned to avoid accepting the conclusions reached in studies without carefully considering both the study design and the detailed methods used. We agree that traction research is generally poorly done. Nonetheless, interesting, if not conclusive, research on traction is available, and is cited throughout this chapter.

Effects of Spinal Traction

Correctly performed, spinal traction can cause many effects. Among these are distraction or separation of the vertebral bodies, a combination of distraction and gliding of the facet joints, tensing of the ligamentous structures of the spinal segment, widening of the intervertebral foramen, straightening of spinal curves and stretching of the spinal musculature.

The relative degree of flexion or extension of the spine during the traction treatment determines which of these effects are most pronounced. For example, greater separation of the intervertebral foramen is accomplished with the spine in a flexed position during the traction treatment, whereas greater separation of the disc space is achieved with the spine in a neutral position.

In the lumbar spine, studies show that a minimum force of up to 40-50% of the patient's body weight on a friction-free surface is necessary to cause vertebral separation.[17,39] In the cervical spine, Judovich found that a force of 25-45 lbs (11-20 kg) was necessary to demonstrate a measurable change in the posterior cervical spine structures.[38] Jackson confirmed this finding.[36] In another comprehensive work, Colachis and Strohm demonstrated that a force of 30 lbs (13.6 kg) produces separation of the cervical spine.[10] There is no evidence that mid and lower cervical spine separation occurs at forces less than 20 lbs (9 kg).

Other interesting effects have been reported in the literature. Manual traction with forces of 30 and 60% of the patient's body weight has been shown to immediately improve straight leg raise testing in subjects with and without back pain.[59] Traction has been theorized to reduce pain by relieving pressure on the dorsal root ganglion or mechanically stimulating large diameter myelinated nerve fibers, thereby silencing ectopic discharge. Improved nerve conduction could result from improved blood flow or alleviation of mechanical compression resulting from traction.[44] One study reported reduced flexor carpi radialis alpha-motoneuron excitability with manual cervical traction, providing evidence of a neurophysiologic rather than a mechanical response to traction.[4] Lower motoneuron excitability suggests manual traction may improve motor function by modifying the involuntary activation of muscle. Harris suggested that cervical traction may reduce myoelectric activity of the upper trapezius,[32] but a subsequent study by different authors failed to confirm his finding.[37] DeLacerda actually saw an increase in upper trapezius EMG activity during the pull phase of intermittent cervical traction.[19] This effect increased with a greater angle of cervical flexion. In a study using 25% of the body weight, investigators found a significant decrease in C5-6 paraspinal EMG activity during the pull phase of intermittent traction.[91] The effects of spinal traction on the intervertebral disc are discussed below.

Indications for Spinal Traction

Herniated Nucleus Pulposus with Disc Protrusion

Spinal traction is indicated for the treatment of herniated nucleus pulposus (HNP).[15,16,31,32,33,35,36,38,39,48,54,55,56,57,67,71,73] There is evidence that a disc protrusion can be reduced and spinal nerve root compression symptoms relieved with the application of spinal traction. Mathews[56] used epidurography to study patients thought to have lumbar disc protrusion. He applied static traction forces of 120 lbs for 20 minutes and showed that the protrusions were flattened and that the contrast material was drawn into the disc spaces, indicating a suction or "decompression" effect. He also found recurrence of the bulging defects later (Fig 12-1).

Gupta and Ramarao[31] also used epidurography to demonstrate reductions of lumbar disc protrusions in 11 of 14 patients treated with 60-80 lbs of force. The force was applied for intermittent periods every three to four hours for 10-15 days. Extension principles were also used. Clinical improvement was noted in the patients in whom defects were reduced (Fig 12-2).

A study by Onel et al is particularly intriguing.[67] This study used computed tomographic investigation to evaluate the effect of static horizontal traction on disc herniations. The effects of 45 kgs traction (99 lbs) were evaluated in 30 patients with lumbar disc herniations. The force used was 65 to 81% of the subject's body weight. Results showed the herniated disc material retracted in eleven (78.5%) of the median, six (66.6%) of the posterolateral and four (57.1%) of the lateral herniations (Fig 12-3). The clinical improvement in the median and posterolateral herniations was far better than in the lateral herniations.

Onel concluded that since the widening of discal space under the effect of traction causes a decrease in intradiscal pressure,[61] the decreased intradiscal pressure "sucks back" the herniated nuclear material. Furthermore, the widening of the intravertebral disc space causes a stretching of the anterior and posterior longitudinal ligaments. Since the median and posterolateral herniations are located anterior to the posterior longitudinal ligament (PLL), the PLL may help to push the herniation back into place. Therefore, the effect of traction on HNP may be due partly to the suction effect of the decreased intradiscal pressure and partly to the pushing effect of the PLL.

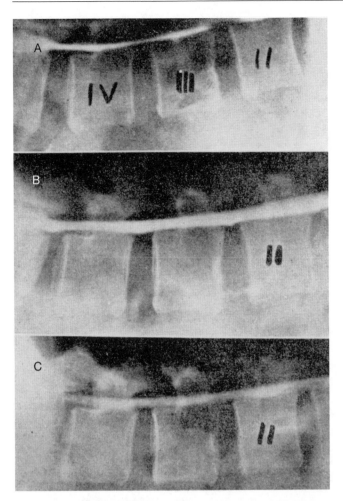

Figure 12-1: A) L2-3 disc protrusion before traction; B) The disc protrusion is being reduced with traction; C) The protrusion partially returns after traction is released (from Mathews).[56]

Onel described two cases in which the traction increased both the amount of herniated nuclear material and the patient's symptoms. These two patients had fragmented discs, which were probably out of reach of the suction effect of the traction. One patient who noted no improvement had a calcified disc. Overall, clinical improvement was noted in 28 of the 30 subjects in the study. The two unimproved subjects underwent subsequent surgery.

These studies show that traction can separate lumbar vertebrae and cause decreased intradiscal pressure with a resulting suction force. In addition, this suction force can draw material from the epidural space into the disc space. It appears that any anatomical correction produced is unstable. Thus, if patients are not carefully treated with a total management regimen, traction alone is unlikely to be successful. The patient must be carefully monitored as the traction treatment is administered.

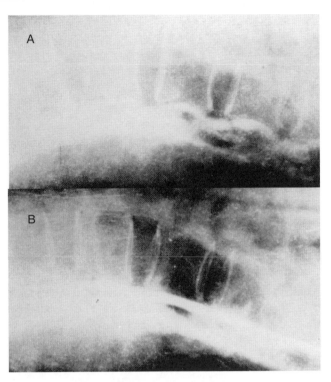

Figure 12-2: A disc protrusion being reduced by traction. A) Before traction; B) During traction (from Gupta and Ramarao).[31]

Several recent studies have documented good results using traction to treat cervical radiculopathy.[9,12,24,34,42,60,64,74] A wide variety of study designs were used, and none of the studies had control groups. Traction forces used in these studies ranged from 5 to 55 lbs. One MRI study showed either complete or partial reduction of HNP in 21 of 29 patients who received 30 lbs seated traction with an inflatable traction device.[9]

Traction treatment is often uncomfortable, but it should not be painful. The patient must be comfortable enough to relax so that the treatment can be effective. For both cervical and lumbar HNP treatment, the rules of centralization and peripheralization of the patient's symptoms (discussed in Chapter 5, *Treatment by Diagnosis*) must be followed closely. Distinguishing between central symptoms and peripheral symptoms is extremely important and should govern all treatment activities, including the application of spinal traction, spinal mobilization and exercises.

As with all conservative treatment approaches for HNP, patient education and a gradual, cautious return to activities are necessary if the traction is to be successful. Once the disc protrusion is reduced by spinal traction and spinal nerve root symptoms have been relieved, the rest of the principles discussed in Chapter 5 must be applied.

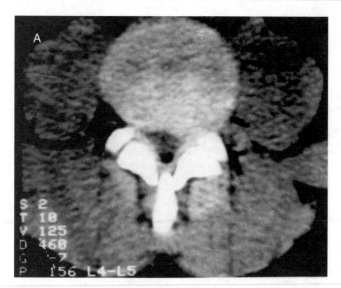 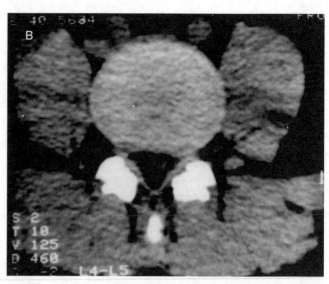

Figure 12-3: A disc protrusion being reduced by traction. A) Before traction—a left lateral HNP at L4-5 with invasion of the neural foramen by herniated nuclear material; B) During traction—regression of the herniated nuclear material from the discal space and neural foramen (from Onel, et al).[67]

Degenerative Disc or Joint Disease

In one of the few controlled trials studying cervical traction, Zylbergold and Piper showed that patients receiving traction had significantly better outcomes than a control group.[94] Improvements were noted in range of motion, need for further treatment and medication use. Most of the patients in this trial had diagnoses of degenerative disc disease.

It is our experience that patients with degenerative disc or joint disease often experience dramatic pain relief when treated with traction. What phenomenon accounts for this pain relief? Although traction can cause separation and widening of the intervertebral foramen and intervertebral disc space, the effect is temporary. If traction is applied to a patient with a narrowed intervertebral foramen or to one who has osteophyte or ligamentous encroachment, the disc space and intervertebral foramen are obviously not restored to their original size and structure.

Therefore, the relief such patients experience must be explained using a different theory. We already know that the pathology seen on x-ray or in CT scans does not necessarily correlate to the degree of symptoms present.[2,29,43,50,51,52,88,90] Many people have narrowing of the disc space and intervertebral foramen without signs and symptoms of spinal nerve root impingement, or even neck or back pain. Asymptomatic patients in whom degenerative changes or osteophytes have been present for some time may have a sudden onset of symptoms related

to a certain activity or position. A very fine line must exist between cases in which encroachment or irritation of the spinal nerve root or other tissues occurs and does not occur. The traction treatment must somehow move, separate or realign the segment in such a way as to relieve the impingement or irritation. Other pain control mechanisms discussed earlier may play a part. Goldish speculates that the degenerated disc may benefit from traction because lowering intradiscal pressure by traction may affect the nutritional state of the nucleus pulposus.[30]

Joint Hypomobility (Soft Tissue Stiffness)

Traction may be regarded as a form of mobilization since it involves the passive movement of the disc and facet joints by mechanical or manual means. Any condition of joint hypomobility may respond favorably to traction. One argument against using traction for mobilization is that it is nonspecific and simultaneously affects several segments. However, when traction is applied to a series of spinal segments, each segment receives an equal amount of traction. If the force applied is sufficient to mobilize the involved segment, it is irrelevant that other segments are also receiving the same amount of traction unless, of course, traction is contraindicated at those other segments. If this is the case, a more specific technique of joint mobilization should be selected.[70, 76]

We believe that traction is the treatment of choice for patients who need mobilization but cannot tolerate certain manual techniques involving rotation, side bending, flexion or extension. Chronic patients with degenerative disc or joint disease and generalized hypomobility often fit this profile. The chronically stiff patient can often tolerate relatively strong traction forces when, at the same time, manual techniques involving movement into the restricted barriers are irritating and cause exacerbation of symptoms. The more severe or chronic the symptoms, the more likely traction will be the preferred technique.

Facet Impingement (Subluxation)

When facet joints become restricted due to mechanical impingement or subluxation, manual mobilization and manipulation techniques are often used to free the restrictions. Manual techniques that isolate the individual joints are sometimes the best techniques. However, traction is another treatment option. If the spinal segment is "out of alignment", any traction force sufficient to separate the joint surfaces may allow the segment to realign itself, similar to the way traction can be used to realign an extremity dislocation or fracture.

Traction as a treatment for facet impingement or subluxation is relatively ineffective in the thoracic area and it should not be used if traction is contraindicated at any segment that receives the traction force.

Cervicogenic Headache

Cervicogenic headache can be treated successfully with cervical traction. Olson reported success with two difficult cases of headache due to chronic whiplash, using 25-30 lbs home traction with the Saunders Cervical Hometrac® and cervical exercise.[65,66] Both subjects had previously tried physical therapy modalities, exercise, and over-the-door cervical traction with poor results.

Muscle Spasm

Both traction and stretching exercises can relieve muscle spasm. Traction can also decompress or separate painful joint structures. If the pain is relieved by traction, muscle spasm will be relieved as a result of relaxation of nociceptive reflexes.[30]

Contraindications for Spinal Traction

Traction is contraindicated in structural disease secondary to tumor or infection, rheumatoid arthritis, in patients with severe vascular compromise and in any condition for which movement is contraindicated.[92]

Relative contraindications include acute strains and sprains and inflammatory conditions that may be aggravated by traction. Strong traction applied to patients with spinal joint instability may cause further strain. Traction should be avoided if the patient has had recent spinal fusion. Since spinal fusion technique and healing rates vary from patient to patient, the surgeon should be consulted before applying traction if the fusion is less than one year old. Other relative contraindications may include pregnancy, osteoporosis, hiatal hernia and claustrophobia.

Section Two—Lumbar Traction

Bed Traction

Bilateral leg traction and pelvic belt traction are methods used for applying traction in bed. The traction rope is pulled over a pulley at the foot of the bed and free weights are attached. Bed traction is applied for as long as several hours at a time. This long duration requires that only small amounts of weight be used because the patient's skin cannot tolerate prolonged traction at high forces. Thus, it is generally accepted that this form of traction cannot separate the vertebrae when applied to the lumbar spine.[39]

It is often said that bed traction's main purpose is to keep the patient immobilized in bed. However, even when bed traction is applied continuously, the force is not enough to prevent the trunk muscles from moving the spinal segments. The patient is not truly immobilized. Therefore, some authors argue that bed traction is not any better than bed rest alone.[30] No studies report a beneficial effect of bed traction. Deyo's study shows that excessive bed rest can actually be harmful.[23] Therefore, it is increasingly hard to justify the use of bed traction at all, and we consider it an obsolete technique.

Mechanical Traction

Mechanical traction differs from bed traction in that the traction is applied for a shorter duration on a treatment table. Since mechanical traction is not continuous, much higher forces can be tolerated without risking skin breakdown. Traditionally, traction force is applied through a pelvic harness, with a thoracic harness used to provide counter traction to prevent the patient's body from slipping down the table. One traction device uses the patient's upper body strength to provide the counterforce. The patient grips handholds rather than using a thoracic harness. Such a device might prevent adequate relaxation, since it is difficult for the patient to selectively contract upper body muscles without contracting trunk muscles. Ideally, the patient's muscles should be as relaxed as possible while receiving traction.

The simplest form of mechanical traction involves the use of free weights hanging from a pulley system at the foot of the table. In this sense, it is similar to the bed traction described earlier except that shorter durations and heavier forces are used. Mechanical gear or winch systems have also been used. Most methods used today involve a traction machine that is specially made to produce a traction force.

The most common method of applying the traction force involves anchoring a thoracic harness to the upper (head) end of the table. The pelvic harness is attached with a rope to a traction machine at the lower (foot) end of the table. The table is split, and the lower end of the table is on friction free rollers. As the traction machine imparts force, the split table separates, and the lower half of the patient's body is pulled horizontally. Since traditional traction machines are attached higher than the surface of the table, the force is usually pulling upward at an angle. All of the traction force is imparted through the pelvic harness.

Recent advances in mechanical traction tables incorporate a system in which the lower half of the traction table is actively powered. Rather than being attached to a rope, the pelvic harness is attached to the lower end of the table. The traction power source actually pushes or pulls the lower end of the table apart. With this method, the lower half of the patient's body "sticks" to the table as the table separates, until the force is sufficient to overcome its weight. Then, the rest of the force is transmitted through the pelvic harness. Depending upon the force used and the patient's body weight, as much as 25% of the traction force results from the table movement alone. This results in a more comfortable traction treatment for the patient, since less force is transmitted through the pelvic harness. Another advantage is that the pull is in a straight line rather than at an upward angle.

Mechanical traction can be static or intermittent. Static traction is applied with a constant force for a few minutes. Intermittent traction alternately applies and releases the traction force every few minutes or seconds. Many traction machines manufactured in the 1960's and 70's had very short hold and rest times in intermittent traction mode.

With a short hold cycle, many patients were unable to adequately relax. Later machines improved by increasing the hold and rest times to 99 seconds. New traction devices allow even longer hold and rest times—up to 5 minutes. The newer devices allow a wider variety of settings, and in some ways have changed our thinking about optimum protocols to treat various conditions.

Mechanical traction is much less effective if a split table is not used. We consider a split table essential to proper technique. It is also very important that a mechanical traction device maintain constant tension. Any slack developed as the patient relaxes during the treatment must be automatically taken up so that the desired amount of traction is maintained. A three-dimensional (3D) table enhances the effectiveness of mechanical traction. Mechanical traction technique is discussed thoroughly in *Mechanical Lumbar Traction Technique* on page 309.

Manual Traction

To apply manual traction, the clinician grasps the patient and manually applies a traction force. Manual traction is usually applied for a few seconds, but it also can be applied as a sudden, quick thrust. It allows the clinician to feel the patient's reaction.[17,40,70] It is sometimes more difficult for the patient to relax with manual traction than with mechanical traction because the exact amount of force that will be applied cannot be anticipated. A steady prolonged stretch is also more difficult to maintain since the clinician eventually fatigues.

Paris uses manual lumbar traction for treatment of HNP. These techniques are sometimes used with a sudden thrust and can be directed unilaterally.[70] Kaltenborn also describes various manual traction techniques that can be used for spinal mobilization.[40] Manual traction can be used to test the patient's tolerance to traction or to find the most comfortable direction in which to administer the treatment. The clinician either pulls on the legs or lifts the patient by the elbows (Fig 12-4).

Manual lumbar traction is of questionable value in most cases because of the physical difficulty of applying and sustaining forces great enough to be effective for many conditions.

Positional Traction

Positional traction involves positioning the patient's spine using pillows, bolsters, or sandbags to cause a longitudinal pull on the spinal structures. The patient is placed in a side lying position over a rolled pillow or blanket. The roll is typically six to eight inches in diameter and is placed at the

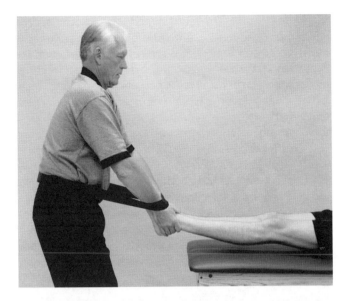

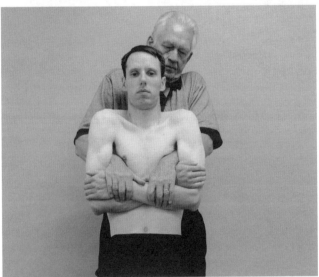

Figure 12-4: Manual lumbar traction techniques.

level of the spine where the traction or separation is desired. The effect is a unilateral stretch of the soft tissue structures, gapping of the facet joints and opening of the neural foramen on the side opposite to the roll. The technique can involve either pure side bending or side bending with rotation (Fig 12-5). The side bending technique can be used to correct the lateral scoliosis (shift) sometimes seen in patients with HNP. Positional traction is inexpensive and can be used at home.

Lumbar Autotraction

Autotraction incorporates a special traction bench composed of two sections that can be individually angled and rotated. Patients apply the traction by pulling with their own arms and can alter the direction of the traction as the

treatment progresses. Treatment sessions can last one hour or longer and are supervised by a clinician.[45,48,62] Autotraction is not as popular as it once was. Most newer traction machines incorporate some sort of mechanical traction device, rather than relying on patient operation of the device.

Gravity Lumbar Traction

With gravity lumbar traction, the patient is stabilized with a specially made vest secured to the top of a bed or table. The patient is then tilted into a vertical or nearly vertical position. In this position the free weight of the legs and hips exerts a traction force on the lumbar spine.[7,30] Gravity lumbar traction with the patient in an upright position has been claimed to be effective in the treatment of HNP. The amount of force that can be applied is limited to approximately 40% of body weight,[7] but there is evidence of distraction of lumbar vertebrae using this method.[83] A moderate amount of physical effort is required from patients. Chest pain caused by the thoracic vest is sometimes a limiting factor. Gravity lumbar traction is recommended only for medically screened, well-motivated patients whose body size and shape allows this form of treatment.[68] The typical protocol consists of one hour of traction twice daily. This protocol is not consistent with the theories of HNP treatment discussed on page 310, which require heavier forces and shorter treatment times. Other disadvantages of gravity traction include difficulty controlling the spinal position (flexion, extension or lateral bending) and force.

Two other types of gravity traction have become popular through commercialization efforts. One technique uses specialized boots that attach to the subject's ankles.

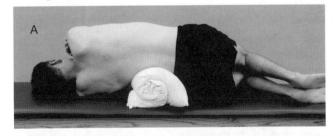

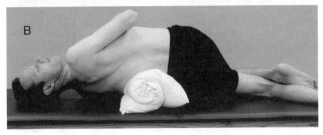

Figure 12-5: Positional traction. A) Left side bending; B) Left side bending and right rotation.

Patients suspend themselves from a frame into a fully inverted position. Another technique involves a device that supports the anterior thighs so that the patient is able to hang inverted with the hips and knees flexed. Both techniques will achieve a traction force of approximately 50% of the total body weight on the lumbar spine.[63] A study by Kane showed significant separation of both the anterior and posterior margins of the lumbar vertebral bodies at all levels as well as increased dimension of the intervertebral foramina using the inversion boot method.[41]

Since higher forces can be achieved, gravity traction in an inverted position may be effective in certain cases. However, there are some risks associated with inverted gravity traction. The inverted position can produce marked changes in heart rate and blood pressure in young adults. There is also evidence of increased ocular pressure and the potential for retinal damage.[47] Inversion traction may be dangerous for hypertensive individuals and those with cardiac anomalies or cerebral vascular disease. In any case, blood pressure, heart rate and patient comfort should be monitored closely during inversion and the patient should be acclimated to the inversion position on gradually.[41]

We believe that gravity traction devices can improve joint mobility and general flexibility, but they do not offer the control of spine position and, in some cases, the amount of force necessary to effectively treat patients with HNP or degenerative disc or joint disease. Most of the gravity lumbar traction devices are portable and can be used for home treatment.

Home Lumbar Traction

Home lumbar traction devices are most useful as an adjunct treatment for those patients who have had successful traction treatment in the clinic. They are most appropriate when a high degree of control and specificity of treatment technique is not required. Patients who require specific positions are better treated with clinical mechanical traction systems that accommodate advanced positioning techniques.

Home lumbar traction is an important treatment consideration when the patient's condition is chronic. Many patients have conditions, such as degenerative disc or joint disease, which are intermittently symptomatic. If traction has been beneficial in the past, it makes sense to give the patient a home option to treat recurrent episodes. One advantage is cost-savings. Another is allowing the patient to begin self-treatment immediately, perhaps lessening the severity of the episode.

Home lumbar traction should also be considered when more frequent treatments are necessary. In today's health care environment, it is typical to see patients in the clinic only 2-3 times weekly. More frequent traction treatments may be indicated, especially for patients who initially benefit from traction, but gradually worsen again through the day. Home lumbar traction allows the patient to obtain more frequent treatments without an unacceptable health care cost.

Some patients may benefit from clinical visits, but live too far away from the clinic to travel. What's more, many patients with lower back pain have increased pain with sitting. The long drive to the clinic sometimes negates any beneficial effect of the clinic visit. Home lumbar traction offers these patients a more effective treatment strategy.

90/90 Traction

For years, 90/90 home traction devices were the only home lumbar traction treatment available (Fig 12-6). These devices require positioning the patient with the knees and hips bent at 90° with a posterior pelvic tilt. A rope attached to a pelvic belt is draped over the top of an A-frame. The patient pulls on the rope to lift the pelvis off the floor. This produces additional posterior pelvic tilt and lumbar flexion.

A study of 90/90 traction showed greater posterior disc distraction than anterior disc compression.[30] However, flexing the hips to 90° alone also produces posterior distraction. Therefore it is questionable whether 90/90 traction devices actually provide significant traction or whether their main effect is simply to flex the lumbar spine. We do not feel 90/90 devices produce a clinically effective traction force, and the flexed posture is actually undesirable for treating conditions like HNP. Home lumbar traction devices are available that can produce significant traction forces with better ability to control the patient's position.

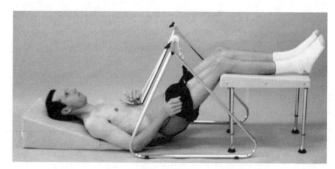

Figure 12-6: 90/90 traction.

The Saunders Lumbar Hometrac®

The Saunders Lumbar Hometrac is one of several commercially available devices that allow traction in a straight-line pull rather than with the hips and knees flexed to 90°. Up to 200 lbs of force can be delivered with the patient lying either prone or supine. Also, a unilateral technique is possible (Fig 12-7).

Mechanical Lumbar Traction Technique

Many clinicians routinely use cervical traction and note the beneficial results in patients with soft tissue stiffness, hypomobility, degenerative joint or disc disease and nerve root symptoms. Yet many do not use traction for treatment of similar conditions in the lumbar spine. We attribute this general attitude to previous inadequacies in equipment and lack of knowledge of effective traction techniques. Disappointment in bed traction caused many clinicians to lose interest in any form of lumbar traction. But with proper equipment and technique, the same satisfactory results that have been experienced with cervical traction can also be accomplished with lumbar traction.

Important Treatment Variables

Force. Theoretically, the traction force must be great enough to cause movement at the spinal segment. Cyriax reported a visible separation with static traction of 120 lbs for 15 minutes.[16] Other studies have reported measurable separation in the lumbar spine at forces ranging from 80 to 200 lbs.[33,46,57] Judovich advocated a force equal to $1/_2$ the patient's body weight on a friction-free surface as a minimum to cause therapeutic effects in the lumbar spine.[39] It is not necessary for the first treatment to be administered at that force, and it must be remembered that the minimum force necessary to cause a measurable separation will not always be enough to produce satisfactory results. Conversely, clinical experience has shown that some patients have pain relief with forces of less than $1/_2$ the body weight. It is important to assess the patient's reaction and results of the treatment after each visit. Adjustments can be made until satisfactory results are achieved.

The forces required to cause damage to vertebral structures have also been studied. In one study, a force of 400 lbs was necessary to produce a rupture of the dorsolumbar spine (T11, T12) in a fresh cadaver.[22] Harris indicated that enormous traction forces were necessary to cause damage to the lumbar spine with the breaking load possibly being as high as 880 lbs.[33]

Friction. A split table is necessary to eliminate friction. As mentioned previously, it is the effective traction force on the spine that is important, and any friction involved must be considered. A split table on frictionless guides essentially eliminates friction (Fig 12-8).[30]

With a traditional traction table using a split surface, all the slack in the harnesses must be taken up before the split table is released. A helpful tip is to begin the treatment with the split table locked. This allows the traction machine to pull all the slack out of the harnesses. If using intermittent mode, allow two or three pulls to take up all the slack, and then release the split table during a rest phase. If using static mode, release the table gradually after the slack has been removed, taking care to avoid a sudden jerk. This can be accomplished by holding or blocking the movement of the table top as the split table mechanism is released, then gradually letting the table apart manually.

When using the newer tables that use an actively moving treatment surface, friction between the patient and table is not an issue. Slack should still be taken out of the harness straps by pulling them taut before beginning treatment.

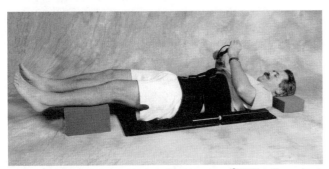

Figure 12-7: Saunders Lumbar Hometrac® (The Saunders Group, Inc.).

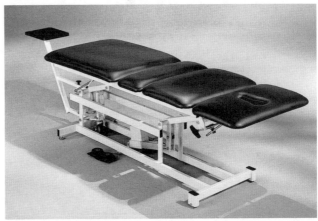

Figure 12-8: A split table is essential for the administration of lumbar traction (Performa Traction Table from Sammons Preston Rolyan).

Relaxation. Patients must be able to relax. The amount of force alone does not determine the effectiveness of the traction treatment. Traction treatment is usually not a *comfortable* experience. However, patients must be able to relax during treatment, or the treatment will be less effective. Cervical traction studies show that narrowing of the intervertebral spaces can actually occur during the traction treatment in patients who are unable to relax.[20] The treatment must not aggravate the condition and patients must feel secure and well supported. It may be beneficial to administer modality treatments before the application of traction. Such agents as ice, heat, ultrasound, electric stimulation and massage are often effective.

Proper Stabilization. The use of a heavy duty, non-slip traction harness is essential. If patients do not feel secure, they will almost certainly remain tense during treatment. A heavy-duty, one-size-fits-all lumbar traction harness system is required (Fig 12-9). Cotton traction belts are not adequate for high forces in terms of strength and stability.

Spinal Position. The position of the spine during traction is an important treatment variable. When using a traditional traction table, the spinal position is controlled with a combination of the patient's position (prone or supine) and the position of the harness straps relative to the angle of the traction source. Sometimes pillows or bolsters are used to impart lumbar or hip flexion. An actively powered traction table with three-dimensional table movement allows better control of the spinal position. Proper setup for both methods is discussed later in this chapter.

The amount of spinal flexion or extension desired will depend upon the disorder being treated and the comfort of

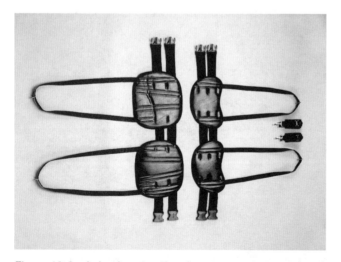

Figure 12-9: A lumbar traction harness system made of vinyl, canvas, and a non-slip surface for the effective administration of lumbar traction (EZ-ON traction belts from The Saunders Group, Inc.).

the patient.[16] In our experience, disc herniation is most effectively treated with the patient lying prone with a normal lordosis. However, this position is not always possible because the patient with acute HNP may not tolerate any position of normal lordosis. If this is the case the treatment must be given in flexion initially with the goal of gradually working toward neutral lumbar lordosis.

Foraminal (lateral) stenosis is usually more effectively treated with the lumbar spine in a flexed (flattened) position initially, with the goal of achieving a neutral lordosis when possible. Soft tissue stiffness/hypomobility and degenerative disc or joint disease may be treated in neutral or some degree of flexion or extension, depending on the goals of treatment. Patient comfort and the patient's ability to remain relaxed during the treatment are important considerations when choosing the most beneficial position and no absolute rule applies. Variations of flexion, extension and lateral bending should be tried to find the most beneficial position for each patient.

There is often a postural component involved with disorders of the lumbar spine. Initially, traction treatments may have to be administered in positions that accommodate the patient's postural deviation. As progress is achieved, the treatment should be administered in positions that encourage a return to normal posture. For example, most patients with disc herniation will have a flattened lumbar lordosis and will be limited in spinal extension. One of the treatment goals will be to return this patient to normal posture. Although it may be impossible to place the patient in a position of normal lordosis initially, one will want to work in that direction as treatment progresses. It may be necessary to give the traction treatment in a position involving some flexion initially. However, as progress is noted and the patient is able to achieve a position of normal lordosis, the traction treatments should be given in a position that helps achieve the normal lordosis.

Mode (Static or Intermittent). The traction mode selected will depend on the disorder being treated and the comfort of the patient. HNP is usually treated more effectively in static mode or with longer hold-rest periods (3-5 minute hold, 1 minute rest) in intermittent mode. Joint dysfunction and degenerative disc disease usually respond to shorter hold-rest periods (1-2 minute hold, 30 second rest) in intermittent mode. Static mode will be relatively ineffective unless the traction machine can take up slack during the treatment.

Time. Treatment time is another important factor to consider. When treating HNP, the treatment time should be relatively short. As the disc space widens, the intradiscal pressure decreases,[61] causing the herniated disc material to be retracted into the disc space. This is theorized to be one of the beneficial effects of traction when treating HNP. The decrease in pressure is temporary, however, because eventually the decreased intradiscal pressure will cause fluid to be imbibed into the disc. When pressure equalization occurs, the suction effect on the disc protrusion is lost. At this point, it is possible for patients to experience a sudden increase in pain when traction is released. We have not observed this adverse reaction in treatments of less than ten minutes in intermittent mode and eight minutes in static mode.

As a general rule, the higher the force, the shorter the treatment time. Often, the first treatment is only three to five minutes long. This gives the clinician a chance to determine the patient's reaction to treatment and plan treatment progression accordingly.

Ramp Up and Ramp Down Phase.   Certain mechanical traction devices can gradually increase the traction force at the beginning of the treatment and reduce the force at the end of the treatment. These features are commonly called ramp up (progressive) and ramp down (regressive) phases or modes. Applying traction with a ramp up/ramp down phase can be equated to a "warm up, cool down" period known to all clinicians. The gradual application and removal of traction forces made possible with these features may enhance the potential effectiveness of traction in certain patients.

Frequency and Duration.   Ideally, some acute or severe conditions should be treated twice daily. We realize this is often impractical in today's health care environment. Unless the patient is hospitalized, the effort to drive to and from the clinic will negate any positive effects of the traction. Nonetheless, initial treatment for some acute or severe conditions should be as frequent as is practical—certainly 3-5 times per week.

On the other hand, we believe in weaning patients from traction treatments as soon as possible. When patients with HNP are able to control radicular symptoms with the home exercise and self-mobilization techniques discussed in Chapter 5, they do not require traction treatments. When patients with painful hypomobility have achieved enough stretching clinically to continue exercise at home, they can be weaned off traction.

Some patients with chronic recurring symptoms will benefit from ongoing traction treatments, but these patients should be transitioned to a home lumbar traction device. There is no reason to continue clinical traction treatments for more than three to six weeks, except in unusual circumstances.

Unilateral Lumbar Traction

For certain patients, lumbar traction involving a pull from only one side of the body has been shown to be more comfortable and effective than regular traction.[5,6,33,62,75] Although the technique seems sound, very little unilateral lumbar traction has been used clinically because of problems with patient positioning and adaptability of equipment.

Some traction setups can be adapted to a unilateral technique by positioning the traction unit at an oblique angle to the table. However, when this is done, the patient's body simply slides to the side of the table and aligns itself with the traction force and the actual angle of pull remains straight. When attempts are made to stabilize the spine to prevent this realignment, the exact area of lateral bending is difficult, if not impossible, to control. For instance, when attempts are made to stabilize the patient with a belt across the torso, most side bending occurs at the segment just inferior to the belt and the exact segment can only be determined by x-ray.

If using a traditional traction table, the unilateral lumbar traction technique we prefer requires use of the heavy-duty traction harness described earlier. By hooking only one side of the harness to the traction source, or by shortening one of the two harness straps, an effective unilateral pull can be achieved. With this method, lateral bending and separation of the vertebrae is uniform throughout the lumbar spine. The technique can be applied in either the prone or the supine position (Fig 12-10).

We have investigated the effects of unilateral traction to determine if vertebral separation occurs, where it occurs and whether a lumbar scoliosis occurs when the unilateral pull is applied. Our investigation examined x-rays of one 200 lb man with no apparent lumbar disorder. The subject was positioned supine and received 100 lbs traction from the right side only. Measurements were taken from the lateral aspect of the inferior edge of the T12 vertebral body to the superior surface of the sacrum at a point adjacent to the lateral aspect of the L5 vertebral body. The unilateral traction produced a separation of 10 mm on the side of the pull and a separation of 2 mm on the side opposite the pull. Lumbar lateral bending of 12° was also observed. The curve was convex on the side of the pull. The separation and curve appeared uniform throughout the lumbar spine (Fig 12-11).

X-ray measurements were taken with the subject in the same position (supine and side bent) but with no traction force. Seven millimeters separation occurred on the convex side and 11 mm narrowing occurred on the concave side of

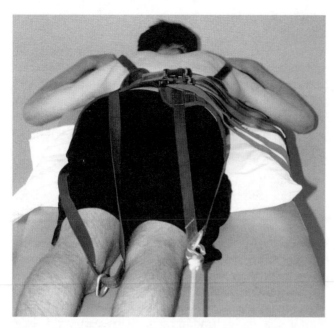 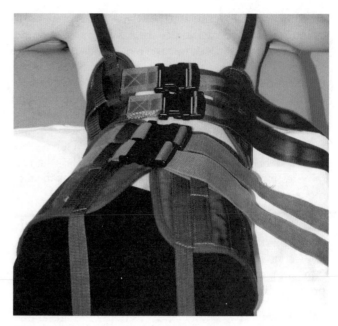

Figure 12-10: Effective unilateral lumbar traction in the prone position. Only the right side of the pelvic harness is attached to the traction force. This results in traction with the lumbar spine convex on the right and concave on the left, or in relative left side bending. The same principles can be used in supine.

the curve (Fig 12-12). Investigation of a subject with a lumbar disorder revealed similar findings (see *Unilateral Facet Joint Hypomobility or Impingement* on page 314).

The general indications and contraindications for applying conventional lumbar traction also apply to unilateral traction techniques. Thorough assessment is necessary, and part of that assessment should involve consideration of the factors that favor the unilateral or the bilateral techniques.

Although there are specific diagnoses for which unilateral traction is particularly useful, unilateral technique can be used for any condition in which traction is indicated. Often, the determining factor is patient comfort and ability to relax with the treatment. A trial of manual traction can be done to determine if the patient is a suitable candidate for traction. The manual traction should be given at various degrees of flexion, extension and lateral bending to find the most comfortable and beneficial patient position.[78] When the disorder is unilateral, the most comfortable position will often be one that does involve some lateral bending of the spine along with traction. It is wise to take advantage of this more comfortable position in these cases.

Four specific instances when unilateral traction may be preferred to conventional traction techniques include:

1. HNP with protective scoliosis or lateral shift;
2. Unilateral soft tissue stiffness, degenerative joint or disc disease;
3. Unilateral facet joint hypomobility or impingement;
4. Lumbar scoliosis caused by unilateral lumbar muscle spasm.[78]

HNP with Protective Scoliosis or Lateral Shift. If a patient has HNP and the protrusion is encroaching upon a spinal nerve root, lateral bending of the spine often offers relief. This is referred to as a *protective scoliosis*. Many musculoskeletal problems involve lateral bending of the spine, and protective scoliosis is only one of several reasons one might see lateral bending. Most patients with protective scoliosis lean away from the side of the symptoms. However, when the disorder involves an HNP with a protrusion medial to the nerve root, the patient may bend toward the side of the symptoms. If the herniation is lateral to the nerve root (most common), the patient will bend away from the painful side (Fig 12-13). In all cases, the patient assumes the position that offers symptomatic relief.[25,85]

When the patient with a protective scoliosis is placed in conventional bilateral traction, the scoliosis straightens as soon as the traction is applied. This may press the herniated disc against the nerve root, resulting in increased pain. The traction does not appear to be beneficial. However, if the scoliosis can be maintained while the traction is applied, the treatment can be applied without increasing the patient's discomfort. Such a technique enhances the chances of achieving the desired results of the treatment.

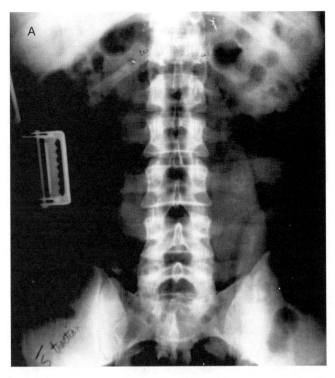
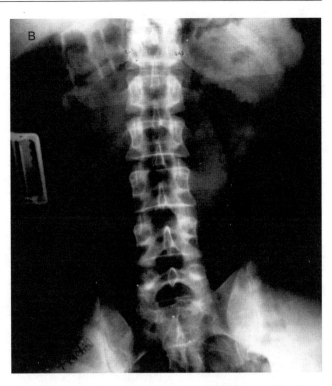

Figure 12-11: Effects of supine unilateral lumbar traction, A/P view. A) No traction force; B) 100 lbs (45.5 kg) force pulling from the right side only. Total vertebral separation from T12 to the sacrum was 10 mm on the right and 2 mm on the left.

A protective scoliosis differs from the condition McKenzie describes as a lateral shift.[58] With a protective scoliosis, the patient places himself in the most comfortable position. A lateral shift is a mechanical phenomenon that occurs when the nuclear gel moves laterally. It is sometimes difficult to distinguish between these conditions clinically, but it is not really critical for treatment planning. In either case, an attempt should be made to manually

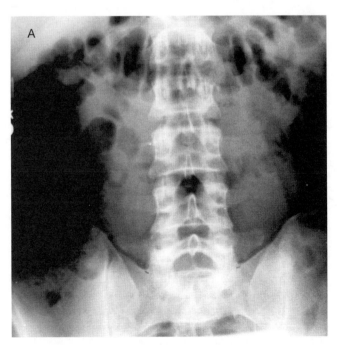
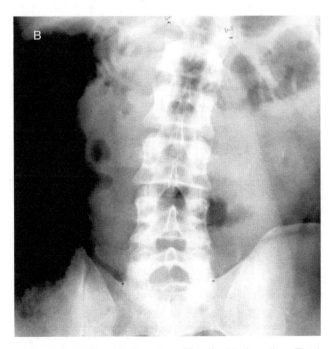

Figure 12-12: Effects of supine left side bending without traction, A/P view. A) No side bending; B) Left side bending. Total vertebral separation from T12 to the sacrum was 7 mm on the right, with an 11 mm narrowing on the left.

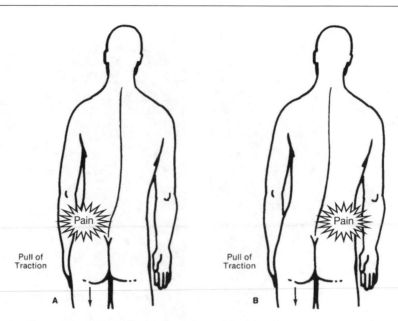

Figure 12-13: A) A patient with a protective scoliosis away from the side of the symptoms; B) A patient with a protective scoliosis toward the symptoms. In both cases, the unilateral pull should be from the convex side of the curve to maintain the scoliosis.

correct the abnormal posture. If manual posture correction results in a centralization of symptoms, the abnormal posture was probably a lateral shift. If manual posture correction causes increased peripheral symptoms, one may be dealing with a protective scoliosis or a severe lateral shift and lumbar traction will be more effective if the abnormal posture is not disturbed.

To maintain the curve for the patient who leans away from the side of the symptoms, the pull should be from the same side as the symptoms. For the patient who leans toward the affected side, the traction pull should be from the side opposite that of the symptoms (Fig 12-13). In either case, the pull is from the convex side of the lumbar curve.

Unilateral Soft Tissue Stiffness or Degeneration. Many patients with chronic back pain have symptoms predominately on one side, with ipsilateral degenerative changes. A range of motion examination reveals stiffness in side bending away from and rotation toward the side of symptoms. While active and passive stretching exercises are often the treatment of choice, unilateral traction can be used to help the patient get started with home exercise.

Unilateral traction provides an effective, relatively general mobilization technique to gently stretch the stiff area. The more painful and chronic the patient's symptoms, the more likely the patient is to benefit from unilateral traction in addition to a home stretching program or mobilization techniques.

Unilateral Facet Joint Hypomobility or Impingement. Conventional lumbar traction can be used as a mobilization technique for hypomobility or impingement. When the pathology involves the facet joints on one side only, a unilateral technique should be considered. The following is a case study of unilateral facet joint hypomobility or impingement involving the use of unilateral lumbar traction.[78]

The subject was a 17-year-old, 155 lb male student athlete. Three months earlier, he had suffered a compression-type fall with the spine extended. The pain was minor at first but had stiffened his spine. Initially, he had not sought medical help. His only complaint was pain with running. The pain was located just lateral to the right L5-S1 interspace.

The x-ray revealed apparent narrowing of the right facet joint (Fig 12-14). Mobility tests revealed hypomobility at the L5-S1 level with the greatest restriction in right rotation and left side bending. Other clinical signs and symptoms supported the presence of facet joint hypomobility at that level. There were no positive neurological findings.

The patient received ultrasound treatment directly over the painful area, followed by intermittent unilateral lumbar traction with a right-sided pull of 100 lbs (45.5 kg) for 10 minutes. An x-ray taken while the traction was being applied showed visible separation of the right L5-S1 facet (Fig 12-14). The patient was nearly symptom free after two treatments, and received a total of four treatments. He

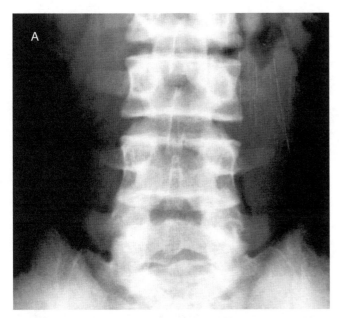

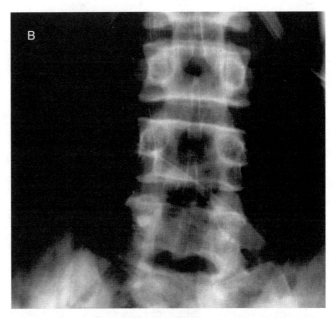

Figure 12-14: P/A radiograph showing a narrowed right facet joint and a position change of right rotation at the L5-S1 interspace; B) Intervertebral separation occurring with a 100 lb (45.5 kg) traction force from the right.

returned to full activities of daily living, including varsity cross-country running, and remained symptom free for several months following the study.

Lumbar Scoliosis Caused by Muscle Spasm. Unilateral lumbar traction can be used to reduce a lumbar scoliosis caused by unilateral paravertebral muscle spasm. The unilateral pull should be from the concave side of the scoliosis (Fig 12-15).[78]

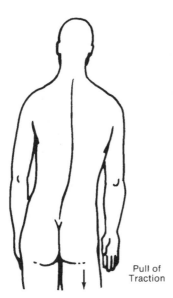

Figure 12-15: A patient with a unilateral muscle spasm causing a lumbar scoliosis. To stretch this condition, the pull should be from the concave side of the curve.

Pull of Traction

Three-Dimensional (3D) Lumbar Traction

The term *three-dimensional traction* refers to using a moveable treatment surface to allow a non-linear traction pull. A 3D traction table's lower half moves in three dimensions: flexion/extension, side bending and rotation. Patients can be positioned in any combination of these positions during traction treatment, and the position can be changed during or after traction treatment. There are two important reasons to use three-dimensional traction: Correction of postural deformities and unilateral soft tissue mobilization.

Correction of Postural Deformities. Postural changes accompany many of the spinal disorders treated by physical therapists. It is sometimes difficult to determine if the abnormal posture is the result of the pathological disorder or if the postural change is the cause of the disorder. Regardless of this relationship, return to normal posture is always one of the treatment goals. For example, the patient with HNP often presents with a flattened lumbar spine and a lateral scoliosis. One of the goals of treatment should be to return this patient to normal posture. However, this is not always possible in the initial course of treatment. Attempts to straighten the lateral scoliosis or restore the lordosis often cause an increase in the peripheral signs and symptoms and a general worsening of the condition. When this is the case, traction is often the treatment of choice if it can be administered so the patient's flexed and laterally shifted posture is not disturbed. Using a traditional traction table, the initial treatment is often given in the prone position with pillows under the lumbar spine to maintain flexion. A unilateral technique pulling from the convex

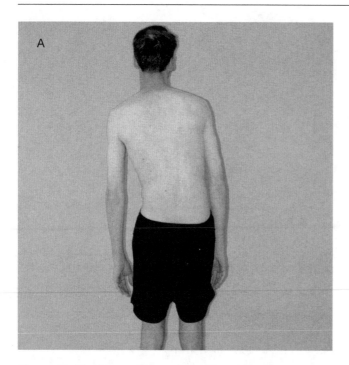
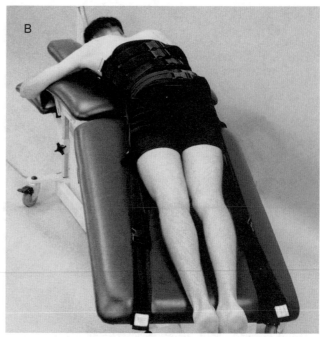

Figure 12-16: Using a 3D traction table with an acute herniated disc. A) The patient initially presents with a flattened lumbar lordosis, left lateral shift, and right lower extremity pain; B) The patient's abnormal posture is initially accommodated by lowering and left side bending the foot end of the table. During treatment, as the patient's lower extremity symptoms decrease, the table position is moved to neutral flexion/extension and side bending. Mild to moderate over-correction into right side bending and extension may be indicated, depending upon severity and acuity. Lower extremity symptoms are constantly monitored and treatment is progressed as long as lower extremity symptoms do not increase (3D ActiveTrac® from The Saunders Group, Inc.)

side of the curve will often allow traction without straightening the protective curve. On subsequent treatments, the amount of flexion and the amount of unilateral pull is lessened as the patient is gradually worked back into a normal postural position.

A 3D table offers an advantage because the table can be initially positioned to accommodate the patient's abnormal posture (Fig 12-16). As the traction force is being administered, the table can be adjusted gradually to return the patient to normal posture. Patients who cannot tolerate conventional traction positions can often tolerate treatment on a 3D traction table. This allows clinicians to treat patients with very acute HNP earlier than might otherwise be possible. Thus, the 3D traction table offers considerable advantage, especially in the ease and convenience of administering the treatment and the ability to treat more severe conditions earlier.

Unilateral Soft Tissue Mobilization. A 3D traction table also offers an advantage when treating the patient with unilateral soft tissue stiffness and/or degenerative joint or disc disease. Rather than using a unilateral pull in a horizontal direction, the 3D table can be positioned to provide a unilateral stretch with a non-linear direction of pull. In the example described on page 314, the patient was limited in both side bending and rotation. If a 3D traction table had been commercially available at the time, the table could have been positioned to stretch both the side bending and rotational components of his stiffness.

The 3D table shown is also pictured in Chapter 10, *Joint Mobilization.* Since a 3D traction table can be used for both traction and general mobilization, it is one of the more versatile pieces of equipment available to the clinician treating spinal pain patients. Generally speaking, a 3D traction table improves comfort and convenience for both the patient and clinician. However, its real value is in treating very severe, irritable conditions that do not respond well to manual techniques, a horizontal traction pull, or a flat prone or supine position. Having a 3D traction table allows one to treat such conditions earlier and more effectively than would be otherwise possible.

Setup Considerations Using a Traditional Traction Table

Applying the Harnesses. Most traditional traction tables use heavy-duty harnesses similar to those shown earlier in Figure 12-9. At first glance, the method of harness applica-

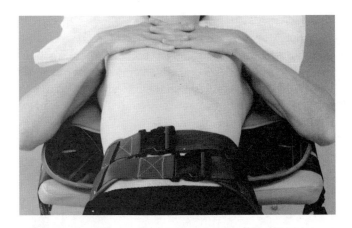

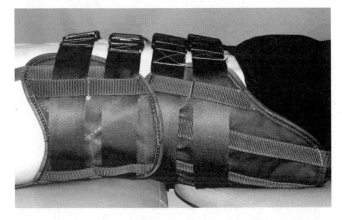

Figure 12-17: The pelvic harness is properly positioned when the top web belt is above the iliac crests and the web belt's top edge crosses at the umbilical line. The pelvic and thoracic harnesses should overlap slightly. Note that the harnesses are placed directly on the skin for optimal technique.

tion may not seem to matter, but careful thought is necessary to achieve optimum technique.

Both the pelvic and thoracic harness surfaces should be placed next to the patient's skin. If the harnesses are placed over clothing, slippage is more likely to occur. Clothing can also take some of the traction force if it is bound tightly under both belts. The pelvic harness should be secured to the patient first. It is properly positioned when the top web belt crosses at approximately the umbilical line. The thoracic harness should be positioned so that it lies on the lateral-inferior chest wall. When properly positioned, the pelvic and thoracic belts will overlap slightly (Fig 12-17).

Depending on the goals of treatment, it can be more or less important to carefully control the position of the spine during traction. If the pelvic harness pulls from the sides only, it is difficult to control the degree of lumbar lordosis. It is much better to use a pelvic harness that can pull from either an anterior or posterior position. The harness is then applied specifically with the goals of treatment in mind. In other words, the pull straps of the pelvic harness are positioned either anterior or posterior, depending upon the patient's position and the amount of spinal flexion or extension desired during treatment. There are four basic options for the position of the patient and pull straps: 1) Supine with a posterior pull; 2) Supine with an anterior pull; 3) Prone with an anterior pull; and 4) Prone with a posterior pull (Fig 12-18).

Lumbar Traction in the Supine Position.   When applying lumbar traction in the supine position, the knees and hips can be flexed moderately for comfort, with a bolster or pillows under the lower legs. If flexion is desired a *posterior pull* should be used. An *anterior pull* will produce a normal to slight extension curve in the lumbar spine. The rope angle to the table should remain relatively in line. This is especially true if heavier forces are used.

Lumbar Traction in the Prone Position.   If the goal is to apply lumbar traction with the spine in a position of normal lordosis or extension, the prone position is probably best.

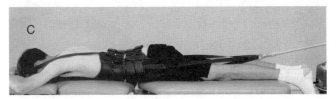

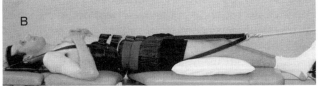

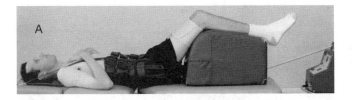

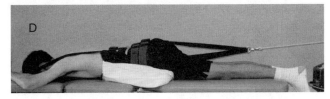

Figure 12-18: Varying methods of applying lumbar traction. A) Supine with a posterior pull; B) Supine with an anterior pull; C) Prone with an anterior pull; D) Prone with a posterior pull.

The harness should be positioned with an *anterior pull*. The patient lies flat on the table and the rope angle to the table is varied to control the exact amount of lordosis.

For patients who cannot tolerate a neutral or extended position, prone traction can be especially effective. Pillows or a 3D table are used to accommodate the patient's preference for a flexed posture. A *posterior pull* is used. Since this type of patient often has significant pain and or muscle guarding, the prone position is excellent for applying modality treatments and the traction can follow without moving the patient. Another advantage of prone traction is that the therapist can palpate the interspinous spaces to estimate the amount of movement that is taking place during the treatment.

Section Three—Cervical Traction

Cervical Traction Using a Head Halter

Certain cervical traction methods use head halters that fit under the chin anteriorly and on the occipital bone posteriorly. Attempts have been made to design head halters without a chin strap (Fig 12-19). Head halters can accommodate both sitting and supine methods. When traction is provided with a standard head halter with a chin strap, force is transmitted through the chin strap to the teeth and the temporomandibular joints become weight-bearing structures. A common problem from administering cervical traction is aggravation of the temporomandibular joints because of the force applied at the chin. The exact amount of force on the chin depends upon the design and adjustment of the head halter, the direction (flexion or extension) of the traction force and the amount of the traction force. Some head halters are better than others. Nevertheless, even when the utmost care is taken to minimize the force on the chin, there often exists enough force to cause an undesirable effect on the temporomandibular joints.[26]

Crisp and others have described patients who experience considerable discomfort in the temporomandibular joints with cervical traction using a head halter.[14,81] This is particularly true if an abnormal dental occlusion exists such as the absence of posterior teeth. In some cases, the discomfort is so great that the treatment has to be discontinued. With advancing age, the tissues become more susceptible to disruption and joint trauma, which, in some cases, may be irreversible.[81] Franks suggests that cervical traction with a head halter and chin strap should be carried out with caution. He reports that, in the older patient particularly, excessive pressure on the jaw can lead to intracapsular bleeding and hematoma in the temporomandibular joint.[27]

Another problem with head halters is that the force applied to the chin tends to cause upper and mid cervical extension. This is undesirable, since most patients with cervical problems have a forward head posture (upper and mid cervical extension with lower cervical and upper thoracic flexion).

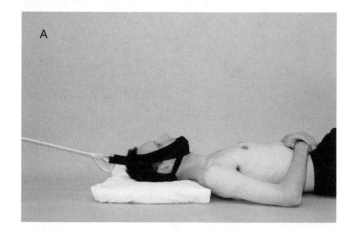

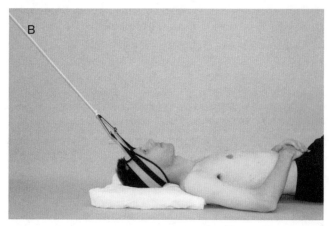

Figure 12-19: Two types of cervical traction head halters. A) Standard head halter (Bird and Cronin, Inc.); B) Supine C-Trax™ TMJ head halter (Therapeutic Dimension, Inc.). Note that the C-Trax halter requires a minimum rope angle of 45° to avoid slipping off, so is not advisable for most traction applications.

The Saunders Cervical Traction Device

The Saunders Cervical Traction Device does not contact the chin or place any force on the temporomandibular joints (Fig 12-20). The device rests on the traction treatment table and is connected to the traction source via an adapter. V-shaped neck wedges are attached to a friction-free carriage. Treatment is applied with the patient lying supine. The neck wedges fit against the back of the patient's neck just below the occipital bone. A strap fits across the patient's forehead to hold the head in position as treatment is applied.

Manual Cervical Traction

Cyriax advocates manual cervical traction and estimates that he exerts forces as high as 200 lbs (91 kg).[17] He often incorporates passive range of motion with the manual trac-

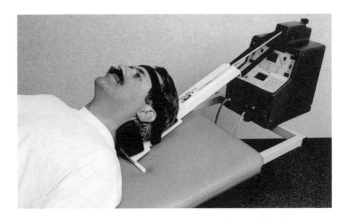

Figure 12-20: Saunders Cervical Traction Device II™ (The Saunders Group, Inc.)

tion (Fig 12-21). A strap (Fig 12-22) or a towel (Fig 12-23) can be used quite effectively to assist with the grip during manual cervical traction techniques. Upper cervical dis-

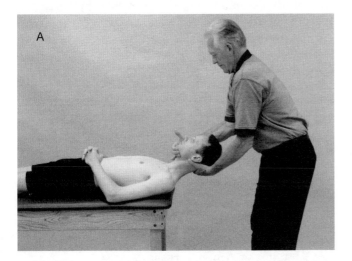

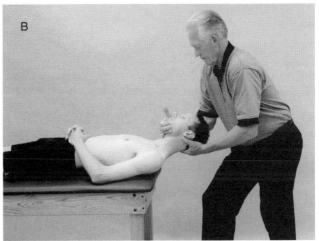

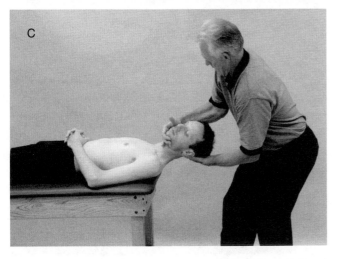

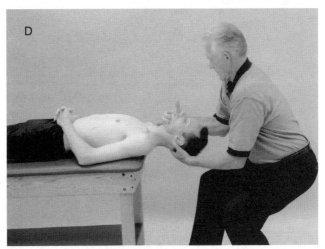

Figure 12-21: Manual cervical traction techniques. A) Traction with a straight pull; B) With right side bending; C) With left rotation; D) With extension.

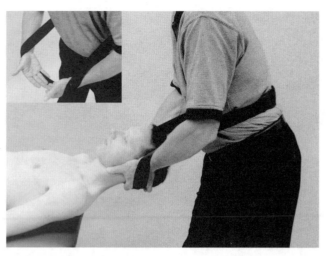

Figure 12-22: Using a strap to assist with manual cervical traction techniques. Inset shows position of strap in hands.

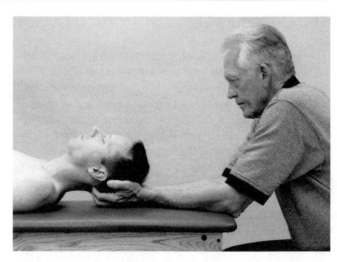

Figure 12-24: Upper cervical distraction, also called inhibitive manual traction or occipital release.

traction (called inhibitive manual traction by Paris) can relax the suboccipital muscles and provide relief of cervicogenic headache (Fig 12-24).[70]

Unilateral Cervical Traction

Unilateral cervical traction is used to direct a stronger force to one side of the cervical spine or to maintain a protective scoliosis. If the traction unit can move relative to the table, placing it at an oblique angle to the table effectively imparts a unilateral pull. However, a stabilization strap must be used over the patient's chest. Otherwise, the patient's body will align with the angle of the rope and the unilateral effect will be lost. An easier alternative involves aligning the patient at an angle to the traction device (Fig 12-25). If a head halter is used, a unilateral effect can be achieved by shortening only one of the two straps that attach the head halter to the traction source.

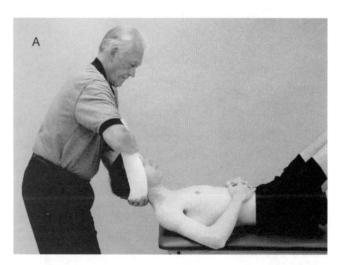

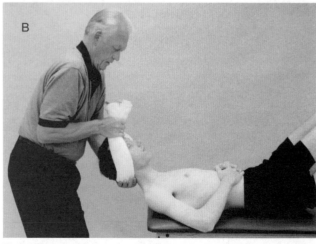

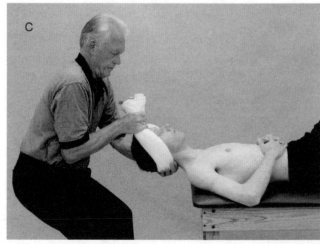

Figure 12-23: Using a towel to assist with manual cervical traction techniques. A) Initial position with elbow sticking out; B) Bringing the elbow to the side to twist and tighten the towel; C) Applying traction by sitting down and leaning back.

Home Cervical Traction

Home cervical traction is typically administered with over-the-door cervical traction devices or with newer devices that do not require head halters. Over-the-door devices use a head halter, rope and pulley system with weights (Fig 12-26). Since supine cervical traction has been shown to be more effective than sitting, the sitting method of over-the-door traction is not recommended. One study reported compression or narrowing of the joint space with cervical traction applied in the sitting position.[20] When the same force was applied in supine, separation was noted. The authors attributed the problem to muscle guarding and inability to relax during the seated treatment. Fortunately, supine over-the-door cervical traction kits are available.

The Saunders Cervical Hometrac is one of two commercially available devices that allow cervical traction in the supine position without a head halter (Fig 12-27). The Hometrac was designed to allow all typical clinical treatment protocols, including delivery of up to 50 lbs (27.7 kg) of force. Both static and intermittent protocols and a unilateral technique are possible.

Over-the-door devices are less expensive than the Saunders Cervical Hometrac, but they have disadvantages. An over-the-door cervical traction device is not appropriate if the patient has TMJ problems or a history of TMJ problems, other jaw or facial problems or claustrophobia. Upper extremity range of motion or strength limitations may preclude the overhead reaching or manual dexterity required to set up an over-the-door device. If the patient requires more than 20 lbs of force, an over-the-door device is not indicated, since they are limited to 20 lbs (9 kg). It is difficult to control the angle of traction or use an intermittent traction protocol using an over-the-door device.

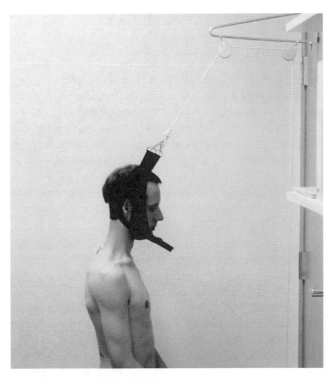

Figure 12-26: Over-the-door home traction treatment.

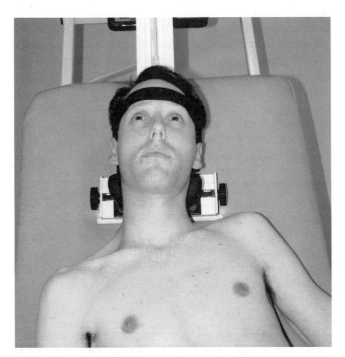

Figure 12-25: Unilateral cervical traction. The patient's trunk is aligned at an angle to achieve a right-sided pull.

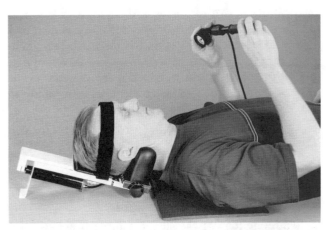

Figure 12-27: Saunders Cervical Hometrac Deluxe® (The Saunders Group, Inc.).

Cervical Traction Technique

Important Treatment Variables

Force. Judovich found that 25-45 lb forces were necessary to demonstrate a measurable change in the posterior cervical spine structures.[38] Jackson confirmed this finding.[36] Colachis and Strohm demonstrated that a traction force of 30 lbs (13.6 kg) produces separation of the cervical spine, and that 50 lbs (22.7 kg) force produces more separation than 30 lbs.[10,11] We have found that 25-40 lbs (11-18 kg) of force for the mid and lower cervical spine is often clinically effective in conditions where a separation of the intervertebral space is desirable.

Examples of these conditions include HNP, interforaminal nerve root encroachment, degenerative disc or joint disease and facet joint impingement. In other conditions where the muscles are primarily affected, less force may be effective. Examples include suboccipital or upper trapezius muscle tension or shortening. Daugherty and Erhard demonstrated separation of the atlanto/occipital and atlanto/axial joints with 10 lbs (4.5 kg) of traction.[18] Therefore, it appears that less force is necessary when treatment is directed to the upper cervical area.

How much is too much? Certainly, patient comfort and clinical response should be the guide. One in vitro study reported that a traction force of 120 lbs was necessary to cause a disc rupture at the C5-C6 level.[22] A more recent in vitro study demonstrated a mean failure load of 128 lbs for a single intervertebral disc and 764 lbs for an intact fresh cadaver.[93] We have successfully used up to 50 lbs without any adverse results when working up to this force gradually. However, we have found that 50 lbs is rarely needed for good clinical results, and our experience and the clinician feedback we have received confirm that 25-40 lbs is typically an adequate and effective force.

Patient Position. We recommend the supine position to facilitate patient relaxation, proper force application and optimum cervical angle. The supine position is favored in the literature.[11,20,32] Cervical traction studies show that narrowing of the intervertebral spaces can actually occur during the traction treatment in patients who are unable to relax.[20]

It is difficult to prescribe the correct amount of force in the seated position. Since the average head weighs 10-12 lbs (4.5-5.5 kg), at least this amount of force would be needed to overcome gravity. However, it is unwise to add 10-12 lbs to the desired therapeutic force, because it may be poorly tolerated, especially since the head halter transmits the force through the TMJ. Finally, it is impractical to control the angle of the cervical spine in the seated position. If patients are told to hold their position "just so", they will

not be relaxed, and it is unlikely they would be able to maintain the proper angle for the entire treatment.

Cervical Angle. Traditionally cervical traction has been performed with the head and neck in some degree of flexion. Some clinicians believe that the greater the angle of flexion, the greater the intervertebral separation in the lower cervical spine. Thus it is a common belief that an angle of 20° to 30° of flexion is best for treating a lower cervical problem. The reference most often cited for the rational is a study by Colachis and Strohm.[10] While this study reports in the abstract and conclusion that, "... the amount of separation increases with flexion of the cervical spine", the clinical relevance of this fact should be questioned when one takes a closer look at the data (Table 12-1).

Table 12-1: Flexion and Separation in the Cervical Spine

Force	Flexion Angle	Posterior Separation	Anterior Separation
	6°	+1.6 mm	+0.3 mm
30 lbs	15°	+2.4 mm	+0.2 mm
	20°	+2.7 mm	-0.2 mm
	24°	+3.4 mm	-0.6 mm
	6°	0 mm	0 mm
0 lbs	20°	+0.7 mm	-0.3 mm
	24°	+1.0 mm	-0.6 mm

While it is true that posterior separation does increase with more flexion, anterior separation *decreases* with flexion. Compression actually occurs at 20° and 24° of flexion. Thus, the commonly held belief that separation is greater with increased angles of flexion is only true when referring to the posterior vertebral bodies. Clinicians must first address exactly what it is that they want to separate when deciding upon the optimal angle of cervical traction. If greater separation is desired at the intervertebral disc space or if traction is being used as a cervical extension mobilization technique, any amount of flexion would render the treatment less effective.

In most cases, clinicians should try to achieve a combination of a posterior and anterior stretch. Since the most common postural problem related to the cervical spine is the forward head posture, treatment goals should be to increase upper/mid cervical spine flexion and lower cervical/upper thoracic spine extension. In other words, the goal of treatment is to decrease the curves of the cervical and upper thoracic spine.

Thus, the ideal traction device will flex the head and neck somewhat, but pull at a relatively flat angle. A 15° angle accomplishes this because the posterior aspect of the head is slightly in front of the posterior aspect of the trunk in a normal standing posture. If the clinician's goal is to increase the space in the intervertebral foramen, it might be tempting to increase the flexion angle beyond 15°. However, caution should be used when increasing the flexion angle for this purpose, since the space available for the spinal nerve in the intervertebral foramen decreases with flexion beyond the neutral or straight position of the spine.[53]

The angle of the rope to the table is not the only factor influencing the amount of flexion or extension administered. In fact, it is probably less important than the choice of head halters or cervical traction devices. If a poorly adjusted or constructed head halter is used, a different

degree of flexion may be imparted, even if the angle of the rope to the table is within the recommended limits.[78]

We recommend the 15° angle of pull for nearly every clinical indication. In some cases, a greater angle may be initially necessary for patient comfort or to accommodate severe postural deformities. Even so, the goal with subsequent treatments should be to obtain as neutral a posture as possible, so the angle should be decreased as tolerated.

Additional Variables. Additional traction variables including the traction mode (static or intermittent), treatment times, use of ramp up and ramp down phases, frequency and duration, are handled the same way as with lumbar technique.

REFERENCES

1. Beurskens A., et al: Efficacy of Traction for Nonspecific Low Back Pain: 12-Week and 6-Month Results of a Randomized Clinical Trial. Spine 22(23):2756-2762, 1997.

2. Bigos S and Battie M. Acute Care to Prevent Back Disability: Ten Years of Progress. Clin Orthop and Rel Res 221:121-130, 1987.

3. Bigos S, Bowyer O, Braen G, et al. *Acute Low Back Problems in Adults.* AHCPR publication 95-0642. Rockville, Md: Agency for Health Care Policy and Research, Public Health Service, US Dept of Health and Human Services; 1994.

4. Bradnam L, Rochester L and Vujnovic A: Manual Cervical Traction Reduces Alpha-Motoneuron Excitability in Normal Subjects. Electromyogr Clin Neurophysiol 40:259-266, 2000.

5. Brodin H, et al: Manipulation av Ryggraden. Scandinavicen University Books, 1966.

6. Brodin H. Manueli Medicine ooh Manipulation. Lakartidningen 63:1037-1038, 1966.

7. Burton C. Low Back Pain. 2nd Edition. Lippincott, Philadelphia 1980.

8. Christy B: Discussion on the Treatment of Backache by Traction. Proc R Soc Med 48:811, 1955.

9. Chung TS, Lee YJ, Kang SW, et al: Reducibility of Cervical Disk Herniation: Evaluation at MR Imaging during Cervical Traction with a Nonmagnetic Traction Device. Radiology 225(3):895-898, 2002.

10. Colachis S and Strohm M: A Study of Tractive Forces and Angle of Pull on Vertebral Interspaces in Cervical Spine. Arch Phys Med 46:820-830, 1965.

11. Colachis S and Strohm M: Cervical Traction: Relationship of Traction Time to Varied Tractive Force with Constant Angle of Pull. Arch Phys Med 46:815-819, 1965.

12. Constantoyannis C, Konstantinou D, Kourtopoulos H, et al: Intermittent Cervical Traction for Cervical Radiculopathy Caused by Large-Volume Herniated Disks. J Manipulative Physiol Ther 25(3):188-192, 2002.

13. Coxhead, C., et al: *Multicentre Trial of Physiotherapy in the Management of Sciatic Symptoms*, The Lancet, 1(8229):1065-1068, 1981.

14. Crisp E: Disc Lesions. Livingstone, Edinburgh 1960.

15. Crisp E: Discussion on the Treatment of Backache by Traction. Proc R Soc Med 48:805, 1955.

16. Cyriax J: The Treatment of Lumbar Disk Lesions. Brit Med Joul 2:14-34, 1950.

17. Cyriax J: Treatment by Manipulation. Massage and Injection. Textbook of Orthopaedic Medicine, Vol 2, 10th edition. Bailliere-Tindall, London 1980.

18. Daugherty R and Erhard R: Segmentalized Cervical Traction. Proceedings, International Federation of Orthopaedic Manipulative Therapists. B Kent, ed. pp. 189-195. Vail CO 1977.

19. De Lacerda F: Effect of Angle of Traction Pull on Upper Trapezius Muscle Activity. J Orth Spts Phy Ther 1: 205-209, 1980.

20. Deets D, Hands K and Hopp S: Cervical Traction: A Comparison of Sitting and Supine Positions. Phys Ther 57:255, 1977.

21. Delitto A, et al: A Treatment-Based Classification Approach To Low Back Syndrome: Identifying And Staging Patients For Conservative Treatment, Phys Ther 75(6):470-489, 1995.

22. DeSeze S and Levernieux J: Les Tractions Vertebrales. Sem Hop Paris 27:2075, 1951.

23. Deyo RA, Diehl AK, Rosenthal M: How Many Days of Bed Rest for Acute Low Back Pain? N Engl J Med 315(17):1064-1070, 1986.

24. Ellenberg MR, Honet JC and Treanor WJ: Cervical Radiculopathy. Arch Phys Med Rehabil 75:342-352, 1994.

25. Finneson B: Low Back Pain. JB Lippincott, Philadelphia PA 1973.

26. Frankel V, Shore N and Hoppenfeld S: Stress Distribution in Cervical Traction Prevention of Temporomandibular Joint Pain Syndrome. Clin Orth 32:114-115, 1964.

27. Franks A: Temporomandibular Joint Dysfunction Associated with Cervical Traction. Ann Phys Med 8:38-40, 1967.

28. Frazer E: The Use of Traction in Backache. Med J Aust 2:694, 1954.

29. Gall E: Lumbar Spine X-rays - What Can They Reveal? Occ Health and Safety 48:32-35, 1979.

30. Goldish G: Lumbar Traction. In Interdisciplinary Rehabilitation of Low Back Pain. CD Tollison and M Kriegel, eds. Williams and Wilkins, Baltimore MD 1989.

31. Gupta R and Ramarao S: Epidurography in Reduction of

Lumbar Disc Prolapse by Traction. Arch Phys Med Rehabil 59:322-327, 1978.

32. Harris P: Cervical Traction: Review of Literature and Treatment Guidelines. Phys Ther 57:910, 1977.

33. Harris R: Massage, Manipulation and Traction. E. Licht, New Haven CT 1960.

34. Honet JC and Puri K: Cervical Radiculitis: Treatment and Results in 82 Patients. Arch Phys Med Rehabil 57:12-16, 1976.

35. Hood L and Chrisman D: Intermittent Pelvic Traction in the Treatment of the Ruptured Intervertebral Disc. J Am Phys Ther Assoc 48:21-30, 1968.

36. Jackson B: The Cervical Syndrome. Charles C Thomas, Springfield MO 1958.

37. Jette DU, Falkel JE and Trombly C: Effect of Intermittent, Supine Cervical Traction on the Myoelectric Activity of the Upper Trapezius Muscle in Subjects with Neck Pain. Phys Ther 65(8):1173-1176, 1985.

38. Judovich B: Herniated Cervical Disc. Am J Surg 84:649, 1952.

39. Judovich B: Lumbar Traction Therapy. JAMA 159:549, 1955.

40. Kaltenborn F: Proceedings of the International Federation of Orthopaedic Manipulative Therapists. B Kent, ed. Vail CO 1977

41. Kane M: Effects of Gravity Facilitated Traction on Intervertebral Dimensions of the Lumbar Spine. Master's Thesis, U.S. Army-Baylor University Program in Physical Therapy, Academy of Health Sciences, Fort Sam Houston TX 1983.

42. Komori H, et al: The Natural History of Herniated Nucleus Pulposus With Radiculopathy. Spine 21(2):225-229, 1996.

43. Kraft G and Levinthal D: Facet Synovial Impingement. Surg Gynecol and Obstet 93:439-443, 1951.

44. Krause M, Refshauge KM, Dessen M, et al: Lumbar Spine Traction: Evaluation of Effects and Recommended Application for Treatment. Manual Therapy 5(2):72-81, 2000.

45. Larsson V, et al: Auto-Traction for Treatment of Lumbago-Sciatica. Acta Orthop Scand 51:791, 1980.

46. Lawson G and Godfrey C: A Report on Studies of Spinal Traction. Med Serv J Can 12:762, 1958.

47. LeMarr J, Golding L and Crehan K: Cardiorespiratory Responses to Inversion. Phys Sportsmed 11:51-57, 1983.

48. Lind G: Auto-Traction: Treatment of Low Back Pain and Sciatica. Thesis, University of Linkoping, 1974.

49. Lindstrom A and Zachrisson, M: Physical Therapy on Low Back Pain and Sciatica: An Attempt at Evaluation. Scand J Rehabil Med 2:37, 1970.

50. Magora A and Schwartz A: Relation Between Low Back Pain and X-ray Changes IV: Lysis and Olisthesis. Scand J Rehabil Med 12:47-52, 1980.

51. Magora A and Schwartz A: Relation Between the Low Back Pain and X-ray Findings II: Transitional Vertebra (Mainly Sacralization). Scand J Rehabil Med 10:135-145, 1978.

52. Magora A and Schwartz A: Relation Between the Low Back Pain Syndrome and X-ray Findings I: Degenerative Findings. Scand J Rehabil Med 8:115-126, 1976.

53. Maslow G and Rothman R: The Facet Joints, Another Look. Bul NY Acad Med 51:1294-1311, 1975.

54. Masturzo A: Vertebral Traction for Sciatica. Rheumatism 11:62, 1955.

55. Mathews J and Heckling H: Lumbar Traction: A Double Blind Controlled Study for Sciatica. Rheumatol Rehabil 14:222, 1975.

56. Mathews J: Dynamic Discography; A Study of Lumbar Traction. Ann Phy Med 9:275-279, 1968.

57. Mathews J: The Effects of Spinal Traction. Physiotherapy 58:64-66, 1972.

58. McKenzie R: The Lumbar Spine. Spinal Publications, Waikanae New Zealand 1981.

59. Meszaros T, et al: Effect of 10%, 30%, and 60% Body Weight Traction on the Straight Leg Raise Test of Symptomatic Patients with Low Back Pain. J Orthop Sports Phys Ther 30(10):595-601, 2000.

60. Moetti P and Marchetti G: Clinical Outcome From Mechanical Intermittent Cervical Traction for the Treatment of Cervical Radiculopathy: A Case Series. J Orthop Sports Phys Ther 31(4):207-213, 2001.

61. Nachemson A and Elfstom G: Intravital Dynamic Pressure Measurements in the Lumbar Discs. Scand J Rehabil Med (Suppl 1): 1, 1970.

62. Natchev E: A Manual on Auto-Traction Treatment for Low Back Pain. Folksam Stockholm Sweden 1984.

63. Nosse L: Inverted Spinal Traction. Arch Phys Med Rehabil 59:367, 1978.

64. Olivero WC and Dulebohn SC: Results of Halter Cervical Traction for the Treatment of Cervical Radiculopathy: Retrospective Review of 81 Patients. Neurosurg Focus 12:1-3, 2002.

65. Olson V: Case Report: Chronic Whiplash Associated Disorder Treated With Home Cervical Traction. J Back Musculoskel Rehab 9:181-190, 1997.

66. Olson V: Whiplash-Associated Chronic Headache Treated with Home Cervical Traction. Phys Ther 77:417-423, 1997.

67. Onel D, et al: Computed Tomographic Investigation of the Effect of Traction on Lumbar Disc Herniations. Spine 14(1):82-90, 1989.

68. Oudenhoven T: Gravitational Lumbar Traction. Arch Phys Med 59:510, 1978.

69. Pal B, et al: A Controlled Trial of Continuous Lumbar Traction in Back Pain and Sciatica. Br J Rheumatol 25:181-183, 1986.

70. Paris S: The Spine. Atlanta Back Clinic. Atlanta GA 1976. Course Notes.

71. Parson W and Cummings J: Mechanical Traction in the Lumbar Disc Syndrome. Can Med Assoc Joul 77:7-11, 1957.

72. Philadelphia Panel Evidence-Based Clinical Practice Guidelines on Selected Rehabilitation Interventions for Low Back Pain. Phys Ther 81(10):1641-1674, 2001.

73. Saal J and Saal J: Nonoperative Treatment of Herniated Lumbar Intervertebral Disc with Radiculopathy-An Outcome Study. Spine 14:431-437, 1989.

74. Saal J, et al: Nonoperative Management of Herniated Cervical Intervertebral Disc With Radiculopathy, Spine 21(16):1877-1883, 1996.

75. Saunders H: Lumbar Traction. J Orthop Sports Phys Ther 1:36, 1979.

76. Saunders H: Spinal Traction: A Continuing Education Module for Physical Therapists. University of Kansas, Independent Study, Division of Continuing Education, 1979.

77. Saunders H: The Use of Spinal Traction in the Treatment of

Neck and Back Conditions. Clin Orthop and Rel Res 179: 31-38, 1983.

78. Saunders H: Unilateral Lumbar Traction. Phys Ther 61:221-225, 1981.

79. Saunders HD: Efficacy of Traction for Back and Neck Pain. Physical Therapy in Perspective 1(2):53-54, 1996.

80. Scientific Approach to the Assessment and Management of Activity-Related Spinal Disorders. A Monograph For Clinicians. Report of the Quebec Task Force on Spinal Disorders. Spine 12(7 Suppl):S1-59, 1987.

81. Shore N, Frankel V and Hoppenfeld S: Cervical Traction and Temporomandibular Joint Dysfunction. Joul Am Dental Assoc 68(1):4-6, 1964.

82. Swezey RL: Conservative Treatment of Radiculopathy. J Clin Rheumatol 5(2):65-73, 1999.

83. Tekoglu I, et al: Distraction of Lumbar Vertebrae in Gravitational Traction. Spine 23(9):1061-1064, 1998.

84. van der Heijden G, et al: The Efficacy of Traction for Back and Neck Pain: A Systematic, Blinded Review of Randomized Clinical Trial Method. Phys Ther 75:93-104, 1995.

85. Waitz E: The Lateral Bending Sign. Spine 6:388-397, 1981.

86. Weber H, et al: Traction Therapy in Patients with Herniated Lumbar Intervertebral Discs. J Oslo City Hosp 34:61-70, 1984.

87. Weber H: Traction Therapy in Sciatica Due to Disc Prolapse. J Oslo City Hosp 23(10): 167-176, 1973.

88. Weisel S et al: A Study of Computer-Assisted Tomography - The Incidence of Positive CAT Scans in an Asymptomatic Group of Patients. Spine 9(6):549-551, 1984.

89. Werners R: Randomized Trial Comparing Interferential Therapy With Motorized Lumbar Traction and Massage in the Management of Low Back Pain in a Primary Care Setting. Spine 24(15):1579-1584, 1999.

90. Witt I, et al: A Comparative Analysis of X-ray Findings of the Lumbar Spine in Patients With and Without Lumbar Pain. Spine 9:298-299, 1984.

91. Wong AMK, Lee MY, Chang WH, et al: Clinical Trial of a Cervical Traction Modality with Electromyographic Biofeedback. Am J Phys Med Rehabil 76(1):19-25, 1997.

92. Yates D: Indications and Contraindications for Spinal Traction. Physiotherapy 58:55, 1972.

93. Yoganandan N, Pintar FA, Maiman DJ, et al: Human Head-Neck Biomechanics Under Axial Tension. Med Eng Phys 18(4):289-294, 1996.

94. Zylbergold R and Piper M: Cervical Spine Disorders: A Comparison of Three Types of Traction. Spine 10:867-871, 1985.

13
SPINAL ORTHOSES

H. Duane Saunders, MS PT and Robin Saunders Ryan, MS PT

Many health care practitioners prescribe spinal orthoses to treat or prevent spinal disorders. In 1970, ninety-nine percent of 3,410 United States orthopedic surgeons surveyed reported prescribing spinal orthoses.[25] A survey of athletic trainers showed that up to 43% of injured professional athletes wear back supports, at least intermittently.[30] While there is no hard evidence of the clinical effectiveness of lumbosacral orthoses, retrospective studies have documented acceptance by patients and improvement of symptoms in 30-80% of cases[1,16,21] and many studies have been performed to try to determine their potential effects.

The literature is relatively favorable toward the use of spinal supports in the immediate post-injury phase, where the goals are to relieve pain and limit movement. However, the prophylactic use of back supports is more controversial. Using back supports to prevent industrial injury has been discussed at length in both medical journals and industrial health and safety publications.

We believe that spinal orthoses, like any treatment intervention, can be used effectively or ineffectively. It is generally agreed that most back disorders are best treated with exercise, patient education, and early activation. Bed rest and excessive avoidance of activity have long been recognized as causing more harm than good.

Therefore, back supports can be used for two very different purposes. In addition to supporting the spine for a short time during the healing process, certain types of back supports can be used to build confidence in the subacute or chronic stages, allowing earlier return to appropriate activity.[9,13] Physical therapists play an important role in determining the need for and selection and fitting of spinal braces and supports.

Spinal orthoses can be grouped into three major categories: *corrective, supportive and immobilizing.* Corrective braces are used in the treatment of disorders such as idiopathic scoliosis and kyphosis and will not be considered here. Instead, we will direct our attention to the spinal orthoses that provide support and/or immobilization for conditions commonly seen by the physical therapist.

Effects of Spinal Supports and Braces

The following potential effects of spinal orthoses have been proposed:

- Reduced sacroiliac joint motion
- Reduced intervertebral joint motion
- Increased motion of intervertebral joints adjacent to those that are immobilized
- Transfer of part of the vertical load from the spine to other structures
- Increased intra-abdominal pressure (lumbar supports)
- Decreased intra-discal pressure
- Decreased venous return from the lower extremities (lumbar supports)
- Control of lordosis or kyphosis
- Patient awareness of correct posture
- Increased confidence or other psychological effects
- Decreased abdominal and/or spinal muscular activity
- Increased spinal muscular activity

Cervical Spine

There have been relatively few quantitative evaluations of the effects of cervical orthoses. Colachis and associates found that the soft collar did little to limit cervical motion and that the more rigid plastic collars were only somewhat more effective.[3] Johnson and associates found that, in general, increasing the length and rigidity of a cervical orthosis improved its ability to restrict motion.[12] The halo vest with skeletal fixation is recommended most for conservative treatment of unstable upper cervical injuries, but newer, non-invasive orthoses have been shown to have potential for limiting motion at C1-2 and C2-3 as well.[27]

The goals of cervical bracing vary according to the patient's problem. Certain cervical muscle and joint injuries may only require gentle support to remind the patient to restrict neck motion or to maintain proper posture. A flexible collar should satisfy these goals. A more rigid orthosis may be necessary to actually limit cervical motion. No orthosis, including the halo vest, restricts all motion.

Another function of cervical collars and braces is to transfer the weight of the head to the shoulders, thus unloading the cervical spine. Although no scientific study supports such an effect, clinical experience indicates that collars and braces that lift under the mandible and occiput do accomplish this task.

Thoracolumbosacral Spine

Back supports and braces have been used for the treatment and prevention of problems in the thoracolumbosacral spine for years. Proponents have cited the following reasons for their use:

Physically Restrict Motion or Movement. The ability of spinal braces to immobilize thoracolumbosacral rotation, flexion and extension has been studied extensively. Norton and Brown showed that lumbar flexion-extension was reduced but not eliminated by many of the braces that they studied. In many cases, however, they found increased motion toward the upper and lower margins of the braces they tested. Braces such as the chairback provided immobilization in the upper lumbar and lower thoracic spine, but considerable increase of lower lumbar movement resulted.[23]

According to Wasserman and McNamee, adequate fixation of the pelvis is essential to achieve restriction of motion in the lower lumbar region. They did find a 50% reduction in rotation at regions in the center of the garments they tested.[39] A comprehensive literature review concluded that there was evidence that lumbar supports can reduce flexion, extension and lateral bending.[33]

For a back brace to physically restrict movement in the lumbosacral area effectively, it would have to be rigid and attach so it would immobilize the pelvis and the lumbar spine. Attempts to secure rigid back braces to the pelvis to immobilize the lumbosacral joint have generally proven impractical or uncomfortable. Thus, it appears that bracing has potential to restrict movements in the thoracolumbar area. However, in the lumbosacral area, physical restriction of movement may not be possible.

Serve as a Reminder to Avoid Undesirable Movements. If a back support or brace effectively limits movement in the lower lumbar spine, it is probably because it serves as a reminder that certain movements, such as forward bending and twisting, are to be restricted. Many individuals report that their back supports help them remember to use good body mechanics. Thus, a properly fitted back support may help individuals avoid certain movements if they are properly educated and motivated about the support's purpose and function.

Help Individuals Achieve Proper Posture. One of the greatest benefits of a properly fitted back support may be the proprioceptive feedback it provides. Wearing a back support increases awareness of the position of the pelvis and lumbar spine. This constant awareness of body position makes it easier for the wearer to avoid undesirable postures.

Increase Intra-Abdominal Pressure to Decrease the Weight Bearing Load on the Spine. Literature reviews of controlled studies have concluded that there is inadequate evidence to support this theory.[24,33] However, non-controlled studies show interesting findings. Early models of back biomechanics predicted that an increase in intra-abdominal pressure relieved the compressive forces on the low back by providing an extensor moment. In the newer models, intra-abdominal pressure functions to stabilize the loaded spine.[37] Nachemson and Morris studied the effect of an inflatable lumbar corset on intradiscal pressure. In all cases studied, there was a considerable (15-28%) decrease in the total load on the disc studied.[20] In another study, Nachemson, Schultz and Andersson found that wearing a lumbar brace significantly unloads the spine in some situations, but has no effect in others. Lumbar spine compression was reduced by about one-third in a task involving trunk flexion.[21]

According to Morris, Lucas and Bresler, the action of the trunk muscles converts the abdominal and thoracic cavities into nearly rigid-walled cylinders.[18] Automatic contraction of the trunk muscles, increasing intra-abdominal pressure and reducing the force on the spine, occurs when lifting weights of 100-200 pounds. Interestingly, an inflatable corset raised the standing and sitting intra-abdominal pressure by 25% but did not change the maximum pressure that was produced during heavy lifting, probably because the trunk muscles were already reducing force during the lifting task. Furthermore, the activity of the abdominal muscles was markedly decreased when the inflatable corset was worn. The authors theorized that either the contracted muscles of the abdominal wall or the external pressure of the corset could act to contain the abdominal contents in a compressed state capable of transmitting the weight bearing force. If back supports do reduce the force on the spine, this unloading effect may be more beneficial and necessary for non-lifting activities than lifting activities.

Since many back disorders are caused by cumulative trauma from activities like prolonged sitting or stooped standing, one can imagine that a relatively constant unloading effect would be of great benefit. Clinically, we find that some patients feel less pain and fatigue at the end of a day when wearing a compressive lumbar support. It makes sense that a back support could be helpful during non-lifting activities, but this has not been demonstrated in controlled studies.

Stabilize the Pelvis and Lower Spine. By increasing intra-abdominal pressure, a back support theoretically acts like the stays and support rings of a barrel. If the support rings are tightened and/or strengthened, the barrel is stabilized. Likewise, when one tightens or contracts the abdominal, trunk and pelvic muscles, the spine is stabilized. A properly fit lumbar support, capable of increasing intra-abdominal pressure, might act in the same way.

One study showed decreased abdominal oblique muscle activity with back support usage during deep squat lifting, suggesting that lumbar supports do have a stabilizing effect.[37] Patients often describe the "stabilized" feeling they have when wearing their back supports.

Sacroiliac Joints

Sacroiliac belts or supports limit motion in the sacroiliac joints by circumferential pressure around the pelvis.[35,4] Most sacroiliac supports have a sacral pad that presses against the posterior sacrum to further limit motion and provide proprioceptive input.

Criticism of Back Supports

There are critics of back supports. A literature review concluded that the relationship between increased intra-abdominal pressure and decreased force in the spine was inconclusive.[25] Some believe that the use of back supports, at least over long periods of time, will create dependency

and weaken the abdominal muscles.[26] At least one study shows that with a back support the abdominal muscles are in a more relaxed state.[18] However, studies done to measure the effect of back supports on back and abdominal muscle strength show there is no weakening effect.[10,19,31,32,36]

Proponents argue that a properly fit back support may actually have a strengthening effect in some cases. If a support decreases pain and helps patients achieve proper posture and avoid potentially harmful movements, they may recover faster and become active sooner. The early activity will actually strengthen the muscles rather than letting them weaken.[5,13,20,30]

The inability of back supports to stay in proper position has long been a criticism of lumbosacral supports and braces in general. If the back support rides up above the iliac crests, the lumbosacral area (where most back problems occur) may not be supported sufficiently. While the problem of a support or brace riding up may not be significant when an individual is relatively inactive, it often becomes a problem during recovery as the patient becomes more physically active. It is also a problem if a back support is to be used for back pain prevention in an active individual. The attachment of a back support to a pair of elastic athletic shorts effectively solves this problem (see Fig 13-16 on page 337).

Indications For Spinal Bracing

In general, any patient with a musculoskeletal disorder who might benefit from immobilization, unloading of compressing forces on the spine and/or postural correction may be a suitable candidate for a spinal support or brace.

In 1970, Perry found that opinion among orthopedic surgeons was divided concerning indications for braces, but that the majority of orthopedists did prescribe a support for treatment of post-operative fusions, spondylolisthesis and pseudoarthrosis.[25] The chairback brace was the most commonly prescribed device for these conditions.

Interestingly, less than 25% of the orthopedists surveyed prescribed supports for acute strain, post-operative discs, disc syndromes and chronic situations. When they did prescribe supports for these patients, the lumbosacral corset was the device most often chosen. More recent statistics on back support usage by clinicians could not be found. Current research on back supports appears to be focused on the use of back supports in industry.

Pain, Muscle Guarding and Spasm

The unloading/stabilizing and proprioceptive effects that a back support may offer can alleviate pain and reduce muscle guarding and spasm.

Acute Sprains and Strains

Acute sprains and strains need protection from undesirable movements and activities. At the same time, proper posture must be achieved for normal healing to take place. Some activity is desirable to maintain strength and fitness; the healing process is actually stimulated by careful movement and activity. Back and neck supports may help relieve acute pain and promote better healing posture, thus allowing safe movement and activity sooner. Since soft tissue injuries heal rapidly, the use of a spinal orthoses for this purpose should be of short duration. Usually, a week or so is sufficient; certainly six to eight weeks is the longest treatment time, even in the most severe cases.

Post-Surgical Fusion, Laminectomy and Discectomy

Many surgeons prescribe a support such as a lumbosacral corset or chairback brace after lumbar fusions and laminectomies, and a cervical support such as a soft collar, semirigid collar or four poster brace after cervical fusions and laminectomies. It is less common to use them following discectomies. The goal with such supports is to immobilize the area, to relieve pain and to remind the patient to restrict movement. Such supports are normally used for short periods — a few days to a few weeks.

Congenital or Traumatic Joint Instability

Congenital defects and severe injuries resulting in spinal joint instability can be problematic for the patient who attempts to lead an active life. In such cases, a back support or brace may let the patient participate in a vocation or in activities that otherwise would result in chronic pain and discomfort. Patients should be advised to use such support only when they need the protection. It is also wise for these patients to exercise regularly to maintain adequate strength of the spinal and abdominal muscles. Since no orthosis can completely immobilize the spine, the beneficial effect of the support is probably due to the unloading/ stabilizing effect and the reminder to use good posture and body mechanics, and not to an actual restriction of movement.

If a spondylolisthesis is unstable, it can be a constant source of aggravation. Spondylolisthesis is frequently associated with hyperlordosis of the lumbar spine. In a hyperlordotic state, the shear forces between the two segments that are slipping apart are greatly magnified. Reduction of the hyperlordosis can reduce the shear forces. Spondylolisthesis can be managed with a support that lifts the abdomen upward and posteriorly. This moves the center of gravity posteriorly and reduces hyperlordosis.

Preteen children who participate in sports that require excessive lumbar lordosis (i.e., gymnastics) and teenagers who participate in contact sports are more frequently found to have spondylolysis.[5,6,7] Such patients can be treated with a brace that provides pain relief and/or maintains the spine in lumbar flexion during the healing phase.

Herniated Nucleus Pulposus (HNP)

Using a back support for treatment of herniated disc involves reducing factors that increase the compressive load on the disc. There is some evidence that spinal supports can reduce intradiscal pressure in both the sitting and standing positions.[20] Rotation and forward bending also increase intradiscal pressure and spinal bracing can help restrict these movements. Furthermore, a spinal support can remind the patient to avoid these movements and to maintain correct posture (lumbar lordosis) during recovery.

Cervical supports may also unload the disc by transferring the weight of the head onto the shoulders, but research has not confirmed such claims. Nonetheless, a cervical support can help maintain the proper head and neck posture required during recovery of herniated disc syndrome.

Postural Backache (Lumbar Hyperlordosis)

Postural backache caused by weak abdominal muscles and excessive lumbar lordosis is most effectively treated with postural correction and abdominal strengthening exercises. Extreme cases may require a lumbosacral support, chairback brace or a Williams brace. When a support or brace is prescribed, an exercise program should accompany it.

Fractures

Various types of fractures of the spine are often treated with braces or supports. A halo vest is typically used for unstable upper cervical spine injuries. The halo vest consists of a plastic jacket attached by four rods to a metal ring fixed to the head with screws in the skull. Innovations in non-invasive cervical bracing have improved the immobilizing effect of certain styles of braces, but halo vests are still the treatment of choice for unstable upper cervical spine injuries.[28,34] Even the halo vest does not totally restrict cervical movement. In general, the upper cervical and lower lumbar spine are the most difficult to immobilize and fractures in these areas will be the most difficult to support with bracing. The fact that the brace reminds patients to restrict movement and maintain correct posture is often beneficial.

Compression fractures occurring in the upper lumbar and lower and mid-thoracic spine are often treated with braces. The goal of a bracing program for compression fractures is to keep the injured part of the spine in extension and to prevent flexion, thus keeping the vertebral body space as wide as possible and allow the vertebral body to heal with as much height as possible.

The Jewett® and Cash™ hyperextension braces are probably the most commonly used braces for treatment of compression fractures. Their sole function is to prevent flexion of the upper lumbar, lower and mid-thoracic spine and to remind the patient to maintain an extended posture.

While the hyperextension braces treat compression fractures effectively, it has been our experience that some patients (especially geriatric) cannot tolerate their rigid natures. In such cases, a Taylor™ brace or dorsal-lumbar corset may be a reasonable alternative. They offer less rigid support, but at least they offer some support and serve as reminders to the patient to avoid flexion. An added benefit of either of these supports is that they may decrease the vertical weight bearing force on the spine by increasing the intra-abdominal pressure. The hyperextension braces do not provide this effect.

Since most compression fractures occur in geriatric females and are associated with severe osteoporosis, supports may have a role in prevention. Active extension exercises should be performed concurrently to enhance muscle strengthening, improve posture and prevent the trunk musculature deconditioning that is apt to occur when a sedentary person uses a back support.

If the patient is instructed to avoid slumping into the brace and to maintain correct posture while in the brace, the patient may actually strengthen the postural muscles. For example, the shoulder straps of a Taylor or dorsal-lumbar corset should act as reminders to the patient to hold herself in correct posture. Their function is *not* to pull the shoulders back and hold the patient straighter. Likewise, the lordotic curve in a chairback brace is a reminder for the patient to stand and sit while actively maintaining the lordosis. This concept of "active bracing" is what the Milwaukee brace uses in the treatment of scoliosis. Patient education and compliance are the keys to appropriate use of bracing to prevent compression fractures.

Degenerative Joint/Disc Disease

Degenerative joint and/or disc disease is often associated with soft tissue hypomobility (stiffness). Treatment for hypomobility of the spine should be directed toward mobilizing the restricted joints and tight muscles. In some cases, however, any mobilizing activity may tend to aggravate rather than relieve the pain and discomfort. The patient will report that any attempt to increase activities is accompanied by another flare up. In such cases, a support may at least allow the patient to participate in activities that would otherwise be too aggravating.

Spinal segment instability is sometimes associated with degenerative joint/disc disease, and may respond favorably to treatment with a spinal support.

Prevention

Much of the debate about back supports takes place in the business/industrial arena, where back supports are sometimes used to prevent occupational injuries. In 1994, the National Institute for Occupational Safety and Health (NIOSH) recommended against the use of preventive back supports in industry, stating there is not enough evidence of their effectiveness.[22]

A 1996 study involving over 36,000 Home Depot employees[14,15] concluded that the use of back supports is effective in preventing low back injuries at work. They reported a significant drop in injury rates after a policy requiring back supports was implemented.

Other clinical trials, however, have concluded that back supports had no effect in decreasing low back injury rates, and some of the methods used in the Home Depot study have been criticized.[32,38] Despite the conflicting reports of back supports' effectiveness, they continue to be used in industrial settings for prevention. In 1995, approximately 4 million industrial back belts were purchased.[38]

Although recent literature reviews[11,17,33] decry the low quality of back support research published, interesting claims can be found. Walsh and Schwartz reported less lost time from work due to back injury after employees attended back school and wore a back support.[36] There was a statistically significant difference compared to control groups having either back school only or no intervention at all. Businesses have reported considerable reductions in workers' compensation costs after implementation of back injury prevention programs that involved the use of back supports and lifting belts.[8] While these reports are not scientific studies, they do merit consideration.

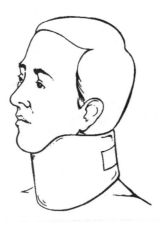

Figure 13-1: Soft cervical collar.

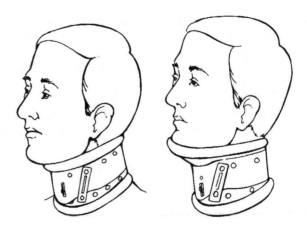

Figure 13-2: Hard cervical collars.

Injury prevention by external protection is common in sports medicine. Pads, helmets and supportive taping are routinely used in many sports. The use of a back support for the *industrial athlete* could be considered in the same way.

Types of Spinal Orthoses

Numerous commercial spinal orthoses are available, and it is impossible to illustrate them all. In this section, we will show at least one example of each of the major types of orthoses used by physical therapists. Where appropriate, general fitting guidelines will be given. The orthoses illustrated include:

- Cervical Soft (Foam) Collars
- Hard (Plastic) Collars
- Semi-Rigid Cervical Collars
- Two- and Four-Poster Braces
- Minerva Cervical Brace
- Dorsal-Lumbar Corset
- Semi-Rigid Dorsal-Lumbar Braces (Taylor™ and Knight-Taylor)
- Hyperextension Braces (Jewett® and Cash™)
- Lumbosacral Corset
- The Semi-Rigid Lumbosacral Braces—Chairback, Knight™ and Williams
- Lumbar Support or Belt
- Sacroiliac Joint Supports

Cervical Soft (Foam) Collars

Soft collars have very little, if any, immobilization effect. They do serve as a reminder to limit head and neck motion, especially flexion (Fig 13-1).

They do not provide forces to position the head in certain postures. However, if they are properly positioned under the mandible and occipital line, they partially unload the cervical spine by supporting a portion of the weight of the head. They are sized according to neck circumference and height. Exact measurements will depend upon the desired head and neck position and expected function.

Hard (Plastic) Collars

Hard collars serve basically the same function as soft collars, but do so with greater immobilizing and supporting effect. Most collars are adjustable. A chin support (plastic cup) may be added to the hard collar for additional support. These braces are also sized according to neck circumference and height (Fig 13-2).

Semi-Rigid Cervical Collars

The Philadelphia collar is a molded plastic, semi-rigid orthosis designed to provide support effects similar to the other cervical supports described in this chapter. It is sized in small, medium and large (Fig 13-3).

The Philadelphia collar is lightweight and may be more comfortable than other cervical orthoses. This collar may also serve as a foundation for cervical casting. Several similar cervical orthoses are available on the market (NecLoc™, Stifneck™, Miami J™, Aspen™). Their efficacy in restricting cervical motion has been studied, and comparative results vary.[2,29] It is generally accepted that semi-rigid support braces are significantly more effective than the soft collar and may be nearly as effective as the more rigid four-poster cervical brace in controlling flexion-extension between the occiput and third cervical vertebrae.

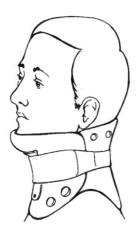

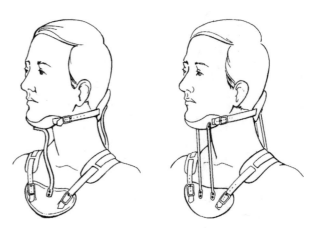

Figure 13-3: The Philadelphia collar, an example of a semi-rigid cervical orthosis.

Figure 13-4: Two- and four-poster cervical braces.

Two- and Four-Poster Braces

The two- or four-poster brace applies forces under the chin and occiput to restrict flexion and extension of the head and cervical spine. One variation is called the SOMI (Sterno Occipital Mandibular Immobilizer).

The two- and four-poster orthoses include an anterior section consisting of a sternal plate, one or two uprights and a chin support, and a posterior section consisting of a thoracic plate, one or two uprights and an occipital support. The two sections are connected by flexible straps between the chin and occipital supports and by over-the-shoulder straps between the thoracic and sternal plates.

The uprights are adjustable for height and position of the chin and occipital supports. They are made of aluminum with leather or plastic padding of the parts that touch the body. A thoracic extension may be added to provide increased support and rotatory control. However, this may impart undesired thoracic movement to the cervical spine. Fine adjustments to the fit can be made and they are more rigid than the soft or hard collars (Fig 13-4).

These braces can effectively restrict flexion in the mid-cervical spine, but they are only partially effective in restricting lateral bending and upper cervical flexion-extension. This brace is sized small, medium and large.

Minerva Cervical Brace

The Minerva brace adds a forehead pad to firm sternal, shoulder, chin and occipital supports to give greater control over flexion-extension and lateral cervical movements than other cervical braces. Its stabilizing effect

has been shown in cadavers (Fig 13-5).[28] Still, the halo vest is thought to be the treatment of choice for instability of the upper cervical spine, since its attachment to the skull tends to ensure better immobilization when fitted and used properly.[28,34]

Dorsal-Lumbar Corset

The dorsal-lumbar corset is sized according to hip measurement and is available in several lengths and developments (Fig 13-6). Development is the difference between waist size and hip size. For example, a size 36" (hip size) with a 6" development will have a 30" waist. The typical women's lumbosacral corset will have a 6-8"

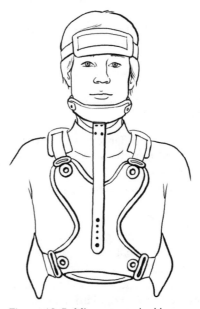

Figure 13-5: Minerva cervical brace.

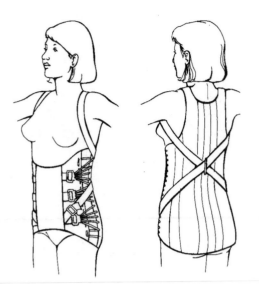

Figure 13-6: Dorsal-lumbar corset.

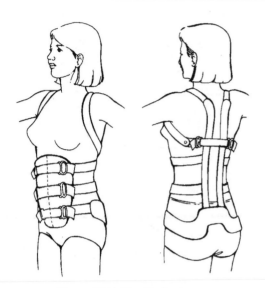

Figure 13-7: The Taylor brace

development, whereas a man's corset will have a 1-2" development.

The dorsal-lumbar corset provides immobilization and support to the lower and mid-thoracic spine. The shoulder loops remind the patient to stand and sit up straight. They are not effective in holding the patient straighter and, if they fit too tightly, they will irritate the underarms.

The dorsal-lumbar corset is used for treatment of compression fractures and osteoporosis for patients who do not require or who cannot tolerate the more rigid support of a Taylor or hyperextension brace. Dorsal-lumbar corsets are also used for other conditions of the lower and mid-thoracic spine, such as sprains, strains and degenerative joint/disc disease.

Semi-Rigid Dorsal-Lumbar Braces (Taylor™ and Knight-Taylor)

The Taylor brace is similar to the chairback brace, except that the posterior uprights extend into the mid-thoracic region and there are straps that loop around the shoulders. The thoracic band may be absent (Fig 13-7).

The Knight-Taylor brace is similar to the Taylor with the addition of lateral uprights and a full corset-like front (Fig 13-8). It is somewhat more rigid and restricts lateral bending better than the Taylor. They are sized similar to the dorsal-lumbar corset and serve the same function, except that they provide a more rigid immobilization effect.

Hyperextension Braces (Jewett® and Cash™)

The hyperextension braces, Jewett and Cash, provide a three-point fixation system consisting of posteriorly-directed forces from the sternal and suprapubic pads and an anteriorly directed force from the thoracolumbar pad. This fixation system causes hyperextension and restricts flexion in the thoracolumbar spine. The pads achieve control of flexion; the frame should not contact the patient (Fig 13-9) and (Fig 13-10). With the patient seated in the prescribed posture and the orthosis properly adjusted and aligned, the sternal pad will have its superior border ½"

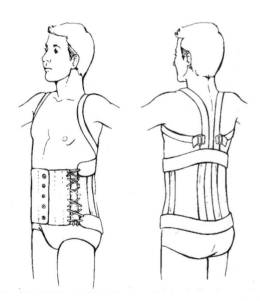

Figure 13-8: The Knight-Taylor has a corset-like front and restricts lateral bending somewhat better than the Taylor brace.

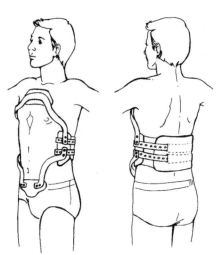

Figure 13-9: Jewett hyperextension brace

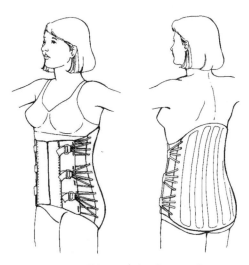

Figure 13-11: Women's lumbosacral corset

inferior to the sternal notch and the suprapubic pad will have its inferior border ½" superior to the symphysis pubis.

Hyperextension braces are normally sized by height, hip circumference and chest circumference.

Lumbosacral Corset

Lumbosacral corsets are usually sized according to hip measurement and have a taller back than front. Most manufacturers feature styles with several different heights and developments. Most lumbosacral corsets have removable metal stays that fit in pockets along the length of the spine.

The women's garment is usually made to cover more of the buttock area. The stays should be bent to contour to the convex curve of the buttocks as well as concave (lor-

dotic) curve in the lumbar spine. A proper fit will help keep the corset from riding up during activity.

The lumbosacral corset is similar to the dorsal-lumbar corset with less height in the back and without the straps that loop around the shoulders. The most common lumbosacral corsets are made of a Dacron® or cotton material, have a snap or zipper front, have 4-6" of size adjustment in the side panels and are washable. Some are made of elastic material and have front closures (Fig 13-11) and (Fig 13-12).

When fitting a woman's lumbosacral corset, it is important to choose a garment that does not crowd the breasts in front when the patient is sitting. The corset should come down onto the buttocks as far as possible if the lower lumbar spine is to be supported. The bottom front of the corset should just touch the angle of the hip when the

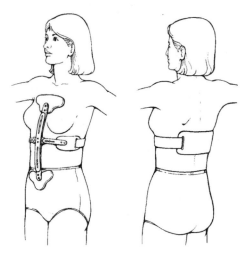

Figure 13-10: Cash hyperextension brace.

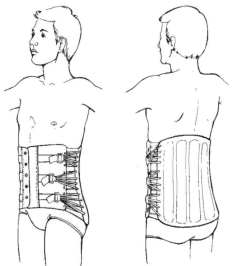

Figure 13-12: Men's lumbosacral corset

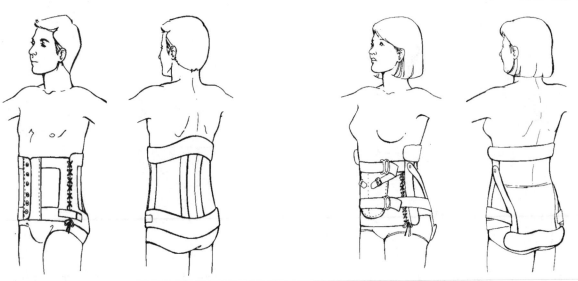

Figure 13-13: Chairback semi-rigid lumbosacral brace.

Figure 13-15: Williams semi-rigid lumbosacral brace.

patient is sitting. The front is always closed from the bottom up. The corset should be put on the patient and adjusted to the proper size and position before the metal stays are shaped and put into place. If possible, the stays should be shaped to the patient's normal standing lordosis.

It is difficult to alter or physically control the lumbar lordosis with this type of support, but the corset can serve as a reminder of correct posture and the patient can alter his lordosis actively. The lumbosacral corset is a flexible support and restricts movement relatively ineffectively, but it can serve as a reminder to the patient to avoid movement and to maintain correct posture.

If the patient is in acute discomfort, the corset should be donned and doffed while lying down. If the condition is

severe, the support is worn at all times when the patient is out of bed. In other cases, the patient may only wear the support while doing activities that might cause aggravation. The support is seldom worn while lying down or resting. While the lumbosacral corset is effective when the patient is relatively inactive, it becomes uncomfortable and tends to ride up as the patient becomes more active.

The Semi-Rigid Lumbosacral Braces—Chairback, Knight™ and Williams

The chairback brace consists of two posterior uprights, pelvic and thoracic bands and a pie pan abdominal support anteriorly (Fig 13-13).

The Knight spinal brace is similar to the chairback with the addition of lateral uprights and a full corset-like front (Fig 13-14). It is somewhat more rigid than the chairback.

The Williams brace provides a three-point pressure system consisting of a posteriorly directed force from the pelvic adjustment strap and anteriorly directed forces from the pelvic and thoracic bands (Fig 13-15). This pressure system tends to limit lumbar extension and reduce lordosis. The brace also tends to limit lateral bending. The brace is made of metal covered with leather and has a corset front. This brace must fit relatively tightly to be effective. This can become a problem because patients often cannot tolerate the brace for very long. It is difficult to keep in place when the patient is active and especially when sitting.

The semi-rigid braces effectively restrict movement in the thoracolumbar region but are not necessarily effective in restricting mobility in the lumbosacral area. One study demonstrated increased lumbosacral movement with the

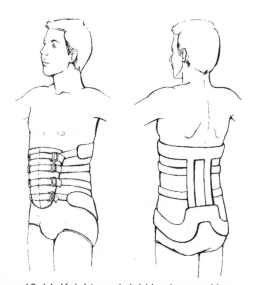

Figure 13-14: Knight semi-rigid lumbosacral brace.

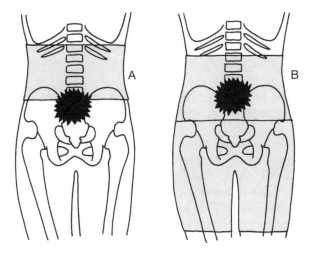

Figure 13-16: A) Many traditional lumbar back supports do not stay in place over the lower lumbar segments; B) Attaching the back support to an athletic short keeps the support in place.

semi-rigid lumbosacral brace during moderate to vigorous activity.[23] Unless the goal is to physically restrict movement in the upper lumbar and lower thoracic area, the semi-rigid brace has no more to offer than a lumbosacral corset. They are usually not as comfortable, are more expensive and have the potential to actually increase mobility at the lumbosacral spine. Therefore, they would rarely be the correct choice for support of the lumbosacral spine.

The semi-rigid braces are fitted according to hip size and length from the mid-sacral to the lower thoracic spine. They are made of metal covered with leather or vinyl. They are somewhat cooler to wear than the lumbosacral corset.

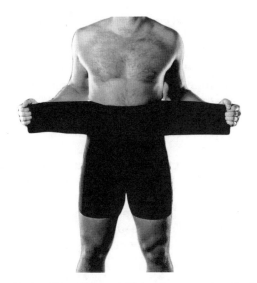

Figure 13-17: The S'port All® back support, attached to athletic shorts (The Saunders Group, Inc.)

Lumbar Support or Belt

Many types of lumbar supports or belts are available. Leather weight lifting belts have been popular for many years; now variations are becoming popular in industry. Most are made of fabric and elastic with Velcro® or buckle closures. Many have flexible metal or plastic stays or a plastic panel in the back to provide some additional stabilization. Some feature adjustable side pull straps and some even have an air bladder that can be pumped up to make the garment fit tighter and conform to the shape of the body better. They are fitted by waist size.

Since it is nearly impossible to keep these types of supports or belts down over the iliac crests, especially when the wearer is active, it is questionable if any support or stabilization is afforded to the lumbosacral area. Perhaps they are beneficial because they serve as a reminder to the wearer to practice proper posture and good body mechanics. Some studies show that lumbosacral supports increase intra-abdominal pressure, however, these studies were done using a corset with a wider front panel than many of the supports and belts described in this section.[1,4] Whether the narrower supports and belts that ride up above the pelvis and fail to cover the entire abdominal area have this effect has not been studied.

The difficulty of supporting the lower lumbar spine with a back support or brace has been discussed. Part of the difficulty lies in keeping the back support in its proper position. Stabilizing the pelvis and lower spine is vital because many back injuries occur in the lower two segments of the spine and some "back problems" actually occur in the pelvis. If the back support rides up above the iliac crests, the back support is not supporting either the pelvis or the lower two segments of the spine (Fig 13-16).

Attempts to keep back supports and braces from riding up have included ideas such as groin straps, garter belts and crotch inserts. All have proven to be impractical and/or uncomfortable and irritating. A back support attached to elastic athletic shorts provides a satisfactory way to comfortably keep a back support in place. Because it is combined with an elastic athletic short, the back support stays in place to stabilize the hips and pelvis as well as the back (Fig 13-17).

The one-piece back support/athletic short is non-restrictive and will not slip out of place with vigorous movement. It is constructed of paneled elastic that conforms to body shape and has tapered side pulls. The attached elastic athletic short offers graduated support for the quadriceps, hamstring, groin, pelvis and abdominal areas. This garment is fitted by waist size.

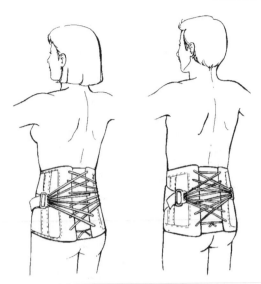

Figure 13-18: Sacroiliac support—Wide style.

Sacroiliac Joint Supports

The sacroiliac belt partially stabilizes the sacroiliac joints and symphysis pubis by providing circumferential support around the pelvis. It is fitted by hip size. It must fit relatively tightly below the tops of the iliac crests to accomplish the goal of stabilization. A removable sacral pad can help patients who benefit from gentle pressure or proprioceptive feedback on the sacrum.

Sacroiliac supports are used post-partum, post-traumatic injury and for hypermobility of the sacroiliac joints. Various sacroiliac supports and belts are available commercially; two types are shown here (Figures 13-18 and 13-19).

The back support shown in Figure 13-17 can also be used to support the sacroiliac region, by moving the adjust-

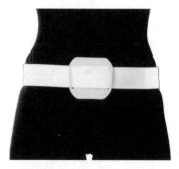

Figure 13-19: Sacroiliac support—narrow belt style (The Saunders Group, Inc.).

able back support lower on the hips. This type of support may be especially useful for athletic patients, because excessive movement tends to make the other SI supports ride up.

Total Management of the Spinal Orthosis Patient

A spinal orthosis is seldom effective in mechanically correcting posture. Its effectiveness comes from reminding the patient to actively maintain the desired posture. For this reason, small corrections are often possible but one should not expect a brace to hold a patient in a posture that he cannot actively assume with some degree of ease. The therapist should have the patient assume his optimum posture, then the brace should be fitted to conform to that posture.

It is often desirable to explain to the patient the effects of the various braces and supports being considered, then fit each of them to the patient and let the patient make the final selection. A brace hanging in the closet that the patient will not wear is not going to help.

When the patient's condition is very acute, the support should be worn at all times except when recumbent. The support must be put on and taken off while the patient is lying down by rolling to the side, placing the support against the posterior spine, rolling back onto the support and fastening the support in front.

Most thoracic and lumbar orthoses are more comfortable with a cotton undershirt or t-shirt worn underneath. This also helps absorb perspiration and keeps the support clean longer.

Back and neck supports play an important role in the treatment and prevention of low back disorders. While they do not restrict physical mobility effectively (at least in the lumbosacral area) they do provide a beneficial effect by unloading and stabilizing the spine and providing proprioceptive feedback to the wearer. These beneficial effects may also help relieve pain, which helps the patient become active sooner, thus speeding the recovery from a back injury. Whether or not back supports can prevent injuries is controversial, but we believe they have a role to play in prevention.

Finally, if an individual tries to substitute a back support for exercise, proper posture and good body mechanics, its use is potentially harmful. Therefore, one must always view a back support as an adjunct to treatment and prevention, not as a substitute for any of the other important principles of proper back care.

REFERENCES

1. Ahlgren S and Hansen T: The Use of Lumbosacral Corsets Prescribed for Low Back Pain. Prosteth Orthop Int 2: 101-104, 1978.
2. Askins V, Eismont FJ: Efficacy of Five Cervical Orthoses in Restricting Cervical Motion. A Comparison Study. Spine 22(11):1193-1198, 1997.
3. Colachis S, Strohm B and Ganter E: Cervical Spine Motion in Normal Women: Radiographic Study of Effect of Cervical Collars. Arch of Phys Med Rehab 54:161-169, 1973.
4. Damen L, Spoor CW, Snijders CJ, et al: Does a Pelvic Belt Influence Sacroiliac Joint Laxity? Clin Biomech 17:495-498, 2002.
5. Feeler L: Weight Lifting. In The Spine in Sports. S Hochschuler, ed. Hanley and Belfus, Philadelphia PA 1990.
6. Flemming J: Spondylolysis and Spondylolisthesis in the Athlete. In The Spine in Sports. S Hochschuler, ed. Hanley and Belfus, Philadelphia PA 1990.
7. Garry JP, Shane J: Lumbar Spondylolysis in Adolescent Athletes. J Fam Pract 47(2):145-149, 1998.
8. Golden, D: Support Belts Can Bolster Prevention Programs. Back Pain Monitor 9(4): 49-64, 1991.
9. Holm S and Nachemson A: Variations in the Nutrition of the Canine Intervertebral Disc, Induced by Motion. Spine 8:866-873, 1983.
10. Holmstrom E and Moritz U: Effects of Lumbar Belts on Trunk Muscle Strength and Endurance: A Follow-Up Study of Construction Workers. Joul Spinal Disorders 5(3):260-266, 1992.
11. Jellema P, van Tulder MW, van Puppel MN, et al: Lumbar Supports for Prevention and Treatment of Low Back Pain: A Systematic Review within the Framework of the Cochrane Back Review Group. Spine 26(4):377-386, 2001.
12. Johnson R, et al: Cervical Orthosis. Joul Bone and Joint Surg 52A:1440-1442, 1970.
13. Kirkaldy-Willis W: Supports and Braces. In Managing Low Back Pain, 2nd edition. W Kirkaldy-Willis, ed. Churchhill Livingstone, New York NY 1988.
14. Kraus JF, McArthur DL. Back Supports and Back Injuries: A Second Visit with the Home Depot Cohort Study Data on Low-Back Injuries. Int J Occup Environ Health 5(1):9-13, 1999.
15. McIntyre DR, Bolte KM, Pope MH. Study Provides New Evidence of Back Belt's Effectiveness. Occup Health Saf 65(12):39-41, 1996.
16. Million R, et al: Assessment of the Progress of the Back-Pain Patient. Spine 7: 204-212, 1982.
17. Minor SD: Use of Back Belts in Occupational Settings. Phys Ther 76:403-408, 1996.
18. Morris J, Lucas D and Bresler M: Role of the Trunk in Stability of the Spine. J Bone and Joint Surg 43A:327-351, 1961.
19. Nachemson A and Lindh M: Measurement of Abdominal and Back Muscle Strength With and Without Low Back Pain. Scand J Rehab Med 1:60, 1969.
20. Nachemson A and Morris J: In Vivo Measurements of Intradiscal Pressure. J Bone Joint Surg 46A: 1077-1092, 1964.
21. Nachemson A, Schultz A and Andersson G: Mechanical Effectiveness Studies of Lumbar Spine Orthosis. Scand J Rehab Med 9(suppl):139-149, 1983.
22. NIOSH Back Belt Working Group. Workplace Use of Back Belts: Review and Recommendations. Publication No. 94-122. National Institute for Occupational Safety and Health, 4676 Columbia Parkway, Cincinnati, OH 45226.
23. Norton P and Brown T: The Immobilizing Efficiency of Back Braces. J Bone and Joint Surg 39-A (1): 111-139, 220, 1957.
24. Perkins MS, Bloswick DS. The Use of Back Belts to Increase Intraabdominal Pressure as a Means of Preventing Low Back Injuries: A Survey of the Literature. Int J Occup Environ Health 1:326-35, 1995.
25. Perry J: The Use of External Support in the Treatment of Low Back Pain. J Bone Joint Surg 52A:1440-1442, 1970.
26. Quinet R and Hadler H: Diagnosis and Treatment of Backache. Sem in Arth and Rheu 8:261-287, 1979.
27. Richter D, Latta LL, Milne EL, et al: The Stabilizing Effects of Different Orthoses in the Intact and Unstable Upper Cervical Spine: A Cadaver Study. J Trauma 50(5):848-854, 2001.
28. Richter D, Latta LL, Milne EL, et al: The Stabilizing Effects of Different Orthoses in the Intact and Unstable Upper Cervical Spine: A Cadaver Study. J Trauma 50(5):848-854, 2001.
29. Sandler AJ, Dvorak J, Humke T, et al: The Effectiveness of Various Cervical Orthoses. An In Vivo Comparison of the Mechanical Stability Provided by Several Widely Used Models. Spine 21(14):1624-1629, 1996.
30. Saunders RL and Saunders HD: The Use of Back Supports for Athletes. Am J Med and Sports 5(2):158-163, 2003.
31. Stamp J, Chock K, and Penrose K: Acute and Chronic Effects Of Pneumatic Lumbar Support On Muscular Strength, Flexibility And Functional Impairment Index. Sports Training Med J 2:121-129, 1991.
32. van Poppel MN, Koes BW, van der Ploeg T, et al: Lumbar Supports and Education for the Prevention of Low Back Pain in Industry: A Randomized Controlled Trial. JAMA 279(22):1789-1794, 1998.
33. van Poppel MNM, de Looze MP, Koes BW, et al: Mechanisms of Action of Lumbar Supports. A Systematic Review. Spine 25(16):2103-2113, 2000.
34. Vieweg U and Schultheiss R: A Review of Halo Vest Treatment of Upper Cervical Spine Injuries. Arch Orthop Trauma Surg 121(1-2):50-55, 2001.
35. Vleeming A, Buyruk HM, Stoeckart R, et al: An Integrated Therapy for Peripartum Pelvic Instability: A Study of the Biomechanical Effects of Pelvic Belts. Am J Obstet Gynecol 166:1243-7, 1992.
36. Walsh N and Schwartz R: The Influence of Prophylactic Orthosis on Abdominal Strength and Low Back Injury in the Workplace. Am J Phys Med Rehab 69: 245-250, 1990.
37. Warren LP, Appling S, Oladehin A, et al: Effect of Soft Lumbar Support Belt on Abdominal Oblique Muscle Activity in Nonimpaired Adults During Squat Lifting. JOSPT 31(6):316-323, 2001.
38. Wassell JT, Gardner LI, Landsittel DP, et al: A Prospective Study of Back Belts for Prevention of Back Pain and Injury. JAMA 284(21):2727-2732, 2000.
39. Wasserman J and McNamee M: Engineering Evaluation of Lumbosacral Orthosis Using in Vivo Noninvasive Testing. In Proceedings of the Tenth Southeast Conference of Theoretical and Applied Mechanics. Cincinnati OH 1980.

14

BASIC SPINAL EXERCISE

H. Duane Saunders MS PT and Robin Saunders Ryan MS PT

Section One—General Exercise Principles

When lay people think of physical therapy, they probably think of exercise. Targeted exercise rehabilitation is one of the most important services that physical therapists provide. Physical therapists must be skilled at prescribing correct exercise programs, and must also function as educators and motivators to help patients follow through with their programs.

Section One of this chapter discusses exercise philosophy. We emphasize the need for individualized exercise prescription and give general guidelines for frequency, intensity and duration of exercises are given. We also outline basic exercise ideas for three common clinical conditions.

In Sections Two through Six, we illustrate some of our favorite exercises. Some of these exercises are the "old standbys" that every clinician will recognize. Others may be new to some readers or may be used in a different way.

The exercises are categorized as follows:

- Section Two—Cervical Exercises
- Section Three—Upper Back Exercises
- Section Four—Lumbar Exercises
- Section Five—Hip Exercises
- Section Six—Miscellaneous Exercises (including neural tension and functional exercises)

We do not intend to compile a complete library of exercises for spinal conditions. Instead, we want to provide a basic framework from which the clinician can expand. The reader should refer to Chapter 15, *Advanced Spinal Reha-* *bilitation and Prevention*, for additional discussion about exercise rehabilitation.

Designing the Exercise Program to Fit Individual Needs

No two back injuries are identical, so it is a mistake for the clinician to prescribe the same exercises for every patient with back or neck pain. The physical therapy evaluation thus becomes the most important part of exercise prescription.

Each patient varies in his response to exercise. In many cases, a patient can progress quite rapidly. Other patients may not progress to the more aggressive exercises for several weeks or at all. The patient's response to exercise may have very little to do with the original diagnosis. For example, some patients with minor sprain/strain injuries progress more slowly than expected, while some patients who initially have severe symptoms or pathology are able to progress quite rapidly. Therefore, the therapist's careful reassessment of both subjective and objective findings at each patient visit is very important.

Frequency, Intensity and Duration of Exercise

The *duration* of exercises is almost always more important than the frequency or intensity. Patients should be taught early on that they should expect to perform a certain amount of spinal exercise for the rest of their lives. This point is especially true in the case of chronic or recurring symptoms.

The therapist should become skilled at finding out how much each patient is willing to participate in his own recovery. If the patient is only willing to invest five minutes per day, a 20 minute exercise program will not be helpful. The patient will become impatient and stop performing *all* of the exercises. In the big picture, it is much more meaningful for the patient to continue a few critical exercises for months or years rather than perform 15 exercises for only a few weeks.

Even if the patient enthusiastically performs a full battery of exercises while he is attending therapy sessions, he may be less motivated when he is no longer being supervised. If the therapist senses that the patient will have trouble maintaining the program after discharge, he should help the patient comply by shortening or prioritizing the exercise list. For example, the patient who has a tendency toward stiffness in extension should know that passive and active extension exercises are the most important items on his list.

The *frequency* of exercise varies depending upon the patient's problem and individual circumstances. If the exercise is designed to increase flexibility or reinforce postural awareness, it should be done frequently throughout the day. As the patient improves, the frequency can be decreased to a maintenance level (as little as a few times per week).

If the purpose of the exercise is to improve strength or conditioning, daily exercise is initially appropriate. As the patient improves and the exercises become more challenging, the frequency can decrease to three or four times per week. The patient should be told at the beginning that the frequency can decrease later as improvement is noted. This gives the patient a goal toward which to strive.

The *intensity* of exercise also varies depending upon individual circumstances. Generally, the patient should start out mildly and increase gradually. Stretching exercises are usually done gently and for relatively longer periods of time (20 seconds to a minute or two). It is usually desirable to have the patient perform relatively fewer repetitions more frequently through the day (3-5 repetitions every 1-2 hours).

Strengthening or conditioning exercises should usually be performed to fatigue. However, symptom response may initially prohibit this goal and common sense must prevail. A good rule of thumb is to start with 5-10 repetitions of a moderately challenging exercise. As the patient improves, 20-30 repetitions may be necessary to achieve the same level of fatigue or symptom response. If the patient can perform more than 20-30 repetitions of a strengthening exercise, the exercise should be modified to

make it more challenging. As more challenging exercises are added, the previous, less challenging ones should be discontinued so that the patient feels he has graduated to a new level. Table 14-1 gives general guidelines for exercise repetition, hold period, frequency and intensity. These should be modified as needed to accomplish specific goals and to fit the patient's schedule and lifestyle.

Table 14-1: General Exercise Guidelines

Exercise Type	Reps	Hold Period	Frequency
Stretching (Flexibility)	3-5	20-60 sec	3-5x/day Gentle, static hold
Strengthening (Power)	6-12	Slow, steady motion	3x/week Moderate to heavy
Strengthening (Toning)	15-30	5-10 sec	1-2x/day Light to fatigue
Conditioning (Aerobic)	N/A	20-30 min per session	3x/week At target heart rate

The choice of exercises and the ultimate intensity of the exercise program should be based entirely upon the patient's functional goals. It is a mistake to say that certain exercises should *never* be done or *always* be performed a certain way. To illustrate this point, consider the conclusions of the following research article. Callaghan, et al, studied several different active back extension exercises, with a goal of determining their effect on extensor muscle activity and joint compression. They found that an exercise involving active prone trunk extension with arm and leg raising (the "superman" position in Figure 14-30) required very high muscle activity levels and resulted in substantial joint loads. They concluded that, "their use is unwise".[2]

While we find their information useful, the conclusion is disturbing. If the authors meant, "their use is unwise for patients in whom substantial joint loads are contraindicated," then we can agree. However, if they meant that the superman exercise is inherently dangerous and should always be avoided, we disagree.

Many work or recreational activities place great compressive loads on the spine. To fully rehabilitate a patient who wants to participate in such activities, aggressive exercise is necessary. At some point in rehabilitation, each patient should be subjected to stresses similar to or greater than the stresses that his desired function will require. This may mean having him perform exercises that cause increased compressive stress, muscle strain and even shear forces. The best exercise program for each patient is highly individualized. The skilled clinician will choose appropriate exercises based on the patient's ability and functional goals, ensure that he is capable of performing them safely and monitor progression closely.

The therapist should pay close attention to signs and symptoms, but may react differently depending upon the acuity of the patient's condition. For patients in the acute and subacute phases of injury, caution should be used with any exercise that causes pain to peripheralize or results in pain lasting longer than a few minutes after the exercise session.

If the patient does not tolerate the exercise well, the exercise technique should be reevaluated. The exercise may still be appropriate, but the patient should perform it with less intensity, fewer repetitions, in a shorter arc or in a different position. There are many alternatives to discontinuing the exercise entirely.

In certain instances, the therapist may decide to proceed cautiously with a more aggressive program even if the patient has continued peripheral pain. The therapist and patient may find that more aggressive exercises do not actually cause the symptoms to worsen dramatically, even though the symptoms peripheralize. The peripheralization may be temporary and non-progressive. If this is the case, the benefit of progressing the exercises may outweigh the drawback of the negative symptom response. On the other hand, progressive neurological deterioration is always a contraindication for exercises that provoke symptoms.

Exercises for conditions involving adverse mechanical neural tension (thoracic outlet syndrome, adherent nerve roots, etc.) can increase symptom peripheralization. Mild to moderate increases in symptoms are acceptable and often necessary, provided the symptoms decrease a few seconds or minutes after the exercise is complete and are not progressive. Since conditions involving AMNT are often highly irritable, the exercise prescription should initially err on the side of caution, progressing to more aggressive stretches as tolerated.

For patients in the chronic phase of recovery, the therapist should monitor symptoms but not rely solely on symptom reports to determine the appropriate rate of exercise progression. Sometimes, patients' symptom complaints are excessive compared to their objective findings. For example, some patients may complain of severe pain but have functional movement, decent strength, and normal pulse, blood pressure and respirations. Such patients should generally be encouraged to continue exercising through their symptoms.

Table 14-2 gives examples of exercise combinations for three common clinical conditions. An inexperienced clinician could use these as a starting point, but will quickly find that customization is needed for maximum patient benefit.

Table 14-2: Basic Exercise Ideas for Common Clinical Conditions.

Upper Cervical/Anterior Chest Tightness; Interscapular Weakness; Thoracic Outlet Syndrome

    Upper Cervical Flexion/Side Bending (Fig 14-2)

    Standing Scapular Retraction (Fig 14-16)

    Corner Stretch (Fig 14-5)

    Resisted Scapular Retraction Progression (Fig 14-17)

    Upper Limb Tension Mobilization (Fig 14-48 through Fig 14-50, as indicated)

Discogenic Low Back Pain; Low Back Pain Related to Flexion Postures

    Shift Correction (Fig 14-21)

    Prone Extension Stretching (Fig 14-27 and Fig 14-28)

    Prone Extension Strengthening (Fig 14-30 and Fig 14-40)

    Lumbar Stabilization Exercises (Fig 14-33 through Fig 14-39; selected ball exercises in Fig 14-41)

    Practice the "Power Position" (Fig 14-47)

Facet Joint Pain; Low Back Pain Related to Hyperextension Postures (Pregnancy, Spondylolisthesis)

    Knees to Chest (Fig 14-22)

    Prayer Stretch (Fig 14-23)

    Abdominal Exercises (Fig 14-32)

    Lumbar Stabilization Exercises (Fig 14-33 through Fig 14-39; selected ball exercises in Fig 14-41)

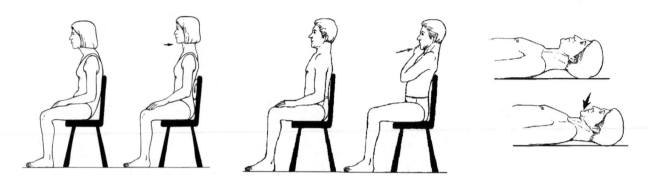

Figure 14-1: Head back, chin in. These exercises both stretch and strengthen to help correct forward head posturing, stretch tight suboccipital muscles and upper cervical joints, correct cervical herniated nucleus pulposus (HNP) and promote good posture in general. The exercise can be performed in sitting or supine. In supine, a small rolled towel under the occiput may be helpful. In sitting, the patient should start with good lumbar lordosis and sternal elevation, with the scapulae retracted to neutral. From this position, the patient usually only needs to nod the head slightly to effect the head back, chin in posture. An example of overcorrection is shown, and this is sometimes beneficial. However, the patient with a flattened mid cervical lordosis should avoid further flattening by excessively retracting the chin into overcorrection.

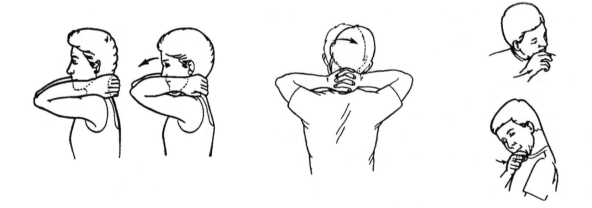

Figure 14-2: Upper cervical flexion, side bending and rotation stretching. Indicated for suboccipital muscle tightness, tension headaches originating from the suboccipital area, tightness of upper cervical joints, forward head posturing, and to reverse stressful positions. For rotation, the neck should be fully flexed prior to the rotation motion. These stretches should be avoided if upper cervical joint instability is present.

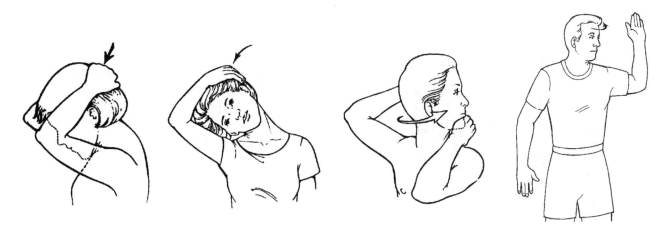

Figure 14-3: Cervical flexion, side bending and rotation stretching. Indicated for soft tissue stiffness, to prevent soft tissue stiffness after injury, to reverse stressful positions and to provide general relaxation or stretching of the cervical musculature. Stretching into end range should be avoided if joint hypermobility, acute joint inflammation or nerve root impingement is present. The stretch on the right is performed against a wall. It is particularly beneficial for stretching and mobilization of the cervicothoracic junction and anterior shoulder musculature.

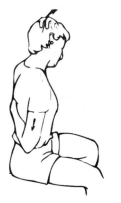

Figure 14-4: Scalenes stretch. It is important that the scalenes stretch is taught correctly. Shoulder depression should be done first and it must be maintained throughout the stretch. Then the cervical spine is side bent just enough to effect a stretch to the scalenes. This stretch is important for scalene tightness, thoracic outlet syndrome or upper limb neural tension caused by tight scalenes. It also helps treat forward head posturing and reverse stressful positioning. It should be performed gently when irritability of the neural structures is present.

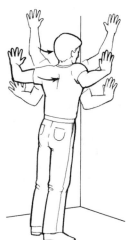

Figure 14-5: Corner stretch for anterior chest. The corner stretch is a good general stretch for the anterior structures of the chest and shoulders. It also stretches the thoracic spine into neutral or extension. It is useful for treating forward head posturing, thoracic outlet syndrome and to reverse stressful positioning. It can be performed with varying degrees of shoulder abduction to change the location and intensity of the stretch.

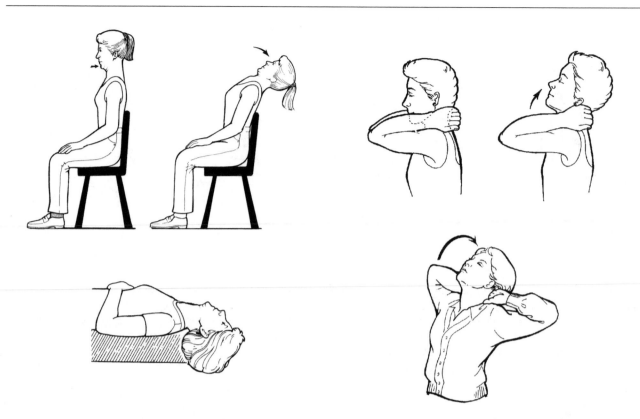

Figure 14-6: Cervical extension stretching. Indicated for limited cervical extension mobility, correction of cervical HNP or reversal of stressful positions. Stretching into end range should be avoided if joint hypermobility, acute joint inflammation or nerve root impingement is present. Sitting or supine cervical extension with a chin tuck should be performed when mid and lower cervical extension is desired, yet the therapist wishes to avoid excessive upper cervical extension. The clinician should ensure that the patient has good technique and adequate muscle control throughout the entire range, or the exercise should be modified to shorten the range. The patient can self-block at any desired segmental level by placing the hands as shown. For many patients, it is particularly beneficial to block at the cervicothoracic junction.

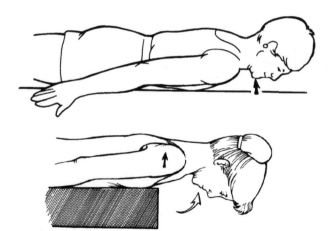

Figure 14-7: Prone chin tucks. Prone chin tucks can be performed on the floor or over the edge of a bed or table. They are indicated for posterior neck weakness and forward head posturing. Prone chin tucks are very useful when performed with the prone scapular retraction exercises shown in Figure 14-17. Prone chin tucks are one of the most important strengthening exercises for most cervical patients.

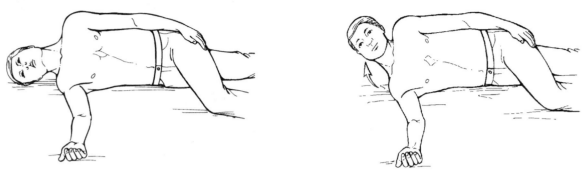

Figure 14-8: Side lying head raises. Important for strengthening the cervical lateral flexors or for general cervical conditioning. Caution should be used with acute cervical HNP, but the patient can progress to this exercise in subacute or chronic stages. Initially, short arcs of motion may be tolerated better, so a pillow should be used. The exercise can be made more challenging by increasing the arc of motion (removing the pillow) and even hanging the head off the edge of a bed.

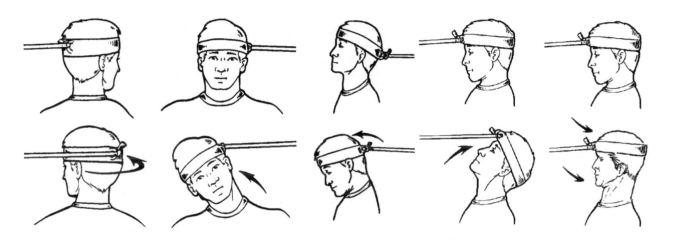

Figure 14-9: Cervical strengthening with elastic tubing. Indicated for strengthening of the cervical spine musculature and general conditioning. The resistance can be varied by changing the arc of motion or adding larger diameter elastic tubing. The patient should be reminded to use slow, smooth movements. Five exercises are shown, in order from left to right: rotation, side bending, flexion, extension, and axial extension (head back, chin in).

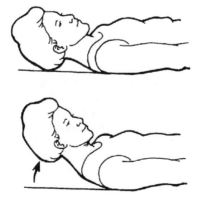

Figure 14-10: Supine neck curls, or chin tucks. This anterior neck muscle strengthening exercise is performed correctly when the chin is tucked into the chest, using the deep cervical flexors, and not jutting upward (which uses primarily the sternocleidomastoid muscle). It is indicated for anterior neck weakness or general cervical deconditioning. Caution should be used with acute cervical HNP, but the patient can progress to this exercise in subacute or chronic stages.

Section Three—Upper Back Exercises

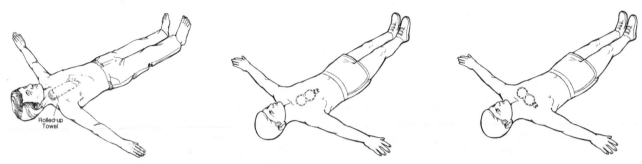

Figure 14-11: Supine thoracic extension over a rolled towel or balls. These stretches are useful for general or specific stretching of tight thoracic segments. It is helpful for forward head, rounded shoulder posturing when actual upper back tightness is a contributing factor. Varying degrees of shoulder abduction can be added to stretch tight upper limb neural structures. The stretch can be made gentler or more vigorous by varying the size and position of the rolled towel. Tennis balls or racquetballs in a sock can also be used for a more specific or vigorous segmental stretch.

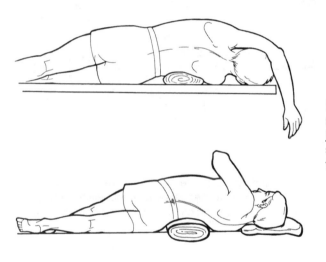

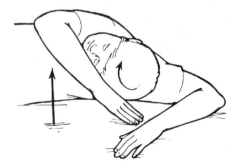

Figure 14-12: Side lying thoracic rotation/side bending over a rolled towel. This stretch is indicated for unilateral thoracic facet joint or general soft tissue tightness. The tight segment(s) should be on the top. The thickness and position of the rolled towel determine the intensity and location of the stretch.

Figure 14-13: Prone thoracic rotation stretching and strengthening. This is a combination exercise because it both stretches and strengthens. It is useful for general cervical and thoracic stiffness, or as a general self-mobilization technique for multilevel rotatory restrictions. The patient should be taught to rotate the thoracic spine by raising the posterior shoulder and elbow upward and backward, and not by twisting the cervical spine excessively, especially when cervical hypermobility is present.

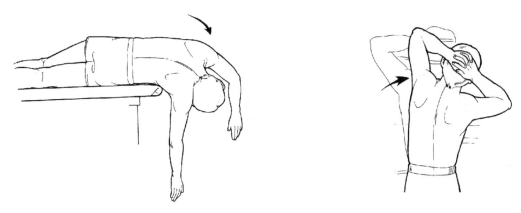

Figure 14-14: Thoracic side bending. The mid thoracic area can be difficult to isolate for stretching into side bending. Here are two exercises we have found useful for stretching interscapular muscles and trigger areas and for self-mobilizing stiff joints.

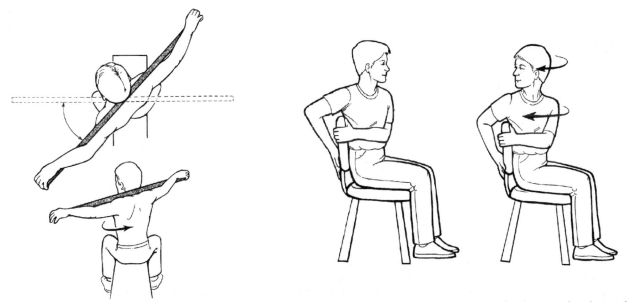

Figure 14-15: Thoracic rotation. These exercises are appropriate when a vigorous thoracic or thoracolumbar rotational stretch is desired in the more functional position of sitting upright. Using the wand minimizes stretching the cervical spine. These exercises should not be done quickly or forcefully.

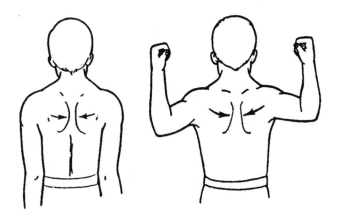

Figure 14-16: Standing scapular retraction. Scapular retraction is indicated as a postural reminder or strengthening exercise to be performed frequently throughout the day. It also gently stretches the anterior chest musculature. It is appropriate for any condition involving the forward head, rounded shoulder posturing. The position of the arms can be varied as desired to make the exercise more specific or functional.

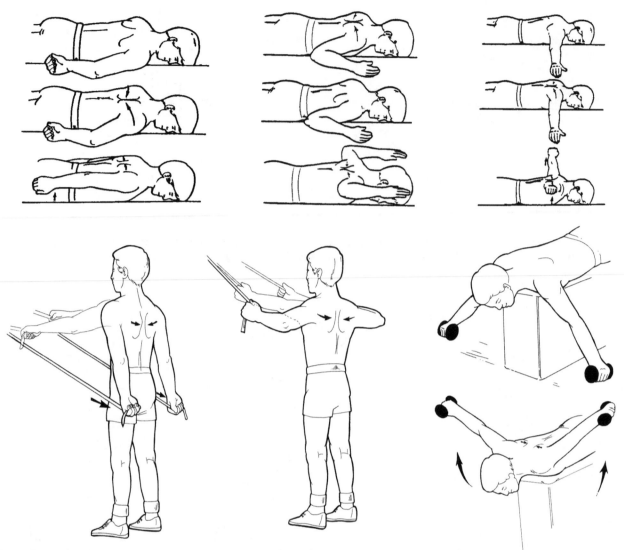

Figure 14-17: Resisted scapular retraction progression. This upper back and interscapular strengthening progression is extremely valuable in the treatment of poor cervical or upper back posture, shoulder girdle dysfunction, thoracic outlet syndrome, or general cervical and upper back deconditioning, and to counteract the detrimental effects of prolonged slumped sitting occupations. The exercises can be performed in prone (with gravity providing the resistance) or in standing. As the arms are held further away from the body, the exercise becomes more advanced. Hand held weights or strong rubber tubing can make this exercise quite challenging.

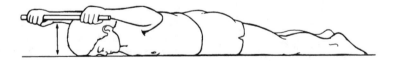

Figure 14-18: Prone shoulder flexion and upper back extension with wand. A challenging exercise for many patients, prone shoulder flexion with a wand is helpful for shoulder girdle and upper and lower back strengthening and conditioning. As the patient improves, cuff weights can be added to the wand.

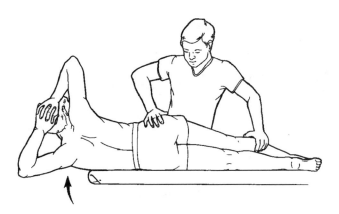

Figure 14-19: Side lying thoracic side bending against gravity. This exercise requires a partner and is for advanced strengthening of the thoracic and lumbar lateral flexors.

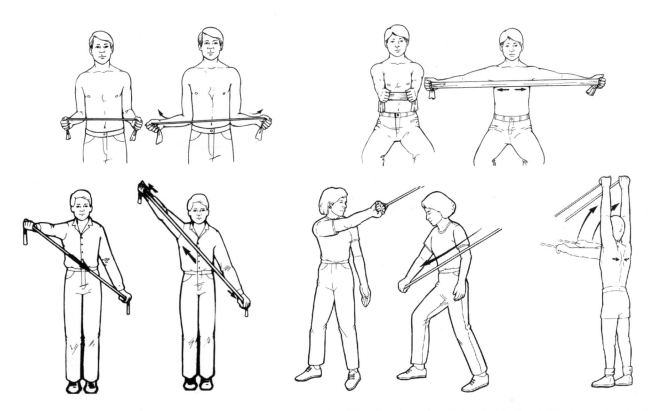

Figure 14-20: General upper extremity tubing exercise progression. Exercises involving diagonal or horizontal flexion and abduction of the shoulders strengthen and condition the upper back. They also help counteract forward head and rounded shoulder posturing and the detrimental effects of prolonged slumped sitting occupations. With co-contraction of the transversus abdominis and multifidus, they can be excellent functional stabilization exercises (see Figure 14-33).

Section Four—Lumbar Exercises

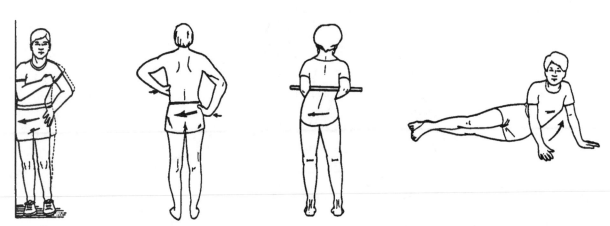

Figure 14-21: Lateral shift correction. Self-correcting an existing lateral shift can be done by performing active and passive lateral shift exercises in the opposite direction. Often, lateral shift correction is necessary prior to performing the passive prone extension progression or other exercises. Sometimes the patient must initially learn in prone or against a wall, but then can advance to more functional shift correction as pain relief and increased kinesthetic awareness occurs.

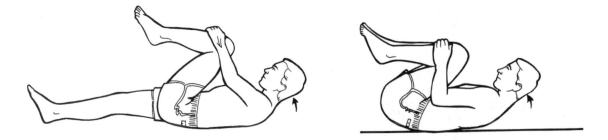

Figure 14-22: Lumbar flexion stretching—knees to chest. The single and double knees to chest exercises are helpful for conditions requiring lumbar paraspinal muscle, spinal interspace or hip flexion stretching. Patients who have a tendency toward excessive lumbar lordosis also benefit. This exercise may aggravate an acute ligament sprain or discogenic back pain, so caution should be used when these conditions are suspected.

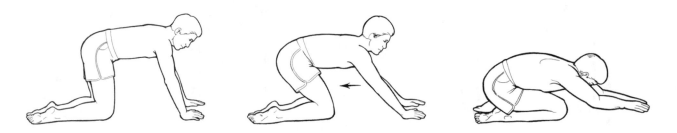

Figure 14-23: Lumbar and thoracic flexion stretching—prayer stretch. Many patients prefer this stretch to the knees to chest stretch because they feel they have more control over the intensity. Since this exercise can aggravate an acute ligament sprain or discogenic back pain caution should be used when these conditions are suspected. The hands can be placed to one side or the other to incorporate a side bending component.

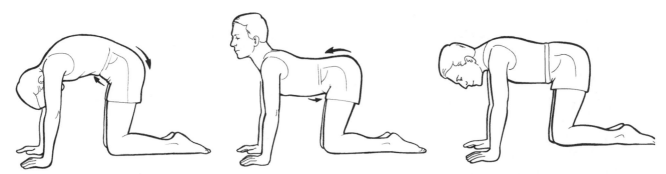

Figure 14-24: Lumbar and thoracic flexion extension stretching—cat back. The cat back exercise can be modified to emphasize either flexion, extension or both. It is a gentle way to teach pelvic rotation or to provide a non-weight bearing flexion/extension stretch to the lumbar and thoracic areas. The hands can be placed to one side or the other to incorporate a side bending component.

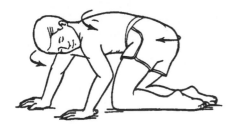

Figure 14-25: Lumbar and thoracic side bending stretching—quadruped "C". The "C" stretch is an effective way to provide a gentle non-weight bearing stretch into side bending. It is helpful for unilateral or bilateral side bending restrictions or lateral shift correction. It can be effective for thoracic as well as lumbar stretching. As the patient tolerates the stretch better, it should be progressed to kneeling or standing, the more functional positions.

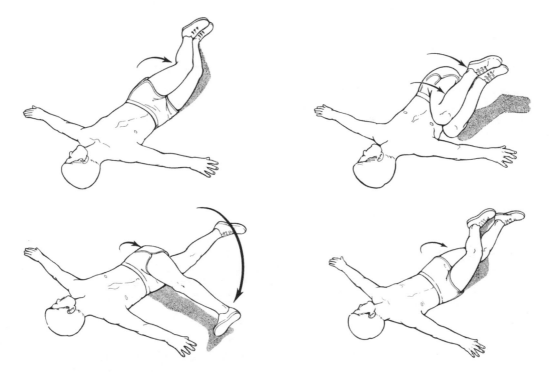

Figure 14-26: Supine lumbar rotation stretching. A few variations are shown. As a general rule, the further the hips and lumbar spine are flexed, the more superior the stretch will be felt. If one or both of the knees are extended, a greater force will be felt because of the longer lever arm. If the patient has trouble relaxing when starting in supine, he can begin in side lying, twisting the upper back into supine instead.

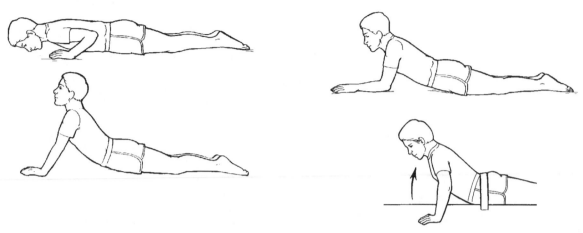

Figure 14-27: Prone extension stretching. If the patient has a flat back posture, is stiff in backward bending or has lumbar HNP, this progression is helpful. The patient should be reminded to let the back relax when pressing upward. Placing a strap across the pelvis will cause a stronger stretch. If a full press up is not tolerated, the hands can be moved further away from the body. The prone on elbows or simple prone position can be a good starting point. These exercises can aggravate a patient with an excessive lumbar lordosis, nerve root impingement, facet joint irritation or a large HNP.

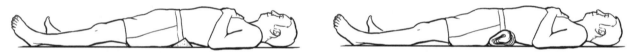

Figure 14-28: Supine extension stretching. If the patient has a flat back posture, but is particularly stiff in the lower lumbar segments, prone on elbows positioning or press ups will not stretch the stiff segments because the motion will tend to occur in the more mobile superior segments. Lying supine over a foam wedge or rolled towel placed inferior to the stiff segment will provide a more specific stretch and augment clinical mobilization treatments.

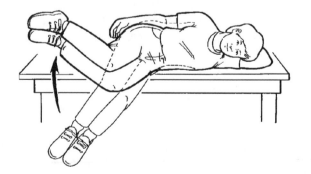

Figure 14-29: Side bending stretching and strengthening. Side lying while hanging the lower extremities off the edge of the bed can provide a non-weight bearing side bending stretch that is more specific to the lumbar spine. Caution should be used when the patient has acute pain or poor muscle control, as this stretch is fairly vigorous because of the long lever arm of the lower extremities. The same motion becomes a lumbar strengthening and stabilization exercise when the hips are rotated up against gravity and back down to provide the resistance. The patient should be reminded to keep the lumbar spine in neutral flexion/ extension and to control the movement carefully. This exercise is advanced and should not be given to a patient who cannot control the movement well.

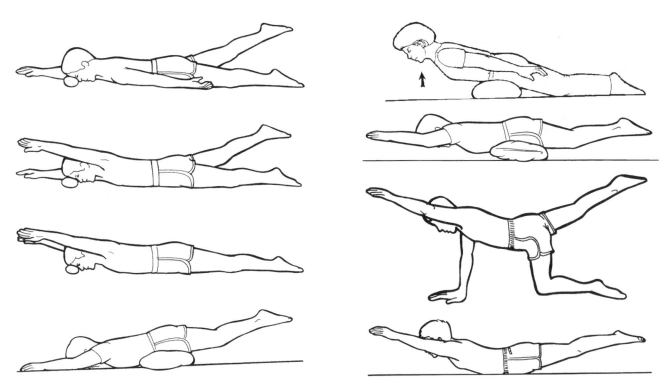

Figure 14-30: Prone lumbar extension strengthening progression. Indicated for strengthening, conditioning and stability of the lumbar spine. As the patient improves, the exercises can be made more advanced by adding both the arms and legs at once ("superman" position), performing them in quadruped or adding wrist and ankle weights. If the patient is limited in extension flexibility or end range extension is not desired, a pillow can be used under the abdomen. The patient should avoid "cheating" during the unilateral variations by bracing with the opposite arm or leg.

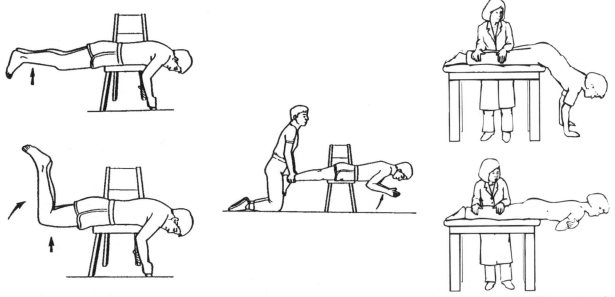

Figure 14-31: Prone lumbar extension off edge of object. A more advanced exercise, prone extension off the edge of a bed, table or chair involves a fuller arc of motion. It can be made more challenging by increasing the arc of motion, extending the arms away from the body or adding wrist weights. A partner, strap or counterweight is required to hold the legs down. The exercise shown on the far right was used in the well-known research study by Biering-Sorenson.[1]

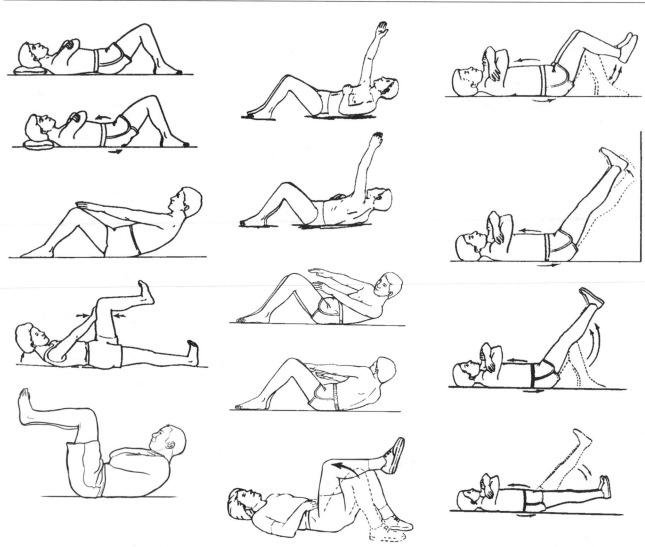

Figure 14-32: Abdominal strengthening progression. There are many variations of the abdominal curl or "crunch." Variations include raising either the trunk or the legs or both; lengthening or shortening the lever arms by changing the position of the arms or legs; and twisting the trunk to the right or left. Many equally effective variations are not shown here. Abdominal curls are indicated for treating excessive lumbar lordosis, weak abdominal musculature and general deconditioning of the trunk. They can be irritating to an acute lumbar HNP and should be introduced gradually once healing begins.

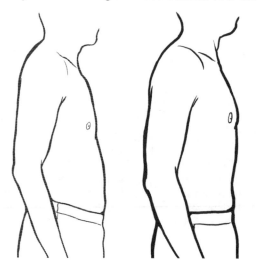

Figure 14-33: Transversus abdominis (TA) and multifidus co-contraction. These exercises are described by Richardson, et al, and are thought to be important in segmental lumbar stability.[5] The patient is instructed to gently "draw in" the abdominal wall and "swell out" the lumbar muscles with an isometric contraction of the lumbar multifidus and the transversus abdominis. The patient should be able to self-palpate muscle tightening medial to the ASIS with no trunk movement at all. Muscle substitution is common, and careful instruction is required to ensure correct technique. Common muscle substitutions include the external obliques, which can be detected by a transverse fold in the upper abdomen, and the erector spinae and rectus abdominis, which cause trunk movement. Exercise progression involves incorporation of the co-contraction into various trunk positions and functional tasks, including the stabilization exercises presented below.

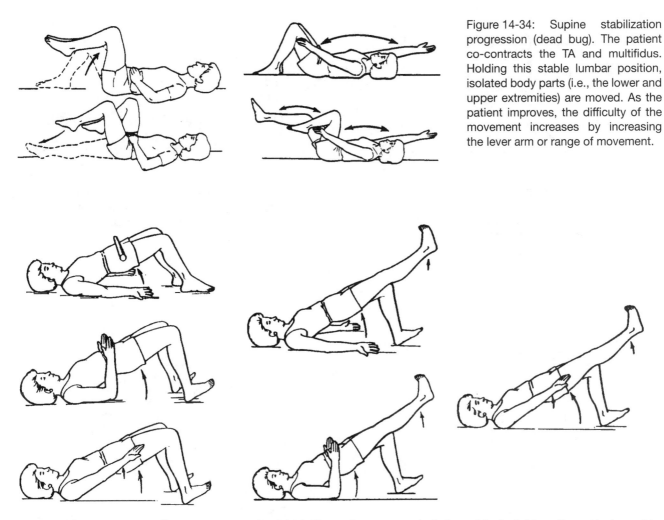

Figure 14-34: Supine stabilization progression (dead bug). The patient co-contracts the TA and multifidus. Holding this stable lumbar position, isolated body parts (i.e., the lower and upper extremities) are moved. As the patient improves, the difficulty of the movement increases by increasing the lever arm or range of movement.

Figure 14-35: Supine stabilization progression (bridging). The patient progressively isometrically tightens the ankle, knee, hip, abdominal, upper extremity and neck musculature, without releasing the other muscles. Holding this stable position firmly, a "bridge" is formed by raising the pelvis. As the patient improves, the exercise can be made more challenging by changing the arm or leg position to decrease stability or increase the lever arm or range of movement.

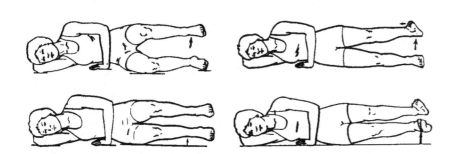

Figure 14-36: Side lying stabilization progression. The patient progressively isometrically tightens the ankle, knee, hip, abdominal, upper extremity and neck musculature, without releasing the other muscles. Holding this stable position firmly, an isolated body part (in this case the lower extremity) is moved to an anti-gravity position. As the patient improves, the difficulty of the movement increases by increasing the lever arm or range of movement.

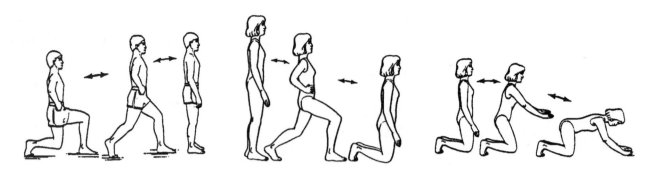

Figure 14-37: Kneeling stabilization progression. The patient progressively isometrically tightens the ankle, knee, hip, abdominal, upper extremity and neck musculature, without releasing the other muscles. Holding this stable position firmly, an isolated movement is performed (for example, the patient slowly rises from the kneeling position). As the patient improves, the difficulty of the movement increases by increasing the lever arm or range of movement.

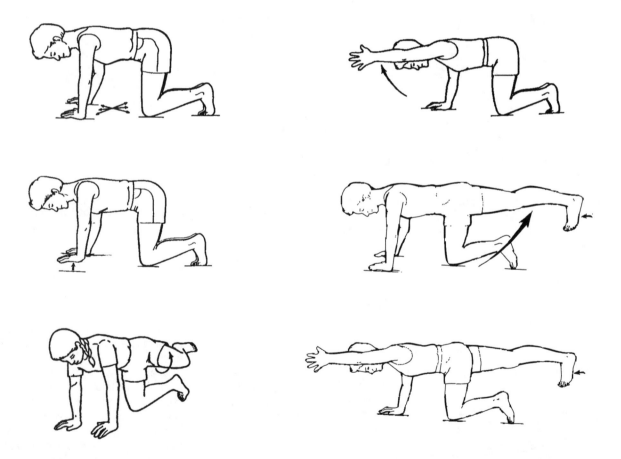

Figure 14-38: Quadruped stabilization progression. The patient progressively isometrically tightens the ankle, knee, hip, abdominal, upper extremity and neck musculature, without releasing the other muscles. Holding this stable position firmly, an isolated body part (in this case the upper extremity) is moved to an anti-gravity position. As the patient improves, the difficulty of the movement increases by increasing the lever arm or range of movement.

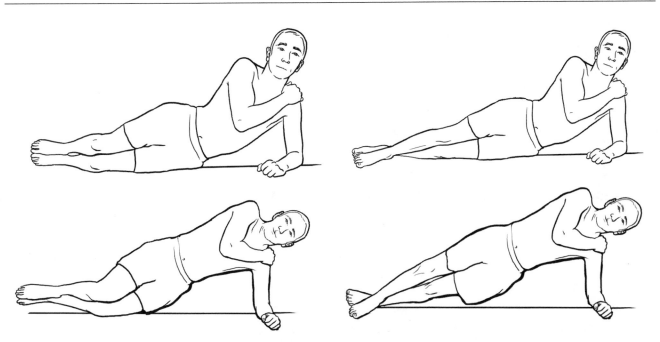

Figure 14-39: Lumbar side bending strengthening (quadratus lumborum). These exercises are described by McGill and are thought to be important for lumbar spine stability.[3] The patient begins in a side lying position supported on the forearm as shown, then raises the hips off the floor. In the simple exercise, the knees are bent. In the more advanced exercise, the knees are straight. McGill describes other variations not shown here.

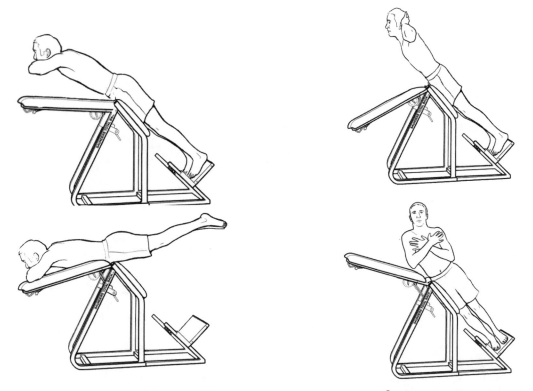

Figure 14-40: Lumbar strengthening on a reclining exercise device (The Total Back® by The Saunders Group, Inc). A reclining board allows multiple angle lumbar extension and side flexion exercise and is advantageous because the intensity of the exercise can be easily adjusted.

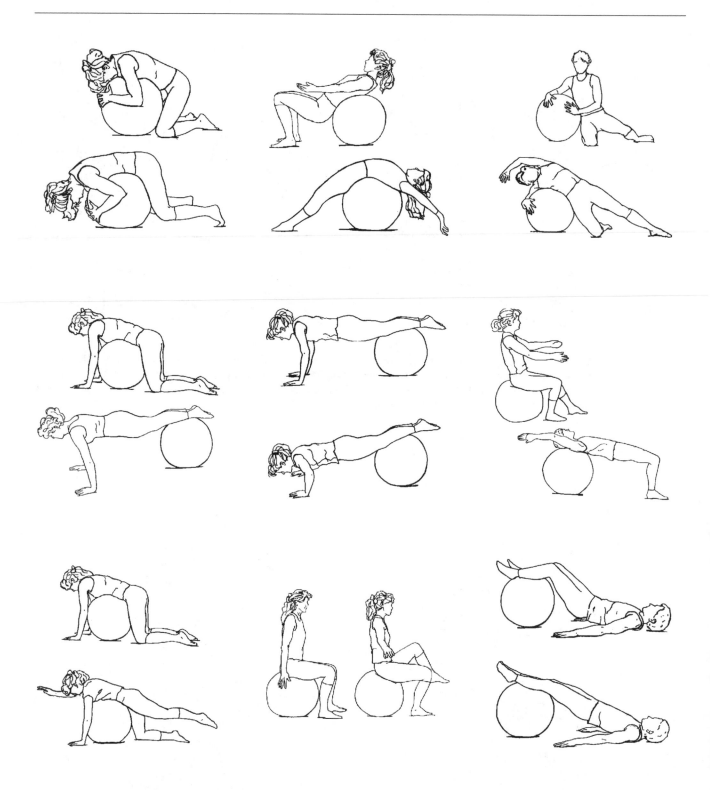

Figure 14-41: Therapeutic ball exercises. Cardiovascular, stretching, strengthening and core stabilization exercises can all be performed very effectively with a therapeutic ball. The three exercises in the top row are for stretching, and the rest are to emphasize trunk stability. For stretching, the patient assumes the starting position shown, then slowly and with control "rolls" into the new position. For stabilization, the patient assumes the starting position shown, tightens the trunk stabilizing muscles, then completes the final movement while not allowing further trunk movement. In other words, the trunk stabilizing muscles tighten to hold a stable "core" while the limbs move as shown.

Section Five—Hip Exercises

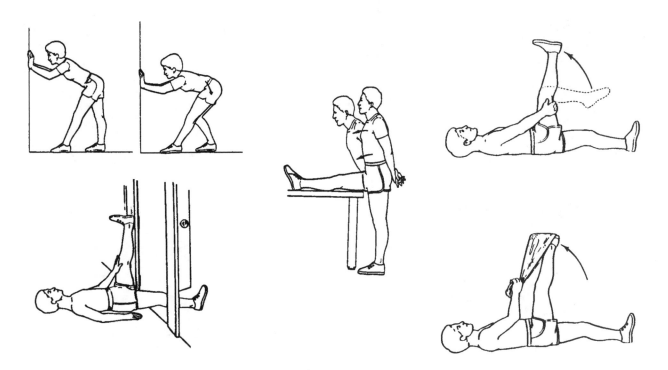

Figure 14-42: Hamstring stretches. Hamstring stretching is indicated when tightness exists or when inadequate hamstring length causes the lumbar spine to perform less optimally during functional activities. Several methods are shown. The hamstring stretches are also indicated for tightness of neural structures such as adherent nerve roots or adverse mechanical neural tension. If a true hamstring stretch is desired, the lumbar spine must be in a neutral, stabilized position during hamstring stretching to avoid transmitting the stretch to the spine. The trunk, head and neck can be flexed, or hip rotation can be added if neuromeningeal stretching is desired. The hamstring or neuromeningeal stretches should be performed gently when an irritable condition exists.

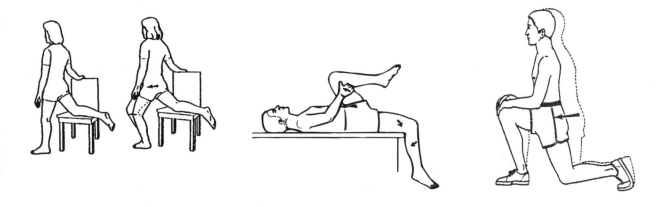

Figure 14-43: Anterior hip stretches. Anterior hip stretching is indicated when tightness of the psoas, rectus femoris, hip joint capsule or other anterior hip structure is present. The patient should be taught to stabilize the lumbar spine to avoid excessive lumbar lordosis, a common substitution pattern with these stretches.

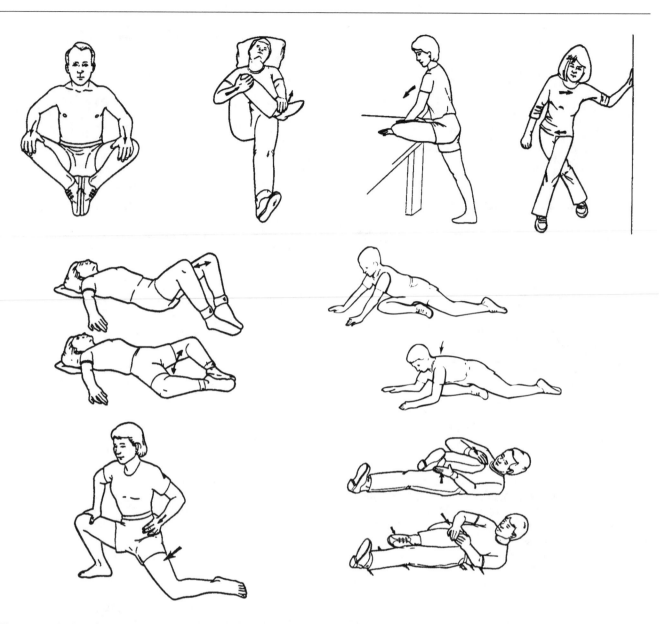

Figure 14-44: Miscellaneous hip stretches. Hip rotation, adduction and abduction stretches are often necessary when tight soft tissues in the hip interfere with normal lumbar soft tissue or joint mechanics. The patient can vary the degree of hip flexion or extension to isolate and modify the stretch as needed.

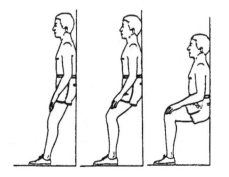

Figure 14-45: Wall slide. The wall slide is a helpful isometric strengthening activity for the quadriceps and hip musculature. Since normative data are available, it is also useful as a test for determining general conditioning.[4]

Section Six—Miscellaneous Exercises

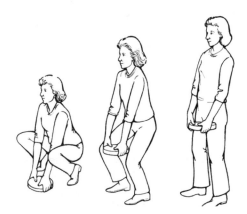

Figure 14-46: Squats. Full or partial squats are very functional exercises for strengthening the hip and back musculature. As the patient improves, he can begin lifting weights or items placed between waist and knee height. As the patient improves further, the weight can be increased and gradually placed lower until the patient is lifting off the floor.

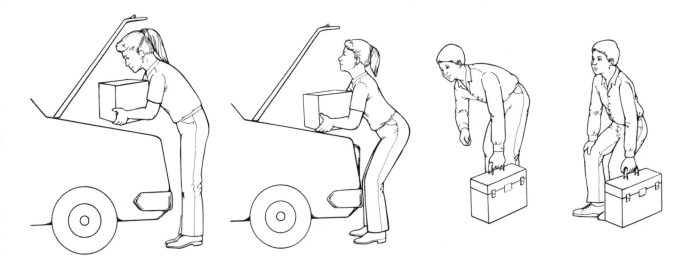

Figure 14-47: The "power position". Practicing the power position causes increased kinesthetic awareness of lumbar and pelvic positioning and helps stretch the lumbar and hip musculature in a functional position. The therapist can provide verbal instruction by saying, "Now power, now weak," in a variety of problem-solving situations such as lifting out of the trunk of a car, bending to pick up a child, etc., to emphasize further that there is a correct and an incorrect way to do almost any activity.

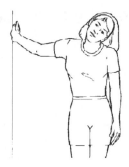

Figure 14-48: Upper limb neural tension mobilization. This mobilization is similar to the ULTT test described in Chapter 4, *Evaluation of the Spine*. Note shoulder external rotation and abduction, elbow flexion and contralateral cervical side bending. The neural tissues are mobilized by stretching the tissue interfaces surrounding them. The intensity of the stretch is varied by the degree of elbow extension and/or contralateral cervical side bending. This mobilization is biased for the median nerve pathway.

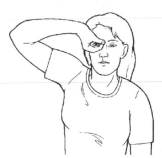

Figure 14-49: Upper limb neural tension mobilization. This mobilization is biased for the ulnar nerve pathway. The neural tissues are mobilized by stretching the tissue interfaces surrounding them. The intensity of the stretch is increased by the patient actively pressing the elbow backward.

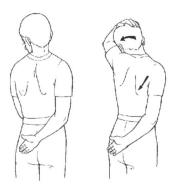

Figure 14-50: Upper limb neural tension mobilization. This mobilization is biased for the radial nerve pathway. The neural tissues are mobilized by stretching the tissue interfaces surrounding them. The intensity of the stretch is increased by the patient actively depressing the shoulder and by contralateral cervical side bending.

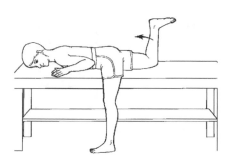

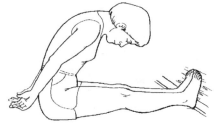

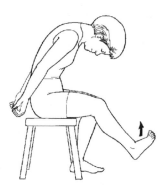

Figure 14-51: Lower limb neural tension mobilizations. The neural tissues are mobilized by stretching the tissue interfaces surrounding them. The mobilization on the left is biased for the femoral nerve, and its intensity is increased by greater knee flexion as shown. The "slump" mobilizations are biased for the sciatic nerve. Their intensity is varied by changing the amount of slump, cervical flexion, knee extension and ankle dorsiflexion in various combinations.

REFERENCES

1. Biering-Sorenson F: Physical Measurements as Risk Indicators for Low Back Trouble Over a One-Year Period. Spine 9(2):106-119, 1984.
2. Callaghan JP, Gunning JL and McGill SM: The Relationship Between Lumbar Spine Load and Muscle Activity During Extensor Exercises. Phys Ther 78(1):8-18, 1998.
3. McGill S. Low Back Disorders. Evidence-Based Prevention and Rehabilitation. Human Kinetics, Champaign IL 2002.
4. McIntosh G, Wilson L, Affleck M, et al: Trunk and Lower Extremity Muscle Endurance: Normative Data for Adults. J Rehabil Outcomes Meas 2(4):20-39, 1998.
5. Richardson C, Jull G, Hodges P, et al. Therapeutic Exercise for Spinal Segmental Stabilization in Low Back Pain. Churchill Livingstone, London 1999.

ADVANCED SPINAL REHABILITATION AND PREVENTION

Robin Saunders Ryan, MS PT and H. Duane Saunders, MS PT

Section One—Spinal Rehabilitation: A Sensible Approach

Our goals in spinal rehabilitation are threefold: To restore or optimize function post-injury, to prevent delayed recovery (e.g., chronic pain syndrome) and to prevent injury recurrence. The role of physical therapy in these goals is clear. Multiple studies have shown that active rehabilitation has a positive effect in treating spinal injuries.[7,16,62,66,69,71,85, 97,105]

Furthermore, it is clear that an excessively passive approach can actually be detrimental. In an oft-quoted study, Deyo, et al compared two days and seven days bedrest for acute low back pain. His study found patients with shorter periods of bedrest had better long-term results.[23] Subsequent studies have shown similar findings.[42,86]

Despite the evidence against inactivity, one still sees patients with acute spinal pain treated with rest, medication and passive modalities for several days or weeks after injury. If the patient does not respond favorably, extensive tests are often performed. If minimal pathology is found, the patient may become suspect in the physician's eyes— maybe the patient is exaggerating the symptoms or doesn't really want to get well. If more significant pathology is found, epidural steroids or surgery may be recommended, "because a trial of conservative care failed."

Commonly, patients appear to improve with a passive treatment approach. However, high recurrence rates and the devastating personal and societal consequences of chronic spinal pain do not permit complacency.[9,27,40,82,94,100] It is common for patients to have a history of minor sprains or strains that appear to improve but recur intermittently. These patients report that each episode is progressively more severe and lasts longer. Patients may believe that each episode is a separate injury. Instead, each episode was probably related to the last, because normal strength, flexibility and biomechanics were not restored after the pain went away.

Common sense tells us that patients with an episode of spinal pain should avoid excessive rest even when in pain. A non-supportive bed, a couch or recliner may place the spine in a position of flexion or side bending, which is undesirable for most spinal conditions. An analogy would be a patient with an anterior talofibular ligament sprain resting the ankle in a plantar flexed and inverted position.

When symptoms are gone, the patient is not necessarily prepared to return to pre-injury activities. The effects of immobilization on soft tissue are well documented.[46,52] After even two weeks of relative inactivity, one must assume deconditioning has taken place. Active exercise to restore the spinal structures to their pre-injury condition is indicated. Often, even this is not enough. The patient's pre-injury condition may have been poor, and may have been a contributing factor to the injury.

Clinicians tend to approach spinal injury rehabilitation different than extremity injury rehabilitation. In general, patients with non-severe ankle, knee or shoulder injuries are initially told to rest the injured body part in a position of biomechanical neutrality. The length of time that rest is advised varies depending upon the severity, but complete immobility for more than one or two days is rarely recommended. Patients are often warned to avoid letting the body part stiffen and are encouraged to perform active, non-resistive exercise even if it is mildly to moderately painful. If the injury requires several days or weeks of relative inactivity, the patient is instructed to perform strengthening or endurance activities to restore the body part to its pre-injury condition—particularly if high physical demands will be required at work or in sports.

Many clinicians tend to be less aggressive with spinal injuries. In general, patients are not encouraged to work through symptoms to the same degree that they are with an extremity injury. Too often, when the symptoms decrease the patient rushes back to work and resumes normal activities without receiving comprehensive instruction or supervised rehabilitation. We believe that these practices contribute to the high rate of reinjury.

There is also a psychosocial justification for aggressive rehabilitation interventions in low back pain. Worker perceptions have been shown to be important predictors of prolonged disability.[32,33,38,51,89,110,111] Rehabilitation interventions can influence worker perception through education, encouragement and confidence building. For some back pain patients, improvements in these non-physical factors appears to be at least as important as physical reconditioning.

Literature Review of Rehabilitation Interventions

Aggressive Physical Exercise

Several clinical trials comparing relatively aggressive exercise to other interventions have demonstrated a positive effect. A supervised fitness program has been shown to be more beneficial for patients with chronic low back pain than education and home exercise.[34,35,53] In a literature review looking at exercise for acute and chronic low back pain, van Tulder, et al concluded that there is evidence for the efficacy of exercise in chronic low back pain treatment.[105]

Manniche, et al reported that intensive trunk exercise was more beneficial than less intense exercise for chronic low back pain.[66] The intensive exercises described in their study did not require the use of specialized equipment and could be performed in a group setting. There is also strong evidence that intensive exercise is more effective than mild exercise in improving functional status and returning to work following first time lumbar surgery.[77]

Other studies have shown a less clear benefit of one type of exercise compared to another. One study showed that both "high-tech" and "low-tech" exercise were superior to passive interventions for treatment of post-surgical low back pain, but that the low-tech exercises were more cost-effective.[97] Another study of patients with chronic low back pain showed several positive effects of three different types of physical exercise. No particular intervention showed a clear benefit over the others. The three types of exercise were: 1) Physical therapist-supervised submaximal isometric exercises with Theraband® and general strength training devices; 2) Specific trunk strengthening machines; and 3) Aerobic and muscle toning exercise classes. Aerobic exercise was much less expensive than the other two interventions, which raised the question of the relative cost-effectiveness of a physical therapist's involvement in exercise.[67,68]

On the other hand, the results of a study by Torstensen, et al showed that medical supervision was both important and cost-effective in patients with subacute to chronic low back pain.[99] Conflicting results about cost-effectiveness may be due to differences between the groups or protocol differences, and caution is warranted when interpreting the results of each study.

In another interesting study, Johannsen, et al compared intensive paraspinal endurance training to less intensive coordination training and found no significant differences in pain, disability scores or spinal mobility between the two groups. The intensive endurance training group had significantly improved lumbar strength, but the improved strength did not appear to affect pain or function.[47]

Multidisciplinary Rehabilitation Programs

Many researchers have studied the effects of a more comprehensive approach to spinal rehabilitation that addresses physical, educational, psychological and behavioral factors using a multidisciplinary team. *Functional restoration* is one term used in several articles. Functional restoration is described as a full-day program lasting from three to six weeks, incorporating intensive physical and ergonomic training with psychological pain management and education.[70] Although good results have been shown with this approach[7,69,71,109], study methods have been criticized[96], and the benefit of such programs has been questioned given their relatively high cost.[6]

Other multidisciplinary programs have been described in the literature. Program comparison is difficult, given that various terms such as functional restoration, Work Hardening, Work Conditioning, and chronic pain programs are used to describe programs that have similar characteristics. Individual programs have reported impressive return-to-work statistics with relatively chronic patients.[4,91,93]

Loisel, et al demonstrated that patients with chronic back pain returned to regular work sooner when they participated in a multidisciplinary program consisting of physical exercise, Work Hardening, a cognitive-behavior approach and ergonomic analysis.[62] Vowles and Gross reported success with a similar program in improving physical capacity for work, and concluded that decreased fear was more important than decreased pain for good outcomes.[109]

Several literature reviews have been published about the use of multidisciplinary biopsychosocial rehabilitation programs in the treatment of various types of problems. Karjalainen, et al reviewed the literature for their use in the treatment of subacute low back pain. They found moderate evidence of their effectiveness, but pointed out methodologic shortcomings in several studies.[49] Guzman, et al's literature review concluded that such programs reduce pain and improve function in patients with chronic low back pain.[41] For treatment of neck and shoulder pain, however, little evidence exists of their effectiveness. The reviewers acknowledge that only two relevant studies were found, and they emphasize that more research is needed.[50]

Education and Cognitive Behavior Intervention

Attempts have been made to study the effects of education apart from physical interventions. In a 1995 review of the literature, DiFabio concluded that education was only effective for treating low back pain when combined with comprehensive rehabilitation.[24] In 1996, a study of 293 patients with acute low back pain showed that an educational booklet was not effective in improving worry, symptoms, functional status or health care use. When nurses combined use of the booklet with discussion and encouragement, patient satisfaction and perceived knowledge improved, but there was still no effect on the other outcome measures.[18]

Subsequent studies have shown more positive results for education when it is geared specifically toward decreasing fears and/or encouraging activity.[45,48,59,109] For example, one study investigated the results of consultation geared toward providing accurate information and encouraging physical activity for patients with subacute low back pain. In a single 1.5 hour-session, patients received individualized body mechanics evaluation and instruction, individualized exercise prescription and education about remaining active. The patient's general physician was given feedback about the session and recommendations for further diagnostic tests, treatment, work and sick leave. The control group patients were treated by their general physicians in the usual manner. The single intervention had a positive effect on symptoms, satisfaction with medical care and sick leave.[48]

Another randomized trial looked at the effects of a six-session cognitive-behavior intervention superimposed on treatment as usual for patients with acute or subacute low back pain. Patients participated in six group sessions with certified behavior therapists. The focus of the sessions was to encourage activity and promote coping mechanisms. Structured discussion of specific topics, group problem-solving and homework were included. The results showed a significant reduction in the risk for development of long-term sick leave and significantly less health care use in the group attending the sessions.[59]

Hsieh, et al compared comprehensive videotape education and individualized exercise instruction to three different manual procedures, and found that there was no advantage to the manual procedures over the educational approach. The population studied was patients with subacute low back pain, and clinicians performing the manual procedures specifically refrained from educating patients about principles taught in the videotapes. The results of this study suggest that patient education is an important component of treatment.[44]

In a 2001 meta-analysis of controlled trials studying back school interventions on back pain patients, the authors concluded that there was evidence of their effect on knowledge and correct back posture and movement, but no evidence of their effect on pain intensity and functional status. The definition of back school used in the analysis included interventions that taught medical information about the spine, specific exercises for the back, ergonomic variables, relaxation techniques, theories of pain and coping strategies, fitness exercises and/or behavior therapeutic elements.[63]

In a separate literature review of back school interventions, authors specifically looked at the effect of back schools on return to work and concluded that they were effective, and that intervention in the subacute phase of low back pain was preferable.[26] Their definition of back school was similar to that used in the meta-analysis.

In both the meta-analysis and the review, the studies examined were not homogenous, in that they included various combinations of the optional elements listed above, and different methods were used to impart the information, including varying lengths and numbers of sessions and a wide variety in the backgrounds of the instructors teaching the classes. When the descriptions of subjects and interventions vary so widely between studies, the conclusions from meta-analyses and literature reviews must be viewed with caution—it is better to read the individual studies.

Some studies have shown that the use of an educational booklet or leaflet to impart information can have positive results.[12,61,84] One study compared the effects of physician endorsement of a self-management booklet to verbal advice from the physician to exercise for patients with a new episode of low back pain. Results indicated that either approach increased satisfaction and improved pain and function. Interestingly, using both approaches together yielded less positive results. The authors concluded that the verbal advice and written information were not mutually reinforcing, perhaps because too much information was given or the information given was not similar enough. In this study, the information in the booklet was specifically geared toward educating patients about the importance of activity and discouraging the development of fear-avoidance behaviors.[61]

Simply advising patients to stay active is probably not enough. While one study showed that maintaining normal activities was superior to back extension exercises for acute low back pain[64], a systematic review of the literature concluded that advice alone has little beneficial effect.[43] Certainly, experience shows that the advice given patients has varying effects depending on individual patient and clinician characteristics. Still, the literature suggests that clinician advice can be a factor in the rehabilitation of patients with spinal pain.

Cognitive Behavior Intervention in a Physical Therapy Setting

Fear-avoidance beliefs in patients with low back pain have been shown to correlate with prolonged disability and work loss.[20,54,104,111] In patients with cervical spine pain, the correlation between fear avoidance beliefs and disability is less strong.[39] George, et al compared a program specifically designed to address fear avoidance behavior with standard care physical therapy.[38] The fear-avoidance program emphasized education and graded exercise that was progressed independent of symptoms. The standard care was based on treatment interventions described by Delitto, et al's treatment-based classification approach.[21] Results suggested that it is important to select patients appropriately for each intervention. Patients did well in the fear-avoidance program only if they had evidence of fear-avoidance behaviors prior to the intervention. Otherwise, they did better with standard care.

Lindstrom, et al studied individuals with back pain who had been off work for 8 weeks. Subjects were assigned to either a control group or an activity group. The control group continued to treat with their own physicians. The activity group took part in an activation program, consisting of functional capacity testing, a work place visit, patient education and an aggressive physical conditioning program. On average, the study group went back to work 5 weeks sooner and had 7.5 weeks less lost time due to back pain over the next two years.[58]

The interventions described by George, et al and Lindstrom, et al both involved aggressive physical exercise and a behavioral approach designed to counteract the effects of fear-avoidance behavior. In both cases, the interventions were performed by physical therapy clinicians—a multidisciplinary staff including clinicians with psychological credentials was not used. No studies have compared a physical and behavioral approach delivered by a physical therapy team to the same approach delivered by a multidisciplinary team. It appears that either team can have good results. It may not be the combination of disciplines, but rather the combination of approaches (i.e., both physical and behavioral components) that is important for back injury rehabilitation.

In fact, one comprehensive literature review looked at physical conditioning programs that include a cognitive-behavioral approach and concluded that there is evidence that these programs can reduce the number of sick days for workers with chronic back pain.[88] Their review did not distinguish between programs that were multidisciplinary and those that were provided by a physical therapist.

Additional Interventions

Reports of various other interventions can be found in the literature. The role of case management and close communication with stakeholders in worker's compensation cases appears to be important.[31,95] A strong case for ergonomic intervention is made, particularly because positive ergonomic change can result in both physical and psychological work stress improvement.[2,78,112]

Combining clinical exercise or functional restoration with progressive return to work appears to be helpful.[25,62] Return to work is seen as part of the rehabilitation process, rather than the end goal. Patients participate in progressive, graded work exposure that is monitored by a clinician.

There is some evidence that a support group and supplementing exercise instruction with video training improves long-term outcomes in patients after lumbar fusion. Both of the interventions described in a study seemed relatively low-cost and simple to administer.[19] There is also evidence that a self-management group led by a trained lay person can decrease disability caused by sub-acute low back pain by decreasing worry and improving confidence in self-care.[108]

One study looked at the effects of teaching problem-solving skills to subjects with chronic low back pain. For the experimental group, problem-solving therapy was added to a rehabilitation program consisting of graded exercise and group education. The control group received only graded exercise and group education. The addition of problem-solving therapy appeared to have a positive effect on decreasing sick leave and improving work status in the long-term.[102]

Our Recommended Approach

Rehabilitation is clearly important following spinal injury, but we do not believe that every patient with back or neck pain needs several weeks of supervised exercise in the physical therapy clinic. While there is some evidence that a supervised program is more effective than unsupervised exercise[34,35,99], there is no clear evidence that lengthy supervision is required or cost-effective for all patients. Each patient's need for supervision is different depending on his ability to understand instructions and his functional goals.

In our experience, patients who have fear, anger, depression or motivation issues require more intense intervention and supervision than patients who have straightforward musculoskeletal problems. To successfully rehabilitate these patients, a multifactorial approach is needed. But providing an intensive therapy protocol for all patients with back pain is not cost-effective.[56] Therefore, it makes medical and economic sense to try to determine which patients need the more intensive, multifactorial approach.

Using the literature as a guide, one would expect acute low back pain patients with fear-avoidance beliefs to be at high risk for delayed recovery.[20,32,33,54,104,111] For worker's compensation patients, there is a correlation between length of time off work and difficulty returning to work following rehabilitation.[4,5] Other factors decreasing the success of rehabilitation programs for back pain include age, gender, availability of work, amount of previous treatment, surgical intervention, back pain severity, receiving compensation and smoking.[4,5] Receiving compensation during injury may affect the reporting of pain and disability in patients with chronic low back pain.[80] Combining all factors, the patient who may be most at risk of a poor outcome is an older man who has severe pain complaints and

has had prolonged time off work. He believes that activity will make him worse, is on worker's compensation, smokes and has poor work prospects. Additionally, he has received a lot of previous treatment including back surgery.

When we see a patient with multiple risk factors, we are more likely to recommend increased frequency or duration of supervised exercise. For work-related injuries, we use aggressive exercise and work simulation with a behavioral approach designed to counteract fear-avoidance behavior, similar to that described by George, et al.[38] We prefer a progressive, supervised increase in real work activities on the job, when possible. We assume a very active role in recommending weekly changes in work restrictions to our referring physicians, and believe that keeping the patient at work is generally preferable to a daily, formal Work Hardening program (see *Work Hardening and Work Conditioning Entrance Criteria* on page 374).

How Acute and Chronic Rehabilitation Differ

We consider any injury older than 10 weeks a chronic disorder from a treatment standpoint, although the definition of "chronic" varies in the literature. After 10 weeks, assuming no new trauma has taken place, any damaged tissue should be stable. In the absence of severe pathology, the patient's continued pain is probably due to factors unrelated to initial tissue damage. It would therefore be a mistake to treat the patient as though he has acute low back pain, even though the quality of the pain may feel the same to the patient.

With the acute patient, much of the focus of education is on what caused the injury to occur, how to relieve the current pain, and how to prevent the next episode. In addition, he is taught that pain with exercise is not necessarily harmful, and a progressive increase in activity will be important in the recovery process.

The patient with chronic pain must be taught the same principles, but may have other problems as well. The patient may have been to multiple practitioners, many of whom have given him conflicting information. The patient is often not interested in preventing the next episode, as a feeling of hopelessness about the current episode may prevail. It is much more difficult to persuade the chronic pain patient to work through stiffness and soreness, as the patient may believe that any pain indicates harm.

With the chronic pain patient, it is important to obtain a detailed history of previous treatment and its effect on the problem. Use of the Fear Avoidance Beliefs Questionnaire

(FABQ) alerts the clinician to beliefs that will interfere with rehabilitation goals, and opens the way for discussion of such issues with the patient.

Patients who have seen multiple practitioners are naturally skeptical; such a patient must be persuaded the new therapist's approach is different, and therefore worth putting a renewed effort into it. If the patient has already unsuccessfully tried many of the ideas the therapist has to offer, the prognosis is poor. If, on the other hand, the patient has never tried an active treatment approach, the prognosis is better.

Many patients will say they tried exercise programs and they either did not help or made the problem worse. It is important to quiz the patient about the specific exercises, and ask the patient to demonstrate them. If the patient cannot demonstrate them, or if the technique is poor, chances are good the patient has not given exercise an adequate trial. Some patients try exercise once, and quit for a variety of reasons. Either the importance of exercise has not been explained, the patient has not had adequate guidance or the patient has a lack of motivation. If the exercise program was inappropriate or incomplete, yet the patient was faithful with the program, the prognosis is good for improvement when the correct exercise program is taught.

The patient with chronic pain often suffers from discouragement, anxiety, fear, lack of motivation and even depression. Often, these problems go away spontaneously when the patient begins to succeed in an appropriate physical rehabilitation program. However, sometimes the problems are more deeply rooted and cannot be helped by the physical therapist alone. It is important that the therapist realize this and be aware of other resources available for such patients. It is irresponsible and detrimental for the therapist to continue to treat the condition as purely physical when the problems that may be interfering with success are nonphysical or only partly physical in nature.

The Importance of Functional Activities

With the advent of Work Hardening and Work Conditioning programs, the importance of functional, job related activities has become well accepted. Unfortunately, body mechanics training and job simulation training are often left to such programs. Clinicians who treat acute and subacute back pain patients also should be concerned with functional activities, work-related or not.

Physical therapists who treat sports injuries know that function must be addressed for the patient to succeed. With the athletic patient, success is usually measured by whether the patient can return to his sport. This also should be the case when dealing with back and neck injuries. Pain relief is not sufficient. The patient should feel comfortable performing hobbies or job activities. This can only be accomplished through emphasis on functional activities during rehabilitation.

It is not necessary for the physical therapy clinic to have a Work Hardening facility for the patient to practice work-related functional activities. Very early on, each patient should practice activities such as picking an object up off the floor, bending to brush one's teeth or reaching into the trunk of a car. These standard daily care activities are followed by more specific occupational activities as the therapist learns more about the patient's required function and as the patient improves.

Ideally, the physical therapy clinic should have an area devoted to practice and progression of common functional tasks like lifting, pushing, carrying and prolonged or repetitive reaching and stooping. Progressive training of these functional activities should not be left to specific work rehabilitation programs. Work simulation should be a tool that every clinician is comfortable using.

Rehabilitation for the patient with back pain thus involves aggressive physical and functional restoration, with behavioral modification and work simulation as needed. Each patient is evaluated for both physical and psychosocial risk factors, and receives the particular interventions required for the best result. Some patients will require multiple visits with relatively intense supervision and coaching, and others will require only a few visits to progress a home program. Even though this concept has not been well-studied for neck pain, we believe the same approach is appropriate.

A small subset of patients will require an even more intensive rehabilitation approach. Formal Work Hardening and Work Conditioning programs are more expensive than supervised physical therapy sessions. However, their cost may be justified when the patient has been out of the work force for a long time. When there is a significant gap between the patient's current physical capabilities and the job goal requirements, or when there are multiple psychosocial or behavioral components present, a more formal approach involving intensive communication with multiple stakeholders (e.g., employer, insurance company, family members, attorney and rehabilitation or vocational counselor) may be appropriate. Section Two defines Work Hardening and Work Conditioning programs and describes our criteria and treatment approach for each program.

Section Two—Work Hardening and Work Conditioning

The Commission on Accreditation of Rehabilitation Facilities (CARF) has outlined specific definitions and criteria for Occupational Rehabilitation Programs (formerly called Work Hardening and Work Conditioning programs).[15] It is worthwhile reviewing CARF's definitions, because it helps one understand the distinction between the simple practice of work simulation activities and the more intense criteria required of a comprehensive program.

According to CARF, an Occupational Rehabilitation Program is individualized, focused on returning to work, and designed to minimize risk to and optimize the work capability of the persons served.[15] CARF further delineates Occupational Rehabilitation Programs into "General" and "Comprehensive" categories. A *General* Occupational Rehabilitation Program is defined as follows:

"... a work-related, outcomes-focused, individualized treatment program. Such a program is usually offered at the onset of injury/illness, but may be offered at any time throughout the recovery phase. The program focuses on functional restoration and returning to work. Goals of the program include, but are not limited to, improvement of cardiopulmonary and neuromusculoskeletal functions (strength, endurance, movement, flexibility, stability, and motor control functions), education of the persons served, and symptom relief. The services may include the time-limited use of passive modalities with progression to active treatment and/or simulated/real work."

CARF defines a *Comprehensive* Occupational Rehabilitation program as,

"...an interdisciplinary, outcomes-focused, and individualized program. Through the comprehensive assessment and treatment provided by occupational rehabilitation specialists, the program addresses the medical, psychological, behavioral, physical, functional, and vocational components of employability and return to work. The simulated/real work used in the program addresses the complexities of the persons served and their work environments."

The American Physical Therapy Association (APTA) has also developed definitions and criteria for Occupational Rehabilitation Programs, and continues to call these programs Work Hardening and Work Conditioning programs.[1] Work Conditioning is defined as,

"...an intensive, work-related, goal-oriented conditioning program designed specifically to restore systemic neuromusculoskeletal functions (e.g., joint integrity and mobility, muscle performance (including strength, power, and endurance), motor function (motor control and motor learning), range of motion (including muscle length), and cardiovascular/pulmonary functions (e.g. aerobic capacity/endurance, circulation, and ventilation and respiration/gas exchange). The objective of the Work Conditioning program is to restore physical capacity and function to enable the patient/client to return to work.

Work Hardening is,

"...a highly structured, goal-oriented, individualized intervention program designed to return the patient/client to work. Work hardening programs, which are multidisciplinary in nature, use real or simulated work activities designed to restore physical, behavioral, and vocational functions. Work hardening addresses the issues of productivity, safety, physical tolerances, and worker behaviors."

CARF's *General* Occupational Rehabilitation Program equates to APTA's Work Conditioning Program, while CARF's *Comprehensive* Occupational Rehabilitation Program equates to APTA's Work Hardening Program. Though there are terminology and other differences between CARF's and APTA's definitions, it is clear that both organizations distinguish Occupational Rehabilitation *Programs* from traditional medical services. A typical physical or occupational therapy clinic will provide individual components that are present in Occupational Rehabilitation Programs. Certainly, simulating functional activities and restoring strength and aerobic capacity are not unusual techniques. However, it is the focus and intensity of such programs, their specific goal-orientation and the involvement of other stakeholders that make them unique and justify calling them "programs".

Despite the existence of CARF and APTA criteria, one can visit many different programs and see several different types of treatment protocols. For example, some programs use quite sophisticated strengthening and conditioning equipment almost exclusively, with very little job simulation occurring. Others use job simulation exclusively with very little exercise equipment present. Some occupational rehabilitation programs have tools, forklifts, warehouse racking or mini-work stations available so actual work is performed. Some programs are run by physical or occupational therapists exclusively, while others involve social workers, psychologists, vocational specialists or other professionals. In the literature, the description of *functional restoration* sounds very much like the Work Hardening Programs and Comprehensive Occupational Rehabilitation Programs just defined.

We prefer the terms *Work Hardening* and *Work Conditioning*, and will use these terms in the rest of this section. Though the following criteria for each program are our own, they are generally consistent with both the APTA's and CARF's guidelines.

One important distinction between Work Hardening programs and Work Conditioning programs is that Work Hardening programs are multidisciplinary, involving personnel specifically trained to address the psychosocial components of rehabilitation. We have already discussed the possibility that multiple disciplines may not be needed to effectively rehabilitate many patients (see *Cognitive Behavior Intervention in a Physical Therapy Setting* on page 370). Nonetheless, we find it helpful to involve a psychologist in our Work Hardening program. His role is to facilitate weekly group sessions and to consult with the physical and occupational therapists regarding psychosocial issues that arise for individual patients.

Another distinction between Work Hardening and Work Conditioning programs is the frequency and length of each session, although this varies because we customize each program to fit individual schedules and goals. Most Work Conditioning patients are seen less frequently (e.g., 3x per week rather than daily) and for a shorter session (e.g., 2-4 hours rather than 4 or more hours). This is because they are often working in a modified job while they are attending Work Conditioning sessions. For these patients, Work Conditioning is designed to "bridge the *physical* gap" between their current abilities and their eventual job requirements. Encouragement, reassurance and problem-solving are also important components of the Work Conditioning program as the patient transitions into more challenging activities on his job.

Work Hardening and Work Conditioning Entrance Criteria

Work Hardening programs should have specific criteria for entering a patient into the program. This ensures that only medically necessary, practical and cost-effective services are provided. In our Work Hardening program, the following six criteria must be met:

1. The patient is unable to return to his optimum level of employment because of pain or dysfunction following an injury or illness.

2. There is a reasonably good prognosis for improved employment capabilities as a result of the Work Hardening program.

3. The patient has a clear, job-oriented goal, and understands the purpose of the Work Hardening program is return to work.

4. The patient's goal is attainable within a maximum of 6-8 weeks.

5. The patient does not have a psychological diagnosis, chemical dependency or symptom magnification that interferes with progress toward the goal.

6. Work Hardening is not medically contraindicated, and the treating physician supports the Work Hardening plan.

For Work Conditioning, the entrance criteria are identical, except that the patient must not have psychosocial issues that require the multidisciplinary services of a Work Hardening program. The presence of psychosocial issues is detected in the evaluation (see *Evaluation* on page 375).

The Work Hardening Trial Period

Sometimes patients who do not meet all the above criteria are appropriate for a short trial of Work Hardening. However, if the patient does not meet all six criteria after a two week trial, he should not continue in the Work Hardening program. It is possible further medical intervention is needed or the patient needs further physical conditioning, psychological counseling or other services before initiating the Work Hardening program. Sometimes, the patient's goal is simply unrealistic. In such cases, the goal should be modified.

By the time a patient becomes a candidate for Work Hardening services, many people are involved intimately with his case. These people include the patient, the family, the employer, the insurer, physicians and a rehabilitation or vocational counselor. All involved parties must support the Work Hardening goal.

At times, patients begin the program uncertain of their goals. Indeed, they may even be convinced they cannot reach a goal, especially if someone else has set it for them. If the insurance company wants the patient to achieve a higher goal than the patient does, for example, the resulting conflict will undermine the success of the program. Such patients will almost always fail a Work Hardening program.

A one or two week trial is often worthwhile. Patients may gain confidence or communication between all parties may be facilitated, thus causing a better result. In our experience, however, improvement must be seen clearly in the trial period for the program to succeed. Continuing beyond the one or two week trial when the goals are still doubtful is almost always unsuccessful.

Work Hardening and Work Conditioning Exit Criteria

Work Hardening and Work Conditioning programs should also have clear criteria for exiting the program. Patients should be discharged when any of the following conditions are met.

1. The patient meets the goals of the program
2. The patient plateaus or stops progressing toward the goals
3. The program becomes medically contraindicated
4. The patient wishes to discontinue the program
5. The patient is noncompliant with the program

An occupational rehabilitation program with clear entrance and exit criteria will have a successful track record. On the other hand, if the program becomes a place to send patients who have "nowhere else to go" or the program indiscriminately takes inappropriate referrals, it will soon gain a reputation for having poor success.

Components of Successful Work Hardening and Work Conditioning Programs

Evaluation. A standardized evaluation should be performed at the beginning of the Work Hardening or Work Conditioning program. The evaluation should test baseline functional abilities, but it does not have to be a formal Functional Capacity Evaluation (FCE).

In most cases, it is not necessary to determine detailed endurance capabilities before beginning an industrial rehabilitation program. Therefore, the evaluation can be less comprehensive and more cost-effective than a formal Functional Capacity Evaluation.

The purpose of the evaluation is threefold:

1. Establish the appropriateness of the client to participate in the Work Hardening or Work Conditioning program by evaluating psychosocial factors, medical condition, musculoskeletal condition and functional tolerance levels

2. Establish a baseline from which progress can be measured
3. Identify other services that may be necessary in addition to or instead of the Work Hardening or Work Conditioning program

The necessary components of the evaluation are as follows:

- Intake Interview - This includes medical history and a detailed discussion of job duties and goals. The physical or occupational therapist also actively screens for fear or anger issues, including an incongruence between the patient's goals and those of his employer, insurance company, case manager, physician or family.
- Psychosocial Evaluation - Developed by our consulting psychologist, this includes written screening tests for depression, anxiety, fear-avoidance beliefs and chemical dependency.
- Neuromusculoskeletal Evaluation
- Baseline Functional Evaluation - The intent is to establish the client's safe maximum tolerance levels for a variety of functional tasks and to determine the limiting factors. This usually includes a standardized list of material handling tasks, as well as static postures and positions and repetitive motion tasks.

The results of the interview and psychosocial screening tests are used to determine the appropriateness of Work Hardening vs. Work Conditioning. If no "red flags" are raised (i.e., the patient does not appear to have issues with anger, fear, anxiety, depression or goal incongruence), then Work Conditioning is recommended. If red flags are detected, Work Hardening is recommended. The only difference between our Work Hardening and Work Conditioning programs is that Work Hardening patients attend weekly group sessions with the consulting psychologist, and more frequent communication is usually required between the staff and the patient's case manager or physician.

At the end of the Work Hardening or Work Conditioning program, the evaluation is repeated to compare pre- and post-rehabilitation abilities. The client's function as it relates specifically to job tasks should be well documented. In addition to the standardized job tasks, performance of specific job duties important for an individual client should be addressed. The final report should be in a format easily understood by the client's physician, employer, insurer and case manager, and its primary purpose should be to specify abilities for return to work.

Program Standards. Consistent methods and standards are essential to the success of industrial rehabilitation programs. The methods and standards established should be described in writing. In addition to outlining entrance and exit criteria, the standards should address such issues as guidelines for written communication (format, content and timeliness), adequate progression in the program, how to identify and address inappropriate illness behavior such as symptom magnification, how often to have patient/staff meetings, how to train new staff, how to evaluate the success of the program, how to ensure quality of the program, and many other issues. Each Work Hardening or Work Conditioning program will have its own issues that are of greater or lesser importance. The methods and standards will probably evolve as the program grows and develops.

Staff. The most important asset of a Work Hardening or Work Conditioning program is its staff. A staff whose members are experienced, creative, enthusiastic and have good communication skills is essential. A program investing in its staff members will always be successful, even without expensive, sophisticated equipment. Occupational rehabilitation staff members must be specialists. They cannot rotate through various departments in a physical therapy clinic or hospital and still be able to give their patients the consistency needed. Many excellent Work Hardening and Work Conditioning seminars and workshops are available to train staff in the many issues and techniques unique to these programs. Staff members should also have a basic understanding of worker's compensation law in their state. Often, this understanding comes with experience, but talking with case managers, attorneys and colleagues who work with worker's compensation clients is extremely helpful.

For daily exercise and job simulation activities, an appropriate staff to patient ratio is 2:10 (one physical or occupational therapist and one assistant or aide per ten patients). As described previously, we use a psychologist for weekly group sessions and miscellaneous consultation. Social workers or others professionals specifically trained in psychological issues also can be used.

Equipment and Space. Work simulation and basic exercise equipment are also a must. The exercise equipment does not have to be fancy or expensive, since the patient will not have this equipment available when he is discharged from the program. The patient should instead use equipment available at home or in a health club, where the patient will hopefully exercise after discharge. The exercises should be individually designed for each patient's problems and situation.

The work simulation equipment must adequately simulate job tasks. Computerized printouts are less important than real life activities. An unfortunate myth exists regarding the objectivity of computerized testing and exercise equipment. Some therapists and referral sources feel they need computer-generated numbers to determine whether patients are improving or whether they are giving forth good effort. This is certainly not true. An experienced therapist can document objective changes in a patient's status without the use of a computer. That same therapist can determine the consistency or inconsistency of a patient's effort by close observation. Effective documentation is the key. Some computer data are actually misleading, because they appear to be objective, yet they are not easily applied to a real situation on the job.

Adequate space is important. The actual square footage required will vary depending upon the caseload. Patients must have enough room to perform their exercise and job simulation tasks. Usually, 2,000-3,000 square feet will accommodate 10-15 patients, depending upon the tasks they are performing.

Measuring the Success of Work Hardening and Work Conditioning Programs

Since the main purpose of Work Hardening and Work Conditioning programs is to facilitate return to work, return to work should be the ultimate criteria for success. However, many factors can cloud the issue and make it difficult to determine whether a program was truly successful or not. For example, many clients will not have an immediate job to which they can return. These clients will enter vocational training programs or proceed with job search. They are successfully controlling their symptoms, have stopped medical treatment for their problems, and are ready to "get on with their lives." They may have successfully met their goals, but it may take them time to find suitable jobs. If return to work is the only criterion for success, it appears these cases were unsuccessful.

On the other hand, a temporary, unsuccessful return to work does not indicate success. If a program only keeps statistics about its immediate results, the statistics may be very misleading. For this reason, the following statistics should be kept. The data should be collected at three months (to give time for case closure) and one year after concluding each client's Work Hardening program.

- Percentage of clients working, and whether they are working in same job or a different job and with the same employer or a different employer.

- Percentage of clients involved in job search or vocational rehabilitation.

- Of those who are not working or involved in job search or vocational rehabilitation, what is the reason?

A program can track its true success by carefully analyzing these statistics. The results can then be used to market the program. Individual Work Hardening programs may wish to track additional statistics that apply to issues unique to their settings. The above statistics represent the minimum amount of information that should be considered.

Section Three—Industrial Back Injury Prevention

Literature Review of Back Injury Prevention

Prevention of back and neck injuries before they occur is known as *primary prevention* in the literature. Primary prevention strategies can be grouped into two main categories: 1) Changing the work; and 2) Changing the worker.

Changing the work generally refers to interventions that reduce the physical demands of work, such as ergonomic redesign or changes in work flow or pace. *Changing the worker*, on the other hand, refers to interventions that attempt to change worker behaviors. Examples include training in lifting technique, safety education, the use of back supports and encouragement of exercise.

Primary prevention is difficult to study, and the results of published studies are not necessarily applicable to environments outside those studied. Multiple factors have been correlated with high rates of injury:[113]

1. Individual factors including a person's weight, muscle strength and smoking
2. Biomechanical factors such as lifting mechanics and postures
3. Psychosocial factors such as job satisfaction and job control

Many attempts have been made to study the effects of changing one or more of the risk factors. Results have been mixed and are inconclusive. Literature reviews summarizing the results of interventions and discussing the difficulties of researching primary prevention are available.[30,37,60,103]

Our Recommended Approach

Despite the mixed results and lack of consensus in the literature, American companies persist in seeking solutions to the back injury crisis. This is because back injuries account for more than 24% of all work-related musculoskeletal disorders[101] and represent a staggering cost. A new breed of consultant has been born out of this need for solutions—the back injury prevention expert.

Companies are interested in hiring consultants because there are individual reports of impressive results, even though randomized trials have not proven one method more effective than another. For example, Tomer, et al reported 67% abatement in back liability claims and a 70% reduction in lost workdays after introducing an injury prevention program at Lockheed Missiles and Space Company.[98] In a massive undertaking at Southern Pacific Transportation Company, 39,000 employees participated in an education and training program. The low back injury rate decreased 22% and there was a concomitant 43% decrease in lost workdays two years after training was initiated.[92]

Three years after introducing a training program at American Biltrite, Fitzler and Berger claimed a 90% reduction in back injury claims, a 50% reduction in lost workdays and a ten-fold reduction in workers' compensation costs.[28,29] In her study of eight different industries, Melton reported a decrease in lost work days with associated reductions in medical insurance premiums. Although an increase in the reports of lower back pain was noted, those reporting showed an 86% reduction in lost time days.[75] All of these interventions involved worker training, sometimes called "back school", and most of the studies described additional interventions such as ergonomic involvement, fitness consultation and changes in management practices.

Back injury prevention consultants can come from many different backgrounds, including fitness, medical, ergonomics and business. Because the cause and prevention of back injuries is complicated and multifactorial, the most qualified consultant is one who understands the complexity and provides a comprehensive solution. Medical providers can be effective consultants, as long as they become competent in the areas that are traditionally nonmedical (e.g., management strategies and ergonomic design) or direct their clients to additional resources so that a comprehensive injury prevention program can be developed and implemented.

Back injury prevention strategies encompass four major areas that overlap: 1) Management Practices; 2) Ergonomics; 3) Education and Training; and 4) Fitness. If a prevention consultant addresses any of these areas without considering the other areas, he has provided the client with a short-term solution at best, and has caused new problems at worst. For example, if employees are given ergonomics awareness training without making sure management is willing to make changes in the workplace, frustration or even open hostility may result.

Management practices are of great importance. If management personnel do not support the prevention process, attempts to take proactive steps in the other areas will be futile. Therefore, strategies to help management develop a comprehensive, prevention-oriented philosophy and a way to handle injuries when they do occur are paramount.

Addressing ergonomics is crucial for both biomechanical and psychosocial reasons. In addition to improving the workplace, positive ergonomic interventions help show that the employer cares about its workers.

Education and training is the vehicle used to impart critical information about effective back and neck injury prevention strategies to all stakeholders. Everyone in the company, hourly employees, supervisors and upper management, must be part of the educational process. In some cases, it seems that upper management needs more education than the hourly workers! In such a company, an intervention that attempts to train workers to use "proper" body mechanics will likely backfire.

Finally, a serious look at fitness is important to overall preventive strategy. No matter how well a company performs in all other areas, injuries will still be a problem if members of the work force are not fit to perform the critical physical demands of their jobs. Fitness is often a difficult area to address because how well individuals take care of themselves is usually outside company control. However, there are many things employers can do to facilitate on-the-job fitness and to motivate and educate individuals to practice healthier lifestyles away from the job.

Interventions in management practices, ergonomics, education, training and fitness overlap significantly. It is possible that the conflicting results of interventions reported in the literature have to do with varying degrees of integration between these critical factors in a given work environment.

Management Practices

There are many actions that a company's upper management can take to create an environment in which active and effective injury prevention can thrive. Not all the actions discussed are easy to implement. Many companies may initially resist the consultant's efforts to take a serious look at the effect management policies and attitudes have on their workers' compensation costs. Many companies want a quick fix, such as a body mechanics training session or an ergonomic analysis.

It has been our experience that successful injury prevention involves a multi-faceted plan that may require a willingness to change the way the company operates. The following discussion is not intended to be comprehensive—many books about management practices to prevent and manage injuries and improve employee morale have been written. Instead, we will list some of the more common steps that progressive employers are taking to decrease injury and severity rates and the effect injuries have on their profitability.

1. Job rotation—Rather than work exclusively on one repetitive task, employees rotate to different stations. This increases variety and reduces exposure to repetitive actions or sustained, awkward positions.

2. Job enlargement—Employees perform more and different tasks in the manufacturing process. This practice also promotes variety and lessens risk.

3. Job enrichment—Employees are given job goals, but are allowed more choices in how to accomplish those goals. This practice promotes teamwork, problem-solving, shared responsibilities and increased control over pace.

4. Reduced pace—Employers reduce the required production pace.

5. Work place exercise—Stretch breaks or exercise breaks are incorporated into the work day.

6. Disability accommodation—Employees with disabilities or injuries are truly accommodated and become productive members of the workforce.

7. Encouragement of early injury reporting—Employers need to know about symptoms early, when they are easiest to treat.

8. Modified duty programs—Injured employees are given productive, temporary jobs that encourage early return to work.

9. On-the-job Work Hardening—Programs that allow for progressive return to work gradually ease the injured worker into unrestricted duty while maintaining co-worker relationships and support.

Gaining Support. For back and neck injury prevention to be successful, management must support it. Top management is motivated by bottom line profit. If they can be convinced injury prevention will increase the profitability of the company, they will support it. Presenting the results of positive studies and testimonials from satisfied clients will help them make the decision to implement a prevention strategy. Once they buy in, top management support involves approving funding for projects and clear communication of policies, including written directives.

Getting department managers and supervisors to buy into the program may be a different story. Often, managers and supervisors live within their own departments and have somewhat misguided ideas of their ultimate role in the company. A production manager or engineer, for example, is expected to produce a certain product as quickly and efficiently as possible. If a new assembly line design or work procedure improves efficiency by 5%, he will think it is a good idea and want to implement it as soon as possible. What if the new design or procedure also increases the risk of back and neck injuries?

The question really gets down to who pays for what. The improved efficiency will add to the bottom line of the production department. But who will pay for the injury? If the production department manager is held accountable to a safety or workers' compensation budget, he will immediately see that improving efficiency while sacrificing safety is not necessarily a good idea. On the other hand, if the health and compensation department at corporate headquarters pays for the injury, the production department manager may not see the same bottom line effect that the company president would. Of course, one of the goals of a comprehensive injury prevention program is to facilitate company-wide understanding of these concepts.

All levels of the management team must be vocal and visible in their efforts to decrease and manage injuries. In other words, management cannot simply give "lip service" to injury reduction, but must be seen as an active champion and facilitator of the entire prevention process.

Providing Authority. In addition to supporting the back and neck injury prevention process, top management must provide authority for implementation, establish accountability and delegate responsibility to appropriate team members to put into effect the recommended policies and procedures.

This may require a major shift in the current corporate culture. However, if management has done a good job of selling the program to department managers and supervisors, then establishing accountability and creating new responsibilities for certain team members can be a smooth process.

Changing Attitudes. Making department managers and supervisors accountable for injuries occurring in their departments and rewarding good safety records will help change the attitude from reactive to proactive. The direct supervisor's attitude in particular should be addressed because he is usually the most visible representative of management in the injured worker's environment.

When injuries do occur, the supervisor's initial reaction and behavior during follow-up are critical. Verbal and nonverbal communication may convey to the injured employee that he is not trusted and that the supervisor does not care about his welfare. Without support and training, this supervisor may turn a minor problem into a costly confrontation. To avoid this situation, supervisors must be taught to do the following:

1. Eliminate problem workers before they have an injury. The workers' compensation system sometimes pays for the mistakes made because an effective employee evaluation system is not in place. Workers who take advantage of their employers by demonstrating low productivity, poor quality work, and high absenteeism can be expected to take advantage of the workers' compensation system, too. Companies with an effective employee hiring and evaluation system can eliminate injury problems before they occur.

2. Understand the nature of back and neck injuries, so that they can be leaders in injury prevention.

3. Convey a positive attitude. Supervisors should treat injured workers with the same respect they would expect if they were injured. Helping find solutions is everyone's responsibility.

4. Solicit employee involvement. Supervisors should routinely seek suggestions and ideas from the workers so they feel they are a part of the solution. They should ask employees to critique the back and neck injury training programs and the prevention process in general. Employees need to know that their concerns are heard.

Establishing Work Procedures and Rules. All companies have work rules and procedures, but they are not always fully understood or enforced. It is essential to clarify safety rules and work procedures, to gain consensus and support, and to make sure everyone understands what is expected.

Medical Management. Business and industry can rapidly improve their work injury statistics through more efficient medical management. Management can be proactive in the following ways:

1. Encourage early, aggressive treatment of reported injuries. When an individual reports an injury or the first symptoms of a cumulative trauma problem, management should encourage early conservative care geared toward reducing symptoms and combating fear-avoidance beliefs.

2. Find competent physicians and therapists. A company must work with competent physicians and therapists if they are going to implement an effective medical management program. They must actively seek physicians and therapists who practice the principles of treatment and management described in this chapter (an emphasis on exercise and education). Then, they must make clear to these medical providers their expectations.

3. Encourage employees to see designated medical providers. Employers cannot afford to allow their employees to be treated by physicians and therapists who do not support their injury prevention and management philosophy. Workers' compensation laws vary from state to state and a company does not always have total control over this situation. Our experience has shown that companies with an organized, positive, proactive medical management system are able to direct most injured workers to the providers selected.

4. Provide appropriate modified duty and on-the-job Work Hardening and make sure medical providers understand it. It is essential that the company's medical providers do everything possible to return the injured workers to appropriate work. Return-to-work is important to prevent prolonged disability.[79] Management and all employees must understand that return-to-work is a treatment issue not a production issue. Returning injured workers is cost-effective in the long run, even if little or no productive work is accomplished short-term.[17,74,76,79,83]

A common mistake that has been made with return-to-work programs is that they have been used in isolation as the only method of treatment or rehabilitation. In such cases, the injured worker is likely to stay in a status quo situation for weeks or months at a time. One should never think of return to modified duty as the sole means of treatment or rehabilitation. The return-to-work process should always involve education and exercise to improve physical capacity and counteract fear-avoidance beliefs.

5. Make sure medical providers consider ergonomic factors in the treatment plan. The medical provider must have a basic knowledge of the interaction between the work setting and the employee's abilities. An ergonomic change may be the most important treatment of all. Even if the patient has symptom relief, return to the same job without ergonomic changes may cause the problem to recur.

Claims Management. A corporate claims management philosophy should emphasize the following objectives:

- Regular contact with an injured employee
- Effective communication with medical providers

To accomplish the above, companies should have specific, written claims management policies. The policies should clearly outline a sequence to be followed every time there is an employee incident that may result in a lost time injury. Injured workers need to be managed as well as treated. The medical providers treat the individual, but the company manages the case. It is no longer appropriate to rely entirely upon the doctor's opinion about the injured worker's care and management. Obviously, the workers' compensation insurance company will be involved in case management to some degree, but it is still necessary for company management to know medical management principles (if for no other reason than to make sure their insurance carrier is doing a good job).

Injured workers must not be allowed to continue ineffective treatment. If progress is not being made with a certain treatment approach, a case manager should be assigned to monitor medical care and inquire whether additional methods of treatment and rehabilitation should be considered.

Eventually, the injured worker will achieve maximum benefit from medical treatment. Too often, cases go on and on from one physician to another, with very little, if any, progress. If the employee has had adequate evaluation and appropriate treatment and rehabilitation, has had multiple medical opinions, and an unusual amount of time has lapsed since injury, he has probably achieved maximum benefit from available medical care. The case should be settled. The employee may return to a permanent job within his restrictions at the present employer, or may have to be placed outside the company. Keeping a case open that should clearly be closed is damaging for both the employee and employer.

The key to long-term success in managing injured employees is developing a positive, open line of communication between the supervisor and injured worker. If employees genuinely feel that management cares about their well-being, a positive atmosphere of cooperation results.

Ergonomics

Ergonomics is the science of designing workplaces, machines and tasks with the capabilities and limitations of the human body in mind. By applying the basic principles of ergonomics, the company and its employees can take many steps toward a safer, more productive work environment.

The best ergonomist is the employee doing the job. Therefore, a major part of an ergonomics program is educating the workers and front line supervisors about the basic principles of ergonomics. Once these basic principles are understood, the employees can return to the workplace and recommend needed corrections.

Worksite evaluation and redesign can also be performed by experts who are trained in industrial engineering and ergonomics. If specific problems are found that cannot be corrected by application of the basic principles of ergonomics, an industrial engineer specializing in ergonomics may be needed. However, simple and inexpensive modifications can often be made to greatly reduce the risk of back and neck injury.

A worksite evaluation or ergonomic survey of the work area is performed for two reasons: 1) to familiarize the prevention team with the work tasks and work procedures so that any educational programs presented can be customized to address the specific problem areas and 2) to identify problem areas that can be redesigned or modified to prevent injuries.

When conducting an ergonomic survey, it is important to note good examples as well as bad. Most of the information gathered in the ergonomic survey will be incorporated into the education sessions later. Positive information will be just as important as negative information as the process unfolds. It is also important for the prevention team to be familiar with the company's injury records before the worksite evaluation begins. This helps focus attention on possible problem areas.

Some basic design principles must be understood before performing a worksite evaluation. With these principles firmly in mind, the worksite evaluation should begin by reviewing an activity or job believed to be more physically stressful than others. All the jobs in the work area should then be carefully reviewed. Examine the positions employees assume or maintain as work is performed.

Back pain can result from many different sources. Be sure to consider more than just the heavy lifting jobs.

Potential problem areas include:

Work too low.   In our experience, the problem of working at surfaces that are too low is the most common problem found in business and industry. If the work is too low, an employee will be forced to stand or sit with the head and neck forward, shoulders slightly rounded, and the low back in a forward bent position. Try to find ways to reduce the need to bend forward. Can the work be raised or tilted toward the worker? Ideally, the work station should be adjustable.

Work too high.   Continuous working at or above shoulder level can be very stressful. Look for tasks that cause the elbows to exceed a 45° angle away from the sides or front of the body, and attempt to lower the work height or raise the worker. This can often be accomplished by using raised work platforms, rearranging storage areas or by providing stair platform ladders that are safer than step ladders.

Work too far away.   Regardless of whether the worker is standing or sitting, repetitive forward reaching at arm's length is very stressful. All work should be performed in a manner allowing efficient use of the arms and shoulders, without creating a long lever arm that transfers excessive force to neck, arms and back. The least stressful work position involves working between shoulder and waist level, with the elbows at a 90° angle and angled <45° away from the sides or front of the body.

Work activities in confined areas.   If there is limited space for employees to maneuver and move objects, they will often twist to accomplish the task. Try to provide enough floor space so the employee can pivot when lifting or moving an item. In some cases, it helps to place some items far enough apart that the employee must turn and step, rather than twist. Swivel chairs help workers who are sitting. Conveyors, chutes, slides and turntables can be used to change the direction of material flow. Always allow for proper clearance through doorways and down aisles.

Prolonged standing on hard surfaces.   A foot rail, box or stool can allow workers to slightly elevate one foot and reduce stress. Rearranging the work so the employee alternates between standing and sitting tasks, or allowing a brief stretching break periodically throughout the day also may reduce fatigue. Rubber floor mats and proper footwear also reduce the strain on the legs and the back.

Sitting or standing in a static positions.   When work requires intense concentration or does not allow movement, the back and neck can become fatigued or tense. It is important to provide some movement to relieve the stress that occurs.

Sitting with the back unsupported. Sitting is even more stressful if the worker slouches. A high stool with no back or foot support is common, and should be discouraged. Sitting jobs should be designed so that 90° angles can be maintained at the elbows, hips and knees. Chairs and stools should provide support for the lower back and allow the feet to rest on the floor or a foot support comfortably. The head, shoulders and hips should all be aligned in an erect, well-balanced position.

Frequent manual material handling. Manual tasks should be reduced or eliminated by using lift tables, lift trucks, hoists, work dispensers, conveyors and similar mechanical aids when possible. To eliminate the lifting and reaching tasks completely, materials can be delivered to the worker by roller ball caster tables, automatic conveyor systems or other means. Follow three principles of task design for manual material handling: 1) minimize the weight or bulk; 2) minimize the vertical and horizontal lifting distances; and 3) provide sufficient time for stressful tasks.

Awkward or oversized loads. Manual handling of an awkward or oversized load can be dangerous. Employees should be encouraged to ask for help or use an assistive device if they are unsure of their ability to handle a load safely.

Miscellaneous hazards. Pieces of metal, paper and liquid spills on the floor are all potential hazards for trips, slips and falls. One should always note these conditions on an ergonomic survey. Is proper non-slip footwear being used? Is absorbent material readily available if there is a spill?

Education and Training

Almost all aspects of effective back and neck injury prevention involve education and training. Effective dissemination of information is essential if policies addressing ergonomics, fitness and management are to succeed. Basic background information about back and neck injuries must be familiar to all stakeholders to prevent miscommunication and enhance cooperation.

Though the required elements of back and neck educational programs are controversial, one thing is clear: Education to prevent fear and encourage activity after injury is key. In addition to providing information about how back injuries occur and how to prevent them, workers should be told what to expect if an injury does occur. Being proactive may help prevent the formation of fear-avoidance behavior. This has not been studied, but the theory has a sound basis in the literature.

In addition to dispelling myths that perpetuate fear and activity avoidance, we believe that basic facts about anatomy and the causes of injury are pertinent and helpful. We also teach about ergonomics, exercise, and the importance of a healthy lifestyle. Although training lifting techniques is controversial, we teach workers the concept of a neutral spinal position, and encourage them to maintain this position in all postures—standing, sitting, walking, reaching and lifting (see illustrations in Chapter 14, *Basic Spinal Exercise,* on page 363).

An educational program must be flexible and meet the needs of each company. We have found that a basic program should consist of two to four hours of instruction, consisting of a combination of lecture and demonstration, with high quality audiovisual materials that incorporate examples of the actual work place. Ideally, a maximum of 30 participants should be included in each session to facilitate more personal interaction and interactive problem-solving.

Common myths about back injuries must be abolished at the outset. Back and neck injuries have been difficult to prevent and to treat in the past because of three incorrect assumptions: 1) Back and neck injuries are caused by a single event such as lifting a heavy weight; 2) When there is no pain, there is no problem; and 3) When there is pain, there is a big problem.

Before proceeding with the rest of the training session, workers should be taught the following instead: 1) Most back and neck injuries are caused a variety of cumulative factors that can be controlled; 2) The absence of pain doesn't mean that you're taking good care of your back; and 3) After a back injury, the presence of pain after a few days does not mean that further injury is occurring. These basic concepts helps set the stage for self-responsibility in injury prevention and the encouragement of early activation if injury does occur.

We teach simple anatomy and function of the back, in order to show the potential strain that results from awkward positions and movements. We also discuss basic pathology of back and neck injuries with regard to stressful postures. We briefly discuss various methods of treatment, but emphasize the body's natural capacity for healing. Participants should be taught that what they do to manage their injuries is almost always more important than what their physician or therapist does.

Even when a company makes every effort to eliminate stressful, repetitive or prolonged positioning and heavy material handling, there will still be times when the employee's choice of technique will make a big difference. Therefore, employees are taught the concept of a neutral spinal position, and are encouraged to maintain this position in all postures—standing, sitting, walking, reaching and lifting. Additionally, they are taught how to reverse stressful activities through positional changes and exercise.

Participants should be encouraged to review their personal standards of fitness, nutrition and stress control. The harmful effects of smoking and its relationship to back pain should be emphasized. Fitness should be encouraged to improve psychological and physical tolerance to pain and stress.

During the program, participants participate in a simple flexibility and strength evaluation and exercise session. Each participant is given a customized set of exercises that may help improve his spinal fitness. For example, prone passive extension, hamstring length and the tests described by McIntosh, et al are tested in small groups (see photos and description in Chapter 4, *Evaluation of the Spine,* on page 82). Proper body mechanics and posture techniques are practiced, and several case scenarios are discussed to encourage group problem-solving. Each participant receives a booklet outlining the main points of the course.

We have had considerable success teaching the above principles in several industrial companies. In our experience, however, the best results depend not on "proper body mechanics," but a multitude of factors, including management commitment and worker beliefs and attitudes.

Fitness

Many stressful or repetitive movements will be unavoidable. If the worksite cannot be modified, workers can be taught specific stretches to counteract stressful movements or positions. These stretches can be performed during short breaks that take place naturally in most jobs.

There is considerable evidence to implicate poor fitness and unhealthy lifestyles as risk factors for back injury.[3,8,11,13,36,87] Therefore, it seems logical that one important aspect of a back and neck injury prevention program is to help individuals identify deficiencies and assist them in efforts to improve their levels of physical fitness.

One study reported a decreased rate of all types of injuries, including back injuries, after an intensive wellness program was instituted at an offshore petroleum unit. The wellness program incorporated fitness training and education geared toward back injury prevention, nutrition and smoking cessation. Study authors reported a significant cost savings and good return on investment.[65]

It is important to emphasize that many work situations are like athletic events: they require a certain level of physical fitness, strength and flexibility to "stay in the game". Many people attempt to work at jobs that require considerable physical labor and involve stressful positions, but they make little or no effort to keep their bodies in the physical condition required to do these jobs.

It is true that most individuals work hard at their jobs and it is sometimes difficult for them to think that they should exercise when they are already tired from work. However, hard work and exercise are not always accomplishing the same thing. In most work situations, we get too much of one type of activity or exercise and usually not enough of another. Many people work hard all day, yet are still very stiff and are in poor cardiovascular condition. An exercise program should emphasize the type of exercise that is lacking at work. For example, if an employee spends a lot of time flexing (forward bending) at work, he should emphasize extension (backward bending) exercises at home and during breaks at work.

To test that theory, one interesting study looked at the effect of prone lumbar extension and extension-oriented education on incidence of back injury in military conscripts. Subjects were taught to avoid lumbar flexed positions and were instructed to perform 15 repetitions of passive prone extension exercises every morning and afternoon while they were in military service (8 to 10 months). Compared to a control group who received no intervention, subjects in the study group reported fewer instances of back pain and medical care use in the year following the intervention.[55]

Business and industry have a lot of options when it comes to fitness. The importance of exercise and other healthy lifestyle behaviors can be incorporated into a preventive educational program. A certain number of individuals will become motivated to exercise or make other positive lifestyle changes through attending such a program. However, it is unrealistic to expect that an educational program will have a positive effect on every employee. Some companies are taking the issue of fitness much further and are encouraging on-the-job exercise programs. Positive results for both employee and employer have been reported.[107]

REFERENCES

1. American Physical Therapy Association: 1111 Fairfax St N, Alexandria VA 22314. Occupational Health Physical Therapy Guidelines: Work Conditioning and Work Hardening Programs. http://www.apta.org/Publications/occ_health/workconditioning

2. Amick BC, Robertson MM, DeRango, et al: Effect of Office Ergonomics Intervention on Reducing Musculoskeletal Symptoms. Spine 28(24):2706-2711, 2003.

3. Anderson C: Physical Ability Testing as a Means to Reduce Injuries in Grocery Warehouses. International Joul of Retail and Distribution Management 19(7):33-35, 1991.

4. Beissner KL, Saunders RL and McManis BG: Factors Relating to Successful Work Hardening Outcomes. Phys Ther 76(11):1188-1201, 1996.

5. Bendix AF, Bendix T and Haestrup C: Can it be Predicted Which Patients with Chronic Low Back Pain Should be Offered Tertiary Rehabilitation in a Functional Restoration Program? A Search for Demographic, Socioeconomic and Physical Predictors. Spine 23(16):1775-1783, 1998.

6. Bendix T, Bendix A, Labriola M, et al: Functional Restoration Versus Outpatient Physical Training in Chronic Low Back Pain. A Randomized Comparative Study. Spine 25(19):2494-2500, 2000.

7. Bendix AF, Bendix T, Labriola M, et al: Functional Restoration for Chronic Low Back Pain. Two-Year Follow-Up of Two Randomized Clinical Trials. Spine 23(6):717-725, 1998.

8. Biering-Sorenson F: Physical Measurements as Risk Indicators for Low Back Trouble Over a One-Year Period. Spine 9:106-119, 1984.

9. Bigos S and Battie M: Acute Care to Prevent Back Disability: Ten Years of Progress. Clin Orthop and Rel Res 221:121-130, Aug 1987.

10. Biering-Sorenson F: Physical Measurements as Risk Indicators for Low Back Trouble Over a One-Year Period. Spine 9(2):106-119, 1984.

11. Boyer M and Vaccaro B: The Benefits of Physically Active Workforce: An Organizational Perspective. Occupational Medicine 5:691-706, 1990.

12. Burton AK, Waddell G, Tillotson KM, et al: Information and Advice to Patients With Back Pain Can Have a Positive Effect. A Randomized Controlled Trial of a Novel Educational Booklet in Primary Care. Spine 24(23):2484-2491, 1999.

13. Cady L et al: Strength and Fitness and Subsequent Back Injuries in Firefighters. Joul of Occ Med 21:269-272, 1979.

14. Callaghan JP, Gunning JL and McGill SM: The Relationship Between Lumbar Spine Load and Muscle Activity During Extensor Exercises. Phys Ther 78(1):8-18, 1998.

15. CARF-Commission on Accreditation of Rehabilitation Facilities. 101 North Wilmot Road, Suite 500 Tucson, Arizona 85711. http://www.carf.org

16. Carpenter DM and Nelson BW: Low Back Strengthening for the Prevention and Treatment of Low Back Pain. Med Sci Sports Exerc 31(1):18-24, 1999.

17. Centineo J: Return-To-Work Programs: Cut Costs and Employee Turnover. Risk Management (Dec) 44-48, 1986.

18. Cherkin DC, Deyo RA, STreet JH, et al: Pitfalls of Patient Education. Limited Success of a Program for Back Pain in Primary Care. Spine 21(3):345-355, 1996.

19. Christensen FB, Laurberg I and Bunger C: Importance of the Back-Cafe Concept to Rehabilitation After Spinal Fusion: A Randomized Clinical Study With a 2-Year Follow-Up. Spine 28(23):2561-2569, 2003.

20. Crombez G, Vlaeyen JWS, Heuts PHTG, et al: Pain-Related Fear is More Disabling than Pain Itself: Evidence on the Role of Pain-Related Fear in Chronic Back Pain Disability. Pain 80:329-339, 1999.

21. Delitto A, Cibulka MT and Bowling RW: A Treatment-Based Classification Approach to Low Back Syndrome: Identifying and Staging Patients for Conservative Treatment. Phys Ther 75:470-485, 1995.

22. Deyo R and Bass J: Lifestyle and Low Back Pain: The Influence of Smoking and Obesity. Spine 14:501-506, 1989.

23. Deyo R, Diehl A, Rosenthal M: How Many Days Of Bed Rest For Acute Low Back Pain? N Engl J Med 315:1064-1070, 1986.

24. DiFabio RP: Efficacy of Comprehensive Rehabilitation Programs and Back School for Patients with Low Back Pain: A Meta-Analysis. Phys Ther 75(10):865-878, 1995.

25. Durand M and Loisel P: Therapeutic Return to Work: Rehabilitation in the Workplace. Work 17:57-63, 2001.

26. Elders LAM, van der Beek AJ and Burdorf A: Return to Work After Sickness Absence Due to Back Disorders—A Systematic Review on Intervention Strategies. Int Arch Occup Environ Health 73:339-348, 2000.

27. Ferguson S and Marras W. A Literature Review of Low Back Disorder Surveillance Measures and Risk Factors. Clin Biomech 12:211-26, 1997.

28. Fitzler S and Berger R: Chelsea Back Program: One Year Later. Occupational Health and Safety 52:52-54, 1983.

29. Fitzler SL, Berger RA: Attitudinal Change: The Chelsea Back Program. Occupational Health and Safety 35:24-26, 1982.

30. Frank JW, Kerr MS, Brooker A, et al: Disability Resulting from Occupational Low Back Pain. Part I: What Do We Know About Primary Prevention? A Review of the Scientific Evidence on Prevention Before Disability Begins. Spine 21(24):2908-2917, 1996.

31. Friesen MN, Yassi A and Cooper J: Return-to-Work: The Importance of Human Interaction and Organizational Structures. Work 17:11-22, 2001.

32. Fritz JM and George SZ: Identifying Psychosocial Variables in Patients with Acute Work-Related Low Back Pain: The Importance of Fear-Avoidance Beliefs. Phys Ther 82(10):973-983, 2002.

33. Fritz JM, George SZ and Delitto A: The Role of Fear-Avoidance Beliefs in Acute Low Back Pain: Relationships with Current and Future Disability and Work Status. Pain 94(1):7-15, 2001.

34. Frost H, Klaber Moffet JA, Moser JS, et al: Randomised Controlled Trial for Evaluation of Fitness Programme for Patients with Chronic Low Back Pain. BMJ 310(6973):151-154, 1995.

35. Frost H, Klaber Moffett J, Moser J, et al: A Fitness Programme for Patients with Chronic Low Back Pain: 2 Year Follow-up of a Randomised Controlled Trial Pain 75:273-279, 1998.

36. Frymoyer J and Cats-Baril W: Predictors of Low Back Pain

Disability. Clin Orthop and Rel Res 221:89-98, 1987.

37. Gatty CM, Turner M, Buitendorp DJ et al: The Effectiveness of Back Pain and Injury Prevention Programs in the Workplace. Work 20:257-266, 2003.

38. George SZ, Fritz JM, Bialosky JE, et al: The Effect of a Fear-Avoidance-Based Physical Therapy Intervention for Patients with Acute Low Back Pain: Results of a Randomized Clinical Trial. Spine 28(23):2551-2560, 2003.

39. George SZ, Fritz JM and Erhard RE. A Comparison of Fear-Avoidance Beliefs in Patients with Lumbar Spine Pain and Cervical Spine Pain. Spine 26(19):2139-2145, 2001.

40. Guo HR, Tannaka S, Halperin WE, et al: Back Pain in US Industry and Estimate of Lost Work Days. Am J Public Health 89:1029-1035, 1998.

41. Guzman J, Esmail R, Karjalainen K, et al: Multidisciplinary Rehabilitation for Chronic Low Back Pain: Systematic Review. BMJ 322:1511-1520, 2001.

42. Hagen KB, Hilde G, Jamtvedt G, et al: The Cochrane Review of Bed Rest for Acute Low Back Pain and Sciatica. Spine 25(22):2932-2939, 2000.

43. Hagen KB, Hilde G, Jamtvedt G, et al: The Cochrane Review of Advice to Stay Active as a Single Treatment for Low Back Pain and Sciatica. Spine 27(16):1736-1741, 2002.

44. Hsieh C, Adams AH, Tobis J, et al: Effectiveness of Four Conservative Treatments for Subacute Low Back Pain. Spine 27(11):1142-1148, 2002.

45. Indahl A, Haldorsen EH, Holm S, et al: Five-Year Follow-Up Study of a Controlled Clinical Trial Using Light Mobilization and an Informative Approach to Low Back Pain. Spine 23(23):2625-2630, 1998.

46. Janda V: Muscles, Central Nervous Motor Regulation And Back Problems. In The Neurological Mechanisms in Manipulative Therapy. IM Korr, ed. Plenum Press, New York NY 1978.

47. Johannsen F, Remvig L, Kryger P, et al: Exercises for Chronic Low Back Pain: A Clinical Trial. J Orthop Sports Phys Ther 22(2):52-59, 1995.

48. Karjalainen K, Malmivaara A, Pohjolainen T, et al: Mini-Intervention for Subacute Low Back Pain. A Randomized Controlled Trial. Spine 28(6):533-541, 2003.

49. Karjalainen K, Malmivaara A, van Tulder M, et al: Multidisciplinary Biopsychosocial Rehabilitation for Subacute Low Back Pain Among Working Age Adults. A Systematic Review Within the Framework of the Cochrane Collaboration Back Review Group. Spine 26(3):262-269, 2001.

50. Karjalainen K, Malmivaara A, van Tulder M, et al: Multidisciplinary Biopsychosocial Rehabilitation for Neck and Shoulder Pain Among Working Age Adults. A Systematic Review Within the Framework of the Cochrane Collaboration Back Review Group. Spine 26(2):174-181, 2001.

51. Keough JL and Fisher TF: Occupational-Psychosocial Perceptions Influencing Return to Work and Functional Performance of Injured Workers. Work 16:101-110, 2001.

52. Kirkaldy-Willis WH: The Pathology And Pathogenesis Of Low Back Pain. In Managing Low Back Pain, 2nd edition. W Kirkaldy-Willis, ed. Churchhill Livingstone, New York NY 1988.

53. Klaber Moffet J, Torgerson D, Bell-Syer S, et al: Randomised Controlled Trial of Exercise for Low Back Pain: Clinical Outcomes, Costs and Preferences. BMJ 319:279-283, 1999.

54. Klenerman L, Plade PD, Stanley M, et al: The Predication of Chronicity in Patients with an Acute Attack of Low Back Pain in a General Practice Setting. Spine 20:478-84, 1995.

55. Larsen K, Weidick F and Leboeuf-Yde C: Can Passive Prone Extensions of the Back Prevent Back Problems? A Randomized Controlled Intervention Trial of 314 Military Conscripts. Spine 27(24):2747-2752, 2002.

56. Lemstra M and Olszynski WP: The Effectiveness of Standard Care, Early Intervention and Occupational Management in Worker's Compensation Claims. Spine 28(3):299-304, 2003.

57. Lindstrom I, Ohlund C, Eek C, et al: Mobility, Strength and Fitness after a Graded Activity Program for Patients with Subacute Low Back Pain. A Randomized Prospective Clinical Study with a Behavioral Therapy Approach. Spine 17:641-652, 1992.

58. Lindstrom I, Ohlund C, Eek C et al: The Effect of Graded Activity on Patients with Subacute Low Back Pain: A Randomized Prospective Clinical Study with an Operant-Conditioning Behavioral Approach. Phys Ther 72:279-293, 1992.

59. Linton SJ and Andersson T: Can Chronic Disability Be Prevented? A Randomized Trial of a Cognitive-Behavior Intervention and Two Forms of Information for Patients with Spinal Pain. Spine 25(21):2825-2831, 2000.

60. Linton SJ and van Tulder MW: Preventive Interventions for Back and Neck Pain Problems. What is the Evidence? Spine 26(7):778-787, 2001.

61. Little P, Roberts L, Blowers H, et al: Should We Give Detailed Advice and Information Booklets to Patients with Back Pain? A Randomized Controlled Factorial Trial of a Self-Management Booklet and Doctor Advice to Take Exercise for Back Pain. Spine 26(19):2065-2072, 2001.

62. Loisel P, Abenhaim L, Durand P, et al: A Population-Based, Randomized Clinical Trial on Back Pain Management. Spine 22:2911-2918, 1997.

63. Maier-Riehle B and Harter M: The Effects of Back Schools—A Meta-Analysis. Int Joul Rehabil Res 24:199-206, 2001.

64. Malmivaara A, Hakkinen U, Aro T, et al: The Treatment of Acute Low Back Pain-Bed Rest, Exercises or Ordinary Activity? N Engl Joul Med 332(5):351-355, 1995.

65. Maniscalco P, Lane R, Welke M, et al: Decreased Rate of Back Injuries Through a Wellness Program for Offshore Petroleum Employees. Joul Occ Environ Med 41(9):813-820, 1999.

66. Manniche C, Lundberg E, Christensen I, et al: Intensive Dynamic Back Exercises for Chronic Low Back Pain: A Clinical Trial. Pain 47:53-63, 1991.

67. Mannion AF, Muntener M, Taimela, et al: A Randomized Clinical Trial of Three Active Therapies for Chronic Low Back Pain. Spine 24(23):2435-2448, 1999.

68. Mannion AF, Taimela S, Muntener M, et al: Active Therapy for Chronic Low Back Pain. Part 1. Effects on Back Muscle Activation, Fatigability and Strength. Spine 26(8):897-908, 2001.

69. Mayer TG, et al: Objective Assessment Of Spine Function Following Industrial Injury: A Prospective Study With Comparison Group And One Year Follow Up. Spine 10:482-493, 1985.

70. Mayer T and Gatchel R: Functional Restoration for Spinal

Disorders: The Sports Medicine Approach. Lea and Febiger, Philadelphia PA 1988.

71. Mayer T, et al: A Prospective Two Year Study of Functional Restoration in Industrial Back Injury. JAMA 258:1763-1767, Oct 2, 1987.

72. McGill S. Low Back Disorders. Evidence-Based Prevention and Rehabilitation. Human Kinetics, Champaign IL 2002.

73. McIntosh G, Wilson L, Affleck M, et al: Trunk and Lower Extremity Muscle Endurance: Normative Data for Adults. J Rehabil Outcomes Meas 2(4):20-39, 1998.

74. McReynolds M: Early Return to Work. Clinical Management 10:10-11, Sept/Oct 1990.

75. Melton B: Back Injury Prevention Means Education. Occupational Health and Safety 52:20-23, 1983.

76. Nachemson A: Work for All: For Those With Low Back Pain as Well. Clin Orthop and Rel Res. 179:77-85, Oct 1983.

77. Ostelo R, de Vet H, Waddell G, et al: Rehabilitation Following First-Time Lumbar Disc Surgery. A Systematic Review Within the Framework of the Cochrane Collaboration. Spine 28(3):209-218, 2003.

78. Pransky G, Benjamin K, Hill-Fotouhi C, et al: Work-Related Outcomes in Occupational Low Back Pain. A Multidimensional Analysis. Spine 27(8):864-870, 2002.

79. Ratzliff J. and Grogrin T: Early Return to Work Profitability. Professional Safety 11-17, Mar 1989.

80. Rainville J, Sobel JB, Hartigan C, et al: The Effect of Compensation Involvement on the Reporting of Pain and Disability by Patients Referred for Rehabilitation of Chronic Low Back Pain. Spine 22(17):2016-2024, 1997.

81. Richardson C, Jull G, Hodges P, et al. Therapeutic Exercise for Spinal Segmental Stabilization in Low Back Pain. Churchill Livingstone, London 1999.

82. Riihimaki H, Wickstrom G, Hanninen K, et al: Predictors of Sciatic Pain Among Concrete Reinforcement Workers and House Painters: A Five-Year Followup. Scand J Work Environ Health 15:415-423, 1989.

83. Ritzel D. and Allen R: Value of Work. Professional Safety 23-25, Nov 1988.

84. .Roberts L, Little P, Chapman J, et al: The Back Home Trial. General Practitioner-Supported Leaflets May Change Back Pain Behavior. Spine 27(17):1821-1828, 2002.

85. Rosenfeld M, Seferiadis A, Carlsson J, et al: Active Intervention in Patients with Whiplash-Associated Disorders Improves Long-Term Prognosis. Spine 28(22):2491-2498, 2003.

86. Rozenberg S, Delval C, Rezvani Y, et al: Bed Rest or Normal Activity for Patients with Acute Low Back Pain. A Randomized Controlled Trial. Spine 27(14):1487-1493, 2002.

87. Schonfeld B, et al: An Occupational Performance Test Validation Program for Fire Fighters at the Kennedy Space Center. Joul of Occ Med 32:638-643, 1988.

88. Schonstein E, Kenny D, Keating J, et al: Physical Conditioning Programs for Workers with Back and Neck Pain: A Cochrane Systematic Review. Spine 28(19):E391-E395, 2003.

89. Schultz IZ, Crook JM, Berkowitz J, et al: Biopsychosocial Multivariate Predictive Model of Occupational Low Back Disability. Spine 27(23):2720-2725, 2002.

90. Scientific Approach to the Assessment and Management of Activity-Related Spinal Disorders. A Monograph For Clinicians. Report of the Quebec Task Force on Spinal Disorders. Spine 12(7 Suppl):S1-59, 1987.

91. Scully-Palmer C: Outcome Study: An Industrial Rehabilitation Program. Work 15:21-23, 2000.

92. Snook SH, Campanelli R, Hart J: A Study of Three Preventive Approaches to Low Back Injury. Joul of Occ Med 20(7):478-481, 1978.

93. Stratton Johnson L, Archer-Heese G, Caron-Powles C, et al: Work Hardening: Outdated Fad or Effective Intervention? Work 16:235-243, 2001.

94. Strong J, Large R, Ashton R, et al: A New Zealand Replication of the IPAM Clustering Model of Low Back Patients. Clin J Pain 11:296-306, 1995.

95. Sullman MJ and Biggs HC: The Impact of an Industry-Based Rehabilitation Programme. Work 17:49-55, 2001.

96. Teasell RW and Harth M: Functional Restoration. Returning Patients with Chronic Low Back Pain to Work-Revolution or Fad? Spine 21(7):844-847, 1996.

97. Timm KE: A Randomized-Control Study of Active and Passive Treatments for Chronic Low Back Pain Following L5 Laminectomy. J Orthop Sports Phys Ther 20(6):276-286, 1994.

98. Tomer GM, Olson C, Lepore B: Back Injury Prevention Training Makes Dollars and Sense. National Safety News (Jan) 36-39, 1984.

99. Torstensen TA, Ljunggren AE, Meen HD, et al: Efficiency and Costs of Medical Exercise Therapy, Conventional Physiotherapy and Self-Exercise in Patients with Chronic Low Back Pain. Spine 23(23):2616-2624, 1998.

100. Troup J, Foreman T and Lloyd D: Back Pain in Industry: A Prospective Study. Spine 6:1-6, 1981.

101. U.S. Bureau of Labor Statistics, Lost-Worktime Injuries and Illnesses: Characteristics and Resulting Time Away from Work, 2000, USDL Number 02-196, Washington DC, 2002.

102. van den Hout JHC, Vlaeyen JWS, Heuts PHTG, et al: Secondary Prevention of Work-Related Disability in Nonspecific Low Back Pain: Does Problem-Solving Therapy Help? A Randomized Clinical Trial. Clin J Pain 19(2):87-96, 2003.

103. van Poppel MNM, Koes BW, Smid T, et al. A Systematic Review of Controlled Clinical Trials on the Prevention of Back Pain in Industry. Occup Environ Med 54:841-847, 1997.

104. Vlaeyen JWS, Seelen HAM, Peters M, et al: Fear of Movement/Reinjury and Muscular Reactivity in Chronic Low Back Pain Patients: An Experimental Investigation. Pain 82:297-304, 1999.

105. van Tulder M, Malmivaara A, Esmail R, et al: Exercise Therapy for Low Back Pain. A Systematic Review Within the Framework of the Cochrane Collaboration Back Review Group. Spine 25(21):2784-2796, 2000.

106. van Tulder M, Ostelo R, Vlaeyen JW, et al: Behavioral Treatment for Chronic Low Back Pain: A Systematic Review within the Framework of the Chchrane Back Review Group. Spine 26:270-281, 2001.

107. Voit S: Work-Site Health and Fitness Programs: Impact on the Employee and Employer. Work 16:273-286, 2001.

108. von Korff M, Moore JE, Lorig K, et al: A Randomized Trial of a Lay Person-Led Self-Management Group Intervention for Back Pain Patients in Primary Care. Spine 23(23):2608-2615, 1998.

109. Vowles KE and Gross RT: Work-Related Beliefs About Injury and Physical Capability for Work in Individuals with Chronic Pain. Pain 101:291-298, 2003.

110. Waddell G, Main CJ, Morris EW, et al: Chronic Low Back

Pain, Psychological Distress, and Illness Behavior. Spine 9:209-213, 1984.

111. Waddell G, Newton M, Henderson I, et al: A Fear-Avoidance Beliefs Questionaire (FABQ) and the Role of Fear-Avoidance Beliefs in Chronic Low Back Pain and Disability. Pain 52:157-168, 1993.

112. Warren N: Work Stress and Musculoskeletal Disorder Etiology: The Relative Roles of Psychosocial and Physical Risk Factors. Work 17:221-234, 2001.

113. Winkel J and Mathiassen SE: Assessment of Physical Work Load in Epidemiologic Studies: Concepts, Issues and Operational Considerations. Ergonomics 37:979-988, 1994.

INDEX